The Cat Repair BOOK

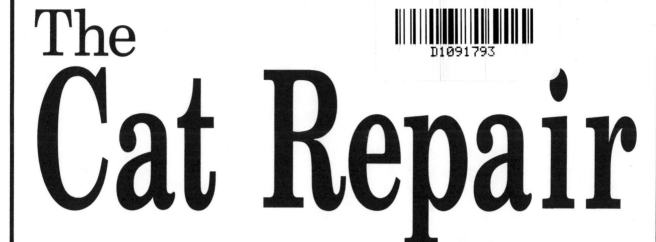

RUTH B. JAMES, D.V.M.

A Do-It-Yourself
Guide for the
Cat Owner

Alpine Press
Mills, Wyoming

Inquiries should be addressed to Alpine Press
P.O. Box 1930
Mills, Wyoming 82644

Published by Alpine Press
P.O. Box 1930
Mills, Wyoming 82644

Final Editing by Harvel Alishouse, D.V.M.
Keith E. James D.V.M.
Kris Brandt Riske

Cover Photo by Ruth B. James, D.V.M.

Interior Photos by Ruth B. James, D.V.M.

Custom photo processing by Norm and Evelyn Grant,
Grant's Photographic Restoration, Tempe, Arizona, 85281

Drawings by Linda Whitehouse

Typesetting by Dan Hashberger and Bruce Studer
Endeavor Books, Casper, Wyoming, 82604

Printed by Cushing-Malloy, Inc.
Ann Arbor, Michigan 48107

Printed in the United States of America

Library of Congress Catalog Card Number 95-076772
ISBN 0-9615114-2-7

To

FRANCIE and JOHNNIE

Who Died

To

LINDA MERRY, D.V.M.

My Dear Long-Time Friend

First Woman President of the
American Animal Hospital Association

Fellow Cat Lover

DISCLAIMER

To help insure the reader's understanding of some of the medical descriptions and techniques in **The Cat Repair Book**, brand names have occasionally been used as examples of particular medication or equipment. However, the use of a particular trademark or brand name is not intended to imply an endorsement of that particular product, or to suggest that similar products offered by others under different names may be in any way inferior. Nothing contained in this book is to be construed as a suggestion to violate any trademark laws.

Although every effort has been made to present scientifically accurate and up-to-date information based on the best and most reliable sources available, it should be understood that the results of medical treatments depend upon many factors, including proper diagnosis, which are not under the control of the author or the publishers of this book. Therefore, neither Alpine Press nor the author assumes responsibility for and make no warranty with respect to results that may be obtained from the procedures herein. Neither Alpine Press nor Dr. Ruth James shall be liable to any person for damage resulting from reliance on any information contained in **The Cat Repair Book** whether with respect to diagnosis, drug dosage, treatment procedure, or by reason of any misstatement or inadvertent error contained herein.

Also, it should be noted that neither the author nor Alpine Press manufactures, packages, ships, labels, or sells any of the drugs or equipment mentioned in this book. Accordingly, neither can be held responsible for results that may be obtained with products manufactured by others.

The reader is encouraged to carefully read and follow the label directions provided by the manufacturer for any product which may be used. If there is a conflict between instructions contained in the book and those provided by the manufacturer, those provided by the manufacturer should be followed.

ACKNOWLEDGMENTS

So many people have contributed to the writing of this book that I can scarcely hope to thank them all. Thanks are due Dr. Keith James who read as much of the manuscript as his busy schedule allowed. My thanks to Dr. Harvel Alishouse, without whose careful attention to detail and valuable suggestions, the book would have been much the poorer. Kris Brandt Riske edited the book with a sharp (and readily wielded) pencil, and has added immeasurably to it. For her help and suggestions I am truly grateful, even if I didn't always take her advice.

Thanks to my valued book wholesalers and readers, who have demanded that I write this book. Their continuing enthusiasm and support have helped to make my previous books successful; they have my unceasing gratitude.

Many of my friends have offered love, support, and continuing encouragement through the long process of writing. Howard Walworth keeps my head in the clouds and my feet on the ground with his ideas and friendship. Frank and Sharon Chapman, Joyce Flora, and JoAnn Milne provided the quiet hideaways where the book was started. Phill Morrison, Sue Achenbach, Marilyn Wright, Elizabeth Scott, and Jerry Buk offer ongoing encouragement. Sue McConaughey made many long drives to deliver edited chapters. I would also like to thank Jim Bradley and Sherry Leman for handling my mail as it chases me in my travels.

Mike Komorowsky and Sherry Leman provided computer equipment at critical points in the writing. Thanks to all those who so graciously shared their cats and themselves for photos. Dr. Gaylord Welch at the Beverly Animal Clinic and his helpful staff provided some truly special fur-footed characters from their resident group of felines. Casper Metro Animal Control Director Pat Bergen kindly loaned their facilities, staff, and animals for photos. It's sad to think that for some of the cats, this photo was their last.

I am also thankful for the teachers who have helped to shape my thinking, and to the clients and animals who have taught me so much. If I have omitted someone who has helped me, it has been because of my imperfect memory, not because of any desire to do so.

Lastly, and far from least, Richard Smith warms my heart and supports my ongoing efforts. Mere words cannot measure his contribution to my life. For him, I am truly grateful.

CONTENTS

INTRODUCTION

My first book, *How To Be Your Own Veterinarian (sometimes)*, was written to help horse owners save money on their veterinary bills. It was aimed at helping them tell the difference between problems they could treat themselves and those which needed the services and expertise of a veterinarian.

Somewhere between the tenth and eleventh printings of that book, customer demand reached a point where it could no longer be ignored. Readers were asking that I write a similar book for dog owners, telling them how to avoid problems and save money on medical care for their dog. The result was *The Dog Repair Book*. Next, the cat owners demanded equal time, so here it is: *The Cat Repair Book*.

As with the previous books, this book tells the cat owner how to treat simple problems at home. I have discussed the ailments for which veterinary diagnosis and treatment are essential. And, I have tried to distinguish clearly between the two extremes. Not incidentally, I hope to save you, the cat owner, some money with this knowledge. If I can save each person who buys this book just one veterinary visit, it will have paid for itself. If I can also prevent the heartache of losing the cat you love, and save that animal some pain and suffering, the time I have devoted to writing it will have been well spent.

When you get this book, please read it at least lightly from cover to cover. In doing this you will come to know my thinking on treatment of injuries and illnesses, and also which problems are considered minor or which need veterinary help immediately. This first reading will give you an idea of how to begin and where to look for specific information when your cat is ill or injured. It should also point out many ways to keep your cat healthy.

I have tried to emphasize preventive measures which may be taken to keep many problems from occurring so that you may never need to treat them. Many illnesses are in large part preventable, but may be nearly incurable or permanently damaging once they have occurred. Preventive medicine is the least expensive form of veterinary care—and the most effective in the long run!

Chapter 1

HELPING YOUR VETERINARIAN TO HELP YOU

- *What Can A Veterinarian Do For You?*
  - *Hospitalization*
- *Finding A Veterinarian*
- *Getting Acquainted*
- *A Second Opinion*
- *A Few Additional Hints*

WHAT CAN A VETERINARIAN DO FOR YOU?

He or she can provide routine care for your cat, including checkups, immunizations, and routine surgery such as spaying and neutering. As with your car, maintenance of your cat is much cheaper than repair. Your veterinarian also can serve your cat's emergency needs for accidents and illnesses and provide hospitalization.

Because of its cost, hospitalization should be reserved for serious problems or extensive diagnostic procedures. Some problems can be handled on an outpatient basis much as they are with humans. You bring the cat in first thing in the morning and take it home at night, even if the cat is still slightly sedated. You provide part of the cat's aftercare in return for a greatly reduced veterinary bill.

Why does veterinary treatment cost what it does? When you or a family member go to a doctor, the doctor provides an office, receptionist, and some routine instruments. A hospital provides X-ray machines, nurses, and all other services. In contrast, a veterinarian provides his or her own hospital and all the equipment, including X-ray machine, anesthetic equipment, pharmacy, and nursing and technical assistants. He or she also provides diagnostic tests, whether in-house or from an outside laboratory. He or she may offer electrocardiograms (EKG's or ECG's) to examine the heart, electroencephalograms (a similar test for the brain), and other sophisticated tests. Maybe we should wonder not why veterinary care costs what it does, but how your veterinarian can provide so much value and care for so little cost!

However, you should feel you are receiving value for your money. Feel free to discuss fees with your veterinarian. How much will tests or treatment cost? If your veterinarian can't give an exact figure, ask for a high and low range. Some clinics ask whether you want minimum, average, or no-holds-barred treatment. Give this some thought. What can you afford? If your veterinarian won't provide an estimate, find one who will. You have a right to it! If you can't afford to pay all at once, ask what arrangements for payment can be made. Does your veterinarian offer charge accounts or take payments or credit cards?

If you can't afford treatment, what are the alternatives? Are you really unable to afford it or do you choose not to? Don't expect free treatment any more than you would from another health professional. In some areas, animal welfare groups offer free or low-cost care to those who truly cannot pay. Some of these clinics are not non-profit, nor are they inexpensive. Check their financial policies. Local veterinary societies may have members who perform some pro bono (free) work each year. Your own veterinarian may not, but another one might. The last choice, if all else fails, is euthanasia to end the pet's suffering (see Euthanasia).

Before you make a final decision, discover what outcome can be expected. Is the cost of treatment consistent with expectations for length and quality of life? If, for example, there is only a 30% chance the cat will live for only three or four months while suffering in pain, $2,500 for treatment may be unrealistic. Even if you can afford it, do you really want to inflict so much pain and suffering on your cat to keep it alive for so brief a time?

HOSPITALIZATION

If your cat needs hospitalization, you should expect realistic information from your veterinarian, including what treatment will be needed and what it will cost. Ask your veterinarian for an evaluation of your cat's potential for recovery and whether your cat might suffer. Communication should be open in both directions.

Some clinics keep cats and dogs together in the same ward. This is good from a disease control point of view, as a cat is less likely to catch a disease from a dog than from another cat. As long as dogs are not caged above them, most cats are not upset. Other clinics provide separate rooms for cats. If this is important to you, look for such a clinic. Most cats with a serious illness or injury rest well in a clinic.

Pet insurance is available in some areas. Like health insurance for humans, it works through the principle of risk sharing. Most policies pay only for surgery or severe illness. As with any consumer product, shop carefully and be sure to read the fine print. Get references. Does the plan have a good payment history? Would it be better to put a sum away each month in a savings account? If you never need it for your pet, you still have it for other uses. We have all seen how health insurance has worked (or not worked) for humans. The jury is still out on insurance for pets. If you keep your cat indoors it has far less chance of needing medical care than one that runs loose.

FINDING A VETERINARIAN

Your cat is perfectly healthy. Why do you need a veterinarian now? Because it's easier to find one before you need him or her in the confusion of an emergency. Most important, you can decide if the veterinarian is the right one for you and your cat and develop a rapport before the confusion of an emergency. Taking your cat in for a checkup or vaccination is a good way to get acquainted.

Many veterinary practices treat small animals only, while "mixed" practices treat both large and small animals. In rural areas, the veterinarian who treats your cow or horse may also care for your cat. This is a great convenience for the rural resident with several cats and dogs, as one visit from the veterinarian does double duty. Let your veterinarian know that you want him or her to examine your cats so he or she can bring appropriate vaccines or medication. Some veterinarians especially enjoy working with cats, and you may be happiest with one who is a cat lover.

In small-animal practices, you have a choice of a house-call practice or a clinical practice. A house-call practice is convenient if you are homebound, work at home, or have small children. The house-call veterinarian may or may not have access to a hospital for surgery and treatment of severe ailments.

Your pet may receive more personal attention from a hard-working solo practitioner (a veterinarian who practices alone). The drawback is that the veterinarian is human, and cannot be on call 365 days a year. You may be referred to an emergency clinic or to a veterinarian who is covering the practice when your veterinarian has taken time off or is attending continuing education.

A group practice is one in which a number of veterinarians work in the same facility. They may take turns on night and emergency call. Each veterinarian may have a specialty in addition to taking his or her share of routine cases. Some may be full-time specialists who do nothing but work on eyes or bone problems, for example.

Your veterinarian may refer you to a specialist who may be on the staff of a group practice or may have a small clinic of his or her own. Expect to pay substantially more for this veterinarian's services. As with any veterinarian, do not hesitate to discuss how much care will cost. A referral to a specialist really means your veterinarian wants your cat to have the best possible care. Return to your regular veterinarian after the specialist has finished treating your cat.

The American Animal Hospital Association (AAHA) is a group of veterinary hospitals which meet certain stated and enforced standards. AAHA hospitals must meet facility, equipment, personnel, and laboratory criteria.

An AAHA "Animal Hospital" or "Animal Medical Center" is a full-service veterinary practice which can provide examination, diagnostic services, and treatment, and is equipped to house and nurse patients. These hospitals may have "Satellite Clinics," which treat most animals on an outpatient basis, while sending cases needing more intensive care to the main hospital. An AAHA "Central Hospital" has a full range of veterinary services, including 24-hour nursing and specialty consultation. An "Emergency Hospital" takes care of animals when the other hospitals are closed, and after treatment, you can expect to visit your regular veterinarian the next morning. In this book, the words "hospital" and "clinic" have been used interchangeably when suggesting that your cat be examined by a veterinarian.

All AAHA hospitals must maintain careful records on all animals they treat. They must provide examination facilities, pharmacy for animal medications, laboratory for routine tests, radiology services, anesthetic and surgical facilities, routine dental services, nursing care, and certain standards of housekeeping and maintenance must be met. They must have a medical library of basic textbooks and current periodicals. They must either provide adequate emergency services or have a referral procedure to send after-hours cases to another hospital. Some AAHA hospitals offer specialty services or have veterinarians on staff who are board-certified in specialties such as ophthalmology (eye care), or orthopedics (bone and joint care). An AAHA certification of the hospital assures you that the veterinary clinic and its practitioners are current in their medical knowledge and that the clinic facility meets tough standards.

Many veterinarians choose not to be members of AAHA, yet still have current medical knowledge and a good facility, while providing top-notch care. To find one, talk with your friends or neighbors. Ask WHICH veterinarian they use, and WHY they like him or her. Or, ask a member of your local cat club. If you are planning to move to a new area, ask your veterinarian to refer you to a veterinarian in your new location, as he or she may know someone personally. While you may not stay with this new veterinarian if your personalities do not mesh, it is a place to start.

You may find a veterinarian through the Yellow Pages. The advantage of this method is you will know if he or she specializes in certain animals, such as birds or fish. The disadvantage is you have NO idea of his or her qualifications or ability.

GETTING ACQUAINTED

Ask for a clinic tour if you want to see the facility. Do so at a time convenient for the veterinarian and the staff. This will give you an idea of what the veterinarian can do for you and your pets.

When you call for advice, give the veterinarian as much factual information as you can when first discussing the illness. You are better acquainted with your cat than your veterinarian. Because it will be your everyday observations that initially spot a problem, don't play down this vital part of the preliminary diagnosis. On the other hand, don't jump to conclusions. Many veterinarians are asked to treat "worms" when the problem is diarrhea or another illness. Tell your veterinarian what your cat is DOING and how your cat looks, not what you think the problem is. As he or she becomes familiar with you and your cat, it will become apparent how astute you are in dealing with your pet and its problems. He or she will then have a better idea of the questions to ask to sort out the information you provide. Facts that seem unimportant to you may be essential to an accurate diagnosis. What looks minor to you may become meaningful after further examination, observation, and laboratory tests.

Don't be afraid to give your impressions of change—the cat is acting better or worse, feeling stronger or remaining the same. This is especially important in treating diseases which take some time to heal. If a problem is not responding to one medication, it may be necessary to change to another. Feel free to call the veterinarian and ask if the cat should be improving more rapidly. He or she can either give you information over the phone or decide that your cat needs to be rechecked in person.

Wait until you are at the clinic to give the cat's detailed medical history. Most veterinarians prefer to have it while looking at the pet, and information communicated over the phone may be forgotten by the time the cat arrives at the clinic. Give any information which comes to mind, even if you don't think it is relevant.

It is important to be honest with your veterinarian.

How long has the problem existed? Are there factors contributing to the problem that he or she should know about? Have you given the animal any medication? Can you administer pills? If you can't, your veterinarian can recommend another way to treat your cat. He or she may have you bring your cat in daily for treatment, change from pills to liquid, or show you how to give pills to your cat.

Is your cat a grouch? Let the veterinarian know so that assistants who are experienced in holding or treating grouchy cats can help. This may save you or your veterinarian from being accidentally bitten, an event that is not the way to win friends. Say something diplomatic such as "My cat sometimes scratches," rather than "My cat hates vets." Sometimes this dislike is due to the animal's previous experience. Or, it may be because the cat is sensitive to the smells of other animals or to medication odors present on the veterinarian's hands and clothing despite the best of sanitation procedures. Some cats probably even dislike the disinfectants which veterinarians use to clean their hands.

A SECOND OPINION

Don't be afraid to get a second opinion on your cat's problem. As with human doctors, veterinarians are not all-knowing. If your veterinarian is confident in practice, there should be no objection to your doing so. If he or she objects, you probably need to find a new veterinarian.

When should you get a second opinion? Get it when you have serious questions about the first opinion, when suggested treatment seems unreasonable in terms of trouble or cost, or if expensive surgery is recommended as the only cure. If the two agree, the diagnosis is probably correct. If the second opinion is different or opposite, DO NOT automatically assume that the first one is wrong and the second one is right. The truth may be the other way around. When the two are very different, GET A THIRD ONE!! Take the cat to a university clinic or specialty hospital and be prepared to pay for extra tests. If you have a well-defined problem, such as an eye ailment, go directly to the appropriate specialist. You can probably trust the recommendations, especially if the veterinarian is board-certified.

A FEW ADDITIONAL HINTS

Take your cat to the veterinarian when it first becomes ill. In the wild, a cat that shows signs of illness becomes easy prey for larger predators. For this reason, cats try to hide the fact that they do not feel well. By the time your cat looks ill, it probably is! Cats are not prone to faking illness. Take the cat to the clinic if it has diarrhea more than one day; vomits, sneezes, coughs, or gags repeatedly; or strains while urinating. Have your cat checked if it has watery, reddened eyes; rough, dull coat; is tired or sluggish; or does not eat for more than one day. First, however, make sure that a neighbor or another member of the household is not feeding your cat.

Please, please, take your cat to the veterinary clinic in a pet carrier or box, in a harness with a leash, or in a pillowcase. If you don't have one, most clinics will loan you a cat carrier. Go in and get it BEFORE you take your cat out of the car—for the safety of both you and your pet. And, use it to return the cat to your car. I once saw a client carry her cat back into the clinic after it jumped from her arms. It had dashed into the street and was hit by a car. Nothing could be done to save it.

Make sure you understand the veterinarian's instructions for care and treatment BEFORE you leave the clinic. If you are not sure, don't hesitate to ask him or her to repeat them or to jot them on paper. Most veterinarians would rather go over instructions an extra time than try to recall what was said when you call two days later. If you don't know how to treat the cat, ask for a demonstration.

Carry out treatments as instructed, even if it means getting up in the middle of the night. Correct timing can be important, especially with certain antibiotics. Keep a sheet of paper handy to record the cat's temperature, feed consumption, bowel movements, etc. Jot down questions to ask the next time you call the clinic. This will make the call brief and efficient. If your veterinarian has asked you to call with a progress report, ask what number you should use and the best time of day to call. It's often worthwhile to call, even if you haven't been asked, to report the animal has recovered. Veterinarians like to hear good news, too.

If your cat does not show improvement within a reasonable time, call your veterinarian. He or she may wish to change the medication and may be able to do this over the telephone. Or, it may be necessary for you bring the cat in for reexamination. Don't let the problem go and then complain because the veterinarian didn't "cure" your cat. If you and your veterinarian work as a team, your cat is the winner!

If you call a veterinarian to treat an animal which has been examined or treated at another clinic, be sure to tell him or her about the first treatment. Some medications can mask symptoms or cause others to develop. If the previous veterinarian has made an erroneous diagnosis (which everyone can do), it will save time for the second veterinarian if he or she knows what was said and what treatment was given. Discontinue any medication given by the first veterinarian. Failure to do so may result in a conflict between the old and new medication. In some cases, it may confuse the diagnosis by complicating signs of the disease, while in others it may actually be dangerous.

In some cases, advice in this book may conflict with that given by your veterinarian. If this occurs, be sure to take your veterinarian's advice, because he or she has the advantage of examining your cat and working "face to face" with the specific problem.

Chapter 2

FELINE CARE AND TRAINING

THE NEW KITTEN OR CAT

Make sure that you want a cat before you inflict yourself on that cute ball of fur. Cats don't need to be walked, but you do need to change the litter box often. For the most part, their maintenance is much more affordable than dogs, although both animals have similar ongoing needs for veterinary care.

Cats are malleable, far more so than dogs. Especially when adopted when young, they adapt to their owner and his or her personality. Some people always train their cats to be loving, while others consistently end up with aloof felines. Except for highly selected purebreds, YOU will have more influence on the cat's personality than will its heredity. That is not, of course, true with an older cat whose personality is already set. In that case, you may be able to change your cat slightly, but for the most part have to take the cat as it is. What you see is what you get, and you will not be able to change it very much. A calm older cat may be a good idea if you have a house full of delicate glassware or similar valuables, as the cat will be settled and less likely to get into trouble.

Rare breeds of cats may have very small gene pools, and may have a higher incidence of antisocial or peculiar individuals than "alley cats." Most Siamese, for example, are loving cats, but a few bloodlines produce felines that are aggressive or excessively timid. You may find these to be unsuitable pets. If you can see the cat's immediate relatives, you may have a better idea of how your kitten may develop and whether its disposition will mesh with yours.

Cats are not a suitable gift for someone unless you ABSOLUTELY know that the individual wants one. Even then, it's a lot better to let the person, whether a child, an oldster, or someone in between, pick his or her own pet. Having the right chemistry between owner and pet is critical to the human-animal bond. An example of the wrong approach is the person who says, "My mother lives alone, and she really needs a cat." You don't surprise someone with the 12- or 15-year commitment that goes along with a pet because you feel that someone else needs it. It's just not fair to the person or the animal.

It's also not fair to a cat to give it to children in order to "teach them responsibility." The cat may end up neglected, or you will end up taking care of the cat and resenting it. Make sure YOU want the cat. Be honest about your motives.

If you have recently lost a cat, it may also not be fair to look for a cat "just like Fuzzy." You are NOT replacing the pet that has died. Just like a human, that cat was a unique individual, and another will not be just like it in looks or mannerisms. You are getting a NEW pet. In fact, it's often easier when the new pet does NOT look like the deceased one. That helps to keep you from having unrealistic expectations. Choose another breed, or another color within the same breed. Give the new pet a chance to be its own quirky self.

If you already have a number of cats, consider what bringing in one or more new animals may do for the existing social order. Stress is one of the most serious factors causing illness in cats, and mixing cats of different ages from different backgrounds is stressful to them. Poor sanitation and poor nutrition caused by overcrowding are serious stresses. Felines can live with many subclinical diseases for years that cause illness when stress is added. The cats may appear to be happy and content, then become ill or die. If cats in your household are consistently spraying urine, defecating outside the litter box, or grooming and chewing themselves to baldness, these may be first signs that you have too many to be comfortable in the available space. Stress from overcrowding can lead to cannibalism, reproductive failure, fighting, and a variety of neurotic behaviors. It is also one of the main causes of house soiling and furniture clawing. Please, please don't keep too many cats. They are truly better off dead than to be continuously upset, malnourished, or unhealthy because the owner cannot afford vaccinations, good food or adequate veterinary care. When taking in strays, there is a division between "softhearted" and "softheaded."

Some people view pets as totally disposable, like a grocery sack, and feel comfortable getting rid of them when they are no longer cute. This leads to huge numbers of two- to five-year-old animals being put to death in shelters. At the other extreme, some people view keeping the pet to the end of its natural lifespan as a sacred duty, even though it may not be a suitable or enjoyable pet. Somewhere between these two extremes, there should be a happy medium between the differing values.

Cats may fall into two distinct categories. Some are very sociable and require a lot of contact with humans. These are ideal, affectionate pets for most owners. Others are aloof and tend to be more self-sufficient, needing play and/or predatory activity more than they need contact with people or with other cats. They make good barn cats, and they also work well for people who don't want or need a close, cuddly "lap cat." Cats that have not been socialized to humans during the first eight weeks of age may never be very friendly. These cats may be ideal for an isolated situation with few people and no other animals. You can sometimes tell which type your kitten will tend to be by watching it with its littermates and seeing how it reacts to humans. The kitten that comes bouncing out of the group toward you has a better chance of being sociable than one who hangs back, runs away, hides from you, or claws and spits when handled.

The runt of the litter may be intimidated enough by its littermates that it may never socialize well with humans or other cats. Some cats are very timid, and have inherited this trait. They tend to dislike being picked up, are very stiff when held and less playful than normal, and do not seem to care about people. They are fearful of noise and movement. A cat like this may become a pet if you work intensively with it, and initially, tranquilizers may help it to accept human contact. However, you might be much happier putting the same effort into a cat with more potential to be the kind of pet you would truly enjoy.

On rare occasion, cats that have been anesthetized will become afraid and timid. You can usually bring the cat back to its normal personality, but it will take diligent and gentle handling.

A cat that is not very friendly can occasionally be changed if you work at it, especially if it is young. Give the cat frequent small meals of tasty food. Call it to you each time, using the same words and tone of voice. Make the cat follow you to the kitchen or feeding area. Gradually increase the amount of time and handling you devote to the cat, but do not chase it or corner it, as that will only make it try to get away from you. You may also lie with the cat in a resting place that it finds comfortable, such as the sofa. If the cat is really shy or wild, it may be necessary to cage it for a week or two to slowly accustom it to human contact.

An older cat that comes from a shelter or pound may or may not become a suitable pet. It may be best to look upon the first couple of weeks as a "trial" period to determine if the cat fits you and you fit the cat. Most shelters allow you to return the animal if it doesn't work out. The cat may be homeless because it slipped out of the house and became lost, or was kicked out because it was unwanted or its owners were moving. On the other hand, the cat may have been in the shelter because it urinated on the bed or clawed the baby. Take in an older animal with open arms and an open heart, but keep an open mind about it until you know that it is going to adapt to your household and family situation. If the cat doesn't fit, the kindest thing you can do is to return it to the shelter.

It is also possible to acquire a cat from a shelter and have it become very ill from a disease contracted there or before going there. Be aware of this when you go to the shelter. Some shelters will treat the animal at no charge. Others will take back an animal that becomes sick. How many dollars are you willing to spend if the cat becomes ill?

If you already have cats, consider that a new cat may bring diseases into your household. Feral or stray kittens pose the greatest risk to your existing cats. Adult cats are safest, especially if they are tested for feline leukemia before you bring them home. Ideally, along with available testing, isolating a new cat completely for six weeks will provide nearly complete protection for your present pets. Bringing home a cat that is already ill or incubating a disease may sign a death warrant for one of your current favorites. Introducing a kitten to a home where adult cats are infested with external or internal parasites can be hazardous to the newcomer.

Kittens born to a household pet are usually quite healthy. In contrast, kittens from a cattery are often exposed to a number of diseases from the time they are born. By the time they are six weeks old, many have had one or more illnesses, and many die before they are four or five months old. In addition to greater exposure, purebred cats often have less hereditary resistance to disease than do their "alley cat" counterparts. Purebred cats, even if not very healthy, may be carefully treated and nursed through diseases. For an extensive listing of congenital defects in cats see Hoskins, 1995. The feral feline often has genetic resistance, coming from true "survival of the fittest."

Some breeds have special hereditary weaknesses or diseases. Norwegian Forest Cats, for example, have an inherited metabolic disease, called glycogen storage disease. Kittens are born dead or die, "fading" shortly after birth. The few that survive begin muscular and skeletal degeneration around five to seven months of age, dying around twelve to fourteen months old (Fyfe, 1995).

There are some dispositional differences between breeds. Ones that have been domesticated for long periods of time, such as the Siamese, have different behaviors and personalities than barn cats that have randomly reproduced through the ages.

Consider getting two kittens or a pair of compatible adult cats if you are busy or are away at work much of the time. They will keep each other company, and tend to stay out of trouble better than a single cat—a bored single cat can think of all sorts of mischief. Cats in couples also adapt to moves and changes in their household better than a single animal. Two elderly cats that have been together much of their lives may live longer and happier lives than the solo pet. The disadvantage is that when one of a closely bonded pair dies, the other may be distraught and suffer a personality change, which sometimes may be permanent. Having two cats can give you double the love, too.

Male or female? If unaltered, female cats may be very vocal when in heat, while males will tend to wander in search of females. If neutered or spayed, the dispositions and personalities of both sexes are quite similar, and they are equally affectionate. There is more difference between individual cats than between neutered males and spayed females.

Selecting a healthy kitten will go a long way toward a happy start for your new pet. Whether it comes from a humane shelter or pound, from a pet shop, from the neighbor's backyard, or from a prize-winning cattery, its home surroundings should be clean and free of unpleasant odors. Because good sanitation goes a long way toward a good start in life, shop somewhere else if the place smells bad.

The kitten should have bright eyes that are clear and free of drainage or matter. If the cat is white and the eye color is blue, chances are good that it will be deaf. It may make a good pet, but will require special care and consideration not needed with a cat that can hear. The nose can be damp or dry, but should not be draining or cracked. The mouth should be a normal pink, neither white and pale, nor an angry red.

If you are looking for a show cat, the teeth should meet perfectly. An undershot or overshot bite can ruin its chances for a championship. Teeth need not be perfect for a pet cat, although a misaligned canine tooth which threatens to penetrate a lip or damage the roof of the mouth might need correction later in the cat's life.

The ears should be normal in color and free of drainage or unpleasant odors. The kitten's body should be in normal physical condition, and it should be lean, but not thin or bony under its coat. Its stomach should be firm, not bloated and soft.

Look under the kitten's tail for signs of diarrhea. Redness, drainage, hair loss, or filth on the fur may be a sign of intestinal infection or worms. Determine the kitten's sex while you are observing the area. A female kitten will have sex organs that appear flat. If you examine them closely, you can see a tiny slit in the genital area, and the two openings are close together, much like an upside-down exclamation point. A male kitten's genitalia appear to be more puffy or protruding, and the rounded openings usually have a space between them. Looking at one kitten, it may be difficult to tell what it is. Compare all the kittens in the litter and you will begin to see the differences between them, assuming that you have at least one of each gender.

Notice the kitten's disposition and get acquainted with the kitten by offering your fingers. A curious and interested kitten that comes over to see what is happening is usually well-adjusted. The kitten that fluffs its tail, hisses, and backs away, or acts excessively withdrawn or shy is usually a poor choice. It may just be timid, but chances are good that it is ill. At any rate, a shy kitten is a particularly poor choice for a household with children. You can test the kitten's playfulness by pulling a piece of string across the floor—a playful one will quickly attack it. This animal will make a happy, lively pet.

If your kitten or cat is registered, be sure to get a copy of its "papers," the certificate you will send to the registry to document your ownership. This is important if you want to show the cat or produce registered kittens. It is best to take care of this when you purchase the cat, to be sure everything is in order.

It is a good idea to get two or three days' of whatever food the kitten is eating so you don't have to change its diet at this stressful time in its life. If possible, get a piece of cloth from its bed, as it will have the scent of the mother and littermates on it; this will help comfort the kitten in its new home. Get a few ounces of soiled litter from the litter box the kitten has been using and put it in the new litter box to help the kitten start using it. Use a clay litter without scent so the cat will learn to go to its own odor in the box. Whatever litter you are using, don't change it while the cat is learning to use the box. If you have a covered litter box, it may work better to take the lid off while the kitten is learning to use it.

It is also a good idea to have a new kitten tested for feline leukemia before you have it immunized. A kitten (or cat) that tests negative may be negative, or it may be a latent carrier that will later become positive. A positive cat may be a true positive or a cat that will eventually become negative on testing. A cat that is positive should be tested again in four months. A positive result on a second test generally means a life expectancy between five months and three years.

Kittens are cute and cuddly. However, for the first few days, your new kitten may be frightened. It is probably away from its mother for the first time, and in new surroundings with strange people. Handle your kitten gently and as little as possible. Let the kitten rest or sleep at will. Try to avoid bright lights and loud noises. Don't allow children to overwhelm the kitten with their exuberance or to maul it or drag it around. Don't let them grab the kitten roughly, or pick it up by the nape of its neck. Rather, teach children to place one hand firmly under the kitten's chest, and the other under its hindquarters.

A new kitten may cry for several days, including standing in the middle of a room, tightly closing its eyes, and screaming at the top of its lungs. The kitten is simply trying to call its mother and siblings because it is lonely and frightened. This crying is perfectly normal and will stop when the kitten realizes no other cat will come to its aid. The crying may last for a day or up to a week, but it will eventually stop.

The kitten needs a private, secure place to call its own. You can buy all sorts of kitty cuddlers and cat baskets. Be aware, however, that the kitten may prefer a corner of your closet or your underwear drawer. A cat carrier or airline crate, or even a smallish cardboard box with ventilation holes cut in the side, will make a good "den." Line the bottom with soft towels or rags. You can shut the kitten in when you have visitors so that no one steps on it, and it will learn to enjoy the security of the crate. Then, when you need to take the kitten to the veterinarian, it will already be familiar with the carrier. If the kitten does not use the crate, it may be in a location where the kitten does not feel secure. Move it around until you find a place that it likes. If the crate has been previously used, wash it thoroughly to remove the smell of other cats or animals. When you open the crate to let out the kitten, make sure all doors and windows are closed. Cat doors and fireplace chimneys should be closed to prevent the kitten from running into them in panic. Open the door or raise the lid slowly and quietly so you don't alarm the kitten. It is sometimes easier to put a cat into a carrier or box rear-end first.

Introduce your new kitten to one room at a time. This allows it to gradually learn the surroundings. It will help the kitten to remember where its litter box is so that it doesn't become confused or lost.

A shallow cardboard box can be used for a disposable litter box, especially if lined with a sheet of plastic or a garbage bag. Or, you can use a plastic or enameled pan. Cover the bottom with a layer of clean, dry sand or commercial kitty litter. Change the litter and scrub the pan every day or so. Box training is usually easy. Just put the kitten in the box and show it how to paw, moving its front feet in a scratching motion. Put the kitten in the box soon after it awakes, about fifteen minutes after it eats, and after it has been playing. If the kitten can reach the box quickly, and if it is clean, soon it will be using it consistently.

In the beginning, keep the litter box close to where the kitten sleeps. After the kitten is accustomed to using it, you can gradually move it to its permanent location. If you have another litter box in use elsewhere in the house, it's still good to have one close to where the kitten will need it most frequently. It's unfair to expect the kitten to toddle to the litter box in the far corner of the basement when it spends most of its time in the kitchen with you. Do not put the litter box near the kitten's feeding place. The kitten may not like eating in its bathroom and may seek a toilet spot elsewhere in your house or not eat enough food because of the unpleasant surroundings.

A kitten will scratch and claw instinctively. This both sharpens and cleans its claws and marks its territory. Offer the kitten a scratching post from the beginning so that it does not get in the habit of clawing or climbing on your furniture, carpeting, or drapes (see below).

Play is important for your new kitten. In fact, it seems to be a full-time job as each day is a new adventure in its life. Play helps the kitten develop intelligence, coordination, and relationships with both humans and other animals. It's also important for its physical development. Contact with the mother cat before the kitten is weaned will give it socialization to the feline world. Play with humans after it is weaned will help it be more curious, self-confident, happier, and more emotionally stable.

Get a toy for your kitten—a toy mouse, a small rubber ball, or any other small, safe plaything. Or, make a small knot of fabric or a crumpled piece of paper. Toys and play help keep the kitten active and reinforce bonding. Inspect all toys, even "cat toys" from the pet shop, to make sure they do not have any small parts which could come loose and be swallowed or any sharp edges which might cause injury. If you use a crumpled cigarette pack, the cellophane

can cause damage inside the stomach if it is swallowed. Aluminum foil can cause blockage in the intestines. Don't allow any cat to play with either one, and take them away if it starts chewing. Give the kitten plenty of love, attention, and affection.

Normal, healthy cats may be awake as little as one-third of the time. The rest of the time they are sleeping, more or less soundly. Very young kittens and older cats may sleep even more of the time. It is not known why cats need about twice as much sleep as other mammals, but they tend to sleep when their stomachs are full and when they feel completely content and safe. Cats may "catnap" briefly or drop into a deeper sleep where they have rapid eye motions (REM sleep). During deeper sleep, your cat's muscles twitch, its legs may move as if it is chasing something, and its mouth may chomp, perhaps as a mouse is captured in a dreams. The muscles are generally relaxed while this is happening.

HOUSEBREAKING

We don't really "train" or "housebreak" cats. They are instinctively clean, and if offered an area that is suitable to them, they will nearly always use it, almost automatically. In the wild, a cat would naturally bury its urine and feces to help avoid attracting predators that could cause harm. Cats will not normally eliminate where they sleep, eat, drink, or hunt. For this reason, the litter box should be well away from the cat's food, water, and bed. Cats usually select an area because of its texture and/or odor.

A kitten may learn from its mother how to use the litter box. The instinct to cover waste is strong enough that most kittens will scratch and cover from about four weeks of age if loose material is available, even if an adult is not around to set an example. If this has not yet been learned, show the kitten the litter box from the first day, even if the kitten seems too young to use it. Take the kitten to the box fifteen or twenty minutes after eating and put the kitten in it.

If there is an accident outside the box, put the kitten's nose near the mistake (not in it) and firmly say "No!". Put the solid matter in the litter box, along with the kitten and move its paw to cover the waste with litter. Do this every time the kitten makes a mistake. Most kittens learn to use the litter box in only a few lessons.

Litter box user styles vary. Some cats barely cover their waste, while others may throw litter for several feet in all directions after using the box.

If you want the kitten to be an outdoor or in/out cat, you can use garden soil for litter. As the kitten learns to use the litter box, gradually move it closer to the door or pet door until you can move it out onto the step and into the garden.

Many types of cat litter are available. These range from plain clay to clay with odor masking and control substances to clumping and scoopable types to corncob and grass litters that can be flushed down the toilet. Some cats prefer cedar bark or chips, and these help keep the odor under control. However, chips that fall off the cat's feet elsewhere in the house may be a reminder of the litter box, encouraging the cat to soil in the wrong place. Baking soda can be added to cat litter to control odor—about one part soda to three or four parts litter. You can also put a layer in the bottom of the box before adding litter. Litter made from recycled pelleted or shredded newspaper is free of dust and sharp edges and is ideal for use after surgery for declawing or for everyday use.

The choice of litter is up to you, the litter purchaser. Keep in mind, however, that cats have strong individual preferences for the type of litter used. Some absolutely will not use scented or chlorophyll-type litters. Others like or dislike the feel of a particular texture or product on their feet. Occasionally, cats prefer different products such as shredded newspaper, potting soil, or playbox sand. If you use shredded paper, don't use magazine paper, as it is slick and not very absorbent. Make the strips fairly thin, and remove them after every use or at least once or twice a day. Plastic litter box liners are available, but may be more trouble than they're worth; cats claw through them, urine seeps underneath, and the result is a smelly mess.

About one to three inches of litter work best for most cats. If there is too much, the cat will sink into it. If there is too little, the cat may be unable to "bury" its waste. Find the amount which makes your cat happiest.

Kitty litter can be used in your garden as a soil conditioner, mulch, compost, or fertilizer. However, don't dispose of any type of kitty litter in an area where you plan to grow root vegetables or where children may play. Also be aware that the odor of used kitty litter in the garden may draw outside cats to use the same area as a toilet.

Cats are normally very clean animals and they are very sensitive to odor. If the litter box smells bad, the cat won't use it; this may be the start of urination or defecation elsewhere in your house. The best way to control the odor and keep the cat using the box is with thorough and frequent cleaning.

Many owners change the litter box only once a week. This may not be often enough for your cat's sensitive nose. Some people find it convenient to keep the litter box in the bathroom, where the fecal material can be scooped out daily and flushed down the toilet. The entire box should be changed every four to seven days. If you use a clumping litter, the clumps should be scooped out daily. Some cats may be even happier if this is done twice daily.

When cleaning and washing the pan, the choice of cleaning product is important. Use a mild dish detergent or a bleach solution. Strong cleansers with heavy odors may make the cat avoid using the box. You can also deodorize the litter box by emptying it and putting it out in bright sunlight for 30-45 minutes on a regular basis.

If you have only one or two cats, a single litter box is probably fine, depending on where it is located, how often you clean it, and how well the cats get along together. In multiple-cat households, territorial battles often occur. You may not see the fighting, but you may see the results in puddles or piles elsewhere in the house where one or more cats keep others from using the litter box. A good rule of thumb is to have one litter box per cat. If you have ANY problems with inappropriate elimination, try putting out an extra litter box, in a different location, with a different type of litter. Some cats prefer to have two litter boxes, using one for urination and one for feces. Litter box location is important, as cats usually prefer a private bathroom. Put the box in a quiet place, away from household noise and traffic. Just make sure it is not too difficult for older cats and kittens to get to it. If you have several litter boxes, put them in several different places to make for easy access.

Another consideration is the type of litter box. A small kitten may have trouble climbing into a box meant for an adult cat. A box with low sides can easily be made from a cut-down cardboard box, or you can use a shallow cake pan or cookie sheet. This will work well until the kitten is large enough to use a regular box. Low boxes also are good for elderly cats that have trouble climbing in boxes with high sides. A very large cat may not fit in some boxes made for the average cat; buy an oversized litter box. Some cats are perfectly happy with a plain plastic kitchen dish pan. These are inexpensive enough that they can be replaced if damaged. Over time, any plastic litter box will react with urine, forming odors that many cats find unpleasant. Get a new litter box every year or two.

Some cats will use covered or hooded litter boxes, which are great for cats that kick litter. One of these litter boxes, especially when it has a charcoal filter, can greatly reduce cat box odors. Other cats seem to be bothered by the confined space or odors held inside the box and refuse to use them. Owners of unneutered male cats may be happier with a box with a rim, which keeps the cat from spraying the floor or walls.

A new type of litter system is The Dry System™ (The Sweet "P" Corp., 610 Buffalo Ave., Niagara Falls, NY 14303). It is a litter box with a slotted bottom, underneath which is a pullout tray with an absorbent pad. The litter granules are coated and non-absorbent, so they last for six months or more. Pieces of fecal material are easily scooped out of the granules. Urine goes through to the pad, where it dries. Pads are changed weekly, and the granules are rinsed. The pad system makes it easy to detect blood or crystals in the cat's urine; it also allows the owner of a diabetic cat to easily collect urine for glucose testing.

You might like to screen your litter box or put it in a private place, both for your cat's comfort and feeling of security and for your own esthetics. If you have a tub or shower you aren't using, this is a perfect spot—private, safe, and easily cleaned. Place the litter box on a towel or rag which extends a foot or so beyond it. This will act as a floor mat to remove litter from the cat's feet before it leaves the area. A lower cupboard also works to conceal a litter box. Use one that has a latch the cat can open or put a pet door in it, but don't do this in the kitchen—it isn't sanitary. You also can put a pet door in a door leading from the house to the garage and put the litter box there. Some cats will tolerate a fabric, cardboard, or wooden "privacy screen" hiding the litter box.

Some cat owners have trained their cats to use the toilet. You can buy a cat toilet-training device, or you can use a child toilet trainer. Start by putting the cat's litter box next to the toilet. Raise the box two inches each day, putting the litter box on a level, sturdy stack of blocks or books. Once the box has been raised to the same level as the toilet seat, place the toilet-trainer above the litter box for two or three days until the cat is using it comfortably. Then remove the litter box and put the trainer on the toilet seat for another two to four days. You should then be able to remove the trainer as the cat will be using the toilet. Make sure all the people are trained, too—to leave the lid open so the cat can use the toilet! Not all cats can be trained to use the toilet, so if you have given it a good try and the cat doesn't want to do it, don't force it—it won't work anyway.

When a cat urinates outside its litter box or in a different part of the house, it usually indicates the area is more attractive. It may have a more suitable texture, it may have an odor from another cat eliminating, or it may be cleaner than the litter box, more secluded, or further away from an eating or sleeping area. The cat may be emotionally upset because there has been some sort of disturbance in its environment, and may urinate outside its litter box to mark its territory. This may be caused by the addition or loss of an animal or human from the household. Other cats outside the house, or disturbances such as construction, also could upset the cat.

Thoroughly cleaning the carpet may help remove the odor; however, this may not keep the cat from using the area. Something about the area was attractive to the cat before it started using it, and this attraction may remain after it is cleaned. On the contrary, cleaning the spot may make it even more attractive: ever notice how a cat will rush to use a freshly cleaned litter box?

Carefully evaluate the cat's situation to try to determine why it is soiling in places other than its litter box. It is usually easier to change the environment than to train the cat. Some cats just don't care where they eliminate, and this can be very difficult to correct. Changing the location of the litter box or cleaning it more frequently may correct the problem. If not, consult your veterinarian, who may be able to offer suggestions or refer you to a feline behaviorist.

It can be difficult to remove cat urine odor from carpet or other fabric. Vinegar and detergents (such as Ivory liquid) will effectively remove odor from carpet on a temporary basis, but it is not permanent. Woolite Rug Cleanser (spray foam) and Scope mouthwash remove the odor, but leave the carpet smelling like the product. Several effective cleaners are made specifically for removing cat odor from carpets: Feline Odor Neutralizer spray, Cat-Off and Outright Pet Odor Eliminator. For housebreaking problems, see Urinary Chapter, Feline Inappropriate Elimination section.

TRAINING YOUR CAT

Much of what is viewed as misbehavior in cats is actually their natural behavior. The cat that climbs on your kitchen counter is merely playing the part of a small furtive mammal sneaking through the underbrush. Climbing to a vantage point allows the cat to look for prey and to more easily avoid larger predators who would enjoy having it for dinner.

Cats can be trained to do simple tricks such as sitting up. Tricks are easiest for the cat to learn when they are related to natural instincts involving prey or food. Training sessions should be kept short—the cat's attention span for this sort of "work" is about five minutes. Repeated short sessions will allow the cat to understand what you want and to fix the new learning in its memory.

If you don't want a cat on your table, train it to stay off. Merely hiss/spit loudly when the cat attempts to climb up there, just as another cat would do. You can also shout "No!" in a nasty loud voice. Or, you can squirt the cat with a water spray bottle, throw a "shake can" (a can with a few pebbles inside) so it lands nearby, or use a jangly, noisy piece of small-sized chain. Another technique is to throw your car keys or a shoe so that they land near (not on) the cat, startling the cat out of the behavior.

It may be helpful to put mousetraps on the counter. If you are worried about the cat's foot being snapped, place them upside-down so they will spring and startle but not snap onto the cat. If you're still worried, "Snappy Trainers" are available. They are mousetraps with a piece of plastic to avoid injury. Use plenty of them so the cat can't just tiptoe around them. Some cats are deterred by two-inch strips of double-sided sticky tape or duct tape placed sticky-side up. Do NOT use flypaper instead of the sticky tape! A few mothballs will help keep the cat out of areas where it may be harmed or do damage to valuable belongings, such as closets and planters. These methods have the advantage that they also work when you are not present. Meanwhile, make another high perch that is legal for the cat—perhaps a carpeted spot on the end of a bookshelf, a cat "tree," or one high surface where the cat IS allowed.

You CAN teach cats to stay off tables and food preparation surfaces, at least most of the time. Keep training—consistently. Most cats are never completely reliable when tempting food is exposed and you are out of the room. Take that into account. It may be easier to lower your expectations than to train the cat. I keep a hanging wrought iron bird cage in my kitchen. I put meat in it to thaw, or anything else I don't want the cats to get and know they can't resist.

To keep the cat off your upholstered furniture, set regular spring mousetraps on it. There is also a "Pet Trainer" which sounds a loud noise when touched or jiggled. This may be enough to startle some cats off a sofa, chair or counter.

The cats that we invite into our lives accept us as "mother." This may be what makes it possible for what would be a solitary animal in the wild to form a social bond with humans. Kittens (and even older cats) that accept humans as "mother" mimic the human's behavior. When the cat is viewed as learning from humans, our opinion of their behaviors may change, making us less inclined to feel the cat is being "mean or spiteful."

If your cat is a kitten, training is usually much easier than for an adult cat that has grown up elsewhere. However, behavior modification techniques often work even with the adult cat. I call it the "carrot and stick" method. One of my cats reached a point where he was screaming, not just meowing, as he sat by the table during our meals. When he yowled, I would gently "bop" the top of his ears. The other part of this method, the "carrot" part, is the difficult one. It's easy to ignore the animal when it is being quiet. This is, however, very counterproductive. This is precisely the time at which the cat MUST be recognized favorably. So, I made special efforts to pet him and praise him ONLY when he was quiet. In about a week, I had a quiet cat who could again be allowed near the dinner table.

Occasionally, a cat will meow or howl until it is fed or held. This may even happen in the middle of the night. The demanding behavior is reinforced if you reward it by feeding or holding the animal. Discourage this behavior by ignoring the cat, spraying it with a squirt bottle, or blasting it with a hair dryer. Give attention only when the animal is quiet.

Think about the training program before you begin. What are you trying to do? How can you (gently) punish the cat for bad behavior? How can you reward the good behavior? In some cases, you can redirect the behavior, such as moving a clawing cat from your drapes to its scratching post. When used with a kitten or young cat this may be especially successful. Whatever training you are trying to do, it is very important that all members of the household treat the cat the same so that it is disciplined promptly and consistently each time it misbehaves. Also make sure that all household members agree on what is right and wrong.

Female cats, neutered males, and kittens that have plenty of food and shelter, can live happily together in groups. Cats who live by themselves without support from humans, as feral felines do, have less resources available. For this reason, they are usually solitary except at mating time and when the queen is raising a litter of kittens. The kittens stay with their mother from birth until they are about six to twelve months of age, then go off on their own to set up hunting territories. Cats become sexually mature around six to nine months of age, but may not assume their complete adult personalities until they are two to four years old. At this point, one cat may start fighting with others with whom it has previously lived in harmony. This may occur with either males or females, and sometimes happens even if the cats are neutered. Some cats are more territorial than others, and this may also cause fighting. Nine out of ten cases of aggression between male cats are cured by neutering. Your veterinarian may use hormone treatments for a fighting male cat if you don't want to neuter him at the moment.

Aggression between cats can be a problem. It is common when one mature cat is placed in a home which already has one or more established adult cats, or it may occur when a strange cat comes into your cat's yard. It can happen gradually when one cat becomes the aggressor and starts a fight which escalates as the "victim" is attacked. If two of the cats are intact males, the fighting may be violent. As with many wars, it usually begins with taunting and screaming between the parties. Fluffed hair

coat and tail, arched back, and hissing or spitting are next. It may escalate to full-scale warfare with clawing and biting. There are two choices for resolving the battle of the hormones. You can neuter one or both parties to the conflict or completely separate them. When one cat runs away, it does not necessarily stimulate other cats to run, too. Cats do not show the submissive behavior of dogs. Given a chance, the subordinate cat will run rather than fight or submit to the dominant animal.

Aggression can also occur accidentally. One cat may be sleeping near another when they are startled awake by a loud noise. They may instinctively start fighting with each other. Redirected aggression may occur when two cats are playing with each other and a dog strikes a nearby window. The cats are unable to attack the primary target (the dog), and instead attack each other.

Be careful during a cat fight. You can be badly clawed or bitten by trying to referee a cat fight or separate the combatants. Take care of your own safety first. You can toss a blanket, folded into quarters, over one of the cats. Or, perhaps you can insert a broom between them or hose them down with water. Do NOT allow the cats to fight it out because this will only make the problem worse. Even if the fight has occurred by accident, it may be difficult to smooth over the relationship between them. Keep them separated so they cannot see each other until you can bring them together under supervision.

Play and feeding are positive experiences that can be used to reinforce favorable feelings between the two animals. Feed the cats in adjacent rooms, but where each cat can see the other. Then, feed them with one at each end of a hallway or on opposite sides of a room. They will associate the feeding with good feelings about each other. Pet them and praise them for good behavior. Continue the petting and praise while moving the feed dishes closer together until the cats can be allowed to eat without fighting. The speed of this process should be gauged by the reactions of the cats.

Most of the time, we do not know why a cat that has been loving and normal toward its companion suddenly becomes territorial and begins fighting. Drugs may help to suppress the behavior in some cats. In others, the behavior cannot be successfully managed, and the cats must to be separated. For some, the only cure is to find a new home for the aggressor. Most of them will not adjust to a home with another cat, but will be quite happy to be the only cat in a new household.

Aggression toward humans can be a real problem. The cat may bite or scratch one or more persons. It is natural for a cat to do so when frightened. This may happen if it is cornered or picked up by a stranger, or when upset by commotion in the household. Then, after the cat has bitten or scratched, the person may drop the cat, hit it, or let out a shriek, all of which further frighten the animal.

Allow the cat to hide if it is uncomfortable with visitors, allowing it to make the first move. Most cats will eventually come out of hiding as their curiosity gets the best of them and they become accustomed to the presence of the stranger. Ask the visitor to talk to the cat, then gradually pet it. Wait to pick up the cat until it is completely comfortable with the contact. Better yet, wait until the cat comes to the lap of the visitor sitting on the sofa. It can also be helpful to feed the cat only when visitors are present (assuming you have frequent visitors!). At first, feed the cat only when strangers are in the house. Then, feed the cat in the same room, and then when someone is standing or sitting near the cat. If the cat enjoys being petted, ask the visitor to pet the cat while it is eating. Then you can begin waving arms, legs, jackets or other objects which previously frightened the cat.

Normal cats almost never attack without warning. Respect the cat when it is growling, its teeth are bared and its ears are flattened against its head. A cat that is the low man on the social totem pole may cower, flatten itself to the floor, and show these same behaviors. Don't approach it when it is doing this. If you MUST handle the cat, cover it with a blanket or shuffle it into a box or carrier with a shovel or piece of cardboard.

A cat that was raised by itself may never have learned how hard it can bite without hurting its littermate. If you are raising an orphan, it is your responsibility to teach it this social rule, either by gentle discipline or by ceasing play when it bites too hard. Tap the cat firmly on the nose when it bites you.

It is natural for a cat with kittens to be aggressive. She should be disciplined only gently, if at all, for this behavior—she is just taking care of her family. Instead, keep children and strangers away from her for the first week or two after the kittens are born.

Some cats remain fearful no matter what is done. Rather than forcing strangers upon them, it is best to just let these cats hide when visitors arrive. If you have guests for several days, shut the cat in a quiet room with food, water, and a litter box. If you can't do this, tranquilize the cat for its comfort and safety, as well as that of your guests.

The cat may act as if your legs, feet or hands are its prey. Cats normally play by stalking, chasing, pouncing on the prey, and biting it. This is accompanied by ferocious faces, and may be directed at an imaginary mouse, another pet, or a human. One of my friends suffered a painful bite on her bare big toe when their cat (who had been badly teased by her children) leaped from under the sofa and attacked her. Cats usually end this game by leaving. Let the cat go. Continuing to pursue it may cause real aggression. Instead of leaving, some cats become defensive, growling, spitting and biting hard. Relax and ignore the cat, giving it time to cool down. It may be useful to step into another room for a few minutes, closing the door to leave the cat alone.

Young cats may make a ritual of aggressive play. The animal may attack only one person in the household, always under a similar situation, such as when the person comes in the front door or steps into the hallway. Be aware that this may escalate into a pull-no-punches attack, and the behavior is best stopped before it becomes a habit. Cats that play too roughly with humans may have been played with roughly by people or may not have had enough play with other kittens. Channel the cat's energy in other directions. The easiest cure is to get another active young cat and let them play with each other. If you don't want to do that, be sure the cat has plenty of hard play. Active games such as chasing a ball, rope or crumpled piece of paper will allow the cat to wear off some energy and redirect the aggression. Play aggression is usually easy to manage, and drugs should not be needed.

Some cats may suddenly bite or scratch when being petted, while otherwise seeming content. They seem to reach a threshhold of annoyance or overexcitement, beyond which they lash out, jump away from you, run a little distance and sit down, perhaps while grooming. This behavior may be seen when they are petted too much, and they will usually give warning signs before attacking—tensing body, twitching tail, ear flattening, growling and narrowing the eyes.

It has been suggested that cats that strike are responding sexually to being petted by a human. During mating, the male cat bites the female's neck, and the female strikes at him with her claws out. When a human rhythmically pets a cat, he or she may be doing what the cat considers sexual stimulation and it may be responding accordingly. Another theory is that the cat enjoys the stroking so much that it falls asleep, awakens suddenly, feels trapped, and fights its way to freedom. By the time it is in the middle of the floor, the cat realizes where it is, and starts grooming itself to feel apart from its actions.

When the cat claws or bites a human, the instinct is to jerk the hand away and let out a shriek. At this point, the cat may switch from a sexual mode to a predator mode, and may seriously begin to bite and chew. The proper response is the one that is hardest—freeze! Don't try to pull away—that only stimulates the pet to try to hang onto the "prey" that is trying to get away. Stop petting the cat until it relaxes. Remain absolutely still and quiet until the cat opens its jaw and loses the glassy look in its eyes. Either the cat will let go of you, or it will relax enough that you can gently and slowly free yourself from it. Cats that persist in either of these behaviors may benefit from hormone treatments.

The same sort of reconditioning used with pleasurable experiences can be used with play aggression. When the cat attempts to strike your hands or legs, tease it into playing with a toy. You can pet the cat for short periods of time, stopping before you push it into annoyance. Stroke the entire body instead of just the head, neck, and back. Pet its chest, chin, and sides. Often, you can gradually desensitize the cat to where it will tolerate handling. It just takes time and work. Be sure not to reward the cat for inappropriate behavior. When it tries to bite or scratch, stop petting it immediately. Food is perhaps the best positive stimulus. Do not withhold regular meals, but schedule treats and conditioning sessions before the regular dinnertime. Do not hit the cat, as this may make it even more aggressive and afraid of you.

Alternatively, some cats that bite humans respond well to firmer discipline. You can tap the cat firmly on the end of its nose when it tries to bite, saying "No!" at the same time. You may also hiss/spit sharply in its face as another cat would do. Squirting the cat with a water spray bottle may be effective, as may throwing a "shake" can (don't hit the cat with it). It also may help to divert the cat by encouraging it to hunt and "kill" a catnip toy. You can put the toy on the end of a string or fishing rod so that you can move it around and encourage the cat to chase it. Wild games like this are best played in the early evening when the cat would begin its hunting if it lived in the wild. One cat owner calls this activity the "night crazies." Some cats that attack humans are play-deprived and will respond well to these periods of activity. It also may be helpful to acquire another cat to give the first one company and interaction. Most of these cats can be retrained with consistent, firm discipline by everyone in the household, unless the animal is unbalanced. Yes, there are a few cats that are mentally unbalanced and will not be helped by behavior modification or medication.

Some biting cats respond well to hormone treatment, rapidly becoming normal and loving while on medication. Unfortunately, they usually revert to their nasty selves when taken off the medication. This medication also has side effects which may include diabetes, so it should only be used temporarily, not as a substitute for training. If you think medication could help your animal, consult your veterinarian (after you have exhausted behavioral corrections).

Cats that have been normal and suddenly or gradually become aggressive toward humans should have a complete physical examination. Rabies must be ruled out if the cat spends time outdoors. A lack of thyroid hormone can cause a bad temper and attacks that can easily be corrected with a proper dosage of thyroid hormone. The cat will need this treatment for the rest of its life, as the attitude usually returns if treatment is stopped. Epilepsy may cause some cats to become nasty, and cats with urinary tract problems, abscesses under the skin, infected or ulcerated teeth or gums, or other illness may become aggressive if they are pushed to be sociable when they don't feel well.

Redirected aggression occurs when a cat is prevented from attacking its primary target. Instead, it attacks a nearby person. The most common cause is anger at another cat, especially if two males are involved, and castration may completely cure the problem. Strange people, cats or dogs visiting the house, or visits to strange places may initiate aggression, which is then aimed at the nearest person. The odor of a dog on a visitor's clothing may be enough to set off the cat. The cat may remain upset for quite some time. A cat that was threatened outdoors by another cat twenty minutes earlier may suddenly attack its unwitting owner when picked up. Avoid approaching a cat that has suddenly become aggressive. Look for a reason. Wait for the cat to calm down and approach you. If you must handle the cat, use a blanket or heavy gloves. Try to avoid stress for the cat, and punish its unwanted behavior.

Occasionally, a cat will tolerate its owner but no other humans. If the cat does not seriously attack you, you may be willing to put up with the behavior. You can shut the cat in another room when visitors are in the home or warn others to leave the cat alone. Life has enough problems without spending time and effort on humoring a sociopathic cat. If the cat continues its attacks (vicious ones, not playful attacks), it should be euthanized. Don't pass the cat on to someone else or take it to a shelter where it may hurt someone before its flaw is discovered. It would be a tragedy to have a child blinded by being scratched by this sort of cat.

Your cat may have a difficult time when a new baby comes into the house. It is often assumed that the cat is "jealous" of the new baby, when in reality, it may have trouble understanding the turmoil and changes within the house—emotional changes in the humans and new furniture and decorating. Allow the cat to explore the baby's room before the child is placed in it. If possible, bring something home from the hospital with the baby's smell on it, such as a blanket. Allow the cat to inspect it and sleep on it if it wishes, allowing it to become familiar with the odor. When you bring the baby home, remember to spend plenty of time with your pet. An older cat that has never been around children may take some time to adjust to a new baby, so don't leave the cat alone with the baby until you are sure the relationship is going well. Meanwhile, don't scold the cat when it comes near the baby out of curiosity. If you do, the cat will resent the baby. Instead, give the cat attention when it is near the child so it will associate pleasant feelings with it.

Introducing a new adult cat or cats into a household with an established clique of felines (or even one established feline) can be a traumatic experience for the cats and the humans in the area. It can be one of the most difficult behavioral problems imaginable. If at all possible, try to keep them from fighting at first, as this can create an unfavorable start which may take years to overcome. Confine the newcomer(s) in the basement or spare bedroom and allow the established cat(s) to have the rest of the house. If both cats are new to the household, confine them in separate areas. Although each cat may show an aggressive display at the other cat's door, this is okay, if it is not excessive. Then, allow each animal, one at a time, into the common areas of the house for short periods—a half-hour or so at a time. Do NOT allow either cat into the other one's "private" area, but only into areas they will eventually share. It may take anywhere from a few days to several weeks for the new cat to feel comfortable in its new house. When the new cat appears to feel at ease and the old cat no longer attacks the basement door, you can begin to bring them together.

Do something good for one of the cats within sight of the other. For instance, instead of feeding it in the bedroom, feed it in the common area within sight of the other cat. Pay attention, play with, or feed whichever cat is feeling more uneasy. With two people, one can play with the established cat while the other feeds the newcomer. Do this for ten to fifteen minutes twice a day. If any of the cats shows signs of aggression, discipline it with a firm "No" while tapping it on the head with one finger. Try not to yell or frighten the cat, as this may make it associate unpleasant things with the newcomer or with your presence in the situation. It may take as much as two months of this patient introduction to get the two animals to accept each other so that they can live permanently together. The investment in time and effort can save you from a year (or a lifetime) of spitting and fighting, and urinating or marking behavior.

When training cats to accept each other, be sure NOT to reward aggression. Instead, they should be mildly punished. Be careful not to frighten them and be consistent. Give them as much security as possible, and try to make their situation as routine and predictable as you can. Do not put the cats together without supervision until they get along well together. Above all, be patient and don't be in a hurry. You are making an investment in their future together and your family's comfort in living with them.

Aggression of cats toward other pets can sometimes be decreased by gently disciplining the cat. However, it is usually difficult to make life completely safe for a guinea pig, pet rat, or other small rodent. Cats have a tough time resisting temptation, and having a natural prey animal puttering around the house is more than most felines can resist. A cat may be well-trained, and appear completely compatible with the other pet, but may be unable to avoid chasing or attacking the animal when you are not present. Cats are natural predators and, even if by accident, usually play for keeps. For that reason, it is best to make sure your cat is out of the room before you (or your children) feed, play with, or observe a small pet. Even if you are in the room, a cat can suddenly lunge for, and kill, a small rodent or bird, before you can react. Remember, in the wild they do that for a living, and the instincts are still there in the household tabby! Also, some cats can be jealous, and may attack the animal BECAUSE you are paying attention to it rather than to them. A cat may learn to live in harmony with a rabbit that is about its size, but until the rabbit reaches that size, it could be in danger from your cat.

The best method is to make sure that the rodent or other pocket pet is safely confined in a cage of its own, and that the door to the room is closed except when a human is present. Small snakes are also tempting to cats, as they wriggle in a most enticing manner, almost asking to be batted by feet and claws. While the cat may not eat the snake, it may easily "play" it to death. Large snakes may turn the tables, and veterinarians occasionally hear of a large python or boa constrictor that makes lunch of the household feline. A small pet bird is easy prey for the cat when it slips out of its cage. Conversely, a large pet bird such as a parrot or cockatoo could easily put out a cat's eye or tear up its face.

Some cats will go fishing in an aquarium, and can either catch the fish and kill them, or pursue them until they die of anxiety. Or, the cat may playfully bat them out of the tank to die on the tabletop. Make sure the top is securely fastened or heavy enough that the cat cannot lift it, and that fish in an aquarium, or reptiles or rodents in glass tanks, have plenty of hiding places. It is stressful to a rodent to be watched through the glass by what must

appear to be a giant, interested predator. Fish can actually die of fright when harassed through the wall of the tank because they have no place to hide. Diligent separation of the species is the safest course for all animals involved.

Occasionally, a cat will suck on its own fur, tail, or paw. It may also suck on a human's or another cat's skin or hair. This usually happens when the cat is weaned from its mother too early (usually less than six weeks of age and occasionally up to eight weeks of age). It may also occur when a kitten is starved or malnourished, leading it to suck on its littermates, a furry toy, another animal (the family dog) or itself. Sucking may disappear on its own by the time the cat is about two years old. If the tail is not becoming raw or reddened from the sucking, the problem may be more annoying than harmful. To try to stop it, use continuous, consistent, gentle discipline. Sharply tell the cat "No!" when you notice chewing, spray water on the cat with a squirt bottle, or spray deodorant or perfume in front of the cat (not in its face!) while saying "No!" Also, try putting hot sauce or spray deodorant on its tail or on your skin. If the cat is sucking on you, bop it on the end of its nose, as this will help "wean" the cat just as its mother would. The habit may be modified even if it's not cured if you and everyone in the household will consistently discipline or divert the cat every time the behavior is seen. Hormone treatment may help the most persistent cases.

Wool sucking is a peculiar behavior seen in a few cats, especially some Siamese, Himalayan and other oriental breeds. It may be hereditary. The reason for this behavior is unknown; perhaps it's like gum chewing in humans. In some cases, the cat may be attracted to the odor from human sweat glands which is left on clothing, and it may occur when a cat sees a human as its "mother." When the cat is not allowed to suck on you, it will lick or chew at the corner or edge of a woolen sweater or blanket (occasionally the cat may suck on other materials, including cotton and synthetics). The cat salivates continuously, working itself into an emotional frenzy. Kittens that are removed from their mothers too early may become cats with this habit.

In many cases, the cat cannot be cured of wool sucking. Some may even stand on their hind legs in a closet, chewing on all wool clothing they can reach. Keep all attractive articles of clothing and bedding away from such a cat. If you can't do that, spray it with Bitter Apple, peppermint oil, perfume, or any other unpleasant substance. Change the spray from time to time, because some cats become accustomed to the flavor and begin chewing again. It may be necessary to give the cat a mild tranquilizer until the chewing episode passes, because if the behavior isn't controlled, the cat may eat enough of the material to have a fatal obstruction. If you reprimand the cat, it may just become a "closet" sucker, chewing frantically on a wider variety of objects than it did previously. It will also tend to hide or do it when you aren't around. If left alone and ignored, some of these cats will outgrow the behavior; others may be helped with thyroid hormone. A desperation treatment, which may work when nothing else does, is for your veterinarian to remove the cat's upper canine teeth. The cat may suck and leave a damp spot, but is unable to shred the material.

Some cats may become addicted to eating strange materials such as thread or string or plastic shower caps, a condition called "pica." They may eat corn, cardboard, paper, brooms, brushes, and items such as hearing aids, which may penetrate the digestive tract or cause an obstruction. These depraved appetites were once thought to be caused by vitamin deficiencies, but this is an unlikely cause if you are feeding a well-balanced commercial cat food.

It is a good idea to have the cat checked by a veterinarian to make sure there is no physical reason for its peculiar appetite. If not, look for psychological problems. Is there a reason for the cat to be annoyed or upset? Has there been a change in the environment? While it's not a cure, one solution is to cat-proof your home by having all members carefully keep the attractive items out of reach of the cat. If necessary, you can put the cat in a cage or crate when someone is not directly with it. You can also discipline the cat when you see it chewing a forbidden object. The best punishment is one the cat cannot associate with you, such as a spray of water or a noise other than a shout. You must correct the cat EVERY time it chews something it shouldn't. Many cats eventually outgrow pica.

A few cats seem to be hyperactive, a condition also known as hyperkinesia. The cat may dash madly around the house, or crouch down on the floor by a window and suddenly jump high into the air, all for no apparent reason. This behavior is usually seen in cats that are normally very active, but it also may occur when the owner is at work all day and the cat is home by itself. The cat may be trying to get attention in one of the few ways it can. This activity doesn't usually cause problems unless the cat is clawing the curtains. If you want to stop the behavior, you may be able to do so by gently scolding the cat when it acts this way. Then, be sure to reward it with lavish praise and petting when it is being still and quiet. It would be possible to keep the animal lightly sedated with a tranquilizer, but this isn't a very good alternative. Or, you could acquire another lively young cat to keep the first one company. A very young kitten may be overwhelmed by the cat's enthusiasm, so a three- or four-month-old cat may be the best choice.

Cats naturally enjoy play, whether with each other or with their human companions. Kittens play with each other and with their mothers. Some cats will play with toys such as catnip filled balls or mice. Others enjoy small objects such as walnuts, hard candies, or marbles—at least until they roll them under the furniture or down the heat vent and lose them. This self-directed play is usually brief, however, compared to the play they enjoy with humans. Some cats will learn to fetch and retrieve a crumpled ball of plastic wrap. A child-sized fiberglass fishing pole will allow you to cast out a cat toy on the end of the line, an activity that is fun and good exercise for the cat, and that will hold attention much longer than a self-play toy. Whatever you use, don't give your cat string, twine, or yarn as a toy. They can be fatal if swallowed.

Drug therapy for behavioral problems may include tranquilizers, anti-anxiety drugs, anti-depressants and hormones (progestins). Most of those do not result in permanent cures, but they may combine well with environmental changes and behavior modification. The drugs are then gradually withdrawn.

More pets are sent to animal shelters because of incurable behavioral problems than for any other reason. People acquire the animal, are unable to cope with things it is doing, and then get rid of it. If you have a cat with a behavior problem, it may be curable. Begin by having the cat examined by a veterinarian to be sure there are no health problems, and then ask the veterinarian for suggestions to change the animal's behavior so that you can live with it. If this does not work, ask him or her to recommend a behavior specialist. Some veterinary clinics and many veterinary schools have behaviorists on staff. One example is Ontario Veterinary College's Small-Animal Behavioral Service. It deals with many different problems and is said to have a 72% success rate. Or, you can write to ALPO Petfoods, P.O. Box 2187, Lehigh Valley, PA 18001 for a list of behavior specialists. It may also be worthwhile to check your library for books which may suggest alternate methods.

SCRATCHING

Kittens scratch instinctively. It helps them to sharpen their claws and shed the worn, outer layers. Scratching also may exercise the cat's claw muscles, as well as stretching its leg muscles. It seems to have some social uses, because cats that live in the wild or run free tend to reach high up in a conspicuous place, leaving noticeable scratch marks. They are probably marking their territory. The cat may be more prone to do this in the presence of another cat, or in an area where it or another cat has urinated. Secretions from its feet may leave a scent marker at the same time. Older cats may scratch as a dominance gesture in the presence of other cats, and its significance may be similar to that of urine marking.

Indoors, the cat may scratch your sofa or climb on your drapes just as it would on a tree outdoors. Unfortunately, the cat can't tell the difference between the corner of your sofa and a scratching post; once it has started scratching an object, it will usually continue, renewing the scent and scrapes as it would outdoors. It is often helpful to place the scratching post near where the cat sleeps, as many cats scratch as soon as they arise.

There are three basic ways of stopping the cat from causing damage by scratching. You can make it more difficult for the cat to scratch by changing its environment, use rewards or punishment to change its behavior, or change its claws by trimming, using claw covers or declawing. The sooner you stop the behavior, the easier it is to prevent it from becoming an ongoing habit.

Begin by offering the cat an attractive scratching post, a foot or two taller than the cat standing on its hind tiptoes.

Commercial scratching posts are available, from plain to elaborate palaces and trees. Or, you can make your own by tacking or gluing a carpet scrap to a piece of wood. Many cats prefer the firm texture of the back of the carpet rather than the soft carpet that is usually on a post. Also, using the top surface of the carpet may encourage the cat to claw your carpeted floor. Or, you can wrap sisal or hemp rope around a piece of wood or heavy cardboard. This can then be tacked to the wall on a doorway or convenient section of wall. A scratching post with a corner or rounded surface is attractive to many cats because they can scratch both sides at once. Some cats like to scratch on pieces of wood and will be perfectly happy with a tree limb with the bark still on it. Others are glad to have wooden or cork fishing floats. Place the scratching post near where the cat sleeps, because most cats like to mark their territory close to their sleeping place. The cat also needs to feel that the marking will be noticeable—there's no point in marking its territory where it can't be seen (McKeown, 1988).

You should acquire a scratching post at the same time you acquire the kitten or cat. Teach the cat by using the post yourself. Scrape your fingernails down the post, then praise the cat when it copies your action. Or, you can start with the scratching post lying on the floor and move it to vertical as the cat learns to use it.

The scratching post should be solidly set on a firm base or anchored so that it will not sway or tip. The cat may not use it if it moves or wobbles. If the post is tall and falls over, it may injure the cat. Size may also be important. In general, smaller cats prefer posts that are smaller in diameter, while larger cats prefer larger posts. In one house, I had a floor-to-ceiling scratching post that allowed cats to climb to ceiling level and then step onto a carpeted bookshelf. My cats loved it!

It is unfair to punish your cat for scratching the furniture or clawing the drapes if you do not provide a suitable, "legal" place for scratching. The cat will continue scratching, and find a time and place to do it when you are not around. It is a good idea to put the post in a prominent area, as the cat may not bother to look for it in an out-of-the-way corner.

Watch where your cat scratches, and try to match an area it prefers. Some cats would rather have a horizontal scratching board than a vertical post. If you use a horizontal board, be sure it will not fall over and injure the cat, or move around when it tries to scratch. Tack a spring toy to the post or board to entice the cat to use it. Rubbing catnip on it will attract some cats, and others like a post best when its covering is tattered and shredded. If you are removing a damaged piece of furniture, use a piece of its covering on the post to encourage the cat to use it. Since it may be used as a marking signal between cats, this makes it more visible. Don't be too hasty to replace the covering until it totally falls off or until the cat loses interest in the scratching post.

When the cat starts to scratch furniture, scold it with a firm "NO!" Then take the cat to the post, gently stretch its forelegs upward, and run its claws down it. It may be helpful for you to make scratching movements with your fingers along the post while the cat is watching. Make this a pleasant experience rather than a punishment. Try putting a scratching post in front of a piece of furniture or corner where the cat is already scratching, or in place of it.

Meanwhile, make the environment less attractive to the cat. You may want to temporarily remove valuable furniture, or you may need to put plastic or foil on it until the cat is trained, keeping it from scratching in the interim. Nylon netting works with some cats who dislike getting their claws caught in it. Pinning pieces of orange peel to furniture where the cat is trying to scratch it will stop some of them. Once the cat is using its post much of the time, sticky tape or mousetraps may help keep it away from furniture.

It is important for every cat to have one or more accessible, attractive scratching posts. Most learn quite easily that you want them to use the scratching post.

The cat may cause damage with its claws in ways other than scratching. It may "dig out," using its hind claws to get traction as it runs across a table, bookcase, or other smooth surface. The cat may cause damage as it climbs a screen door, or lies on its back and pulls itself along the underside of a sofa with its claws. None of these is true scratching behavior, and cannot be corrected in the same way. The only way to change these behaviors is to make the area inconvenient or unattractive so that the cat no longer travels across or under it. Cover the area with slick plastic until the cat learns to avoid it.

You may choose to change the cat's claws. Keeping them trimmed will not keep the cat from clawing the furniture, but it may decrease the damage it causes. If this is not enough, the cat can be declawed or have nail covers applied to its claws.

DECLAWING

To declaw or not to declaw: That is the question. I prefer not to declaw my own cats because I feel that cats with claws walk more normally. I rely on a scratching post and training to keep they from tearing up furniture or damaging the drapes. But, I have very good luck in training cats, and can usually convince them to see things my way. If you train your cat not to claw the furniture, drapes, and humans in its world, it saves you the costs and risks of surgery. I do NOT feel, however, as some humane organizations and a few veterinarians do, that declawing is cruel.

Some veterinarians recommend declawing for all cats. For some, this comes from a sincere conviction that the declawed cat makes a better pet. For others, it is a revenue-producing measure. THINK before you have YOUR cat declawed. Is it what you really want or need to have done? Do not have it done as a routine procedure. Do it because it is right for you and for your cat. Many cats never develop undesirable clawing behavior, and all cats should not be declawed just because a small percentage of them claw the furniture. Studies have shown that there are rarely any behavioral problems because of declawing, and for many owners, there are real advantages to the declawed animal. A few cats who have been declawed will tend to bite when they are threatened or stressed, perhaps to compensate for their lack of armament. Others seem to be prone to jumping on counters and tables after declawing.

However, when the cat is tearing up your sofa or otherwise damaging your house, it is certainly kinder to declaw it than to send the cat to the shelter or euthanize it because the behavior upsets you. It can also make a cat safer around a baby or small child, where it might scratch or damage an eye, even if by accident. For the problem cat, declawing may be a true, lasting gift as it gives the cat a longer, happier life with its family and keeps it from being euthanized or tossed out into the cruel world as a stray. It's better to be declawed than to be dead.

Declawing can be done at any age, even on young kittens. There is no upper age limit for declawing as long as the cat is otherwise healthy, although convalescence takes a bit longer in older cats. You may want to move food, water, and litter box into the same area to make life easier for the cat during the healing process.

If the cat is to be declawed, it is best to remove only the front claws. This will protect eyes and furniture, while allowing the cat to defend itself (somewhat) against other cats and dogs if outside. Claws make it easy for a cat to run up a tree, but very difficult to get down, especially if it tries to get down headfirst. Most cats climb down a tree tail-first, looking nervously over one shoulder. Declawing the front feet may make it harder for the cat to climb up a tree, but it may make it almost impossible to get down without its front "hooks." If your cat climbs a tree, it may be left sitting forlornly wailing on a branch or end up diving desperately out of the tree to try to return home. Declawing, for many reasons, is best done to the cat that will remain indoors for the rest of its life. If you are expecting the surgery to keep the cat from killing birds, it probably will not do so.

The cat is prepared for surgery as for spaying (see Reproduction Chapter). After the cat is anesthetized with a general anesthetic, and is asleep, its paws will be cleansed. Some veterinarians coat the paws with a depilatory to remove the fur, while others clip the feet with electric clippers. The paws are disinfected and a tourniquet is put above the elbow to reduce bleeding.

Removing the claw also involves removing a part of the third phalanx bone within the foot. This still allows the cat to have normal-looking feet and to walk normally. Some veterinarians remove the entire third phalanx. Their rationale for this method is that the claw can never regrow, which occasionally (rarely) occurs with other methods. This is true. However, many cats that are declawed in this manner do NOT have normal-looking feet. They may also walk tenderly and awkwardly for the rest of their lives. The larger the cat is, the more abnormal its gait will be.

A rarely-used technique involves cutting through the deep digital flexor tendon. The claws are not removed, but the cat cannot use them for scratching. Some people find this preferable to "amputation" techniques. The disadvantage is that the cat's claws must be regularly trimmed for the rest of its life. Don't have this surgery done if you don't want to keep the claws trimmed, because the cat will still scratch and cause damage.

If there is any doubt as to which method your veterinarian uses, ask. Or, ask to see a cat (or two) which the veterinarian has declawed and which is fully healed from the surgery. Or, ask a friend who has a cat that has been satisfactorily declawed for a referral to the surgeon.

As with any surgery, there is some pain for a short time afterward, and everything possible is done to minimize it. The veterinarian may keep the cat for a day or so after surgery to make sure there is no bleeding. When you bring the cat home, make sure that it stays indoors until it is completely healed so that dirt does not get into the surgical area and the cat does not have to defend itself or run away from a dog or cat. You may need to keep the cat inside from two to 14 days, depending on your veterinarian and the procedure used.

Use shredded newspapers, a recycled newspaper litter, or other box filler recommended by your veterinarian until the cat is completely healed. Clay fillers may have tiny particles which can enter the surgical areas and cause irritation. Do not go back to your clay filler until the cat's feet are completely healed—usually one to two weeks. A few cats may refuse to use shredded paper litter and become constipated; they may use pelleted newspaper litter if it is offered. Some cats will not use any type of paper litter, and may begin soiling somewhere other than the litter box. Keep an eye out for this behavior after declawing, and change the litter situation to correct any problems before they become permanent.

Do not encourage the cat to play or otherwise be active. It may be necessary to restrict or confine the cat to keep it from running and jumping until healed. Keep other cats, dogs and children from annoying the cat and, if necessary, shut the cat in a separate room to keep them from bothering it. Everyone should be VERY careful not to step on the cat's toes. This is one of the most common complications after this surgery.

If the cat has any bleeding, pus or other drainage, odor, swelling, or lameness, return the cat to your veterinarian to be checked. If a few small spots of blood are seen, don't worry. Some cats will walk with a slight limp or hold one foot up for more than a few days after surgery. When these cats are examined, they may not show any sign of infection or pain. Your veterinarian may give the cat a low dose of a corticosteroid, to which these cats usually respond within 24 hours. If infection is found, the area will be cleaned and the cat will usually be given antibiotics for a few days.

Some veterinarians bandage the feet, while others send the cat home with feet unwrapped. The surgical area is often sealed with tissue glue rather than being sutured. If the cat comes home with its feet bandaged, make sure the bandages stay clean and dry. If the bandage gets wet, take the cat back to the veterinarian to be rewrapped. If the feet become wet in the evening, don't go to an emergency clinic, but to your veterinarian first thing in the morning. The cat's feet may be tender for a week or two after surgery.

On rare occasions, a claw may regrow after the feet have healed. Return the cat to your veterinarian to have it removed, or have this done if the cat is being anesthetized for teeth cleaning or other surgery.

A substitute for declawing is a soft plastic covering such as Soft Paws® (Smart Practice, P.O. Box 29222, Phoenix, AZ 85038-9222). These covers, sized for kittens or adult cats, are glued onto the cat's claws to reduce damage due to clawing. First, the cat's nails are trimmed. Then, the covers are safely and easily attached to the cat's claws with a quick-setting, nontoxic glue. At first, the cat may lick or shake its feet, and may try to chew at the caps or pull one or two of them off its nails. However, after a short adjustment period, the cat becomes accustomed to wearing the nail caps. The only disadvantage is that the coverings fall off every four to six weeks when the claw sheaths are shed, or more often if the cat is outdoors. Then, they need to be replaced. If you don't mind attaching new ones from time to time, these covers may be good for you and your cat. It is a good idea to have your veterinarian apply the first set of covers so you can see how it is done and how your cat will react. Your veterinarian can apply new sets of nail covers when needed; do-it-yourself, take-home kits are available from your veterinarian if your cat is cooperative.

Claw covers are a good choice if you don't want to declaw your cat for any reason. They are ideal for cats that are normally outdoors but must be inside temporarily, such as when they are ill or because of a move. They can also be used on older cats or cats in poor health who may be poor candidates for surgery. Covers are completely safe and harmless to cats. If the cat accidentally swallows one, it just passes through.

INDOORS OR OUT

Keeping your cat indoors at all times is the safest. It may add five to seven or more healthy, happy years to its life. This decision is best made when you first acquire a kitten, because if you never allow it outside, the cat will never know it is missing anything. It will not want to go outside, and there will be no fuss or crying. Outdoor cats live an average of three to five years, while a strictly indoor cat may easily live 17 years or more. Indoor cats tend to be more affectionate and to have a closer relationship with their owners than do cats who are trying to survive in the cold, cruel world outdoors.

In the city, outdoor cats are exposed to traffic, and cars kill and maim many cats every year. In cold climates, cats often climb up under the hood of a vehicle to sit on the still-warm engine after it has been driven. When the owner comes out to start the car, the cat doesn't have time to move, or doesn't know that it needs to do so. When the engine is started, the cat panics and often runs headlong into the fan or belts. Some cats survive the encounter. Others do not. In winter, thump on the car hood before you get in your car, honk your horn, and wait a few seconds before starting your engine. This will awaken your outdoor cat (or your neighbor's cat) and give it time to move before you start your car.

The free-roaming cat may encounter other cats who may fight with it or carry disease. The cat can easily pick up fleas in its travels, bringing them back to keep your other pets and your home continually infested. It can also pick up parasites, such as tapeworms, by eating rodents and insects. Occasionally, malicious humans (especially children) may harm a free-roaming cat. Even their innocent attentions may be fatal to the cat if it runs into a street to escape. Harm can be done by poison or traps, especially those set by people who love birds, or who don't want cats digging in their flower beds. Or, you may lose your pet to someone who takes in "that poor little kitty" begging on the doorstep.

The roaming cat may eat a rodent that is dying because it has been poisoned by rat poison, and thus becomes poisoned itself. In suburban and rural areas, cats make good food for hawks and coyotes. In some areas, owls make it almost impossible to keep a white or light-colored cat that roams outdoors. The cat's coat is like a restaurant beacon to the night-hunting bird. Encounters with poisonous snakes also may be fatal.

Cats that roam lawns and gardens can come into contact with many toxic pesticides. Because the poison may be slow-acting, the cat may be well along toward death when it is finally detected. Licking sweet-tasting anti-freeze from a driveway or gutter where it has been drained may fatally poison the cat. Keeping the cat indoors can lead to a much longer, healthier life (and cheaper in terms of veterinary care costs!). For every outdoor cat that lives to eight or ten years of age, there are dozens that don't survive the perils.

Cats that are allowed outdoors will instinctively hunt, for sport or food or both, because they are natural predators. They will do this even if well fed on the finest of foods. Putting a bell on a cat does not keep it from killing birds and animals because wildlife does not associate a ringing bell with the attack that follows. Also, many cats learn to walk gently to keep the bell quiet.

The hunting cat may bring you mice, gophers, or birds. This is a natural behavior. It is an attempt to share the wealth with you and help care for you as part of its family. The cat also may be asking for a bit of praise for its hunting prowess. A few cats will stop hunting a particular prey if you scold them for it. Others will just quit bringing home their trophies. If you want the cat to keep hunting, be sure to laud its efforts with petting and kind words, even if you don't appreciate half-dead mice being dragged in through the cat door. Or, the cat bringing in a live mouse and turning it loose in the kitchen! Declawing does not keep a cat from killing—it will merely bat down prey with its paws. If you want the cat to stop hunting, or prevent it from killing birds, keep the cat indoors.

Opinions vary as to how much damage outdoor cats cause to the bird population. Only the most skillful of cats are successful bird hunters; however, cats who start hunting birds are almost impossible to stop. You may scold or squirt the cat when it brings you a bird, but this may only keep the cat from catching birds when you are nearby. If you want a cat that doesn't hunt birds, get a kitten whose mother does not hunt them. Or, you can acquire a kitten around six weeks of age and keep it indoors until it is more than a year old.

Cats do not have any particular NEED to be outdoors, and many of them live their entire lives safely and happily indoors. If you live in the city and move to the country, there is still no reason to make your cat live outside. It can quite happily spend the rest of its life indoors. Indeed, it may be quite upset at having to learn about the hazards of the wilds.

A cat that is outdoors part of the time can sometimes be trained to stay in your yard, especially if you stay around when it is outside and hiss at that cat or spray it with water when it tries to leave. If the cat is unattended for long periods, don't expect it to stay in your yard. The cat doesn't know that particular area is "yours," and its idea of territory may extend far beyond your yard.

Cats can be trained to stroll on a leash so you can safely take them for a walk. Wait until your cat is at least four-months-old, and get a harness that fits the cat's chest snugly and comfortably. Let the cat wear it around the house, starting with a few minutes and working up to a whole day. Do this when you are at home, keeping an eye on the cat. If possible, don't remove the harness when the cat seems annoyed with it, but take it off when it ignores it. When the cat is accustomed to the harness, attach a lightweight leash or piece of rope and let the cat drag it around. Make sure it does not become caught on anything. After a few days, sit on a chair and hold the leash, letting the cat walk around you. Do this several times a day for five to ten minutes, for a week to ten days. When the cat is comfortable with this, walk around the house, leading the cat with gentle quick tugs. Praise the cat when it follows, petting it lavishly. When the cat has learned to walk comfortably around the house with you, take it outdoors, safe from harm or loss.

Cats who live indoors are much happier if neutered. It's no fun to live with a female that is yowling and climbing the curtains and rolling on the carpet for months on end because she is in heat. It's also no fun for an intact male to be teased by tom cats that walk around the outside of his house, howling challenges and urinating on bushes, walls, and windowsills where he can smell the odors. He can also catch the scent of a female in heat on the wind, and this may cause him to urinate in your house, out of frustration or from a need to mark his territory against imagined intruders. For the comfort of both cat and owner, spaying and neutering are great ideas. The only reason to keep an intact cat, either indoors or out, is if you have definite plans for breeding it.

Some people worry about the cost of keeping a cat indoors. There are a few costs at the beginning. The cat will need a litter box. A scratching post is a necessity, but you can easily make that yourself if you don't want to buy one. Purchasing litter is an ongoing expense, but if you are near open spaces, your cat may be willing to use sand or topsoil instead of commercial litter. You will save enough in veterinary bills (because your cat lives a

healthier life) to more than pay for any additional costs of keeping it indoors.

If you wish, you can make life positively luxurious for your indoor cat by building a screened porch. It can be built on legs out from one of your windows, similar to a bay window. Put a weatherproof roof on it and a mesh or hardware cloth floor. Then put a cat door through your wall or window so the cat can go in and out at will. If you wish, put the litter box out there so that stray bits of litter will fall through the wire and out onto the ground. The porch will keep litter box odors outside, and you can build a door into the outside wall of the enclosure for changing the box. However, don't forget to change the litter just because it's outside. The porch allows your feline(s) to enjoy sunshine and fresh air without exposure to harm.

With indoor cats, there is a realistic limit to how many you can have in the household. Too many cats will lead to continuous fighting, urine marking, and soiling in places other than the litter box because they feel they don't have enough space.

If you live on a farm or ranch, or have a business that has a mouse or rat problem, an outdoor or free-roaming cat can serve a useful purpose. Otherwise, it's much more fair to take responsibility for the cat's life in our complex and confusing world. Don't send your cat outside to chance being killed.

It is difficult but not impossible to change an adult cat from an outdoor or in/out animal to a strictly indoor cat. It can be done with time and persistence, consistency among household members, and a deaf ear to its pleas. It is easiest if you ALWAYS keep it inside. The cat will find it hard to understand if you sometimes allow it to go outdoors and refuse to do so at other times. When you first keep the cat in, expect protest. The cat may cry or howl, claw at screens, climb the curtains, try to dart past you every time a door is opened, and generally make a nuisance of itself. Hang in there! What seems hard-hearted in the short term may be the kindest course in the long run as you protect your beloved pet from the hazards of the outside world. This is especially true if you have moved from a rural or suburban area into a town or city. If your cat is a solo animal, it is sometimes helpful to acquire another cat to keep it company. (See above for tips on introducing the two felines to each other.)

Outdoor cats can be safely confined to an unfenced yard by Invisible Fencing® (1-800-538-DOGS), in which an antenna wire is buried around the perimeter of your yard. It can also be used to keep your cat out of the garden or flower beds. A transmitter located in your basement or garage sends a signal to the wire. The cat wears a collar which is activated when it approaches the wire. After a short training period, the cat will not go beyond the allotted area. The good news is that this system works well in keeping your cat on your property without a fence. The bad news is that since there is no fence, the cat may still be attacked by stray cats, dogs, or wild animals that can freely come in across the barrier.

FERAL FELINES

Feral cats are domestic cats that have escaped or been turned out and are now running wild. They may make a living by scrounging in trash cans or eating food set out for pet dogs and cats. Some people may even specifically feed them because they enjoy having them around, much as they do with pigeons. Cities such as Rome have a love-hate relationship with their homeless cats. Whether in rural wilds or deep in the heart of the city, these felines may have been living free for a number of generations, where they form loose groups. Reducing their available food supply by feeding domestic pets indoors may help to reduce their numbers if rodents and birds are not plentiful.

Feral cats can have a large negative impact on wild bird populations. In rural areas, they can greatly reduce the number of pheasant and quail chicks reaching maturity. In cities, they can reduce songbirds to nearly zero.

If you don't want the cats around, or if they pose a health threat to you, your pets, and your children because of rabies in wildlife in the area, disposal can be attempted. In some counties, rabies control or shelter employees may arrange to trap them for you.

If you live far enough out in the country, shooting stray cats with a small-caliber rifle or shotgun can be a safe and humane method of disposal. In most cases, however, removal (whether by shooting or trapping) simply opens up a habitat slot which is quickly filled by newcomers. These cats may migrate in from surrounding housing areas or from being dumped by city dwellers, or by increased kitten survival from unspayed queens who have not yet been caught.

Some shelters or veterinary clinics loan or rent live traps so that the cats can be caught. You can then turn them over to the clinic or shelter for disposal. Use tuna or a similar strong-smelling fish for bait. Do not trap in wet or very cold weather, or when it is hot, as the frightened, excited cats are prone to freezing or heat stroke. Cover the trap with a cloth or towel as soon as you find the cat in it. This helps to calm the cat and keep it from fighting the cage and injuring itself. Cats may scrape their noses and claws on the cage wire. These scratches are usually shallow and heal quickly.

It does not work to feed tranquilizers to stray cats. They leave the area before the drug can take effect, and may be harmed by a dog or person, or get run over by a vehicle because they cannot walk across a road. Tranquilization also is not a good method to capture feral cats if they are eating from a common food source. One cat might get enough to be fatal, while others don't get enough. Also, the cat may just crawl into a remote place where you can't get it.

Do not trap a mother who has nursing kittens unless you can catch them, too. The kittens will die without their mother to care for them. If you accidentally catch a queen who is nursing, release her in the area where you caught her. Catch her again when the kittens are six- or eight-weeks-old.

Feral cats or kittens that have grown up without being socialized can be captured with a humane box-type trap. This will not be detrimental to their opinion of humans. Kittens that are more than nine-weeks-old are likely to mistrust humans no matter how kindly they are treated. If you find a home for such cats, warn the new owner that they are never likely to be sociable or to tolerate much handling. Some of them can be taught to accept some petting if they are handled gently without teasing or rough discipline.

If caught around six to eight weeks of age, feral kittens can sometimes be tamed and placed as pets. If you do not have homes for them, leave them running loose until they are around four-months-old. Then trap and neuter them and turn them loose to return to their companions. Kittens who are trapped too young will have to be bottle fed, which is a lot of work. The one advantage of bottle feeding is that they become very tame. Treat feral kittens with as much respect as you would treat an adult cat. No matter how young they are, they often have grouchy attitudes and can give you nasty bites and scratches.

Another choice, if you wish, is to manage the feral cats as a distinct animal population (Zaunbrecher, 1993). Even if you trap dozens of cats in your area, you leave a vacant habitat which was obviously suitable. New cats will merely move in to fill the ecological niche. The solution is to trap and neuter the cats, and then release them to defend their normal territory against newcomers. This will keep them from reproducing, and will keep you from having to remove an unending flow of newcomers. It also lessens annoying behaviors such as howling, spraying, and fighting among tom cats. The cats also do less roaming, so fewer of them are hit by cars or otherwise injured.

Be sure to tell the veterinarian who is handling the cats that they are wild. If possible, the veterinarian should have a squeeze-sided cage, allowing the cat to be sedated before anesthetizing it for surgery. Upper respiratory infections are common in feral cats, and both external and internal parasites are often found. These should be treated before the cats are neutered. The veterinarian should use dissolvable sutures to avoid the need to trap and handle the cat again. To be sure there are no complications, males who have been neutered should be kept in captivity for at least two days and females for at least three days after spaying. If the cat becomes ill after it is released, it may be difficult to catch it again. Or, it may merely hide and die.

Some colonies of feral cats have considerable kitten loss. As many as half the kittens born in these groups may die of diseases that would be treatable or preventable if they were in captivity. Sick and dying cats are a frequent sight. If the kittens live through their first four to six months, they will probably be immune to most diseases that afflict domestic cats. It is important to vaccinate these cats for rabies when they are neutered or spayed so that they will protect you and your domestic pets by being immune to it.

It is a good idea to test the first half-dozen cats that you capture for feline immunodeficiency virus (FIV) and feline leukemia. This will give you a good idea whether these infections are present in your local population. In most areas, only a small percentage of the cats are infected. If the cats are positive, they should be euthanized to help prevent the spread of the disease. Or, you can isolate them from other cats and retest them in a month. If they are still positive, euthanasia is still recommended, and the other cats should be tested as you catch them. If the tests are negative, it is reasonable to assume that the rest of the group of feral cats is similarly healthy. Any new cats that wander into the group should also be tested and neutered as soon as you can catch them. You can obtain more information on feral felines from Alley Cat Allies, Inc., (202) 686-2210.

THE BARN CAT

Some owners of pampered household felines envision barn living as some sort of feline Hades. In reality, it can be a pretty good life for a rural pet. The cat can also perform a useful service as she and her kin keep mice and other unwanted pests out of animal feed and housing. For many cats that are on death row at a shelter, it sure beats the alternative! As with household cats, barn cats make much more suitable pets if they are spayed and neutered (and healed from the surgery) before being put outdoors. Keep the cat in a carrier or cage, or shut in a stall or feed room, for several days before turning it completely loose in the barn or stable. An outdoor cat can also make a good pet for someone who loves cats but is badly allergic to them, as it often can be petted and held if the person washes his or her hands afterward.

You can also have cats that live inside, along with cats that live outdoors. At one point, I had two indoor cats (they were never allowed outside), and nine outdoor cats (they were never allowed in the house) on my farm. The outdoor cats were just as loved and special as those that lived in the house. All but one would come when called by name (the one who wouldn't come was deaf!).

It is important to keep your barn cats vaccinated. Giving them their normal vaccinations against diseases such as panleukopenia will keep them from dying en masse when epidemics sweep through your area. Keeping all of them currently vaccinated against rabies will protect them against possible rabies transfer from wildlife. It will also protect you and your family, your other pets, and your livestock against exposure to the disease via the cats. Cats are quite easily exposed through animals such as raccoons and skunks. Infected cats can spread toxoplasmosis to each other and to cattle and goats by defecating in animal feeders and on hay or grain. Getting rid of unwanted strays will help lessen this risk.

Pseudorabies is a disease that commonly infects swine. The unexplained death of a cat or dog may be the first sign that the virus is present on your farm. If this disease is diagnosed in your hogs and your pets haven't contracted it, be careful that they don't come into contact with an ill or dead animal. Cats contract it from contact with swine that are infected. They can also contract it by eating uncooked or undercooked pork, or by eating infected rats.

Cats infected with pseudorabies rarely live more than one to two days after signs begin. If you see any signs at all, they may include depression, lack of appetite, restlessness, excessive salivation, abnormal swallowing movements, vomiting, and changes in the voice. The cat may resist having its mouth opened, and may rub, scratch, or chew at itching areas of the skin until they are raw and bleeding. A few cats may have a longer course of disease with depression and swallowing problems but no itching or mutilation. Because these signs look much like those of rabies, handle the cat as if it has rabies until it is proven otherwise. Consult your veterinarian immediately for a definite diagnosis (see Rabies). Pseudorabies is not contagious to humans. If you have hogs, the disease may be a serious problem for you.

If you choose to let your barn cats reproduce, be aware that males will often kill kittens that are not theirs. As with lions, this helps the female come back into heat more rapidly, allowing the male to rebreed the female and perpetuate his own genes. A stray tom cat may be best euthanized or shot rather than allowed to kill your kittens.

CAT IDENTIFICATION

A cat, whether it lives outdoors or indoors and out, should have a collar with at least your name and phone number on it so you can be called if it is found or injured and requires medial attention. Otherwise, your cat may be euthanized in as few as 72 hours by the shelter or pound rather than being treated. A collar with I.D. tag is a good idea even for a permanently indoor cat, as it can slip out when someone opens a door, panic and become lost.

Make sure to use an elasticized safety collar so it will come off if the cat catches it on a tree limb or other obstacle; otherwise, it might strangle. You should be able to slip two fingers between the collar and the cat. However, it should not come off TOO easily. The collar should be tight enough that the cat cannot get a front leg caught through it, which could make it critically tight around the chest. Be sure to adjust it as your cat grows.

You can have your cat tattooed with identifying numbers that are registered with a national registry such as Tattoo-A-Pet™ or, if you prefer, your name or driver's license number put on the animal. Tattoos can be put inside the ears of light-colored cats, or they can be placed inside the hind leg. This can be done very easily at the time the cat is anesthetized for any other surgery such as a spay, or it can be done separately.

Another way to identify a cat is to have a microchip implanted in it. This is a computer-readable chip smaller than a grain of rice which is implanted under the skin of the cat's neck with a quick, nearly painless injection. It can be done by your veterinarian or humane organization, and lasts for the pet's lifetime. Pets that land in a shelter are examined with a reader that is passed over the animal's neck. This identifies its number, which can then be checked against a registry to help insure its return. One such system is made by Anicare™ (1-800-395-5585). This will also help your cat be returned if it is lost after slipping out an open door, or escaping via a natural disaster such as an earthquake or hurricane, or even a tree limb, vehicle or burglar crashing through a window when you are out.

Keep a complete set of clear photos of your cat unless it is solid black or white. Be sure to have right and left side pictures, as well as front and side views of its head if there are identifying markings.

CATS FOR IMMUNOCOMPROMISED PERSONS

Persons who have damaged or suppressed immune systems, are called immunocompromised (IC) or immunosuppressed. This can be because of medication or because of a disease. IC persons include people who have had organ or bone marrow transplants and those undergoing therapy for cancer. People with cirrhosis of the liver and alcoholism, diabetes mellitus, kidney and liver failure, malnutrition, those born with deficient immune systems and some types of cancer can have immune suppression. The most damaging suppression is seen with human immune deficiency virus (AIDS).

Cats are ideal pets for IC persons, and can make a great contribution to their well-being and will to live. For these persons, a mature cat may be a better pet than a kitten because it is less likely to bite or scratch, or to carry cat scratch disease.

It is important to take basic precautions to keep your animal healthy if you are IC. Feed only a high-quality, well-balanced diet. Do not give the cat any uncooked meat or scraps.

Extensive guidelines for pet health for IC persons is given in an article: "Caring for Pets of Immunocompromised Persons" by F.J. Angulo, et al., *Journal of the American Veterinary Medical Association*, Vol. 205, No. 12, 15 December 1994, pp. 1711-1718. You may be able to find this article through your library or through a local veterinarian.

Chapter 3

KNOWING YOUR CAT: THE NORMAL ANIMAL

- *Behavior*
- *Posture*
- *Movement*
- *Voice*
- *Appetite*
- *Digestive System*
- *Skin And Coat*
- *Mucous Membranes*
- *Abdomen*
- *Feces*
- *Urine*
- *Vaginal Discharge*
- *Brain And Central Nervous System*
- *Other Indicators Of Health*
- *Body Temperature*
- *Pulse*
  - *The Stethoscope*
  - *Normal Heart Rate*
- *Respiration Rate*
- *Gut Sounds*
- *Blood*
  - *Anemia*

Repairing your cat begins with knowing your own pet, and knowing what is normal for it. United States Treasury agents are trained to spot counterfeit money by looking at literally thousands of real bills. The same is true of you and your cat. You must know what is normal before you can know what is abnormal. Observe your cat from day to day and note changes that occur. It is extremely valuable to know what is "normal" for cats in general, and for your breed and individual in particular.

Trust your feelings about your cat. Many times, a cat owner takes his or her cat to a veterinarian and says something is wrong with the cat. The owner knows that the cat is "not quite right." The veterinarian cannot see anything wrong. Whatever is wrong is so subtle that the owner, who lives with the cat every day, is the only one who can see a problem. This does NOT mean the veterinarian is incompetent, nor does it mean it is your imagination. It only means that the problem is so subtle that it is not

obvious at this point, and that the cat's problem is not serious, at least not yet. It will either become better or worse. If it gets better, you do not have a problem! If it gets worse, your veterinarian will be able to diagnose the problem and offer a solution for it.

When you see a problem with your cat, take a moment to think before you panic and call the veterinarian or rush the cat to the clinic. If there is a swelling, check for one like it on the other side. An owner will occasionally take a cat to the veterinarian to check a large swelling bulging between the last rib and the hipbone, just below the back area. In many cases, there is one just like it on the other side. And, the cat is probably significantly overweight because the bulge is fat! If you have another cat, check that animal to see if it has the same bulges. In many cases, this will give a clue to the reason for them.

This sort of comparison extends to judging the cat's attitude—is it lying down or sleeping more than normal? Does it seem upset or restless? It is useful to know cat conformation (parts of the cat) so that you can discuss the location of the problem with your veterinarian.

A complicating factor is the feline's small size. It's easy to think the cat hasn't lost much weight, when, in reality, a large percentage of its body weight is gone. A cat that has gone from 10 pounds to 8 pounds has lost 20% of its body weight. This is a SERIOUS weight loss. A drop from 10 pounds to 9 pounds is significant, but can easily go unnoticed. The cat may be into dire weight loss before you see that it is becoming thin. For this reason, you should weigh your cat from time to time so you know its normal weight. Any time the cat is sick, weigh it at the first sign of illness, and again every few days.

BEHAVIOR

The cat's behavior will give you many clues to what might be wrong with it. Is your calm, sedate old Siamese suddenly grouchy, pushing and snarling at your other cat? Is it hissing at the children? Some queens (female cats) become upset and act oddly when they are coming into heat. This behavior can also be seen with back problems—the cat is grumpy because it is hurting. A cat with an abscess beginning under its skin may be upset when the sore area is touched or stroked. Personality changes are also seen with rabies and other diseases which affect the brain or nervous system. Behavior varies from animal to animal and somewhat from breed to breed. Behavior that would be considered peculiar from a laid-back Domestic Shorthair may be considered normal (or at least tolerable) for an Abyssinian.

Determine as much as possible how your cat is affected by stress and environmental changes. Some cats are severely upset by visitors in the household, especially children. When your mother-in-law comes for a stay, the cat may live under the bed for the first week until it becomes accustomed to her presence. This may be hard to explain to the visitor—some people take it personally! You may lessen the affront by telling the visitor that your cat does that with everyone it does not know. It's harder to explain to the cat about your mother-in-law. If she's there long enough, the pet will eventually adapt, although it may take a month or longer. It is normal for many cats to hide when a strange person or animal enters their household. However, if a normally sociable cat suddenly hides for more than 24 hours without a good reason, it should be checked by your veterinarian. This may be the first (and only) sign of illness. A well-groomed cat that stops licking and cleaning itself may be becoming ill. A normally well-mannered cat that suddenly scratches, bites, or howls when handled should also be examined.

Other cats are disturbed when they have to travel. Make a distinction between changes which are temporary (an afternoon visitor) and those which are long-term (moving to a new neighborhood or taking a cross-country vacation). Does the cat settle down after a few days of travel or is it in turmoil for the entire two-week vacation? Does your cat panic only at storms or loud noises? Is it better with another cat for a companion, or is it a confirmed "only cat?" Knowing the answers to these and other questions helps you to spot problems. They will help you to assure an environment in which your cat is comfortable and happy.

POSTURE

Your observation of the cat's posture may be the first clue that something serious is wrong. A cat with a belly-ache, for almost any reason, may stand with a hump-backed posture, and have a "hangdog" (or is it "hangcat") look on its face. Or it may lie down, either on its bed or in an unusual place, and roll and stretch its legs forward and back. The same cat may be restless, in contrast to a healthy cat, that stands or lies quietly

Variations in posture may not indicate a specific disease. If the cat completely refuses to put weight on a foot, this is more specific. It tells you something is wrong with the leg, but not necessarily WHAT is wrong. The problem may be in the foot, knee, elbow or hock, or as high up as the shoulder or hip. It may be anything from a thorn in the paw to a fractured bone, or an abscess which is just beginning to cause pain.

Extreme changes in the animal's normal posture often occur with severe disease problems. Tetanus (lockjaw) is an example of an abnormal posture. While this disease is rare in cats, it still is occasionally seen. The cat may become so stiff and tight with the muscle spasms which accompany the disease that its front legs stick forward and its rear legs push out backward, making the animal resemble a rocking horse. Its head will be pulled up and back, its tail may be rigidly extended, and its ears will be stiffly upright. These signs indicate the condition is nearly terminal, and you are faced with an extreme emergency. Get veterinary help immediately.

MOVEMENT

Movement is closely related to posture. Abnormal movements are among the first signs of injury or disease processes. They can show that the animal is annoyed or uncomfortable. The cat that has its hackles (hairs over the shoulders and along the spine of the back) stiffly raised is either afraid or defensive. This usually goes along with a stiffly fluffed tail and an arched back. A cat that also has its ears pinned back along its head is signaling that something is going on that it doesn't like. Find out what is bothering the cat, and change it before either you or another person or animal are recipients of the threat, or even an outright attack.

Movements such as pawing at ears or shaking the head may indicate a serious problem such as ear mites or a hematoma (blood clot) in the ear flap. Almost all cats routinely lick their paws and wash their faces and ears. Other cats lick their sides, back, and tail out of boredom and keep licking until they cause irritation and sores. It is up to you to compare these movements with your knowledge of your cat's normal actions and decide if what you are seeing is normal.

The sequence of movement of the legs is called the gait. These movements can be compared to previous motions of the same animal, or to similar movements of other animals. The term "way of going" is often used to express the combination of movements which make up the gait. In horses this is very important, because imperfections in the way of going can cause the horse to hit one foot on another leg, injuring itself. Or, one leg may tangle with another, causing the horse to fall down. Because a cat is not expected to carry weight, defects in the way of going (such as limping) are not usually serious. These irregularities can, however, indicate injury in one or more legs. A cat may, for instance, have damage to its radial nerve because it has been hit by a vehicle or otherwise injured. One of its front legs may knuckle over as the cat travels. This is one of the most severe gait problems seen in cats. A cat with a fracture or severe injury in one leg may hold the leg up or drag it. One of the first signs of leg injury may be a change in the animal's way of going.

A stiff gait may also be social in nature, as when two cats, especially toms, meet that are strangers to each other. Each may strut the last few steps to the other cat on the tips of his toes with hackles raised and back arched and stiff. This maneuver helps the cat to appear larger to the stranger, thus intimidating it.

What is a normal gait or way of going for one cat is often completely abnormal for another. You must know what is normal for your cat. A cat that has extra toes often walks differently from a cat with normal, conventional feet.

VOICE

The cat's voice is a means of communication, both with other cats and with humans. A growling or snarling may mean that another cat has entered your front yard. After you and your cat have lived together for a while, you will be able to recognize the "language of meow." "I'm glad to see you," "I'm hungry," "Someone's at the door," "There's a stranger in the yard," "There's another cat out there," and other variations are all recognizable with time. Hoarseness may indicate the cat has been meowing for a long time. This sometimes happens when the cat has been in a boarding kennel or veterinary clinic for several days. Given a bit of rest and time, the voice will return to normal.

APPETITE

How well your cat is eating is one of the best indicators of its overall health. When you are feeding the same carefully measured amount of cat food every day, it is easy to tell when the cat is not eating and may have a health problem. Don't panic if your cat eats lightly at one meal occasionally, but look closely for a cause if a hearty eater suddenly lacks an appetite for several meals in a row. A normal cat should not go without eating for more than a day or day and a half without asking why this is happening. Ask if a neighbor is feeding the cat. Is someone in the household overfeeding the cat at other meals, or giving treats between meals which are ruining its appetite? Is the cat tricking someone into thinking it has not been fed, and thus receiving an extra dinner? Are there any signs of illness?

The cat's level of activity also influences its appetite. Moderate exercise may cause hunger while heavy exercise, such as a life-and-death race with a dog, may leave the cat too tired to eat. Loss of appetite is seen with digestive problems, fever, and severe pain from any cause.

A depraved appetite, in which the cat eats wool or other abnormal substances, is occasionally seen. Make sure you are feeding the cat a nutritionally adequate diet, and that it does not have any vitamin or mineral deficiencies. Have a stool sample checked to see that the cat does not have worms.

An evaluation of the animal's appetite should also include monitoring its thirst. With some illnesses, the cat may stop eating but continue drinking. Cats drink more water than normal with fever, diabetes mellitus, and some digestive system and kidney problems. If your cat is sick and you have an automatic waterer, it is a good idea to shut if off and give the cat water from a bowl or other container so you can measure intake. Make sure the container is heavy enough, or has a bottom wider than the top, so the cat cannot tip it over or otherwise spill it. In this way, you can tell IF the animal is drinking, and how much water it is consuming. You may need to confine the cat if you have several pets so you can tell exactly how much it drinks.

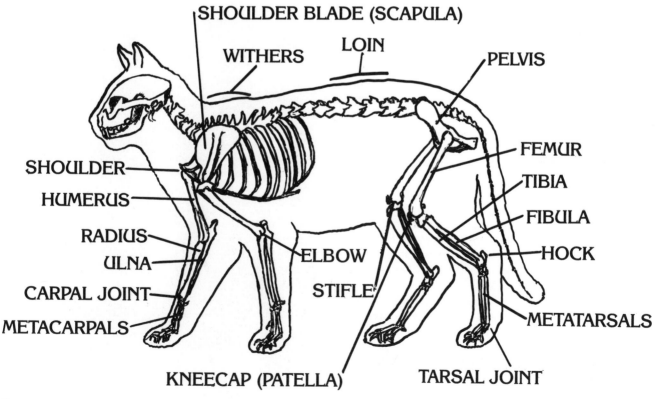

Parts of the Cat.

DIGESTIVE SYSTEM

After you have evaluated the animal's appetite, check the digestive system. Examine the mouth. See that the teeth are normal and that there are no sores, ulcers or foreign bodies on the tongue or gums. Saliva may drip from the mouth with any of these conditions or when the animal has a bone or other foreign object lodged in the mouth. This may also occur with the administration of certain drugs (especially those that are bitter) or when the cat is unable to swallow. If you are in an area where rabies is present, be aware that drooling saliva may be a sign of rabies because the animal's throat is paralyzed and it can't swallow.

SKIN AND COAT

The skin is a good indicator of the cat's health and of the level of care it is receiving. The skin should be clean and healthy, free of dirt and parasites. A small amount of scurf ("dandruff") may be present near the skin of cats that are not regularly groomed. This does not indicate any disease. Cats that are fed good quality cat food will have shiny, bright-looking coats. Long exposure to sun may dry the cat's coat so it looks rough and dull. A normal winter coat (on a Persian, for example), should look healthy even though it is long and furry. It may even shine.

Skin abnormalities can include missing patches of hair, scrapes or bites, sores, or dry, scaly or greasy skin. Contagious disease such as mange, ringworm and lice often involve more than one cat in a household, or more than one cat in the neighborhood if the cats are running loose and trading diseases. Some of these skin diseases, such as ringworm, can even be passed on to the cat's human friends. Warts or tumors may be found, and should be examined closely to determine whether they need to be removed or just watched. A foul odor can occur with skin infections, abscesses, seborrhea and some kinds of mange.

The leathery end of the nose can be an indicator of health. It does not have to be "moist." It can be either dry or damp as long as it is not dried, cracked or coated with mucus or dried discharges. It may appear abnormally pale in a cat that is anemic or has feline leukemia. The skin just above this area is prone to sunburn and skin cancer, especially in cats where it is white or very pale in color.

MUCOUS MEMBRANES

These are the membranes which line the body openings: the nostrils, mouth, eyelids, anus, prepuce (sheath) and vagina. The membranes inside the eyelids (also called conjunctivae) and the membranes of the mouth are good places to evaluate the animal's overall health. This is called "checking the animal's color."

A bright red conjunctival sac may merely mean that the cat's eyes have been irritated by dust or it could mean they are infected. However, if the membranes in the animal's mouth are the same color, this may indicate a serious illness affecting the whole body. A cat with white skin around its eyes may be prone to irritation of the conjunctivae by the sun. It may have red eyes much of the time, especially in summer. A few cats, such as some Persians, have eyelids that sag outward. The exposed pocket collects dirt and is exposed to the elements. It will also be red much of the time. Fortunately, this can be helped by surgery. This is another example of needing to know what is normal for your cat.

A cat that is short of red blood cells (suffering from anemia) or that has suffered blood loss may have very pale mucous membranes. A dark red (or purplish or bluish) color is called cyanosis. It indicates a lack of oxygen in the blood, and is seen with some heart problems and a few poisonings. A yellow coloration is called jaundice or icterus. It usually indicates a liver problem. With some diseases, small hemorrhages or spots of blood may be seen under the membranes. These may be as small as the head of a pin or may be large, irregular blotches. Any of these abnormal conditions may indicate a serious illness, and should be checked by your veterinarian.

Dry membranes may indicate a fever, or may be caused by the administration of certain drugs. Note any peculiar odors in the mouth. Gum infections and plaque and tartar on the teeth can cause foul-smelling breath.

A quick indicator of the state of the cat's circulatory system is its "capillary refill time." Lift the cat's upper lip. Press your thumb firmly against the gum area above its upper teeth, and hold it there for six to eight seconds. Remove it and count how long it takes the bleached-out spot to return to the color of the rest of the gums. It

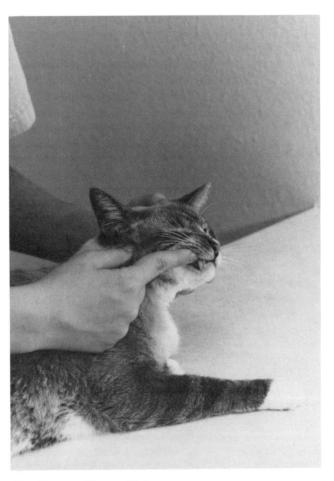

Checking capillary refill time.

should not take more than one second if the cat's circulation is normal. More than two seconds indicates a severe problem.

ABDOMEN

The size and shape of the cat's abdomen depend on a number of factors, including the breed, sex, age and conformation of the animal. It varies with what the cat has been fed. A sagging, enlarged abdomen may be due to an abdominal tumor or an accumulation of fluid in the abdominal cavity. More commonly, it will indicate that an unspayed female cat is pregnant. It may also show that the cat has had little exercise to help keep the muscles toned and in shape. The skin below the abdomen may hang down in an older cat, especially a male, and this flab may sway from one side to the other as the cat walks. While not especially attractive, it is essentially normal for many cats.

FECES

Feces is the technical name for the waste products of the intestinal tract. Manure, dung, stools, scat, or bowel movements refer to the same material. The animal's feces often give important clues to what is going on in its digestive tract. They are normally brownish or slightly reddish, depending on the type of food the cat is eating. Kitten feces may be more yellowish, especially when the kitten is still nursing or fed a milk replacer product.

Normal cat droppings should be well formed but not hard. Hard feces may indicate a lack of water, lack of exercise, or inadequate fiber or bulk in the diet. Very soft feces may be due to food to which the cat is allergic or to excess fat in the diet. Diarrhea may be due to similar food problems or to intestinal parasites or bacterial diseases. Eating spoiled food or getting into garbage may also cause diarrhea. Diarrhea which contains blood or large amounts of mucus or does not respond to simple treatment within two days is a signal to have your cat examined by a veterinarian. This is also true if the animal otherwise appears ill in addition to its diarrhea.

Grayish, foamy-appearing feces may be due to pancreatitis or other disease of the pancreas. Black feces may be due to treatment with bismuth subsalicylate products (such as Pepto-Bismol®). Dark, tarry stools may be due to bleeding in the intestinal tract. If you cannot relate it to anything the cat has eaten, have your veterinarian examine the cat.

Some cat foods produce larger amounts of feces than do others. If excess material in the litter box is your problem, try a cat food with a greater caloric density which will produce less fecal bulk. If the stools become too hard, you've gone too far and need to add some bulk back into the cat's diet.

URINE

Normal feline urine is yellowish and clear. It may be darker yellow if the cat has not had adequate water. Excessive urination may be due to diabetes or adrenal problems. This urine may be very diluted and almost colorless. It may also be a side effect of treatment with certain corticosteroids. If your cat is on medication and shows excessive urination, call your veterinarian and ask about it.

The urine of a healthy cat will not contain any blood or clots. Cats with stones in the kidney or bladder may pass blood clots or reddish urine. Have the cat examined by your veterinarian as soon as possible if you observe reddish urine.

VAGINAL DISCHARGE

Female cats may have a slight discharge when they are coming into heat. This is reddish to brownish as they come into heat, clear during the estrus period, and cloudy to whitish as they are going out of heat. This process is accompanied by swelling of the vulva, as well as other signs. You may not see the drainage because the cat licks it off in her normal cleaning ritual.

Small amounts of pus or whitish drainage in a female cat that is young or not in heat may indicate an infection of the vulva, vagina, or uterus. The cat should be examined by your veterinarian within a day or two.

Large amounts of pus or reddish, greenish, tan, or brownish vaginal drainage may indicate a severe infection in the uterus. This can be life-threatening. The queen should be examined by your veterinarian as soon as possible.

After a queen has had kittens, she may drain material for a week or so. This includes fragments of membranes and fluids which have surrounded the kittens. It may be reddish, brownish, or a horribly colored blackish-green. As long as it is not accompanied by a foul odor, it is normal. If it smells bad or the cat does not feel well, she should be examined by a veterinarian.

BRAIN AND CENTRAL NERVOUS SYSTEM

Since the brain cannot be examined directly, external signs must be relied on to indicate what is going on inside the cat's head and spinal column. Brain problems may first be seen by attitude and mental changes—the animal becomes dopey or sleepy, or may instead be nervous, upset, and excited. Cats with epilepsy may pass out for a long period of time. Problems in some areas of the brain or spinal cord may be shown by a staggering or uncoordinated gait, or dragging one or more feet as the cat walks. Nervous signs may be seen from some poisonings, such as strychnine, lead, and organophosphate insecticides.

Paralysis of a single limb or one group of muscles is caused by an injury to a motor center in the brain, or, more commonly, to a nerve leading to the involved area. Paralysis of the rear half of the body may result from injury to the spinal cord. This can be due to material from a ruptured disk oozing into the spinal canal and putting pressure on the spinal cord. It may also occur with spinal fractures or dislocations.

Paralysis of the entire body may be caused by severe damage to the brain. Or it may be due to physical or nutritional exhaustion, where the animal is too weak and too ill to rise. It often occurs shortly before coma and death.

Coma refers to the loss of consciousness. It may be caused by exhaustion of the body's resources by various disease processes, or by certain poisonous plants or other toxins. It is frequently the last stage before the cat dies, reflecting cardiopulmonary collapse, low blood pressure, and insufficient blood flow and oxygen to the brain and other parts of the central nervous system.

OTHER INDICATORS OF HEALTH

Your observations are extremely important in determining whether your cat is healthy or ill. In addition, you can use some simple tests and measurements to help determine if you have a problem, and to give your veterinarian more information about what is wrong. Use them in addition to evaluating your cat's overall attitude, behavior, and movement to determine whether there is a problem, and, if so, how serious it is. Always check the animal's temperature, pulse and respiration if you think it is ill. Do this before you examine the cat further or move it. If any of these are greatly different from normal (usually higher than normal), do not immediately assume that the animal is ill, but correlate it with other observations on the animal's condition and activity.

Check your cat for dehydration. A dehydrated cat's gums will feel sticky and dry. Gently grasp the skin along the rib cage or at the top of the shoulders. Lift the pinched skin and let it drop. It should immediately spring back into place. In a dehydrated cat, it will stay bunched together or drop very slowly back into place. As with other tests, you should do it occasionally when your cat is feeling well so you know what is normal.

BODY TEMPERATURE

This is one of the best indicators of animal health. For cats, you can use a rectal thermometer made for babies. These thermometers are stubby and thick so they are strong and unlikely to break. Or, you can get a small veterinary-type rectal thermometer with a ring in the end. It can be equipped with a small alligator clip from an automotive store and a short (4 inch (9 cm)) length of heavy nylon thread or fishing line. Anchor the clip onto the hair of the cat's rump, helping to prevent breakage if the cat swishes its tail and pulls the thermometer from its rectum. Thermometers should be stored in a cool place. Leaving one on a south-facing windowsill usually ruins it.

Begin by shaking down the thermometer. The easiest way to do this is to hold it by the upper end between two fingers and the thumb. Shake it downward with a short snapping motion of the wrist. Hold it tightly. Glass thermometers don't bounce when they are flung on the floor! This shaking often has to be repeated 10 to 15 times to move the mercury toward the bulb end. It should be shaken down to about 95 degrees Fahrenheit (F). How low you

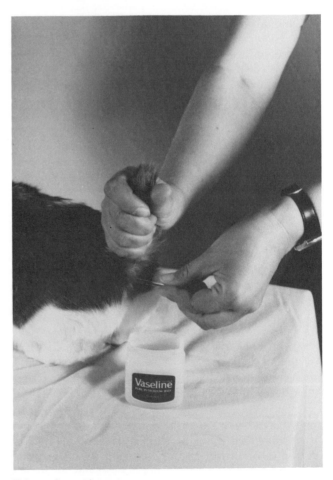

Thermometer with clip.   Taking the cat's temperature.

shake it is not critical unless the cat's temperature is well below normal (hypothermia). If this is the case, shake it all the way to the bottom and see if it comes back up at all. It is helpful to lubricate the thermometer with petroleum jelly or a similar product before inserting it into the cat's rectum.

You can often take the temperature of a calm cat by yourself. Place the cat on a countertop or table that is about waist high. If the cat is not normally allowed on a table or counter, it may be upset. You may be more successful putting it on top of a dresser, worktable, or washer or dryer. A slick surface is to your advantage, as the cat cannot get traction to pull away from you. If you are right-handed, tuck the cat under your left arm, facing toward your back. Hold the cat snugly to your body, but not so tightly that it fights. If you are left-handed, reverse the directions.

It is often helpful to have someone hold the cat's head while you take its temperature. If you are right-handed, hold the thermometer in your right hand. Grasp the cat's tail, if it has one, at the base with your left hand, holding it vertical, or steady the rump with your left hand. Gently insert the thermometer until it is about halfway into the rectum, depending on the size of the cat. It should be inserted at least two inches for all but the smallest kittens. If you don't have a cord on the thermometer, continue to hold it in place. If you do have a cord on the thermometer, clip it to the hair. Either way, leave it in place three to five minutes to get an accurate reading. Stay with the cat during this time to make sure it does not sit on the thermometer and make itself uncomfortable, or worse, break it off, leaving part inside. Unattended cats may also pull it out, dropping it onto the floor and breaking it.

Reverse the procedure to remove the thermometer, unclipping it from the hair and grasping it by the end. Hold the tail with the left hand and gently pull the thermometer straight out. Wipe it with a tissue or paper towel. Read it. After reading, wash it with lukewarm water and a bit of soap. Do not use hot water, as it may break the thermometer. Clean the thermometer with alcohol or other disinfectant before putting it away. Store it dry or in a vial of alcohol.

Normal temperature for the cat is 100.5 to 102.2 degrees Fahrenheit (F), with an average of 101.5 degrees F (38.1 degrees Celsius (C) to 39 C, average 38.6 C).

Normal temperatures may run slightly higher in hot, humid weather, or if the animal has been in direct sunlight or left in a hot vehicle. Under these conditions, temperatures will be toward the high end of the range. The temperature is often elevated if the cat has just been frightened or is excited.

Normal temperatures are usually a degree or so higher in the afternoon than they are in the morning. An elderly cat may have a slightly lower temperature than a younger cat. The cat's body temperature is usually slightly higher one to two hours after a meal. Cats that are in unfamiliar surroundings or handled by strangers may also show an elevated temperature.

Exposure to cold weather or winds or drinking large amounts of cold water may lower the animal's tempera-

ture briefly. A temperature which remains at 99 degrees F (37.2 C) or less may indicate that the cat has been severely chilled and is suffering from hypothermia. Or it may indicate that the cat is going into shock or collapse because of internal bleeding or other causes.

Fever is the term used when body temperature is above normal. An elevated temperature (fever) will be seen from an infectious illness and from sunstroke (heat exhaustion).

It is well worth the effort to take your cat's temperature morning and evening daily for a week or so when you know the animal is healthy and in its usual environment. This gives you a base reading to use later to determine whether the animal's temperature is normal. A cat that is ill will generally be more than one degree above its normal (baseline) temperature for that time of day. Don't worry until a cat's temperature goes over 102.5 to 103 degrees F (39.2-39.4 C) if the day is hot or the cat is excited and there are no signs of illness. Cats may have very high fevers, even off-scale on the thermometer, but these do not seem to cause the sort of permanent brain damage seen with similar fevers in humans. This does not call for extreme measures such as ice baths unless it is due to heat stroke.

Do not be in a hurry to reduce a moderate fever. Fever is one of the body's active defensive mechanisms. The rise in temperature makes the body a less hospitable environment for many bacteria and viruses, helping the body to kill the attacking organisms. When the temperature goes to about 103 degrees F (39.4 C) or persists more than two to three days (or the cat has stopped eating and is becoming weak), then something should be done to reduce it. Of course, you should have been treating whatever is causing the fever all along, but the fever itself is not the problem in most cases—the real difficulty is the disease causing it.

There may be outward signs that the cat is running a fever. The cat may be trembling and sweaty; its skin may feel cooler than usual, the coat may seem to "stand up," and the cat may be humpbacked and miserable-looking. Cats that are running a fever often have little or no appetite. They may be thirsty and depressed. Take the cat's temperature and record it for your veterinarian.

If the cat is shivering, or it is cold or windy outside, it should be brought into shelter and warmed. If you have to keep the cat outdoors, improvise a covering from a burlap bag, scrap of blanket, or old quilt. The cat should have straw or rags for bedding so that it will be warm and not lose heat to the ground or floor if it wishes to lie down.

Again, it is important to remember that fever is not the problem—it's part of the healing mechanism. Your cat's survival may depend on your quickly finding out WHY it has the fever and dealing with that underlying cause.

PULSE

The pulse, which you can feel in an artery, is an intermittent pressure wave caused by the heart forcing blood through the artery. The arteries alternate between expansion and contraction, and it is this pulse that is palpated (felt) and counted. Counting the pulse rate is really counting the number of times the heart beats in one minute.

One of the easiest places to take a cat's pulse is inside its hind leg on the femoral artery. You can lay the cat down to find the proper area (see photo). After you have done this, reach inside the cat's hind leg while it is standing and take the pulse with your fingertips. Another method is to put your hand around the lower part of the cat's chest. Move it around until you can feel the strongest heartbeat. Or you can place the flat of your hand against the left side of the cat's chest, just behind the elbow. With the latter two techniques, you will be counting the actual heartbeats, not the pulses, but the results are the same.

If you have one, a stethoscope can be used to determine the cat's heart rate. Some people check the heart rate by pushing an ear against the chest wall behind the animal's elbow. Try this method if you do not have a stethoscope and cannot feel the pulse in one of the arteries. The heartbeat may be difficult to hear or feel on an obese cat. Signs of heart or circulatory disease include pooling of fluid in the legs and belly (called edema). The cat may have a cough, may faint, or seem weak when exercised and may not have any energy.

THE STETHOSCOPE

A stethoscope is an instrument well worth having to make it easier to hear the sounds of internal organs. Inexpensive stethoscopes are available; you don't need a top-of-the-line model. One key to being able to hear anything with a stethoscope is to find one that fits your ears. Try before you buy! If it doesn't fit in one direction, take it out of your ears, turn it 180 degrees, then try again. Some stethoscopes fit markedly better one way than the other. The earpieces should snugly fit your ears without pressure or pain. They should not be so loose that they rattle around. Some stethoscopes offer two different sides, one flat and the other bell- or cone-shaped. For most users, a stethoscope with only a flat side is sufficient.

After you have found an instrument that fits, the next step is to practice with it. The head of the stethoscope must be pushed firmly into the cat's side. Learn what the squeaking of the animal's hair sounds like against the head of the stethoscope and against its tubing. Then learn how hard you have to push to make firm contact with the cat's chest wall to avoid that noise and get the best sound.

Listen to a spot on the chest wall behind the left elbow for eight to ten seconds. Now, move one to two inches back, up or down. Compare what you hear with the sounds at the previous location. Are they more distinct or more muffled? Louder or softer? Cover a large area behind the elbow to determine where you can best hear the cat's heart. Examine the left side first. Then go to the animal's right side and repeat the procedure. On which side are the sounds clearer? If you'd like to hear lung sounds, listen over the cat's upper chest.

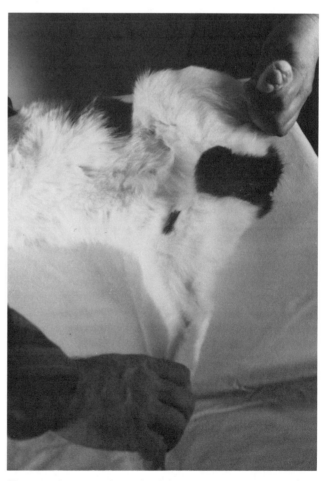

Taking the cat's pulse by feeling heartbeat.

Tape marks area where the femoral pulse can be felt.

When using the stethoscope, the cat should be standing quietly. Don't allow the cat to eat. Rattling tags and other noises should be kept to a minimum. When you are getting used to a stethoscope, have people in the room remain quiet. After you have learned to listen with the stethoscope, you will ignore outside sounds, but it helps not to have them in the beginning.

Using a stethoscope is a skill where practice makes perfect. What at first is an unintelligible bunch of thumps will sort itself out into a distinct pattern of sounds. The loudest one will be a loud "lub," followed by a slightly softer "dub." This pattern is then repeated. Count only the "lubs," or you will get a pulse rate twice as high as it really is. Note the number of "lubs" per minute.

Cats occasionally have what is called a sinus arrhythmia. This gives an irregular heartbeat. If you are listening with a stethoscope, it will sound as if the animal's heart skips an occasional beat. This is normal, as long as the cat does not show fainting or other signs of heart problems. If you have trouble making sense of the heart sounds, ask your veterinarian on your next visit to listen with you and help you understand them.

NORMAL HEART RATE

An adult cat's normal, resting heartbeat varies between 120 and 240 beats per minute, depending on the cat's size and state of mind at the time. A cat resting quietly at home may have a normal heart rate as low as 80 beats per minute. The cat's normal heart rate can vary greatly from one moment to another. A young kitten may have a slightly higher heart rate, around 200 to 250 beats per minute. The pulse is usually slightly faster in the evening than in the morning. The heart rate may be raised by hot weather, exercise, excitement, or alarm. It may be slower than normal with severe exhaustion, old age, or excessive cold. Take the time to determine your cat's normal resting heart rate to establish the baseline. The reading you take at home may be far more accurate than the one taken when the cat is sitting on the hospital table, surrounded by strange sounds and smells.

RESPIRATION RATE

Respiration rate refers to the number of inhalations (or exhalations) per minute—the number of times the cat breathes in (or out). Do not count both in and out, or you will have a rate double what it really is. This is usually easy to count in the cat. Just stand back and observe the ribs moving in (or out). Do this from a distance, with the cat standing comfortably, without excitement. If you have a stethoscope, place it on the underside of the cat's neck, about halfway between the jaw and the chest. You can hear the air moving in and out of the trachea. Again, count it as it moves in OR out, but not both.

The normal respiratory rate for a relaxed, resting cat is around 25 breaths per minute. A cat that is upset or in a strange place such as a clinic may have a very rapid, panting respiration. As with temperature and pulse, respiration is usually faster in kittens. It increases with work, hot weather, overfilling of the stomach and pregnancy. Also, a fat animal will have a respiratory rate well above what is considered normal. Respiratory rate, like the pulse rate, is related to body size, exercise, and temperament. It is often elevated when the cat is examined by strangers, as at a cat show or veterinary clinic.

A cat with pneumonia or other respiratory disease, or with a chest full of fluid due to a disease such as feline infectious peritonitis may try to sleep sitting up. Or, it may raise its head on a pillow, or rest on a slanting surface with its head upward. The cat may breathe with difficulty, with little chest movement, but with its abdomen heaving. Cats with abdominal fluid accumulation also may sleep with the head elevated.

GUT SOUNDS

Another area of examination is open to those with a stethoscope—intestinal sounds. These are the tinklings and bubblings made by gas as it percolates around and through the liquid and solid contents of the digestive tract. By listening to each side of your cat's abdomen for several minutes, you can get an idea of what is normal. This can also be done by putting your ear on its flank. These sounds can be significantly increased when the cat is allergic to something in its food or is about to have diarrhea. What you are listening for is merely whether the sounds are more or less active than is normal for your animal. As with the other tests, you have to know the normal before you can detect the abnormal.

BLOOD

Blood is a fluid tissue consisting of a liquid, called plasma, and numerous cells. It is sometimes considered to be a connective tissue because of its cleansing and communicating functions from one part of the body to another.

Red blood cells are small round discs containing hemoglobin. This chemical can combine with either oxygen or carbon dioxide, whichever is in greater concentration. Because of this characteristic, the cells take up carbon dioxide in the tissues where it is in greatest supply, and move it to the lungs. There, more oxygen is available, so the cells dump the carbon dioxide (where it can be exhaled) and pick up a fresh supply of oxygen to carry back to the tissues.

White blood cells are one of the body's first defenses against infection by viruses and bacteria. The white blood cell component of blood also includes the platelets, which are involved with blood clotting.

Plasma is the term used for the fluid component of unclotted blood. It carries nutrients from one part of the body to another. For instance, it carries fats, amino acids (from the breakdown of proteins in food), and carbohydrates, taking these to cells throughout the body. There, the plasma picks up waste products, dropping them off in the kidneys and liver for removal from the body. Plasma also delivers hormones produced by the glands within the body to other sites where they are needed.

Serum is the fluid portion of the blood which remains after the blood has clotted. Antibodies which prevent disease and infections remain in the serum.

Blood helps control body temperature by moving heat from deeper tissues to the surface where it can be dissipated. It also helps to maintain water balance and a constant pH (acid-base balance) in body tissues.

Approximately 8% of an animal's body weight is blood. Blood transfusions may be given to cats that are in severe shock or have suffered from significant blood loss. Cats do not have antigens against other blood groups as do humans, if they have never had a transfusion, so its first transfusion should not present any problem. If your cat needs a transfusion, let your veterinarian know if it has had one previously.

Blood pressure in cats cannot be measured with a human blood pressure cuff—it simply does not work. Blood pressure measurement in the cat takes special instruments and techniques. It is rarely done except in university hospitals when special monitoring is needed, or in extremely large hospitals during lengthy, unusual surgery.

ANEMIA

A smaller than normal supply of red blood cells is called anemia. Cats may have anemia from a number of causes.

Bleeding, either internal or external, is a common cause. Parasites may suck enough blood to make a cat anemic. These may be external, such as lice, or internal, such as various worms. Or the cat may simply not be producing a normal amount of red blood cells. Autoimmune diseases, in which the cat is allergic to parts of its own system, may cause the cat to be anemic.

Cats that are anemic will have blood with reduced oxygen-carrying capacity. They may have less energy than normal, and may have pale mucous membranes. If the animal is anemic, it is important to find out why. Is there a deficiency of the B vitamins or iron needed to produce red blood cells? Does the cat have worms which are draining blood? Is the bone marrow not producing enough red blood cells? Is a disease process involved? Anemia is seen with some kidney problems and with bone marrow depression. Has the cat recently suffered an injury causing severe blood loss? It is often necessary for your veterinarian to run a number of laboratory tests to determine the exact cause of anemia. Your clue that something may be wrong will be your cat's pale mucous membranes.

Chapter 4

VACCINATIONS AND INFECTIOUS DISEASES

- *What Is Vaccination?*
- *Sample Vaccination Schedule*
- *Feline Panleukopenia (Distemper)*
- *Viral Respiratory Infections*
- *Feline Herpesvirus*
- *Feline Calicivirus*
- *Chlamydial Infection (Pneumonitis)*
- *Feline Infectious Peritonitis (FIP)*
- *Feline Coronavitus*
- *Feline Leukemia*
- *Feline Acquired Immune Deficiency Syndrome (FAIDS, FIV)*
- *Rabies*
  - *Rabies and the Cat Bite*
- *Pseudorabies*
- *Vaccination Related Sarcoma*
- *Lyme Disease*
- *Bubonic Plague*
- *Tuberculosis*
- *Tetanus*
- *Cat Diseases in Humans*

WHAT IS VACCINATION?

Vaccinations are injections which are given to keep your cat from contracting specific infectious diseases. Vaccines do NOT cause the disease. They are special preparations of the disease-causing bacteria or viruses which stimulate the cat's own immune system to produce special proteins, called antibodies, which protect the cat against that disease. Then, if the cat is exposed to the disease-causing organisms, the antibodies neutralize and destroy them within the cat's body. Antibody levels diminish with time. Later vaccinations, called "boosters," stimulate the animal's immune system to "remember" the disease organism and to manufacture more antibodies.

When an animal is exposed to disease before it is vaccinated, it may already be incubating the disease. In this case, vaccinating the cat will have little or no effect and it may contract the disease. This could lead you to believe that the vaccination "didn't work," or that the cat caught the disease from the injection, both of which are untrue. This is especially a problem with cats that are exposed to disease on the street or in a shelter or pound. They are vaccinated, but come down with the illness within a week or two. It normally takes a healthy animal about two weeks to develop an immunity after it is vaccinated. Therefore, the animal in the shelter just hasn't had time to develop immunity. In addition, it may have been malnourished and severely stressed before it was picked up.

Normal kittens get about 95% of their first antibodies from their mother in their first six to twelve hours of life as they nurse her first milk, called colostrum. These antibodies protect the kitten from disease until its own immune system is ready to produce antibodies. When kittens are vaccinated early in life, these "borrowed" antibodies may keep them from producing an immunity to the vaccination by "neutralizing" it. It is difficult to determine exactly when the mother's protection will "wear off." Since it is important not to leave the kitten unprotected from disease and possible death, several vaccinations are given to the young kitten. Although it is possible to test to find out when the maternal protection is gone, these tests are extremely expensive. It's a lot less expensive to vaccinate the kitten several times to make sure it is protected. It is important that the last vaccinations be given around 16 weeks of age, when almost all kittens have lost the antibodies from their mother.

No vaccine can guarantee to prevent disease because there are too many variables involved. The immune system varies from one pet to another, and some cats naturally respond to vaccination better than others. Very young cats have immature immune systems which do not respond well to vaccination. This may also be a problem with elderly cats, or those that are underweight, pregnant, parasitized, or otherwise ill. Stresses such as high summer temperatures may keep the cat from developing an adequate immunity. If an animal under any of these circumstances is vaccinated, it is CRITICAL that it be revaccinated when it returns to normal to be sure that it is protected.

Vaccines sometimes seem to have failed if the cat contracts a disease for which it has been vaccinated. This may be for one of several reasons. The cat may have been exposed to the disease, vaccinated shortly after this exposure, and already been incubating the disease when the vaccine was given. The vaccine which was used may have been a modified live vaccine, which must be kept refrigerated, and improper handling could have rendered it ineffective. The vaccine may have been given by a route via which it is ineffective. For example, a vaccine which is supposed to be given in the muscle may have been given under the skin. A cat that is vaccinated when sick, parasitized, or malnourished may not develop an adequate immunity. And, a cat that is infected with feline leukemia virus, feline infectious peritonitis, or feline immunodeficiency virus may not look ill, but may be incapable of developing an immunity because these diseases cause immunosuppression. Don't take a sick cat to your veterinarian and expect the animal to be vaccinated. It would not help the cat and would only waste your money. Cats that are being treated with corticosteroids also do not develop an adequate immunity.

How important is vaccination for your cat? Respiratory diseases and feline panleukopenia (distemper) are seen in unvaccinated cats. Distemper is often fatal. On the other hand, most cats will eventually recover from respiratory diseases. The vaccines usually combine these diseases, and while you are protecting the cat against distemper, you can keep it from contracting the respiratory diseases (and the expenses and misery that go with them) for little or no extra charge. It is important to vaccinate against them. Most vaccinations are not 100% effective, especially against respiratory diseases and feline leukemia. Cats vaccinated for them can still become ill, although the disease is usually less severe than if they are not immunized. Meanwhile, these infected cats can spread disease to others, and can even become long-term carriers. It is still important to keep your cats away from others that are ill and to avoid bringing new cats into your "herd" without a quarantine period. The best prevention is to keep cats indoors and not to allow other felines to visit your home.

The occurrence of rabies, even in unvaccinated cats, is quite small. However, it can spread to other animals you own or members of your household, with possibly fatal results. Rabies vaccination is VERY important for outdoor cats. Feline infectious peritonitis is seen in less than 1% of unvaccinated cats, and feline leukemia in around 3%. The probability of contracting them is low, but both diseases may be fatal to the cat involved. They are cheap insurance if you can afford them, and may keep you from losing your beloved pet.

So your cat never goes out of your house? Does it still need its annual boosters? Yes, for two reasons. The first is that you can bring some diseases home on your shoes or clothing, merely by walking where a sick cat has vomited, sneezed, or had diarrhea. You will never know what you are bringing home to your beloved cat, and it might be fatal. The second reason is that your cat may be injured or become ill and have to go to a veterinary clinic. There, it may be exposed to some of those same diseases. Or, the cat may accidentally get out the door (or fall out the window!) or may be picked up and taken to a shelter or pound, and be exposed to disease. Annual boosters will keep your cat safe from these disease hazards. While there is a slight risk from any vaccination, it is far less than the risk of NOT vaccinating.

Vaccines for some feline respiratory diseases are given into the nostrils, like nose drops. If you are giving this yourself, mix it using a needle and syringe; then remove the needle and drop the droplets into the nostrils, using only the syringe. Be careful! Some cats object to this treatment.

SAMPLE VACCINATION SCHEDULE

Age: 6-8 weeks—first vaccination
Feline distemper (panleukopenia)
Feline viral rhinotracheitis
Feline calicivirus infection
Pneumonitis (optional)

Age: 10 weeks
Feline infectious peritonitis (optional)

Age: 12 weeks
Feline distemper (panleukopenia)
Feline viral rhinotracheitis
Feline calicivirus infection
Feline leukemia (optional)
Feline infectious peritonitis (optional)

Age: 16 weeks
Feline distemper (panleukopenia)
Feline viral rhinotracheitis
Feline calicivirus infection
Feline leukemia (optional)
Pneumonitis (optional)

Age: 12 weeks to 6 months
Rabies (depending on the law in your area)

Annually: Boosters
Feline distemper (panleukopenia)
Feline viral rhinotracheitis
Feline calicivirus infection
Feline infectious peritonitis
Pneumonitis (optional)
Feline leukemia

Every year to 3 years
Rabies, depending on the law where you live and the type of vaccine that was used

This is a sample schedule. If your veterinarian recommends a different schedule for your area, follow it. This sounds like many shots, but a number of them are combined into a single vaccine and are given in one injection.

Whatever schedule you follow, it is very important that you keep your new kitten away from strange cats until it is about 16 weeks of age and its initial series of vaccinations is complete. Don't take the kitten out around other cats, and don't let other cats come for a visit. The kitten should be kept indoors so that it does not come into contact with strange cats that wander through the yard, or with any discharges from those that stray by. This gives its immune system a chance to mature and become immune to the diseases for which it is vaccinated.

FELINE PANLEUKOPENIA (DISTEMPER)

Feline panleukopenia, also called distemper, is an often fatal viral disease. It is highly contagious. The disease begins suddenly, with the cat showing depression, fever, lack of appetite, diarrhea, and vomiting. Feline distemper affects all felines, up to and including lions. It also can affect ferrets. If you have a pet ferret, it also should be vaccinated against feline panleukopenia. If a number of unvaccinated cats are infected, from one-quarter to 90% of them will die. Feline distemper is completely unrelated to the diseases called distemper in horses and dogs, although canine distemper has killed large cats, including tigers, lions, and leopards in Africa and in zoos in the United States.

The virus is passed directly from an infected cat to one that is susceptible to the disease. The virus can live for long periods of time (up to several years) in carpet, litter boxes, soil, food and water dishes, and any other objects that are contaminated by a sick cat. The disease can also be spread through the air by sneezing or by fleas that carry it from one cat to another. You can bring it home on your shoes from walking where a sick cat has vomited or defecated. It is not killed by common disinfectants, including alcohol and iodine. It IS killed by a 1:32 solution of household bleach.

The incubation period is from two to seven days or longer, but is usually around four days. Some cases progress so rapidly that the cat that was fine last night may be found dead the next morning, making it look like a poisoning. The disease develops within hours—from a depression which may be accompanied by vomiting to coma and death.

The most common form of distemper is seen in populations of feral or farm cats or in shelters, when a large number of unvaccinated cats of different ages are together. The cat may quit eating and become depressed. It will have a fever of 104 degrees F (40 C) or higher.

Vomiting is seen, and a watery, foul-smelling diarrhea develops within one to two days. The diarrhea may be streaked with blood and/or mucus. As diarrhea and vomiting continue, the cat becomes severely dehydrated. Dehydration causes the hair coat to look rough and shabby. The third eyelid often bulges partway across the eyeball. If you feel the cat's abdomen, the cat will exhibit signs of pain. Cats that are not treated for the dehydration may die of shock within one to four days.

A cat with distemper often has a characteristic posture, sitting hunched with the head hanging downward toward the paws. The chin may be resting on the ground, or the cat may hang its head over a food or water dish. It may act like it wants to eat or drink but if it laps a sip or two, will not swallow.

When your veterinarian examines the animal, a blood test will probably be run. This will show the lowered white blood cell count which gives the disease its name, panleukopenia. Toward the end, the cat's temperature will drop. This is a sign that death is close. A coma is followed shortly by death.

To have a chance to survive, cats with panleukopenia must be treated immediately and aggressively. Do NOT give the cat any food or water, especially if it has severe diarrhea or vomiting. Take it to your veterinarian, where it will be treated with intravenous fluids. Diarrhea may hang on for several weeks after the cat is feeling better because of damage to the intestinal tract. This usually disappears with time.

Rarely, mild cases are seen where the cat is not eating and is slightly depressed. The temperature may be slightly higher than normal, and if you feel the cat's abdomen it will gurgle with gas and fluid. The cat will recover with little or no treatment in one to three days, with no complications. Don't, however, count on seeing this type of distemper. Vaccinate and protect your precious cat.

Kittens may be infected while they are still in their mother's uterus; they are born damaged by the disease. This infection usually occurs in mid to late pregnancy, and the queen is rarely ill. Similar damage can happen when the queen is given a modified live virus vaccine while she is pregnant. The kittens may die suddenly after they are born, with no signs of disease. Or, they may show staggering and incoordination when they are two or three weeks old and just beginning to walk. They may fall over, roll from side to side as they try to walk, or twitch the head in irregular spasms. If they can walk at all, they may spread their legs and hold their tails stiff as they attempt to balance. They may walk as if they are stepping over objects when there is nothing in the way. These neurological signs are due to cerebellar hypoplasia. The part of the brain which controls coordination is damaged and does not grow properly because of the infection while the kittens were in the mother's uterus.

These "shaky" kittens appear strong and alert. If they are able to eat, they will mature, but the coordination rarely improves much, if at all. Cerebellar hypoplasia may also be seen (rarely) in kittens that are infected or vaccinated with a modified live vaccine within the first two to four weeks of life. Those that can more or less get around can still make suitable pets.

All cats should be vaccinated against this deadly disease. Antibodies which the mother passes to the kittens in her milk will interfere with vaccinations that are given too early in the kitten's life. That is why several injections of vaccine are given, as this protection "wears off" at different rates, depending on the immune status of the mother cat.

The first injection of distemper vaccine is usually given between six and nine weeks of age. It should be repeated every four weeks after the first shot until the kitten is at least 12 weeks old. It is particularly important that the last injection be given after the kitten is 12 to 16 weeks of age to give a more sure and lasting immunity. If the cat is older than 12 weeks when the first injection is given (and has survived that long), one shot is enough. It's not a good idea to wait until 12 weeks and only give one shot, however. You're betting that the kitten has adequate protection from its mother to be safe for that length of time, and that you're not going to bring the disease home on your shoes.

It is important to give regular boosters to maintain a strong immunity. This is especially important for cats that are kept indoors and do not have a chance for contact with infected cats. This may seem backwards—that your cat is more susceptible to the disease if you keep it well isolated from the ourside world. But it's not. The cat that has had its initial injections gets a natural booster each time it runs into an infected cat (or virus from a location where an infected cat has been). The household pet does not have this advantage. No, that's not a good reason to let your cat run loose. It IS a good reason to give it an annual booster.

VIRAL RESPIRATORY INFECTIONS

Both cats and kittens are attacked by a number of viruses which primarily infect the respiratory tract. These diseases look very much alike and, for practical purposes, it is not necessary for the cat owner to be able to tell them apart. It is enough to suspect that your cat has this type of problem so that you can secure treatment for it. In general, these diseases will remind you of a human "cold."

The first sign may be a mild, clear discharge from the eyes and/or nose. The whites of the cat's eyes may be reddened and swollen, and the lids may be swollen partly or completely closed. If the eyes remain closed for a period of time with the pus lying against the surface of the eyeball, corneal ulcers may occur.

The cat may start sneezing occasionally, with it becoming more frequent and severe over a two to five day period. As the disease becomes worse, the cat's nose may become completely plugged. Because it can no longer breathe through its nose, the cat will breathe with its mouth open. Mouth breathing is uncomfortable for cats, so it may be quite distressed. Because the cat cannot smell, it may stop eating. It may have a clear discharge from its eyes and nose, which later changes to a gummy yellow-green pus. Its eyelids may be completely matted together with dried, crusty pus. Ulcers may occur on the cornea. If untreated, the cornea may perforate or adhere to the third eyelid. Rapid dehydration may be accompanied by pneumonia. Very young kittens may die of dehydration if untreated. The cat may have ulcers on its tongue and around its gums. This pain adds to its unwillingness to eat. The cat may drool saliva, and have a fever as early as the first day after it is exposed to the virus. The fever may persist for seven to 10 days.

Infection rates in a particular group of cats may be nearly 100%. Kittens under six months of age may die from the infection. Adult cats rarely die unless they are infected with feline leukemia or other diseases that reduce the effectiveness of the immune system, or are otherwise ill or malnourished.

Chronic respiratory tract infection may result in cats that are carriers of the guilty viruses. As many as 80% of cats that recover from the acute disease will become chronic carriers that can pass the disease to cats or kittens that are susceptible. These cats may shed virus or have symptoms recur after they are stressed or if they are treated for three or more consecutive days with corticosteroids (such as prednisolone or dexamethasone). Many cats can't be completely cured of upper respiratory disease, and these chronic sufferers (often called "snufflers") may need antibiotics from time to time throughout their lives. Carrier cats may have few or no clinical signs, but they are a major source of infection for susceptible cats. In a large group of British cats that were tested, over half of those that were shedding virus from the respiratory tract

had been fully vaccinated. The vaccination prevented (or lessened) the disease, but did not keep them from being able to pass it along to others (Harbour, 1991).

If you have a group of cats in which kittens are continually infected with respiratory disease, you probably have a cat in the group that is a chronic carrier. Even if virus isolation tests are done, it can be difficult to determine which animal is causing the problem. In a breeding colony, it is worth trying to find the carriers and eliminate them from your program. Intranasal vaccines are available which can be used in kittens as young as eight to 10 days of age if you have a serious problem in your group of cats.

Some adult cats that are chronic carriers will have a pus-filled nasal discharge, and may have uncontrollable fits of sneezing. A few days' treatment with a broad-spectrum antibiotic will give considerable relief from the symptoms, but they return within two or three days after treatment is stopped.

Cats that have had a respiratory tract infection for a long time often have chronic infection in the frontal sinuses (the ones in the cat's forehead, above its eyes). A few cats will also have a middle ear infection. Some cats may have a chronic infection in the mouth and around the teeth, and if this continues, it may result in tooth loss. Cats that are young or middle aged and that have lost several teeth should be suspected of being virus carriers. Cats that have chronic respiratory disease or sinusitis should be tested for feline leukemia or feline immunodeficiency virus, as these may be contributing to the continuing infection. Identification of the particular virus is necessary to confirm that the cat is a carrier.

Most cats that have acute upper respiratory tract infections can be treated at home, especially if they are still eating and drinking on their own. This is usually less stressful (and cheaper!) than hospitalization. If the cat is drooling (an indication of painful ulcers in the mouth), and is not eating, it should be hospitalized. Cats that are hospitalized will be given fluids and are usually fed via a feeding tube into the stomach. The entire recommended amount cannot be fed on the first day, as vomiting or diarrhea may occur. Give one-third of the daily requirement the first day (divided into several feedings), two-thirds the second day, and the full amount on the third day and thereafter until the cat is willing to eat on its own. Some cats can be helped by chemical stimulation of the appetite. Diazepam (Valium®) is one drug which is used. One to two mg given orally will often stimulate the cat to eat within 5 to 10 minutes. Have food sitting in front of the cat when the medication is given. Strong-smelling foods such as sardines may help stimulate the cat's appetite.

Use of a long-lasting nasal decongestant (such as Neosynephrine®) for up to five days may help the cat breathe through its nose. Use one drop in alternate nostrils, one side in the morning and the other side in the evening. Do not use them for more than five days, the limit of their effectiveness. It may also be helpful to put a bit of medication such as Vicks® or Mentholatum® on the cat's nose to help clear the clogged passages. When it can breathe again and smell its food, the cat will usually start eating on its own. Be sure to wipe the cat's nose and eyes several times a day using a soft cloth or tissue moistened with lukewarm water.

Antibiotics are usually given to prevent secondary bacterial infection even if the cat doesn't have a pus-filled nasal discharge. Antibiotics, such as tetracycline or ampicillin, help fight off bacterial infection. Amoxicillin or clavamox are also used, and can be given as tablets or liquid. Vitamins, especially vitamin C, are helpful. The cat may have a poor appetite because of a high fever. It may have enough nasal congestion that it cannot smell its food, or may have ulcers in its mouth which make it painful to eat. B vitamins will help stimulate the cat's appetite. Also, the cat may rapidly move into a state of malnutrition because of fever and stress.

The cat may be fed a highly nutritious product such as Nutri-Cal®. It should be given about 2.5 feet (75 cm) of the gel per day—a few tablespoons are not nearly enough to feed a cat that is not eating. If you are giving a meat-based baby food, the cat should have about two and a half jars each day. A formula can be made for force-feeding the cat by taking 1 can of Feline P/D (Hill's Prescription Diets), 2 ounces of Wesson salad oil, and 10 ounces of water. Mix these in a blender at the fastest speed. If this is too thick to go though a stomach tube, add a bit more water. A 9 pound cat will need about 7 ounces (200 cc) of this mixture per day.

If the cat will not eat, it may be necessary to hospitalize it and give it nutrition and fluids. Some cats that fail to eat will go into fatty liver syndrome. About 35% that have it will die, and those that live may need treatment for as much as six weeks or more. Unless they have a complicating disease or are severely weakened by immunodeficiency, cats rarely die from upper respiratory disease. They die from malnutrition and other complications. As with the human cold, animals that are not seriously ill get well within one to three weeks.

Humidity is very helpful. You can use a vaporizer or nebulizer in a small space, such as the bathroom, 30 minutes twice a day. Take the cat into the bathroom when you take a shower.

Most kittens will recover from acute viral respiratory disease if they are treated promptly and thoroughly. Almost all adult cats will recover if their immune systems are normal. Many of the recovered animals will become chronic carriers that will shed virus to susceptible cats or kittens; thus, vaccination alone may not be enough to prevent outbreaks in a breeding colony or group. Having fewer cats spread over a larger area may help reduce the incidence of respiratory disease. Better ventilation may also be helpful, and more than 12 changes of room air per hour may be needed. Airborne transmission of the virus is important. Even more significant is the spread of virus by inanimate objects such as feed and water dishes, and your own hands and feet bringing viruses home from a household with an infected or carrier cat. Carefully disinfect your hands and shoes if you have been in an area where there is a sick cat. Soak utensils in a 1:32 solution of household bleach in water, rinse thoroughly and allow to dry 24 hours before using. Do not bring any new kittens or cats into the household until at least three weeks after they have been vaccinated for respiratory disease.

Groups of cats with recurring outbreaks should be tested for feline leukemia virus and feline immunodeficiency virus. Cats that are infected should be permanently removed from the household if you expect to raise kittens or introduce new cats without continuing illnesses.

Ongoing vaccination against feline herpesvirus-1 and feline calicivirus help limit the severity of symptoms, but do not completely prevent the diseases in all cats. Give injections at nine and 12 weeks of age, followed by annual boosters. Be sure no vaccine is left on the animal's coat after subcutaneous injections. If a modified-live vaccine is given, the cat may contract the disease by licking or inhaling virus particles from its fur. If you get any of this type of vaccine on the cat, wipe the area thoroughly with alcohol-soaked cotton. Some vaccines are squirted directly into the cat's nose, and there is some evidence that these are more effective than those which are injected.

You should be aware that there is a high probability that a cat that comes from a pound, shelter, or cattery will have an upper respiratory infection. The cat should be vaccinated before bringing it home. If at all possible, it is a good idea to leave the cat, for two to three weeks before you bring it home, with someone who does not have pets. This will give the cat time to develop an immunity. It will also give the cat time to develop any diseases that it might be incubating before you bring it into your "herd." This is especially important if you have a breeding group of registered cats. Vaccinations for most of the upper respiratory infections do not totally prevent the infections. They just prevent the severest form of the disease.

FELINE HERPESVIRUS

Feline herpesvirus, type 1 (FHV-1) is a very common and severe respiratory disease. It was previously called feline viral rhinotracheitis (FVR). Originally, this disease was thought to spread from one sneezing cat to another, however, recent research shows that intimate contact is necessary to spread the virus from a shedding cat to a susceptible one. Eating and drinking from the same dinner plate and licking each other during grooming seem to be the major methods of spreading the disease. It is especially a problem in kennels, shelters, pounds, and pet shops, where numbers of cats are brought together without adequate vaccination. Signs appear one to three days after the cat is exposed to the virus.

A carrier queen can infect her kittens. FHV can cause abortion or reabsorption of kittens in pregnant queens, without the mother having any signs of the disease. The kittens may be born weak and fade away and die several days later. FHV in older kittens is commonly seen when they are around 6- to 12-weeks old, when the immunity from their mother has worn off.

Cats with FHV are miserable, and signs of the disease are unmistakable: runny nose, shaking the head, spasms of sneezing, and salivation. The nasal discharge is clear at first, but may be bloody or pus-filled as the disease progresses. The cat will be droopy, lose much of its appetite, and have a low-grade fever. A few cats may have erosions on the skin, and painful ulcers in the mouth and on the corneas. They seem sensitive to light and squint. If not treated, the ulcers may eat through the cornea, causing blindness. Overall, nasal symptoms are more prominent than those affecting the eyes. Those most severely affected may have a high fever, breathe open-mouthed and gasp for air, and be depressed and stop eating.

FHV usually lasts one to two weeks. Very few cats die from it—they probably just wish they could! Most cats eventually recover fully, although a few go on to develop chronic sinusitis (sinus infection) that is extremely difficult to cure.

Treatment of FHV is aimed at keeping the cat as comfortable as possible, and keeping it adequately fed and watered so that its body can fight off the virus, much as humans do with the common cold. This is not as easy as it sounds. If the cat has a runny nose, it cannot smell food. Therefore, the cat may not want to eat and it may be necessary to force feed or tube-feed it. If the cat will not eat or drink, your veterinarian may have to administer fluids, either intravenously or under the skin.

It is important to keep the cat clean and comfortable. Wipe its nose with a soft cloth dampened with warm water. An antibiotic eye ointment will help make the cat more comfortable. Make sure the ointment does NOT have a corticosteroid in it. An antiviral eye ointment (such as acyclovir) may also be helpful for these cats. This disease can be treated at home, perhaps even better than by hospitalization (and certainly less expensively), if you are willing to give the nursing care that is needed. Severely ill cats may need hospitalization with fluid therapy to treat their dehydration.

Some cats that recover from FHV may be left with chronic infections of the sinuses and nasal passages. They also may be more susceptible to infections in these areas for the rest of their lives. The tear ducts may be damaged so that tears run down the face.

FHV vaccines are available. They give a varying degree of immunity—it is not extremely good, but will give some protection. If the cat does catch the disease after it is vaccinated, it will be much less serious than if the cat had not been vaccinated. Annual boosters are recommended. Some FHV-1 vaccines which contain live viruses may cause upper respiratory disease outbreaks in catteries which did not previously have this disease. This problem varies between brands of vaccine. The use of a killed vaccine avoids this possibility; however, it may also have more side effects. This virus is not the same as herpesvirus in humans, and is not infectious to them.

FELINE CALICIVIRUS

Feline calicivirus (FCV) is another respiratory disease that affects cats. Signs are similar to those of FHV. The cat will have depression and fever and little or no appetite. It may have a runny nose, but it is usually more a clear discharge than the thick mucus of FHV. There may be ulcers on the tongue, the leathery part of the nose, and the lips. These raw, reddened sores make the cat unwilling

or unable to eat. Chronic, red, ulcerated infected areas on the gums are very common with calicivirus infection. Occasionally, the lungs are involved and the cat has pneumonia. Some cats may limp due to muscle or joint pain. This rarely lasts more than two to four days. Overall, the disease is less severe than FHV.

Treatment is the same as for FHV (see above). Vaccine for FCV is usually combined with feline distemper vaccine so that they can be given together. Vaccines are helpful, but do not totally protect against all of the numerous strains of the disease. Vaccination with live-virus vaccine may cause FCV in kittens. Yearly boosters are also needed with this disease. Many adult cats that have recovered from the disease remain carriers.

CHLAMYDIAL INFECTION (PNEUMONITIS)

This feline respiratory disease is caused by *Chlamydia psittaci*, organisms which resemble bacteria. Like the other diseases, this one is spread by sneezing. It may come from carrier cats, especially when they are stressed, and is quite common in catteries as well as among free-roaming cats.

The disease is often seen in kittens and young cats (six weeks to four months old) after the immunity from their mother has worn off. Within five to 10 days after being exposed, the infected cat has runny eyes which may be held partially shut. The cat may start with one eye that is very weepy, but both eyes are eventually infected. Chlamydial infection can occur in tiny kittens, where it delays the opening of their eyes beyond the normal seven to 10 days of age. The eyelids may bulge, and when they are pulled apart, a large amount of gray or whitish material oozes out. It is important that the eyes be opened and treated, or the cornea may be ulcerated and the cat may be permanently blind. The cornea can't tolerate being marinated in pus for more than a day or two. Some cats may have runny noses. Most cats are alert and keep eating. Cats that become more ill or develop pneumonia are often also infected with another respiratory virus.

The eye infection is best treated three or more times a day with tetracycline eye ointment WITHOUT corticosteroids. The ointment should be used for AT LEAST two weeks to help keep the eye infection from coming back when treatment is stopped. A few cats become sensitive to the eye medication. This shows up when the cat improves and then becomes worse as it is being treated. The virus is also susceptible to sulfonamides, but is much less affected by ampicillin, penicillin, or streptomycin. If the cat only has an eye infection, there is no need to treat it with systemic antibiotics, as they are of little or no help for this disease. Cats with respiratory infection can also be treated with systemic tetracyclines. All cats in the household should be treated at the same time for up to four weeks, or two weeks after all signs of clinical illness are gone.

Vaccines against chlamydia can be purchased as separate products. However, it is available combined with distemper, FHV and FCV, which makes it easy and inexpensive to protect the cat against several diseases with a single injection. The chlamydial vaccine is not very effective because the organism does not stimulate a good immunity, especially under conditions of high exposure and stress, as in catteries and shelters. Kittens in high-exposure situations should be weaned around five to six weeks of age and kept away from adult cats that may be carriers of the infection. A 1:32 solution of household bleach will effectively disinfect contaminated surfaces.

Some physicians blame eye infections or "pinkeye" in children on cats. This can happen but is rare. If you touch the cat and then touch your face, you might contract the same eye infection the cat has had. If your cat has this disease, be sure to wash your hands after EVERY time you handle the cat. It is a good idea to keep the cat confined in a crate until the medication takes effect and its eyes and nose have stopped running. When seen in people, it causes a severe conjunctivitis, leaving the whites of one or both eyes reddened and very painful. It may feel as if you have sand in your eyes, and bright light may hurt them. Your physician may give you antibiotics to help treat the ailment.

FELINE INFECTIOUS PERITONITIS (FIP)

Feline infectious peritonitis (FIP) is a viral disease. It is closely related to the viruses which cause coronavirus infection in dogs and transmissible gastroenteritis (TGE) in hogs. It sporadically affects domestic cats as well as some wild felines, and is usually fatal. In groups of cats, such as catteries, shelters, and multiple cat households, as many as 10% of the cats may die. The disease does not seem to spread very readily, and is not easily passed from one cat to another. Exactly how it is spread is unknown, but it is suspected that it spreads via feces and, less commonly, via nasal secretions or urine. The virus may be carried on bedding and feeding dishes, and perhaps on clothing or by insects. Once the cat appears ill, death is nearly 100%. A very few will appear to have the disease and then recover. These animals may contract the disease at a later date if they are stressed, overcrowded, immunosuppressed, or treated with corticosteroids. Many cats that develop FIP have no known contact with cats that are ill with the disease.

FIP is most common in cats between six months and four or five years of age, with most around six months to two years. It can also be seen in elderly cats. Male and female cats are about equally affected. Kittens born to an infected mother are usually healthy, but may later become carriers. Other kittens may be infected, either in utero or shortly after birth, and later develop FIP. The disease is more common in purebred cats, perhaps because they are often raised in catteries where prolonged contact may allow the disease to more easily spread from one cat to another. Some lines of cats may be genetically more susceptible than others. The presence of another disease may make the cat more susceptible to FIP. As many as half the cats infected with FIP are also infected with feline leukemia virus. In experimental infections, the incubation period is short, as little as two to 14 days, but it varies widely with naturally occurring infections.

FIP shows two types of disease in cats. The first is the effusive ("wet") form. Large quantities of liquid form in the abdomen (peritoneal cavity; thus the name, "peritonitis") and/or the chest. The cat's belly may appear to be swollen and rounded. If the chest is involved, it may have trouble breathing because the fluid keeps its lungs from expanding with air. The cat may become fatigued and even gasp if it exerts itself. There may be a fever that goes up and down, lasting from one week to a month or more. The cat may have a poor appetite and weight loss, even as its belly swells. If you feel the abdomen, it is usually not painful. The cat may be droopy and have little energy, and may have a slight discharge from the nose and/or eyes. Some cats may show only the swollen belly but otherwise appear normal until the disease is quite advanced. The mucous membranes may be pale and/or slightly yellowish, and the cat may show alternating diarrhea and constipation. Signs of FIP may be "triggered" by the stress of surgery such as otherwise routine spaying or castration.

This form of FIP may proceed rapidly, with death in a few weeks to several months or longer. The cat gradually becomes less active and eats poorly. It affects about three-fourths of cats with FIP. Younger cats (four to 10 months old) may grow poorly and be chronically ill before signs of FIP are seen.

The second form of FIP is called non-effusive or "dry." This is a smoldering form of the disease, partially controlled by the cat's immune system. It does not produce the fluid, but has growths or lesions throughout the kidneys, spleen, liver, lymph nodes, spinal cord, brain, and eyes. The disease may affect the nervous system, including tremors or convulsions, hypersensitivity, staggering, head tilt, changes in behavior, partial or complete paralysis of the hind legs and urinary incontinence. The same up-and-down fever is seen, as well as weight loss and anemia. Vomiting or diarrhea can occur, and the eyes can appear cloudy or reddened. This form may alternately become worse and improve over a period of many months. It is also possible to see a combination of the two forms of FIP.

This is a difficult disease to diagnose in either form. Currently, there is not a reliable laboratory test for it. Examination of a sample of fluid from the abdomen or chest cavity may be helpful, or organ biopsy may help to positively diagnose FIP in a living cat. Other than that, diagnosis is often made by excluding other diseases that may look like FIP. If your cat shows any of these signs, take it to a veterinarian to be checked.

The prognosis for cats with FIP is poor because no treatment is effective against the virus which causes it. From the time that signs are noticed, cats may die quickly. At best, they rarely live more than four months. All that can be done by treating the cat is to buy a little more time. This is most successful in cats that are not also infected with the feline leukemia virus.

Some cats that are infected with FIP also are infected with feline leukemia. This may be because the leukemia suppresses the cat's immune system, allowing the FIP virus, which had been hiding in the body, to attack at the same time. Others may have the same suppression due to feline immunodeficiency virus.

The only treatment for this disease is with some extremely strong anti-cancer type drugs, which must be given by a veterinarian. They are usually accompanied by corticosteroids. If the lesions are confined to an eye and the sight has been lost, it may be best to remove the infected eye. In addition, large amounts of nursing care will be needed to help cope with the various symptoms as they occur. Do you have the time and money to spend? Are you willing to provide the nursing care that is needed when you might only be buying another month or two? The few cats that have been successfully treated were those that had mild cases and were still eating well. If the cat is already thin and weakened, your chances of making a difference are almost nil.

One vaccine is currently available for vaccination against FIP (Primucell FIP®, SmithKline Beecham Animal Health). The first dose is given after the cat is 16 weeks of age, with a second dose in three to four weeks. Because the vaccine is given at this age, it may not offer adequate protection in high-exposure situations such as catteries where kittens are exposed early in their lives. This vaccination is given into the cat's nose with a dropper. It should NOT be injected! The cat may sneeze or shake its head when the vaccine is given; this is normal. Annual boosters are recommended. Exposure to extremely high doses of FIP virus may overwhelm the immunity and allow the cat to develop the disease. Even if your cat is vaccinated, you should keep it away from known cases of FIP. If you have a cat in your household that has FIP, you should take this into consideration when making a decision to treat or not.

If FIP is present in a cattery, overcrowding should be eliminated. Great care should be given to sanitation and adequate ventilation. The FIP virus is relatively delicate; it dies at room temperature within one to two days. It is also killed by most detergents and household disinfectants. The cats should all be on good nutrition, and stress should be minimized.

Queens with kittens should be kept away from others until their litters are weaned. Kittens of different ages and from different litters should be kept separately. Queens should be selected that have raised large healthy litters, and ones that have weak or sickly kittens should be eliminated from the breeding program, no matter what their bloodlines or other qualities. Newly introduced cats should be strictly quarantined until it is certain they are healthy. All cats with ANY signs of FIP should be immediately isolated (or removed), as should any cats with feline leukemia. After these measures are taken, the remaining cats should be vaccinated for FIP. Only a few of the cats which are naturally infected with the FIP virus ever develop the disease.

FELINE CORONAVIRUS

The virus causing feline coronavirus infection is closely related to the virus causing feline infectious peritonitis. It causes mild intestinal infections in kittens between birth and three months of age. Like FIP, this virus is common in multi-cat households and catteries. Coronavirus causes a mild to moderately severe diarrhea which may last two to six days. A low-grade fever develops, and there may be some vomiting. The kitten is usually droopy, and may quit eating for two or three days. Very few of them die, which is one major difference between this disease and panleukopenia.

The cat should not be given food during the worst phase of the disease. If it becomes dehydrated, a veterinarian may need to give fluids. Antibiotics usually are not needed, and kittens generally recover within two to three days.

Currently, there is no way to prevent this disease, which usually is not severe. It is self-limiting, as the cats recover by themselves. The main point is to distinguish between this disease and feline distemper, which may be fatal.

FELINE LEUKEMIA

Feline leukemia is a cancer or tumor (lymphosarcoma) caused by a virus. It is passed from one cat to another through the saliva, by licking, grooming, biting, or eating out of a common dish over a period of time. Bites that break the skin transmit the virus very efficiently by transferring a large amount of it. It can also be transmitted via urine or feces through a shared litter box, and can spread via blood or tears. The virus only lives for a few minutes outside the cat's body in dry air. For this reason, it is difficult for the cat to contract the disease through contact with an inanimate object.

Less commonly, the virus is passed through the mother's milk or uterus to her unborn kittens. Queens that are coming down with leukemia may infect one or more of the kittens. In some litters, an infected kitten may pass the disease to its littermates, and they may all die.

Feline leukemia is seen in domestic cats throughout the world. At any given time, perhaps 1-2% of our cat population is infected with this disease. Most of these cats will appear healthy, with no signs of disease. Wild felines do not harbor feline leukemia but can be infected when exposed to domestic cats. Rural cats are often free of the disease, but when it is brought in by a stray or dumped domestic cat, most of the cats on a farm or ranch may die of the disease. Infection rates are highest in multiple-cat households and catteries. City cats that live their entire lives in apartments without contact with other cats may have a very low rate of infection. Urban and suburban cats that roam freely may have high rates of infection because of their frequent contact with other cats, some of which will surely be infected with the disease. By the time an outdoor cat is seven to eight years of age, it has usually been infected with leukemia, and either died, become immune, or is permanently carrying the disease. For this reason, leukemia is rarely seen in cats over 10 years of age.

Feline leukemia virus infects the cat through the membranes of the eyes, nose, and mouth. It replicates in the lymph nodes of the head and neck. If the cat is to become permanently infected, the virus spreads to the bone marrow. From there it goes into the bloodstream, finally lodging in various tissues and organs, where it multiplies. Because it is carried in the blood, fleas that have sucked infected blood may pass the virus to other cats. The disease develops slowly, but about 85% of infected cats will die within three to four years.

Exposure to the feline leukemia virus (FeLV) does not always result in the disease. If the exposed cat is healthy and normal, there is about a 40% chance that its body will reject the virus and recover from the infection. These cats become immune to the virus, but will react positively to tests for FeLV. However, not all FeLV-recovered cats will remain immune to reinfection. About 30% of the exposed cats develop a persistent infection and eventually develop clinical signs. In the period before signs are seen, FeLV can be detected by testing, although it may take more than one test to find it.

Another 30% of exposed cats neither develop an infection nor reject the virus. They are called "latent carriers." They usually don't develop the disease, but they may serve as a source of infection for other cats. Their kittens may be born infected with FeLV. Laboratory testing can be done to identify these carriers, but it is painful and complicated. The test involves sampling the cat's bone marrow, and takes up to six weeks.

Some cats are more susceptible to infection by FeLV than others. The immune system in kittens less than four months of age is not fully capable of fighting off disease-causing agents. The immune system in stressed, elderly, or ill cats does not give its normal degree of protection. Queens that have recovered from feline leukemia infection will usually provide enough antibodies in their milk to protect the kittens for the first three months or so of life. Latent leukemia infections may become active in cats that are treated with corticosteroids. Modified live vaccines for feline herpes virus and feline panleukopenia are ineffective as protection against those diseases in cats that already have leukemia; thus, these vaccines should not be used in cats that test positive for feline leukemia. Isolation from diseased cats will protect positive cats better than vaccination.

Cats that are infected with FeLV rarely live more than three years. Many of them will die of other diseases before the leukemia affects them. Cats with FeLV have little resistance to infections by even the commonest viruses, bacteria, and fungi. They may fail to reproduce, or produce weak or dying kittens. They have frequent respiratory tract infections and pneumonia, stomach problems, sores in the mouth, and anemia.

Feline leukemia causes a number of clinical signs, depending on which bodily systems are affected by the virus (and what other organisms are attacking the weakened cat). Leukemia, a cancer of the blood cells, is only one of the many possible outcomes of infection with the leukemia virus. Common signs include depression, weight loss, fever, and loss of appetite. FeLV is one of the commonest causes of anemia in cats. You may first notice that the nose, instead of being a healthy pink, is white as a sheet. About one-third of cats with recurrent abscesses are infected with the leukemia virus. It may also cause obscure signs of central nervous system disease. Immunodeficiency can lead to infection with other diseases, both viral and bacterial. Queens may abort or fail to become pregnant. As many as 70% of weak, "fading" kittens may be infected with FeLV.

Lymphosarcoma, another cancer, is more commonly seen with the FeLV virus than is leukemia. One of the commonest signs of lymphosarcoma is grossly swollen lymph nodes, especially at the shoulder and behind the angle of the hocks. Skin lesions may be seen, including nonhealing lesions or chronic abscesses. Lymphosarcoma can occur in almost any tissue or organ, and it is nearly always fatal. Some cats with lymphosarcoma die quickly, while others die after a long period of misery and deterioration. Lymphosarcoma of the kidney, caused by the feline leukemia virus, is the most common kidney tumor in cats. Diagnosis is made by tapping a few cells from the fluid of the cat's abdominal cavity with a small needle. About 90% of cats with this tumor will test negative for feline leukemia virus, even though they are infected with it.

The FeLV virus dies quickly outside the cat's body (within two or three minutes). It may live up to two or three days in a moist place other than living cells, such as your yard or the cat's cage in a shelter. For this reason, it can be spread by contaminated food and water dishes and litter boxes. It is easily killed by common disinfectants and ordinary household detergents. Although it is unlikely you could carry the virus from one cat to another on your clothing or skin, it is a good idea to wash your hands after handling a cat that doesn't live in your house—before handling your own cats.

Prolonged cat-to-cat exposure is needed to transmit the virus, such as where cats groom each other or use the same litter pan. If all cats in your household test negative for leukemia virus, keeping them away from strange cats will go a long way toward keeping them free from it. This means keeping them indoors or in a fenced yard, preferably where strange cats cannot come into contact with them. It also means not bringing ANY other cats into the household, not even for a visit, unless they have recently tested negative for leukemia virus. Treat even a vaccinated cat as if it were completely at risk and keep it away from other cats—the best of FeLV vaccines are only about 80% effective. Test a new kitten before you bring it home to be a companion for your beloved older cat. The best catteries do not allow new cats to come in without testing AND a one to two month quarantine period.

If you have had a cat with FeLV in your household, after the cat dies or is removed from the premises, wash all the bedding, feed and water dishes, and litter boxes with hot water and soap. Disinfect them with a 1:32 solution of bleach. Wait at least 10 days before you bring a new kitten or cat into the household.

Your lone cat can become infected if it goes roaming and runs into a cat with FeLV. This accounts for the higher rate of leukemia infection in male cats. For this reason, it is especially important that outdoor cats and intact males be vaccinated against this disease. If you must feed stray cats, keep them outdoors and do not allow them in your house. Better yet, find a home for the stray and keep your own cats indoors!

There is no treatment for cats with feline leukemia. Some of the secondary infections such as abscesses and tooth infections can be treated, giving the cat relief from those miseries. Blood transfusions may buy another few weeks or months of life for some cats with anemia. Many medications have been tried, including huge doses of vitamin C, but none have proven effective against the disease. In some cases, interferon treatment may slow the progress of the disease. Cats with vague symptoms, poor appetite, depression, and weight loss may be greatly helped by intermittent small doses of corticosteroids. Chemotherapy may give temporary remission for cats with lymphosarcoma, but it will not cure it.

What happens to a cat that is exposed to leukemia is determined within the first four months after exposure. Cats become increasingly resistant to the virus after one to two months of age.

If there are several cats in a household or cattery, the best way to protect cats that are uninfected is to test for the presence of leukemia virus, using the immunofluorescent test (IFA), and to remove infected animals. ELISA tests that are performed at a veterinary hospital should be confirmed by IFA testing before the cat is taken out of the household. This is because false positives can occur with the ELISA test. About 10% of antigen-positive cats do not have infective virus in their blood (Jarrett, 1991, p. 1279). The IFA test also should be used on ELISA-negative cats that have clinical signs of FeLV-caused disease. Cats that are positive on an IFA test should be considered carriers of the virus in their blood. Current information suggests these animals are infected for life. They can spread the disease to cats around them by grooming and licking, and will contract with the disease later in life.

Remove any infected cats, either by euthanizing them, or isolating them. If infected cats are removed, the remainder of the cats should be kept quarantined, with no other cats coming in or out, and retested again in a month. If any infected cats are found on the second test, they should be removed, and the test repeated in three months. When all cats in the group test negative on two tests given three months apart, they are considered to be leukemia-free. Then, you can vaccinate the healthy cats to give a good immunity. As many as 30% of the cats in this type of environment may be infected or carriers before testing and vaccination are begun. In the Netherlands, feline leukemia has been completely eliminated in catteries by testing and removal of cats that were positive.

A number of blood tests allow the veterinarian to determine if the cat is infected with FeLV. No test is 100% accurate, but most are quite reliable. A blood test that is positive for FeLV does not guarantee that the cat is going to die of leukemia. It merely means it has been exposed to the virus. A negative test does not guarantee the cat won't become infected with FeLV; it just means it is not actively infected at the time of the test. If the cat is exposed to the virus in the future, it could still develop the disease. This is why it is so important to vaccinate against it!

Much of the progress in eliminating feline leukemia has been due to testing groups of cats and eliminating the positive animals. This helped to remove carriers that had spread the infection. It is still a good idea to test new cats before bringing them into your household. Do not rely on vaccinations to prevent feline leukemia because they are not 100% effective.

It is recommended that all healthy cats nine weeks of age or older be vaccinated against feline leukemia. First-time vaccination calls for two doses two to three weeks apart. A third dose may be given two to four months later. After that, the cat should have yearly boosters. Current vaccines seem to be about 80% effective in preventing the disease. A few cats will have reactions after vaccination, including fever, depression, lack of appetite, and vomiting. They should not last more than 24 hours; if they do, consult your veterinarian. The cat may also experience pain at the vaccination site for a few days.

Some veterinarians recommend that the cat be tested for leukemia before it is vaccinated. This is not a necessity before giving the shots, although some veterinarians require it. The advantage of testing before you vaccinate is that any infected cats can be identified and others protected from exposure. After vaccination, it is impossible to tell if a positive test is from infection or vaccination.

There is no harm in vaccinating a cat that already harbors the FeLV virus, but on the other hand, the vaccine is of no help in curing the disease. Inadvertently giving the vaccine to a cat that already has the disease may give you a false sense of security. If you don't want to have the testing done, be aware of these realities, and find a veterinarian who doesn't require it. Then, don't blame him or her for a vaccination failure if the cat contracts the disease.

A negative test only means that the virus is not active in the cat at THAT moment. It may be a cat with a case of FeLV that is dormant, and the disease may surface if the cat is stressed or treated with corticosteroids. Negative FeLV tests do not guarantee the cat is free from the disease and conversely, vaccinations against the disease never give 100% protection. They are, however, far better than doing nothing! In the overall population of healthy cats, only about 2.3% of them, based on IFA tests, are infected with feline leukemia virus (Jarrett, 1991). For this reason, many veterinarians pull a blood sample for testing and vaccinate the cat for FeLV at the same visit.

There is some slight concern among public health personnel that it might be possible for the feline leukemia virus to be transmitted to humans (Hardy, in Holzman, 1987, p. 255). Thus, some veterinarians recommend that cats that are positive on the IFA test be either strictly isolated or euthanized. Studies have NOT proven that transmission to humans can occur.

FELINE ACQUIRED IMMUNE DEFICIENCY SYNDROME (FAIDS, FIV)

So-called feline AIDS (FAIDS) is an immune deficiency syndrome caused by a virus that is somewhat similar to the feline leukemia virus. It is also called feline immunodeficiency virus or FIV. Like AIDS in humans, it allows other diseases to attack, weaken, and eventually kill the cat. Like humans with AIDS, once a cat is infected with FIV, it will never recover from the disease. The virus is only distantly related to that of human AIDS, and is NOT the same disease as AIDS in humans. However, there is hope that

FIV can be used as an experimental model because it affects the cat's body in a similar manner to the way the AIDS virus affects humans. While looking for a cure for FIV, researchers may help find a cure for AIDS in humans. More than 80 different strains of FIV have been found in naturally infected cats. FIV cannot infect dogs, humans, or other animals, as it is not contagious between species. A person cannot give human AIDS to his or her cat, and the cat cannot give FIV to a human.

As many as half the cats infected with feline infectious peritonitis, unhealing sinusitis and chronic pneumonia, and chronic mouth and gum infections are also infected with either the feline leukemia virus or the feline AIDS virus. This has caused an immune suppression. Similar to AIDS in humans, when immune suppression occurs, the other diseases eventually lead to death. Any cat that has a chronic infection which does not respond to normal treatment should be tested for FIV infection and feline leukemia.

Like human AIDS, this disease is primarily spread through blood exchange, especially by the bite of an infected cat. It seems to be more readily spread within two to four weeks after the cat becomes infected. This is, of course, before anyone is aware of the illness. For this reason, the new male cat on the block may be more likely to spread the disease than the ragged old tomcat that has been there for years. Cats with mouth lesions may more easily spread the disease. Casual contact, such as mutual grooming or using common food dishes or litter pans, does not easily spread the disease. Queens that have been recently infected during pregnancy or lactation may pass the disease to their kittens via the placenta or milk. However, other kittens from these same mothers may not be infected (Barr, 1995).

Ideally, kittens less than six months of age from unknown backgrounds should be tested for FIV. If negative, retest in three to four months, as about 20% of cats that test negative are positive. A second negative test means the kitten is negative. If the first test is positive, retest after the kitten reaches six months of age. If the second test is negative, the kitten is probably negative, and the first test detected antibodies from the queen. If the second test is positive, the kitten should either be retested using another method, or rechecked in six months (Sellon, 1994).

It may take eight to 12 weeks after the cat is exposed for the virus to show up on tests. The disease may also disguise itself and fail to show up on tests, so that a cat that tests negative may actually be carrying the virus. Most cases of FIV occur in cats five to six years old. Interestingly, the incidence of FIV in catteries is very low. Infected cats are more of a hazard to free-roaming cats with which they fight than to others in the same household. This is because the disease is transmitted mainly by biting. FIV-positive cats are not usually removed from the household because the disease is not easily spread by grooming or via dishes.

As with human AIDS, the virus itself is not fatal. However, the animal's weakened immune system may allow secondary bacterial infections to infect the cat and eventually kill it. Cats do not usually die immediately, but often live as long as five years or more, averaging around two years (Fleming, 1991). The cat may not even show signs of disease for up to five years after it is infected. Cats do not recover from the infection once it is acquired.

The cat may show signs of chronic infection, such as recurrent sores on the mouth or a recurring cough. Poor appetite, fever and weight loss are common. The cat may have kidney or bladder problems, or diarrhea. Dental disease, abscesses, and toxoplasmosis are also seen. The cat may have cancer of various types, especially cancer of the kidney. It may have swollen lymph nodes and anemia, which may occur when the disease is quite advanced and the animal is near death. The cat may test negative for feline leukemia (FeLV), although a high percentage of cats are infected with both viruses. Other cats succumb to bacterial infections, parasites, yeast infections, and viral infections such as FeLV.

If you have several cats and one is diagnosed with FIV, the others should be tested. If one is positive and the others are negative, you have several choices. You can euthanize the infected cat and retest the others at three and six months, again removing any infected cats. You can quarantine the cat and keep it away from the others for the rest of its life. Or, you can leave them together and take your chances on spread. Since it does not seem to be very contagious, if the cats are not breeding or fighting, there should be little chance of spread—at least as far as is known at the present time. Occasionally, FIV can be spread to very young cats from their mother, perhaps through her milk or via close contact. It may still be a good idea to feed the cat separately. Because of false negatives with current tests, some cats may still be infected, showing symptoms of the disease at a later date.

Manage medical problems as they occur and love the cat until the end of its life. Antibiotics may be used to control secondary infections. Corticosteroids and drugs such as AZT, which is used to treat AIDS in humans, are helpful against FIV, but their benefits must be weighed against their considerable side effects. Supportive measures which may be needed include blood transfusions, intravenous fluids, and high-calorie nutritional supplements.

Feral cats are thought to act as a reservoir for the disease. As with feline leukemia and many other cat diseases, FIV can be prevented by keeping your cat safely indoors and away from strange cats.

RABIES

Rabies is a viral disease which affects warm-blooded animals throughout the world. There are sporadic outbreaks in populations of wild animals. In the northeastern United States it is more commonly spread through foxes, while in the southeastern states it also is seen in raccoons and other animals. West of the Mississippi, skunks are a common reservoir. As of 1991, record levels of rabies in skunks and raccoons were reported, and the numbers of infected animals may still be rising. In 1993, oral baits were used to vaccinate raccoons in New Jersey and Texas in an effort to halt the spread of the disease. Maryland was also severely affected by this outbreak. New York State reported

2747 cases of rabies in 1993 (Krebs, 1994). Rabies has been controlled in foxes in Switzerland by distributing chicken necks injected with rabies vaccine.

Increasing numbers of rabid raccoons have been seen in Virginia, Pennsylvania, West Virginia, and the District of Columbia. These are wild animals living in urban settings in attics, garages, and chimneys. They scrounge meals from dog dishes and garbage cans as well as occasionally eating outdoor dogs and cats. In such intimate contact, it is easy for the outdoor urban cat or dog to come into contact with an infected raccoon.

You can reduce the rabies danger to your cat, your dog, and yourself by not feeding these urban invaders, either deliberately or accidentally. Get rid of trash around your house which can give them shelter, and cover or screen any openings which might house them. Put a screen guard over your chimney and patch holes in your roof. These moves will help reduce the carrying capacity of the habitat, thereby reducing the number of raccoons that can live on it. Locking your garbage to deny them dinner is one of the best defenses against this dreaded disease.

In the southern border states, cats may be exposed to rabid dogs, cats, or wild animals that come across the border from Mexico. Recent droughts and flooding in Texas have pushed coyotes into populated areas where they can easily get food and water. An unvaccinated cat can be bitten by a rabies-infected coyote and bring the disease into your home! The average domestic animal with rabies will expose five times as many people to the disease as a wild animal with rabies (Clark, 1988).

Rabies may be present in bats in some areas, especially California and southern states which border Mexico. They may expose cats that catch them and are bitten in the process. In addition, a bat that is sick with rabies may be on the ground where the cat can easily catch it, instead of flying well out of reach. Any bat caught by a cat should be considered rabid until proven otherwise. Cover it with a blanket or towel and carefully kill it. Don't use a blow to the head on such a small animal, as it will damage brain tissue which is needed for testing. Freezing will work to kill the bat and it can still be tested (this is NOT true of larger animals) (Alishouse, 1996). Take it to your veterinarian to be sent to the laboratory for examination. Handle it with gloves or a towel and don't get bitten in the process!

Rabid bats have been reported in every state except Hawaii. Because only an extremely small percentage of bats are affected, wholesale destruction is NOT justified. Colonies of bats eat literally tons of insects which are otherwise destructive to plants and crops. Only bats in colonies proven by laboratory tests to have rabies should be destroyed. Antibody analysis shows that very few terrestrial animals have been infected with strains of rabies originating from bats (Clark, 1988; Krebs, 1994, p. 1697). It is, however, a good idea to keep bats out of houses, barns, and other places that humans and their animals inhabit. This can be done by screening or sealing up holes where they enter. For safety, avoid handling bats.

Rabies is more often seen late in the spring, into summer and early fall, when wild animals are more active. Domestic animals are more likely to be outside and roaming widely during these seasons, too. Humans are active outdoors and can encounter the wild animals.

To lessen the possibility of rabies exposure to yourself, avoid wild animals that seem ill or are injured, especially in rabies areas. Be very wary of a nocturnal animal (such as a skunk or raccoon, normally not seen during the day) that is out in the daytime. Any animal involved in an unprovoked attack should be considered rabid until proven otherwise. Keeping your cat indoors will almost completely avoid the chance of exposure. If you travel in foreign countries, do NOT stroke or handle dogs or cats; dogs are the major vectors for rabies in most developing countries. Controlling the numbers of feral cats (and stray dogs) goes a long way toward reducing the chances of rabies being transmitted from wild animals to your farm cats or pets.

Cats are susceptible to rabies because of their roaming and hunting habits when they live outdoors full- or part-time. In addition to chasing bats that might be infected with rabies, the cat may be chased by an infected fox, skunk, raccoon, dog, cat, or other animal as it is out prowling. In the United States, there are more cases of rabies in cats than in dogs, and probably because of roaming, male cats are more often infected than females. Cats also coexist comfortably with skunks. One night I walked into the shed on my farm where I fed the cats. There was a cat at the feeder, a skunk, and two more cats, all eating shoulder-to-shoulder. Dogs, in contrast, tend to have confrontations with skunks rather than living happily alongside them. Rabies virus has not been found in skunk spray, so if you or your animals get doused, there is no danger of the disease if there is no other contact (Clark, 1988).

Even worse than the danger that your cat might get rabies from a rabid animal is the possibility that it might get it and pass it on to you! Rabies in humans is almost always fatal. Within 10 days before an infected animal dies, the virus is present in its salivary glands and it shows signs of the disease. This is when you can catch it, if the animal bites you or licks at a scratch in your skin. The 10-day rule is only true of domestic animals. Some wild animals comfortably carry the rabies virus, can pass it on to you, and live on after you are dead from the disease.

If a cat is bitten by a wild animal of any kind, including a bat that has escaped, it should be considered as having been exposed to rabies. If the cat is not vaccinated, it should be quarantined for six months. This may need to be done in a veterinary facility, depending on laws in your state. At the very least, it should be done in a cage or pen where the cat has no direct contact with humans. Food and water should be passed through a door or opening, and you should be careful not to handle the animal until the quarantine period is over. The cat should be vaccinated with an approved rabies vaccine at the time of the bite and again after five months of quarantine or as directed by local health officials.

Ideally, the cat that is bitten by an animal that proves positive for the rabies virus should be humanely and safely euthanized to avoid the possibility that it may get the disease and pass it to a human. While this may be easy to do with a feral or stray cat, it's not an option that many cat owners would like to consider.

Realistically, most cats that are bitten by rabid animals are vaccinated and quarantined. If the cat is bitten by an animal that is confirmed as being rabid and the cat has been vaccinated for rabies within the previous 12 months, it should receive a "booster" shot of rabies vaccine. It should then be confined for 90 days, as described above, according to the laws in your locality. Rubber gloves should be worn while treating any wounds on its body, but the cat should be handled as little as possible.

On rare occasions, a vaccinated pet may develop rabies. This usually occurs in young animals that have had only one dose of vaccine. If your pet (cat or dog) has had a rabies vaccination before six months of age, be sure to get another one after that age, and then keep the boosters current. Rabies may occur in cats that are infected with feline leukemia virus (Wills, 1993, p. 359) and vaccinated with a modified live rabies virus. It may happen if a modified live rabies virus vaccine is given under the skin rather than intramuscularly, or when a rabies vaccine is given that is not approved for use in cats. Some of these cats will show paralysis in the hind legs (where the vaccine was given), while others may progress to "classical" signs of rabies.

Cats without current rabies vaccinations face a much worse fate when bitten by an animal that is known or strongly suspected to have rabies. Euthanasia is again the first choice of public health officials. If you don't agree with this, the cat is kept in strict quarantine for six months. It is vaccinated for rabies one month before being released. This is the best possible reason for keeping your cat's rabies vaccinations current, in addition to the protection it offers you and your family.

There is no reliable method of determining that a live animal is free of rabies. Skin biopsies and other tests have been tried. Currently, they have too many false negatives to be dependable.

The incubation period for rabies in cats varies from nine days to more than 50 days. The cat may have been treated for a wound within the previous six months. In some cases, the wound is severe enough that it is not suspected to be from a bite, and it may already have been infected when first noticed.

The first sign is usually a change in personality. The cat may be depressed or restless. A friendly cat may suddenly become unapproachable or irritable, and may want to hide in a dark place. An aloof cat may become loving. It may cry or howl in an unusual voice, and the cries become more frequent as the disease progresses. Some owners describe an unusual look in the cat's eyes—blank, spooky, staring, wild, or anxious. Contrary to popular belief, cats with rabies only rarely drool saliva from the mouth.

The next stage of rabies may be the "furious" stage. A cat in furious rabies can be a serious hazard to the humans and animals around it. It may grab and bite or chew foreign objects such as branches or furniture. Your legs or those of your dog may be next. Farm cats may attack and bite cows or horses, or may run through the yard chewing on vehicle tires. Rabies may be seen in horses, mules, cattle,

sheep, goats, and swine. Do NOT reach down the throat of any farm animal that appears to be unable to swallow or has a changed voice, as these are two common signs of rabies in large animals. Rabies is also found in groundhogs and woodchucks. It is a significant problem in mongooses in Puerto Rico, and dogs and cats on that island should be vaccinated against rabies (Cappucci, 1994). Rodents, such as squirrels, chipmunks, mice, rats, and rabbits and hares, are almost never infected with rabies, although all of them are susceptible.

The cat may chew at the site where it was bitten, gnawing at its leg without apparent pain until it is shredded and bleeding. It may have muscular twitching and weakness. It may go berserk, running into objects and biting anything it touches until it collapses from exhaustion. The cat may die during a seizure.

If the cat is touched, it may go into violent spasms. It should only be handled with VERY thick leather gloves (cat canine teeth can penetrate most leather gloves). Or, you can use a blanket folded into many layers so that you have no contact with the animal. If at all possible, handle it with a loop of rope on a pole, or by lowering a cage or garbage can over it so that you can avoid touching it.

As the virus causes paralysis of the throat muscles, the cat is unable to eat or drink. A few cats may drool profusely. Just trying to drink will increase the spasms which are occurring in the muscles which control swallowing. Because of this discomfort, the animal may be afraid to drink water. This reaction gave birth to the old name for rabies, hydrophobia ("fear of water").

In some cats, a paralytic or "dumb" stage occurs before the animal dies. The cat may have an abnormal gait, starting in the hind legs, which are described as "wobbly" or "collapsing" (Fogelman, 1993). The cat may be paralyzed, first in the hind end, and then in the whole body. Then the animal becomes comatose, with death usually occurring from two to five days from the first signs of illness. In some cases, the animal may live up to 10 days after the first signs. About one-third of cats with rabies only go through the dumb form of the disease.

If there is any chance that a cat may have rabies, it should be examined by a veterinarian. If the cat is a stray or is unwanted, it should be euthanized, and the head sent by your veterinarian to a laboratory for examination.

If a cat suspected of having rabies is going to be watched, it should be confined for 10 days. If it is healthy at the end of that time, it is considered to have been incapable of transmitting the virus at the time it bit a person or another animal. If it dies during the 10 days for any reason (even if it escapes and is hit by a car), the head should be sent to a laboratory to be checked.

Cats that develop rabies invariably die within 15 days. No treatment is given for two reasons: no treatment is known to work, and treatment might give a false sense of security, allowing the cat to bite and infect other animals or humans with the disease before it dies.

It is as important (or perhaps even more so) to vaccinate your cat for rabies as to vaccinate your dog. A cat that is kept indoors all the time is at less risk, and it's a judgment call as to whether it needs to be immunized (other than to protect yourself legally if it bites someone). If you live on a farm in an area where rabies is a problem, that small injection may be the best life insurance you can buy. While you're at it, vaccinate the dog, too. You can also vaccinate valuable breeding cattle, hogs, horses, and sheep using vaccines approved for these species.

Cats can be vaccinated as young as three months of age. This is a good idea in areas where rabies in wildlife is a problem. Any cat that is vaccinated between three and six months of age should receive a booster when it is over six months of age. This will assure that antibodies from its mother's milk have worn off and that it will develop a solid immunity. Then, boosters should be given every one to three years, according to the laws where you live, and depending on the vaccine which is used.

If you give your own rabies vaccinations, it is CRITICAL that the vaccine be approved for cats. Don't use something for the dog that you had left in the refrigerator. If cats are vaccinated with rabies vaccine that is not made for cats, they may develop rabies.

Unless the package flyer says otherwise, rabies vaccine is usually given deep into the heavy muscles of the thigh, all in one location. Be aware if you give your own vaccinations that it may not be considered valid if the cat bites someone. Most areas require a certificate signed by a veterinarian as proof of current rabies vaccination. Some states do not allow the sale of rabies vaccine to anyone other than veterinarians. Also, having the vaccination given by a veterinarian helps relieve you of liability if the cat bites someone.

Most airlines require that a cat have a current rabies vaccination in order to be shipped by air or taken with you as a carry-on pet.

RABIES AND THE CAT BITE

In 1994, six people in the United States died of rabies (Rhone-Merieux, 1995). If you are bitten by a cat (or any other animal), cleanse the wound using a disinfectant such as povidone-iodine (Betadine®), scrubbing for a minimum of five to 10 minutes. Rabies is not generally a danger if the skin has not been penetrated by a bite or scratch, or by the animal licking an open wound. Consult the animal's owner, if known, to determine its current rabies vaccination status. In some areas, the cat MUST be taken to a veterinary clinic or animal control facility for a mandatory 10-day quarantine. If a cat that has bitten a human—even your own cat—dies within 10 days, it is a good idea to have the brain examined to be certain it does not have rabies. If the cat has not been vaccinated, always have the brain checked. This is especially important in an area where rabies is common. The cat could have rabies but be killed before you are aware of it. Meanwhile, consult your physician to determine if further treatment is necessary. If you have any questions about the advice, consult your county and/or state health department for further information. Tetanus immunization and/or antibiotic treatment for infection may be needed, depending on the bite. Under some circumstances, the physician may advise you to take

a series of rabies injections. Rabies cannot be transmitted by petting or handling an animal.

If you are bitten by a wild animal, the animal should not be confined because the incubation periods are extremely variable. The animal should be killed and submitted for examination, again without damage to the head. Keep it refrigerated, but not frozen, until you are able to get it to your veterinarian. Testing for rabies may not be needed with rodents because of the extremely low incidence of the disease, but check with your veterinarian or physician to be sure. If the wild animal escapes after biting someone, rabies immunization is almost certain to be recommended for the bite victim. Why? Because the animal is presumed to be rabid unless it can be proven otherwise.

Don't be too afraid of taking treatment for rabies exposure—it beats the alternative! Very few persons in recorded history who have developed signs of rabies have survived the disease. You've probably heard about "shots in the belly button." That was an old treatment that is no longer used. One current post-exposure (after the bite) treatment includes a series of five injections of human rabies vaccine, given in the upper arm, and one shot of anti-rabies immune globulin, given at the same time as the first injection.

Don't even THINK of giving yourself an injection of animal rabies vaccine—some of them could possibly cause rabies in a human if deliberately injected in quantity! Also, don't wait to consult your physician. Treatment is much more likely to be successful if started early. About one in five persons who has been bitten by a confirmed rabid animal has developed the disease and died (Connaught, 1992). The incubation period for rabies in humans can vary between five days and two years, but is usually 30 to 90 days (Fishbein, 1987). This allows plenty of time for a preventive vaccination against rabies to take effect.

If you are in a high-risk area for rabies (such as parts of the southwestern and southeastern United States), and have reason to be exposed to wild or possibly rabid domestic animals, pre-exposure vaccine IS available for humans (Imovax®, Connaught Labs, Inc., Swiftwater, PA., 1-800-VACCINE). Three small doses are given within a month to give you an immunity which will help protect against rabies. Then, if you are bitten by a rabid animal, you take two doses instead of an entire series. The first series allows your body to produce an effective immunity with the addition of two injections after a bite. Do not rely on the first series to completely protect you against the disease if you are bitten. You will still need the important booster injections. If the animal is confirmed to be rabid, your doctor may also give rabies immune globulin.

Pre-exposure rabies immunization may be a good idea if you live in an isolated area, or if you are a veterinary assistant, a caver or an archaeologist who frequents caves inhabited by bats, or if there is another reason you might be exposed to any species of rabid animal. There is only a very small risk of reaction to the vaccine. Discuss this with your physician if you think you are a candidate for pre-exposure vaccination.

Some wild animals, especially skunks, raccoons, foxes, and bats, may carry and spread the rabies virus for weeks or months before they show symptoms of the disease. Infections have been shown to last more than two and a half years before the animal dies. Some wild animals can even recover from a rabies infection or remain as healthy carriers. They could bite your cat or dog, or you, and you could contract rabies while the wild animal is still healthy. No rabies vaccine is approved for use in captive wild animals. If a modified live rabies vaccine is given to the animal, it may even cause the disease. For this reason, wild animals should not be kept as pets. That cute little skunk may be fatal to you or a member of your family.

Don't handle wild animals, especially if they approach you, appear ill or are injured. If you have to handle one, use a stick, shovel or heavy gloves to avoid direct contact with it. Any bite by a wild animal, especially skunks, foxes, raccoons or bats, must be treated as possible exposure to rabies. Teach children to leave wildlife, stray animals, and neighborhood pets alone. "Love your own, leave others alone." Tell your children to let you know immediately if they are scratched or bitten by any animal. This does not mean you should panic. It just allows you to contact your physician if you believe it is necessary, and to determine whether someone's pet has a current rabies vaccination.

PSEUDORABIES

Pseudorabies, also called mad itch, Aujezsky's disease, or infectious bulbar paralysis, is primarily a disease of pigs. It can spread to cats via raw pork from infected hogs. Signs are similar to those of rabies, including lack of appetite, drooling, deep depression, muscular twitching, itching, convulsions and coma. These signs in cats or dogs on a hog farm suggest that the disease should be suspected in the hogs. Infected cats are not aggressive. They invariably die, usually within one to two (but up to nine) days after infection. Treatment is not successful. Cats should be removed from farms with infected hogs and kept away until all signs of illness in the hogs have been absent for three weeks.

VACCINATION RELATED SARCOMA

This is a rare side effect of vaccination which occasionally occurs in cats. The incidence is estimated to be one or two per 10,000 cats that are vaccinated. This is a very low incidence and would never show up in vaccine trials. Several million cats were vaccinated before the occurrence of the disease was found. The tumors occur in areas of the body where the animal has been previously vaccinated, such as the upper part of the neck, the back, between the shoulder blades, and the hip. The sarcomas may occur between three months and three years after the vaccine is given. Some veterinarians believe that repeated vaccinations in the same location may increase the risk of sarcomas at that site. It is suggested that there is less possibility of sarcoma development when vaccine is given intramuscularly rather than subcutaneously (under the skin). Cats with vaccination-site tumors were more likely to have been vaccinated with feline leukemia vaccine and less likely to have had rabies vaccine than cats with non-vaccination-site tumors (Hendrick, 1994). All in all, the risk of a vaccine reaction is far, far less than the risk of catching the disease against which the cat is vaccinated.

The occurrence of these side effects is NOT a reason to go without vaccinating your cat. It is just a warning to be on the lookout for unusual lumps and bumps, and to have them checked early. Removal results in a cure for most of these tumors. Vaccine manufacturers are aware of the problem, and vaccines which do not cause reactions should be readily available in the near future (McGill, 1993).

LYME DISEASE

Lyme disease (borreliosis) is caused by a spirochete, *Borrelia burgdorferi*, which is carried by ticks. The organism almost never causes disease in cats, with only a few cases reported. In other animals (and humans), the most common sign is lameness in one or more joints, along with fever, lack of appetite, and lethargy. Cats may be somewhat resistant to the disease, or their grooming may remove ticks before the pests can inject the organism, which takes 12 to 24 hours of attachment.

Cats may carry infected ticks into the house, where they can crawl off the cat and onto you. Avoid this danger by keeping pets indoors in Lyme disease areas, and by religiously controlling ticks on pets and in your house and yard. Insecticide-treated cotton (Damminix®) has been spread outdoors in problem areas. White-footed mice, which carry the ticks, use it for nesting material, reducing the number of ticks they carry. Reducing the numbers of mice had very little effect on the number of ticks, but the cotton treatment was quite effective.

BUBONIC PLAGUE

Cats are especially susceptible to bubonic plague, and they can be a source of bubonic plague for humans. This is mostly a problem in rural parts of the western United States, especially New Mexico and northeastern Arizona. Other recent cases have been reported in Lyons, Colorado (near Boulder), Pueblo and Colorado Springs, Colorado, Jayton, Kent County, Abilene and Dallas, Texas areas, Sequoia National Forest, California, Albuquerque, New Mexico, and Ashland, Montana. Mountain and prairie areas of California and Utah also contain pockets of plague. In cities, rats may act as reservoirs for the disease. Outbreaks of plague may be sharply confined to a particular campground or to a single block in the city. Warm, humid conditions favor flea survival and reproduction. They allow plague-infected fleas to survive longer off the host rodent, and give them a better chance to feed on non-rodent animals.

Plague is carried by rodents, and passed on either when the cat eats an infected rodent, when an infected flea goes from a rodent to a cat (which may even happen as the cat strolls through a prairie dog town or rodent village), or when a cat inhales plague bacteria. Plague can also occur in wild carnivores, especially predators such as bobcats. Coyotes tend to develop antibodies but are not usually seen with the disease. Presence of plague is monitored in Arizona through collection and testing of coyote blood.

Two of the first three human cases of plague in 1993 were exposed by cats, and several cases in 1992 were acquired from cats (CDC, 1993). Cats do not seem to spread plague to humans by carrying infected fleas home. Infected cats pass plague to humans via scratches or bites, even if inflicted during play. Humans can also be infected while treating a cat that has an abscess due to the plague organism. A cat with the pneumonic form of plague can pass it by sneezing, and this is one of the commonest ways it is spread to humans. It is also spread to people via body fluids or by biting. The incubation period in cats can be as short as one to two days. Dogs can be infected with plague (much like coyotes) but they rarely get sick or carry it to humans. However, they can carry fleas and flea-infested carcasses into your yard or house.

Hunters or trappers can contract plague from handling carcasses of predators or rodents that are infected. When gutting or skinning this type of wild animal, impervious gloves should be worn. Avoid contact between fluids from the carcass and your mucous membranes such as eyes, nose, and mouth. Carry a can of household insecticide and spray all carnivore carcasses thoroughly before handling them in any way. All meat from wild game should be thoroughly cooked. Using a dilute solution of household bleach, disinfect all cutting boards and utensils that are used in preparing the raw meat,

The cat may have a fever (as high as 107 degrees F (41.5 C)), poor appetite, and lack of activity. There may be swelling around the eyes, head, or neck, and the cat may sneeze pus or cough blood. Lymph nodes, especially around the head, may be swollen. In a plague area, any cat abscess should be treated with suspicion. Full precautions must be taken, including complete isolation. The cat should be treated by persons wearing caps, disposable masks, and gloves. Cats with pneumonic plague may sneeze, wheeze, cough and drool, and die rapidly. In either case, the cats may die within a few days. A few cases may last up to three weeks before death.

If you live in an area where plague is a problem, the safest course is to keep your cat (and your dog) confined to your house and/or yard to minimize possible contact with the disease. Keep the flea population under control by treating the animals and premises as needed. Treat your cat for fleas at least weekly in a problem area. Flea collars are NOT an adequate safeguard. In an area where plague is a problem, do not allow pets (cats, dogs, or others) to sleep with you or your family members, and keep them out of bedrooms and off beds during daytime hours. Any pets that go outdoors should NOT be allowed in or near sleeping quarters. Spaying and neutering of outdoor pets will help reduce their roaming and chance of contact with infected rodents.

Maintain good rodent control by putting out poisoned bait in places where pets and children can't get them. Eliminate wood piles and trash in your yard which can harbor rodents. When you are camping, do not camp in an area with a number of rodent holes, especially if flies are buzzing around any of the holes. This means that the inhabitant has died and its fleas are looking for new homes.

Bubonic plague in humans is usually acquired by flea bite or by infecting a skin wound with the plague bacteria from a plague-infected carcass. The primary symptom is swollen, painful lymph nodes, especially in the armpit or groin. High fever (up to 105 degrees F), vomiting, and diarrhea are also seen. If this is not treated promptly, it can progress to plague septicemia or plague pneumonia. Septicemic plague usually comes with getting fluids from a plague-infected carcass into skin wounds. Symptoms include high fever, muscle aches, and malaise, and sometimes vomiting and diarrhea. If untreated, it can progress to plague pneumonia, or it may be fatal.

Pneumonic plague can occur secondary to the first two types, or it can be acquired directly from respiratory droplets from a plague-infected cat or human. Symptoms are high fever, difficult breathing, and flu-like symptoms, and sometimes vomiting and diarrhea. It can also be fatal. All of this sounds grim. The bacteria which cause plague can be easily treated with antibiotics, and if caught in time, it is almost always curable. If you have any of these symptoms, especially fever with or without swollen glands, seek medical attention immediately. Humans who have been exposed to plague-infected (or suspected) animals may be given preventive dosages of antibiotics. If you live in another area and have been camping in the southwest, be sure to tell your doctor if you become ill after returning home. Your physician is unlikely to think of plague.

In a plague area, any ill animal, especially a cat, should be checked by a veterinarian immediately. Cats can be treated successfully with antibiotics if you are willing to pay for the isolation and care. If an infected cat cannot be completely isolated (for the safety of the humans around it), it should be euthanized. Humans who have been in contact with the cat need not be hospitalized but should be treated with tetracycline for a week—just to be safe (Rosser, 1987).

TUBERCULOSIS

Cats are slightly susceptible to the strain of tuberculosis most common in humans. They are very susceptible to *Mycobacterium bovis*, the species usually seen in cattle, especially dairy cows. Cats usually contract it via the digestive tract, by drinking unpasteurized milk from an infected cow, or eating raw meat from infected animals. Farmers who have infected cattle should monitor the health of their cats. Cats have a high degree of immunity to the tuberculosis organisms which occur in fowl, probably by natural selection as they have hunted birds through the ages. Tuberculosis-infected cats are usually less than five years of age.

A few cats may become infected through exposure to infected humans, especially those with compromised immune systems. Cats belonging to tuberculosis-infected AIDS patients should be carefully observed so they do not catch the disease and pass it on to other humans.

The incubation period for tuberculosis in cats is around three weeks. Signs may include weight loss, poor appetite, low-grade fever, and dehydration. More than 80% of affected cats show intestinal problems, including diarrhea and/or vomiting. Some animals may have difficulty in breathing, but they rarely cough. Occasionally, blindness may occur when the eyes are affected. Abscesses around the eye, head, or neck, or enlargement of the bridge of the nose may also be due to tuberculosis. Tuberculosis of the skin is occasionally seen, with ulcers, nodules, or flat swellings, especially around the head and shoulders. Infected cats usually die within several days to several weeks. A few may have a slowly-developing disease, but even these rarely live more than a few months. Diagnosis is usually not made in time to treat the cat.

Treatment of cats with tuberculosis is generally not advised because of the danger that it may spread to humans before it is controlled or cured. If you are in a foreign country where tuberculosis is a problem, avoid contact with cats. Infected cats can serve as reservoirs to reinfect cattle on farms.

TETANUS

Tetanus occurs when spores of the bacteria enter the cat's body, usually via large injuries to the limbs, such as trap wounds, or via surgical incisions which are for some reason contaminated. It may also occur with a uterine infection after a cat has kittens. Signs occur two days to two weeks after the initial injury. They are usually most severe in the wounded limb, but progress to involve the entire body. At first, only the injured limb is spastically extended. Later, the cat's entire body becomes stretched and stiffened. The cat will be lying on its side with its back arched, head pulled stiffly back, and the legs stretched outward and backward. With antibiotic treatment and proper supportive care, many cats will make a complete recovery over a period of several weeks. Cats are so rarely affected by tetanus that they are not routinely vaccinated for it.

CAT DISEASES IN HUMANS

As we have mentioned previously, tuberculosis can sometimes spread from an infected cat to humans, as can rabies and bubonic plague. Toxoplasmosis can (rarely) go from cats to humans (see Internal Parasites Chapter). Some types of worms can be spread to humans if the person accidentally eats some cat feces. This is a good reason to keep your child's sandbox covered, and have him or her wear shoes or sandals when playing outside. It is not a good reason to get rid of your cat, as the neighbor's cats will come to your yard even if you don't have a cat. Ringworm is a skin disease that is easily spread from cats to humans (see Skin Disease Chapter). Scabies (notoedric mange) can readily spread to humans.

Tularemia is a disease which cats (and humans) can catch by eating wild rabbits or possibly when bitten by ticks, fleas, or flies which have sucked blood from an infected rabbit. Humans can become infected when bitten by a cat that has recently eaten an infected wild rabbit or that is ill with the disease. Symptoms in cats, which resemble those of plague, include lack of appetite, depression, fever, and enlarged lymph nodes. Jaundice (icterus) may be seen shortly before death. Older cats may either recover or die within five to 10 days, while kittens may

quickly die. Both humans and animals are treated with streptomycin, gentamycin, or another antibiotic, with good results. This disease is another good reason to keep your cat indoors. If tularemia is present in rabbits in your area, be careful when handling barn cats, and do not encourage or allow play during which the animal breaks your skin by clawing or biting.

Cat scratch disease is a disease not of cats, but of humans. Also called cat scratch fever, benign lymphoreticulosis, and bartonellosis, cat scratch disease occurs after a person is bitten or scratched by a cat. It can occur when a cat licks a cut or scratch in the skin. The cat is considered a mechanical carrier of the disease. The real source remains unknown, as it may also be caused by pricking oneself with thorns, splinters, or fish bones, or a similar injury. It is caused by a rickettsial organism, *Bartonella* species (sometimes called *Rochalimaea henselae*). If your child contracts the disease, do not automatically assume that it came from your cat. It may have come from a neighbor's cat, from a stray with whom he or she played, or from a twig or weed puncture. Possibly, it also may be carried by fleas or ticks from infected cats.

Cat scratch disease is the most common cause of swollen regional lymph nodes in children (August, 1988). The swollen nodes, in the area near the bite, may look like symptoms of leukemia, tuberculosis, mononucleosis, and other diseases. In some cases, it is necessary to biopsy the lymph node to tell the difference. Other signs include headache, fever, lack of appetite, and muscle aches. The Centers for Disease Control in Atlanta recently developed a test for the disease. In the worst cases, which are extremely rare, neurological problems may result in severe headaches, convulsions, and even coma. Pneumonia may also occur.

Virtually everyone who contracts cat scratch fever survives. Recovery is within two to three months. Antibiotics do not seem to help in treating the disease. Doctors believe that a person who recovers from cat scratch fever will remain immune to it for life. A syndrome caused by the cat scratch organism, called bacillary angiomatosis, occurs in immunocompromised persons (especially those with HIV), who may require four to six weeks of treatment (also see Koehler, 1994). In these persons the disease may even be fatal.

There is some difference of opinion as to whether cats carry the disease for long periods of time or only briefly. Cats that carry the bacteria in their blood can be treated with doxycycline, which eliminates the infection. There seems to be a high incidence of the disease in cats in the San Francisco Bay area. The cat usually appears to be in normal health, and it does not make a difference whether it lives indoors or outside.

There is no test that will reliably determine if a cat is carrying cat scratch fever. Previously, it was recommended that cats in a household with a case of cat scratch disease be declawed. Since antibiotic treatment has been found to be effective, this is far less important.

If the scratches of a particular cat seem to produce the disease, the easiest cure is to declaw the cat (only if it is an indoor cat). However, most cats only harbor the bacteria for a short period of time, often no more than two to three weeks, so this is unnecessary unless more than one case results from the same cat.

Flea control is also important in a household with a case of cat scratch fever. As many as one-third of veterinarians test positive to the disease without ever knowing that they have been infected, while reactions are uncommon in the rest of the population. There is no evidence of person-to-person transmission. Cat scratch fever is rare, and is no reason to condemn a cat associated with it. Handle the cat gently so that it does not scratch or bite. Wash your hands after petting it, and keep it from licking any open cuts or scratches.

Some physicians recommend that people dispose of the cat when a child is found to have strep throat. If your child has strep throat, it is no reason to do that. Children rarely, if ever, get strep throat from cats. However, transmission of strep throat from people to cats has been documented (Pedersen, 1988, p. 136).

Cat bites can easily cause infection (the same is true of dog or human bites, too!). ANY bite wound should be immediately scrubbed with a germicidal soap or disinfectant such as tamed iodine. Continue washing for three to five minutes, rinsing with plenty of water. If the bite is serious, with a lot of bleeding, apply direct pressure with a sterile dressing and go to the nearest emergency room. Otherwise, consult your family physician as soon as possible and follow his or her recommendations. In most cases, antibiotics will be given for a week to 10 days to make sure there is no infection. Rabies treatment may be a consideration (see Rabies, above). If a tooth stabs through or near a tendon and infection occurs, that part of the hand may be permanently crippled. If the infection is serious enough, the hand may even be amputated. For that reason, any bite which involves a hand should be treated as potentially very serious. Get help immediately!

Incidentally, cat bites often carry *Pasturella* bacteria from the animal's mouth. Consult your physician if you are bitten by a cat, even accidentally during play. In humans, this causes a rapid, painful infection, as above. In birds, however, the infection is often fatal. If your pet bird is bitten by a cat, preventive antibiotic treatment is almost mandatory (Pedersen, 1988, p. 156).

Feline leprosy is a disease caused by an organism closely related to, but not the same as, human leprosy. It is very similar to a leprosy which is seen in rodents, and cats probably catch it from them. The disease is more common in cats in coastal cities. The incubation period may be two to 12 months. The first sign is usually a non-healing painless ulcer, plaque, or sore on the skin. If surgically removed, it usually returns, even though this is the treatment of choice. Feline leprosy is not contagious to humans, or from one cat to another.

Hantavirus is a rodent-carried disease that can infect people. Seen sporadically throughout the world, it gained national attention from an outbreak on the Navajo Reservation in the Four Corners area of the southwestern United States. Cats do not seem to have the disease, but might bring it home to you by carrying an infected rodent into your house. It is a good idea to avoid touching live or dead rodents. Reduce rodent populations around your house and outbuildings. Avoid inhaling rodent-contaminated dust by wearing a dust mask or respirator. Disinfect dead rodents or dust contaminated with droppings by dampening them with a 10% solution of household bleach. Hantavirus does not kill rodents infected with it. Do not camp in areas or buildings which show evidence of rodent infestation, and be very careful not to stir up any dust in these areas.

Chapter 5

THE FELINE GOURMET

FEED COMPONENTS

As has been mentioned previously, cats are not just small dogs. While both come from a common ancestor, they went their separate ways about 30 million years ago. Cats became true carnivores, metabolically speaking. They lost the ability to manufacture certain nutrients. Today, they can obtain these only from their diet, from animal tissue. Substances which cats cannot make for themselves include arginine and taurine (two necessary amino acids), essential fatty acids and niacin. Cats also need high levels of dietary protein and all the water-soluble vitamins.

Protein provides the building blocks for muscle growth and cellular maintenance. Cats are unique in that they use much of the protein in their diet for energy, as opposed to other animals that get their energy needs mostly from carbohydrates. Cats have the highest protein requirement of any of the commonly domesticated animals, needing two to three times more than other animals, including humans. The minimum protein requirement for a growing cat is about 18-20% of its total calories. This may be as much as 30-35% protein on a dry weight basis, to allow for imperfect digestion and utilization. Adult cats need 12-15% protein for maintenance, far higher than the needs of a mature, non-working dog.

This is also the reason why you should never feed cat food to your dog, especially a mature or elderly dog. The high protein levels can severely overload the dog's kidneys. There are two reasons why dogs love cat food. In addition to its very high protein level, extra care is taken to make cat food very tasty to coax the finicky feline to eat it. Conversely, dog food is far too low in protein to keep your cat healthy on a long-term basis. A protein deficiency can hinder growth and reproduction, and the cat may be in poor health and have little resistance to infectious diseases. If necessary, put the cat's food out of reach of your dog(s). It can be placed on a shelf, on top of your clothes dryer, on a counter, or in a box or container the dog is unable to reach.

A cat's protein requirements are best met with protein from animal sources such as fish, meat, meat by-products, dairy products, and eggs. These are easily and efficiently digested. The protein quality is high, providing a well-balanced mix of amino acids. Plant proteins have low nutritional value for cats, and they have poor digestibility and lack many amino acids essential for the cat.

Cats have a special requirement for the amino acid taurine. They make small amounts of it in their bodies, but not enough to meet their needs. Without adequate quantities, the cat may go blind because of degeneration of the retinas. They may fail to reproduce, or produce deformed or stillborn kittens. Any kittens that are born alive will have muscular problems, shown by staggering and spastic paralysis of their hind legs. Severe heart damage may also be seen, where the heart becomes more like a flabby balloon than a muscular pump. Young cats will have poorly developed brains and nervous systems. Small blood clots may occur in the blood vessels, and the immune system may not function properly.

In the wild, cats get taurine from the animals they eat. It is found in most animal tissues, including meat, seafood, and milk. It is absent in almost all plant foodstuffs. Dog food is almost totally lacking in taurine, which is another good reason not to feed it to your cat. A diet with inadequate taurine levels for as little as 10 to 14 days may cause problems. Normal cats need about 50 milligrams of taurine per day. Adequate taurine is now added to all good-quality cat foods, and cats that are fed dry food retain the taurine which they absorb better than those fed canned food.

Taurine supplements can be prescribed by your veterinarian in cases of deficiency. Cats with heart problems should have an oral taurine supplement, in addition to being treated for heart failure. If signs of acute heart failure have not yet developed, this supplementation should be adequate to reverse the changes in the heart muscle. When the cat's heart is stabilized, taurine supplementation should be reduced, as continued dosages at this level cause the cardiac muscle to overgrow (too much of a good thing!). Oral taurine has been successful in controlling epileptic seizures in some cats.

Clam juice has been suggested as a source of taurine. It has some of this amino acid, but to meet its requirements, the cat would have to drink a quart of clam juice each day! Or, it would require 10 tablespoons of minced clams, which would leave very little room for the rest of a balanced diet. On the other hand, tuna is an excellent source of taurine. However, a high-tuna diet can cause other problems. Taurine tablets are a much better choice.

Modern cat foods have taurine added in amounts large enough to compensate for the quantity lost when the food is processed. The food label might say "taurine added." When you read the label, taurine should appear somewhere in the middle of the ingredient list, not toward the end. If it is at the bottom of the list, there may not be enough to meet the cat's needs. Occasionally, cats will have taurine deficiency even when they are fed adequate amounts. The reason for this is unknown.

Cats of all ages also have a unique requirement for the amino acid arginine. With their high protein diets, cats have to get rid of large quantities of ammonia from the protein breakdown. They convert ammonia to urea in the liver and then excrete urea in their urine. This conversion requires the amino acid arginine, which they have to obtain from their diet. If the cat is deficient in arginine, excess ammonia will accumulate in the body after meals. Signs include muscle tremors, depression, incoordination, and even death within a few hours. Most foods contain adequate arginine, so deficiencies are rare. If milk products are fed as the sole protein source, arginine will be low and must be supplemented (Dhein, 1986).

Fats readily provide the cat's main source of energy (calories), and they do well on high-fat diets. Easily digested and absorbed, fats are normal components of cat foods. Fat also helps make a tasty food that is attractive to cats. They like beef and sheep tallow or vegetable fats in preference to butter, lard, or chicken fat (Kane, 1977). Many of them find oils to be palatable. An abrupt change to a high-fat diet, or adding too much fat to the diet may overwhelm the digestive system, causing diarrhea. Gradually increase the amount of fat over a one to two week period. This gives the cat's system time to increase the

amount of enzymes secreted to digest the fats. If you are going to a food with a higher fat content, give less food overall. Otherwise, the cat will gradually become overweight on the increased calories. If the high-fat diet is not well balanced, it may lead to deficiencies, especially in thiamine, iodine, and protein. If the diet is high in polyunsaturated fat, the cat will need higher levels of vitamin E. Given a choice, cats prefer a diet containing 25-40% fat.

Cats also need adequate levels of essential fatty acids as part of the fat portion of their diet. Linoleic, linolenic, and arachidonic acids are essential fatty acids necessary for healthy skin and normal reproduction. These acids are not produced by the cat's body and must be supplied by its diet. Arachidonic acid comes from animal fat and is completely lacking in a cereal or vegetable-based diet. Cats must eat a certain amount of fish, meat, or poultry products to give them the required amounts of essential fatty acids. Surgery may greatly increase the need for linoleic acid (Wolfran, 1978). Fatty acids are usually added to cat food via fish oils, fish meal, and flax seed. Cat foods containing avocado meal and supplements made from grape seed oil claim to provide essential fatty acids.

Carbohydrates come from sugars and starches. They can help provide energy for the cat's body. Cats require fewer calories per pound of body weight than do dogs of the same weight. Adequate energy intake is rarely a problem for cats, while obesity is occasionally seen. Carbohydrates are a very minor part of the cat's diet in the wild, and there is no evidence that they need them. Of all dietary components, carbohydrates seem to be the least important. Conversely, they don't seem to cause harm, and are often used as ingredients in cat foods. The cat's digestive tract is short, and lacks a cecum full of bacteria. Food passes through its system relatively rapidly. All this suggests that the cat is adapted to a high-energy, low-bulk diet (one that is high in fat and protein and low in carbohydrates and fiber).

Normal, healthy cats also have very little need for fiber, and it is not considered a necessary nutrient. It is largely undigestible, being primarily a source of bulk. As such, it can influence the health of the digestive tract by helping other foodstuffs to move efficiently through the gut. Fiber also can provide minerals.

Diets which contain excessive amounts of fiber can give bulky, abundant stools. High-fiber diets are sometimes recommended to help overweight cats lose weight, with the fiber being used to control the level of calories. Some experts feel these diets have not been evaluated sufficiently for exclusive use over long periods of time; however, they may be useful for weight loss over more limited periods of several months. Normal cat foods probably should not have fiber as more than 10% of the dry weight analysis (Brown, 1989).

Cats completely lack the enzyme system to convert beta-carotene in food or plant material into vitamin A. In the wild, they get vitamin A from eating prey that have already made vitamin A from plant material. The fact that cats have NO ability to make this vitamin is another strong clue that plants were never meant to be part of their diet. The vitamin itself must be provided in their diet—cats don't make good vegetarians. When was the last time you saw a cat stalking some berries? Lack of vitamin A may cause infertility, abortion, or kittens born with birth defects such as cleft palates.

An excess of vitamin A is also hazardous to the cat's health. Growths may occur on the bones, especially in the neck vertebrae. These changes may result in abnormal posture and pain. The cat also may show weight loss. Excess storage of vitamin A (and even a toxicity) may occur in cats given large amounts of liver or cod-liver oil. Vitamin A toxicity shows up as pain and stiffness, especially in the forelegs and neck. The cat may look ragged because it is reluctant to groom itself. Eventually, the cat will lose its appetite, lose weight, and have large bony growths at the joints. These skeletal changes are not reversible even when the excess of vitamin A is corrected.

Cats also cannot produce niacin, a B-vitamin, and they need rather large quantities of other B-complex vitamins in the diet. Cats seem to have a very low requirement for Vitamin D, and deficiency is almost never seen.

Cats need more than twice as much thiamine as do dogs. Thiamine deficiency results in downward flexion of the cat's neck, abnormal reflexes, and muscular weakness. This may be a problem in a cat that does not eat for two to three days. After two weeks or more of thiamine deficiency, the cat may salivate, fail to eat, and show weight loss, staggering, and vomiting. Feeding large amounts of raw fish such as herring, carp, catfish, red tuna, bullhead, smelt, and others (or inadequately cooked fish or soybeans) to cats can cause deficiencies of both thiamine and vitamin E. This may even cause death. If the fish or soybeans are cooked, this is not a problem. Thiamine is also destroyed by heat and storage. Thus, cooked homemade diets may be deficient in thiamine. Reputable cat food companies add thiamine to make up for the amount lost in processing the food.

Cats that are given large amounts of fish without vitamin supplementation may end up with a vitamin E deficiency. This is known as yellow fat disease (steatitis). The cat may have a poor appetite, depression, vomiting, and abdominal pain and may have firm, painful lumps under the skin. It may go downhill until it either dies or is euthanized for humane reasons. Reputable cat food companies add extra vitamin E to their all-fish foods to prevent this deficiency. Vitamin E deficiency is occasionally seen in cats on almost any diet for reasons that are not yet understood. Vitamin E, as well as vitamin C, are antioxidants which are thought to help retard aging. Both vitamins are needed together for this effect. Cats can synthesize vitamin C, so it need not be added to their diets.

Cats that have diarrhea or similar digestive upsets may lack adequate vitamins. Your veterinarian may recommend an injection of fat-soluble vitamins and an oral solution of water-soluble vitamins. Vitamin supplementation may also be needed if you are giving the cat old or stale dry cat food, as well as if you are feeding the very cheapest of cat foods. It's less expensive to simply feed a good quality cat food.

Some vitamins are lost when pet food is processed. However, extra amounts are added before processing to make up for this loss, and the food is monitored to be sure adequate amounts remain after it is cooked, as well as to make up for losses which occur between the factory and your cat's stomach. Because vitamins are destroyed by oxidation, especially from heat and light, store food in a closed container in a cool, dark place.

Minerals needed by cats are generally supplied by a normal, good-quality cat food. The residue of minerals left after food is burned is called "ash," which is composed of a number of minerals such as calcium, magnesium, potassium, sodium, phosphorus, and chloride. Early studies of bladder stones in cats recommended low-magnesium ("low-ash") diets, and this has been a concern to some cat owners. Later studies, however, showed that the only time magnesium was a problem was if the urine was not kept acidic. It's a lot easier to produce a food that will keep the urine acidic than it is to remove magnesium from natural food ingredients. Cat food manufacturers have changed their formulas, and magnesium levels should no longer be a problem. The jury is still out on the effects of continuous urinary acidification on bone development, growth, and kidney function. Veterinarians don't yet know if one problem is being cured and another being created.

Calcium helps build strong bones. However, too much calcium can actually retard the cat's growth and cause skeletal abnormalities. It can cause scaly skin and may cause deficiencies in zinc, copper, iron, and phosphorus, all of which can cause other health problems. Phosphorus levels relate to those of calcium, and an excess of phosphorus can cause bone and kidney problems. These minerals and the relationship between them are very important to the cat's health. They are carefully balanced in quality cat foods. Random supplementation of the cat's diet with calcium and phosphorus is NOT a good idea.

Potassium levels in cat food seem to be adequate for normal cats. These levels are also important in regard to acidified diets, because the food (or medication) doesn't acidify the urine—it acidifies the whole cat. In some cats, this eventually results in a loss of calcium from the bones. The ideal balance will produce just enough acidification to prevent the formation of stones in the urinary tract.

Potassium deficiency, called hypokalemia, is a problem in some cats, for unknown metabolic reasons. It is common in cats with chronic kidney disease, and in many cases it is hard to tell whether the potassium deficiency or the kidney disease came first. It also occurs in cats with liver disease, hyperthyroidism, diabetes, vomiting, severe diarrhea, and some central nervous system disorders. Cats that are given medication to acidify their urine or cats that are on a special diet may be short of potassium. Those on intravenous fluids may have low potassium levels, and as many as one-third of cats that are already ill will show potassium deficiency. Any geriatric cat that is ill should be checked for potassium level.

Early signs of low potassium may be subtle. They may be blamed on "old age" or other diseases. Potassium deficiencies can cause muscular weakness, apparent muscle pain when handled, reluctance to walk, crouched posture, and an abnormal stilted gait. An inability to hold the head up is one of the most common signs, as the cat allows it to sag toward its chest.

Inadequate potassium levels may also cause kidney dysfunction, resulting in a vicious cycle. Cats with kidney dysfunction pass excess potassium in their urine, making the problem even worse. Some cats with low potassium will show poor appetite, diarrhea, vomiting, weight loss, ragged hair coat, changed behavior, and general weakness. They may also may be anemic and/or constipated.

Cats with a potassium shortage can be treated with potassium supplements. Severely ill cats are treated intravenously by your veterinarian. This will be followed by an oral potassium supplement. Potassium gluconate is more palatable to many cats than potassium chloride, and tends not to acidify the urine. Some cats that have been treated with potassium gluconate powder will stop eating, but they usually resume when powder treatment is stopped. For these cats, tablets and gels (such as Tumil-K®, Daniels Pharmaceuticals) are available. If one product doesn't work, try another. Diluting oral potassium products half-and-half with water can reduce the stomach irritation, nausea, and vomiting that may occur. Taurine levels may be lowered, and both substances may need to be supplemented for a sick cat. Improvement is usually seen within a couple of weeks. Some cats, especially those with chronic kidney disease, may need treatment for the rest of their lives.

In an emergency, if there is no way you can take the cat with signs of potassium deficiency (especially the hanging head and muscle weakness) to a clinic, you could give it a tiny pinch of "Lite Salt®" or, better yet, "Un-Salt." If the cat is eating, mix it with its food. If not, mix it to a thin slurry with water and drop it in the mouth with a syringe or eyedropper. If this results in improvement, continue it once or twice a day for five to seven days. The chloride component of these products may aggravate the cat's problems if used for long periods of time. An excess of potassium can cause a life-threatening rapid heartbeat, with weakness and collapse, so don't overdo the potassium. Consult a veterinarian at your earliest opportunity to find out why the cat developed the problem.

DO CATS EAT MEAT?

Do cats really eat meat? In the wild, cats do not eat "meat" in the sense that we think of a well-marbled piece of steak. When a cat eats a mouse, it eats the whole animal. The intestines and their contents, which are not "raw" but are partially digested, nutrient-filled vegetable matter, provide fiber and vitamins. Bones are a good source of calcium and other minerals. Hair gives some fiber or roughage in the diet. Internal organs are rich in vitamins. The muscle mass that we think of as "meat" is a minor part of the meal.

A small rodent, such as a mouse, contains about 65-75% water, 14-18% protein, 6-18% fat (35-40% on a dry matter basis), and 1-5% minerals (Kane, 1987). This equates to about 45% of the diet being protein. The enzymes in the cat's liver which promote protein breakdown are permanently set to work at a high level. With a lowered protein intake, these enzymes do not slow down.

They continue converting protein to energy at the same rate as when there is a high protein intake, which can lead to deficiencies of amino acids and nitrogen. This inability of liver enzymes to "gear down" is the reason for the cat's higher protein requirement. No, cats do not eat meat—they eat ANIMALS!

Cat food manufacturers spend a great deal of time and money trying to reinvent the mouse. This isn't totally necessary. Cats simply require adequate amounts (but not too much) of about 40 nutrients. It doesn't matter whether they come in a can or a box, in a pouch, or on four legs racing across your carpet.

TYPES OF CAT FOODS

A suitable cat food is one which provides all the cat's nutrient needs for good health and a long life. Cats have been found to respond first to the odor of their food (Research by The Iams Company)—from the cat's viewpoint, not ours! It is very important to clean the nostrils of a cat with upper respiratory disease to help it to be able to smell and thus increase its appetite.

"Mouthfeel" is important. This is how the food feels in the cat's mouth as it eats, whether sticky, crunchy, or covered with gravy. Some cats prefer the crunchiness of a dry food. Many cats do not like foods with a doughy consistency, and may totally refuse a powdery, dry, or finely textured food.

The actual taste of the food is clearly in third place as a dietary consideration. Many cats prefer frequent changes of flavor and appreciate the large variety of flavors made by cat food companies. Hungry cats, unlike humans and dogs, may continue to refuse a nutritious but unpalatable diet. This refusal may go on long enough for the cat to approach starvation. Cats generally prefer fish over chicken and liver (Houpt, 1981).

The degree of palatability can be used to control food consumption. At one time, I had nine outdoor cats on my farm. When I fed one particular brand of dry food, free-choice, the cats just sat and ate and got fat. They didn't hunt mice and scarcely left the food dish. It was just too tasty. I changed to another brand. They quickly became thin, stood around and meowed continuously. That diet was too unpalatable and they wouldn't eat it. The third brand was "just right." The cats ate enough to maintain good body condition, but not so much that they were obese or lazy.

Many cats seem to prefer food warm or near body temperature, much like that of freshly killed prey. Warmth also helps make the odor more obvious, again increasing palatability. You can either warm the food 15 to 20 seconds in the microwave is usually about right) or let it set out for a short period of time to approach room temperature.

A good quality cat food should allow for efficient use of its nutrients, giving small, firm stools. If your cat consistently has loose stools, or ones that are unpleasantly smelly, try another brand of food, or one of the prescription diets. This makes the cat more pleasant to live with, and the litter box easier to clean. It should be mentioned that feeding one's pet can have more than nutritional significance. Feeding your cat can be a social experience for both pet and master.

PREPARED CAT FOODS

Commercial, prepared cat foods are ready to feed to your cat. Manufacturers of good quality cat foods employ highly trained staff nutritionists. They utilize the latest nutritional research to provide your cat with a balanced and healthy diet. They also maintain kennels where cats are raised through several generations to make sure they grow, reproduce, and age gracefully on the same diet sold to you for your cat.

A cat food should show that it meets all National Research Council (NRC) standards. Or, it can meet AAFCO (American Association of Feed Control Officials) food testing guidelines. Either one (or both) guarantees that the food is adequate for the cat's nutritional needs. Whatever food you use, it should be labeled "nutritionally complete and balanced," or similar wording.

Moisture content in cat food varies considerably. Dry foods generally have 10% or less moisture to prevent mold growth. Dry foods may take in moisture in damp climates and can mold if not stored in tightly closed containers. Canned cat foods will range between 70 and 78% moisture. Some of the water comes from the meats and other materials used to make the food and some is added to rehydrate dried ingredients. Moisture content has no bearing on the nutritional quality of cat food.

Cat foods come in a number of forms: dry meal, soft-moist, canned, and frozen. In the final analysis, the cat food you choose depends on convenience, cost, and what you, your veterinarian, and your cat agree on. Your choices are:

1) Dry cat foods. These are the least expensive foods available; you don't pay for the packaging and transportation of water. Dry foods are convenient to feed. They help clean the cat's teeth as it crunches the pieces, reducing tartar buildup and helping prevent dental disease when compared to soft-moist or canned cat foods. You can leave dry food in a bowl for self-feeding without spoilage.

Low-quality dry foods may not have adequate palatability and digestibility. The cat may not eat enough to maintain good body condition. A cat that is growing rapidly or nursing a litter of kittens may simply not be able to eat enough dry food to maintain good condition, even if the food is of good quality. Dry foods also may spoil more rapidly in humid climates than canned or pouch-sealed semi-moist foods.

Dry cat foods have sometimes been blamed for causing (or at least predisposing cats to) Feline Urologic Syndrome (FUS). This is because dry commercial cat foods are usually lower in digestibility and calories than are canned foods. The cat must eat a larger quantity to meet its energy requirements, increasing the amount of magnesium consumed. In good-quality dry foods, however, the amount of magnesium is regulated so there is an adequate amount, but not an excess. Meanwhile, the food is carefully balanced to keep the cat's urine acidic, helping to prevent FUS.

Dry foods may become rancid when stored for long periods of time. Do not feed the product if it has an off odor or shows mold growth. Food which is stored for more than six months may lose vitamins. If you have to feed "stale" food, give a vitamin supplement along with it. Excessively old food may have lost so much flavor that your cat may not eat it.

Store dry food in a cool, dry place. Almost all dry pet food products, even those from the best manufacturers, can contain eggs of flour beetles. They cause "weevils" in flour and cereals in your kitchen. Pet foods are one of the major ways these pests are brought into houses. Keeping pet food in a can or jar with a tight lid helps avoid this problem. If you have extra freezer space, you can freeze surplus dry pet food. Freezing for one to two months will kill pests. Wash the container occasionally with soap and water between batches of cat food, and rinse it with hot or boiling water.

2) Soft-moist cat foods. These foods are a cross between canned food and dry food. They usually come in convenient pouches and don't need to be refrigerated. Soft-moist foods can be left out for the cat to eat as it wishes.

Soft-moist cat foods are chemically preserved. Part of this is done by reducing the amount of water by adding sugars and propylene glycol. It may also be done by lowering the pH by adding phosphoric and/or sorbic acids. However, the propylene glycol can cause an anemia in some cats. For this reason, soft-moist foods may not be the best choice for continuous feeding, and they should not be fed to cats that are ill. They may best be used as occasional treats. The disadvantage of these foods is that they do not help clean the teeth and they are expensive. Also, they are tasty enough that some cats can easily become obese.

If urine from a cat on a soft-moist food diet is tested with Clinitest® reagent for diabetes mellitus, the cat will appear diabetic even though it isn't. This is because sugars and sucrose in these foods are not completely metabolized in the cat's body and pass through in the urine.

3) Canned foods. They are usually very tasty and digestible. Unlike soft-moist foods, canned foods do not contain any preservatives. They will spoil if left out in the bowl, especially in hot or humid climates. Any food saved for the next feeding must be refrigerated. Cats that eat canned food may not drink much water, as they are getting the necessary amount from their food.

Canned foods come in two major types. Ration-type diets, often labeled "nutritionally complete," or "complete, balanced diet," are made of mixtures of meats and vegetable products. Cooked together in their sterile cans, these can make good long-term diets. Gourmet-type foods are made mainly of muscle meat or fish. These products, by themselves, do NOT make a balanced diet. They must be carefully balanced by adding vitamins and minerals.

Even with additives, gourmet foods are probably a less healthy diet for long-term use than are products made from a variety of foodstuffs. If the label says, for example,

100% beef, that means beef is the entire content of the food. Nothing can be added but trace amounts of preservatives and flavorings. Watch out, because some of these foods are NOT nutritionally complete. At best, it is a poor diet for your cat. At worst, it may cause bone or heart damage, or blindness.

Remember, too, that pet food manufacturers are trying to reach your "hot button" in their advertising. One will push quality nutrition, while another touts a food that looks like "people food." One may push the inexpensive price while a different one tries to appeal to those wanting something "natural." They are also balancing quality nutrition with affordable price. Is the food more appealing to you or to your pet?

PRESCRIPTION FOOD OR NOT?

Prepared cat foods come in three broad categories: the common brands (call them "over-the-counter" brands), prescription foods, and specialty foods. The basic difference between them is that the over-the-counter ones are for cats with no needs other than a maintenance diet, while the others are designed with particular purposes in mind.

1) Over-the-counter cat foods. These are the ones you see at the grocery store, pet shop or feed store. They are produced by companies from one end of the country to the other, ranging from small, local milling companies to major national corporations. You see cats galloping toward them on TV and are faced with ads in many magazines. Foods produced by small mills may be very good, or may be totally lacking in major nutrients. If lacking one or more nutrients, they occasionally may cause nutritional deficiencies in cats. These foods are suitable for adult cats (over nine to 12 months of age) that are in normal health and are not pregnant or nursing.

Generic cat foods (those not associated with a brand name) are available in many grocery stores and at some pet food suppliers. They are usually the lowest-priced foods available, making them attractive to many pet owners. This may be a false savings. People are accustomed to buying generic human foods, but they do not make up one's total diet. If they are lacking a few nutrients, it is no disaster. On the other hand, the generic food makes up most or all of the cat's diet—it is its only source of nutrients. Lack of one or more essential nutrients may lead to an unhealthy cat. Lack of taurine may leave your cat blind and with heart disease.

Major brand foods, even though they may not list taurine as an added ingredient on the label, can be trusted to have adequate quantities of it. Fish-based foods are extremely high in taurine, while meat-based foods require taurine supplementation. It rarely pays to buy the cheapest food available. Foods produced by national corporations are backed by skilled nutritionists and a wealth of research, as well as by long-term feeding trials, to make sure the food is adequate for reproduction and raising successive generations. This is also true of the:

2) Prescription or therapeutic diets. These are available through veterinarians or specialty sources. They are formulated to meet special needs, such as a low-sodium diet for the cat with heart disease, or food lower in certain minerals to aid the animal with bladder stones. Foods also are available for cats with allergies to certain ingredients common in cat foods.

Prescription cat foods are VERY effective when used for the condition for which they were prescribed. They should be fed without any supplementation except as prescribed by your veterinarian, so don't give table scraps or treats unless the clinician approves them. As with any other cat food, make sure the prescription diet you are feeding is "nutritionally complete." This type of food is generally not needed by a normal, healthy cat. They are expensive when compared with other foods. However, for a cat with a heart or bladder condition, or some other problem which can be helped by a special diet, the increase in health and longevity can be well worth the added expense.

Prescription (therapeutic) diets sometimes appear to be "unpalatable." One reason for this may be that they are often introduced when the cat is ill and has a poor appetite. The cat may associate the diet with being ill, thus avoiding it and developing a "learned aversion" to the food. Because of this learning, the cat may avoid the food when it gets well, and it may be nearly impossible to get the cat to eat it. The cat may need to be fed via a feeding tube, or given alternate foods until it is well. If medication is likely to cause gastrointestinal upset, the cat should be changed to a different food to keep it from developing a learned aversion to its usual diet.

3) Specialty diets. These foods are similar to prescription diets in that they are formulated to deal with specific needs. Unlike the prescription diets, specialty diets are not usually used to treat diseases. You will find specialty diets for kittens, for cats subjected to stress, and for elderly cats, among others.

For the average, healthy, non-stressed, sedate mature cat living in comfortable surroundings, a food intended for "maintenance" is quite adequate. My preference is to buy a dry cat food made by a major national manufacturer, in the mid-price range. This is an excellent compromise, giving quality nutrition at reasonable cost.

An extremely cheap food may have been made using poor ingredients or the cost may have been held down by skimping on needed amounts of vitamin or mineral additives. Quality control may not be up to par, and some batches may lack essential nutrients. Also, cheap foods may occasionally contain EXCESS quantities of some ingredients. Since it is much more expensive to remove excess vitamin A, for example, than to leave it in, the resulting food may have more than the "minimum guaranteed analysis" stated on the label. It may even have a dangerous excess. Too much of certain nutrients may lead to health problems far more expensive to treat than the savings in food price. However, if you buy the most expensive food, you may be paying for advertising and fancy packaging, above and beyond the price of adequate nutrition.

PRESCRIPTION FOODS

Precision-formulated cat foods are available for specific ailments. Some of these are:

1) Urinary tract diets. These foods contain precise amounts of high-quality protein. Phosphorus, sodium, and other minerals are carefully regulated, as the diet is formulated to keep the cat's urine acidic. These foods are used for cats that have urinary tract stones or plugs, and may be used to dissolve certain types of stones. They also may be used for some animals with liver disease.

2) Intestinal diets. A bland, highly digestible, low-residue diet is available for cats that have digestive tract problems. It can be used for a cat that has eaten something which has irritated its gut or that is recovering from a disease involving the digestive tract. This food is also useful for cats with colitis. Intestinal diets have low levels of fiber and fat, and are made from ingredients that are nonirritating. They are usually fed in small amounts three to six times a day for seven to 10 days until the cat's digestive tract has healed. For a cat with a chronically sensitive digestive tract, the food may be given for a longer period of time.

3) Heart diets. A diet for heart patients has a number of differences from the ordinary maintenance diet. The major difference is a very low sodium content. This helps decrease the amount of fluid retained in the body, thus reducing the workload on the heart. Heart diets have an increased amount of potassium to compensate for potassium loss caused by diuretic drugs commonly used to treat heart disease. They also have a slightly lower quantity of high-quality protein, and may have a higher quantity of B vitamins. Many cats with heart problems also have kidney and/or liver disease, and dietary management must take these into consideration.

It is often easier to switch the cat to a new diet early in the disease while it is still eating, rather than waiting until the cat is in an advanced stage when it may have a poor appetite. During the transition stage, you may add a small amount of egg, yogurt, or salt-free broth to help change the cat to the new food. It is very important to keep the cardiac cat from becoming obese. Extra weight will put an extra load on its heart, and will accelerate progression of chronic heart failure. An obese cat with heart disease should be given frequent small meals rather than large meals that put a high metabolic demand on its body.

It is imperative that the cat with heart disease have an adequate level of the amino acid taurine in its diet. Dry commercial cat foods should have at least 500-1000 mg/lb (1000-2000 mg/kg) of taurine. Canned cat foods should contain 1000-1250 mg/lb (2000-2500 mg/kg) on a dry matter basis. In some cases, the diet may be supplemented with oral taurine, at 500 mg twice a day.

4) Allergy diets. Foods are available for cats with food allergies. Allergies to foods which the cat has eaten occasionally may show up as diarrhea, or gas and discomfort. More commonly, however, they show up as skin reactions similar to those seen with inhaled substances (see Atopy). Allergy diets are made from ingredients which are not usually eaten by cats; hence, it is unlikely the cat will be allergic to them. Often based on mutton and rice, allergy diets can be fed on a long-term basis. Or, they can be used for a few weeks to stabilize the cat's system as a diagnostic means to identify the food or foods to which the cat is allergic. To use an allergy diet as a diagnostic tool, feed it ALONE—no treats or people food at all! Give the cat distilled water to drink during this test. Feed the diet for three to six weeks until signs of allergy are gone. Different foods can then be added back into the cat's diet, for five days each, until the offending one is found. One company offers allergy diets for cats, both dry and canned, based on lamb, duck, or rabbit and potato (Innovative Veterinary Diets, division of Nature's Recipe Pet Foods (1-800-359-4483)).

5) Reducing diets. A large number of canned and dry foods are available to help the overweight cat lose weight.

6) Special enteral supplements. These include liquid or powdered milk replacer products which can be used for small kittens, whether orphaned or to help supplement them prior to or after weaning. Other products, such as Formula V™ Clinical Care Feline Liquid Diet (Pet-Ag, Inc., Elgin, IL 60120) are high-energy, highly digestible, ready-to-use liquid foods. They can be used for cats that are ill, injured, recovering from surgery, or otherwise malnourished. These products can be lifesavers for an ill cat. Some cats will lap the product, but it can be fed through a syringe or feeding tube to a cat that is unwilling or unable to eat. Be sure to keep leftover food in the refrigerator, but feed it at room temperature or slightly warmed. It may be necessary to add extra water if the cat is not producing adequate urine.

All in all, there are a number of rather amazing foods designed to meet the cat's special needs. They are available through your veterinarian, and can add years to your cat's life, especially if it has kidney or heart disease. Your veterinarian can recommend a diet specific for your cat's ailment. What is right for a heart problem may not be right for another illness, and may even make the condition worse. Thus, your cat should have a complete examination before putting it on one of these diets. Don't give the cat prescription foods because you think it might have a problem.

Most cats will readily eat prescription cat foods. However, if the food is not accepted after one to two days, try a few tricks: 1) Mix warm water with the dry food and let it sit five to 10 minutes before feeding. 2) Warm it before feeding. 3) Mix it with the cat's regular food, gradually changing the proportions over a seven to 10 day period until the cat is eating only the new food. Try small quantities—a tablespoon or so five to six times a day to tease the cat into eating.

SPECIALTY FOODS

Most cat foods are made for the average, mature to middle-aged cat. Considered maintenance diets, they are made for adult cats that live in a comfortable, relatively stress-free environment with little or no exercise. They offer complete nutrition for the least cost. But, if your cat needs them, specialty foods are available.

1) Kitten chows. These were among the first "convenience" cat foods to appear on the market, and are available in all the major types: canned, dry, and soft-moist. This group also includes products such as Science Diet® Feline Growth®, which can be used to give a higher nutrient level to pregnant or nursing cats, in addition to feeding kittens.

Growing kittens require about twice the energy and nutrients of adult cats of the same weight. Their needs can be met by feeding approximately twice the amount of regular cat food. However, it may be kinder to the kitten's digestive system to give a food which is higher in fat and protein. Kitten foods usually have higher quality ingredients than general purpose foods, and, as a result, are easier to digest. They are convenient, but you can achieve the same effect by mixing a good general purpose dry food with a canned meat food.

Kitten foods should NOT be supplemented with random amounts of calcium, phosphorus, bone meal, or other mineral substances. Don't add yogurt, baby cereal, meats, or other foodstuffs. A quality kitten chow made by a major manufacturer does not need any additives. If supplements are needed, your veterinarian will prescribe specific kinds and amounts. When the kitten is large and growing rapidly, its increased intake of food will provide a sufficient quantity of a balanced diet with kitten food alone. Unneeded supplements may cause abnormalities in bone and joint growth. If these continue long enough, it may be impossible to reverse the damage and the cat may never be normal (see also Kitten Feeding, below).

2) Geriatric diets. Old cats accumulate a number of major and minor ailments. In general, they are less active than younger cats and need fewer calories. Their efficiency of protein utilization declines. Because the cat cannot taste or smell as well as it did when it was younger, it is important that the food be palatable.

NATURAL CAT FOODS

Some cat foods are advertised as "all natural." It is open to interpretation as to what is "natural" and what is not. One man's filler is another man's fiber. While these foods may meet the required "analysis," I question whether some of them have adequate quality control to avoid excesses of some ingredients, such as vitamins, which may cause health problems when fed for long periods. Many of the companies producing these foods have not done ANY feeding tests, much less carried the tests through the number of generations necessary to demonstrate the long-term adequacy of the food. There is no evidence that raw food is healthier for animals (or humans) than is a cooked diet. Cooking kills many parasites and bacteria that could otherwise harm or kill the animal. The "natural" labeling may be more a marketing gimmick to separate you from your dollars than sound nutrition for your pet. Besides, your cat has no idea whether it is "natural" or not. Before you buy one of these foods, do enough research to determine if it is really the best for your cat.

Most commercial foods contain several additives. Some of them, such as spices, garlic, and onion, help add the flavor which encourages your cat to eat the food. Others, in very small quantities, help preserve the food against spoilage. Some vitamins, such as A and E, also act as preservatives. Your animal is more likely to become ill from food poisoning because of food spoilage from a homemade food or one without preservatives than to suffer because of commercial food additives. Today, thanks to scientific nutrition, pets live longer, healthier lives than ever before. Many "natural" ingredients such as excessive amounts of salt, protein, phosphorus, and calcium, can be far more harmful than any preservatives or additives used in cat food.

If you are really trying to duplicate the cat's natural diet, feed it mice or similar small rodents, with an occasional whole canary thrown in for variety. These shouldn't be cage-raised mice, as they will have too high a proportion of fat compared to wild mice. However, if you only feed wild mice, you'll need quite a few every day. Then, too, your cat will be exposed to diseases carried by those rodents, such as tapeworms, tularemia, and plague. Our indoor cats live far longer, healthier lives, for the most part, than most outdoor hunters, and are exposed to fewer hazards. Do your cat and yourself a favor and feed it a medium-priced "nutritionally complete" commercial cat food.

MAKING YOUR OWN?

To make your own cat food or not to . . . that is the question. When you use a commercial cat food, you take advantage of the company's nutritional expertise. Also, the balance of protein and calories in good quality cat food is regulated to the cat's needs. Many people who cook for their cats are guilty of feeding too much of the same kinds of foods, which may lead to excesses of some nutrients and deficiencies of others. Even if you feed a variety of home-cooked foods, it's hard to find a menu to meet all your cat's needs. While I certainly don't recommend it, homemade food can be used if you wish to take the time to make it. Recipes for homemade cat foods (for a regular cat food, as well as many specialized diets) are available from Hill's Pet Products, Inc., P.O. Box 148, Topeka, Kansas 66601. Hill's is one of the nation's largest manufacturers of prescription and specialized diets for dogs and cats, and has been in the forefront of research on pets' specialized dietary needs for a number of years.

TABLE SCRAPS

Feeding table scraps should be done only if you do not have access to, or cannot afford, commercial cat food. Table scraps tend to be low in protein, and are usually high in fat and calories, contributing to obesity.

Many cats, especially some of the purebreds such as Persians and Siamese, are prone to digestive upsets when there is any dietary change. Unless the cat has been raised eating scraps and has a cast iron stomach, "people" food can cause severe digestive problems. Curing them may cost far more than you saved by feeding scraps.

Feeding your cat large quantities of meat or fish products may please its palate, but nutritionally it's a disaster. It may encourage the cat to beg for meat. Worse, the cat may refuse to eat its well-balanced cat food and become ill. Excessive meat can cause a depletion of minerals from the bone, with resulting brittle bones and fractures. Giving the little beggar canned tuna or similar meat products is just as unbalanced. You may think you are being kind by feeding meat because that's what the cat likes. In reality, you're not doing it any favors.

When fed large amounts of raw meat, some cats become extremely aggressive, and may actually climb up your legs and body in a sort of feeding frenzy. Raw meat may contain parasites which are hazardous to your pet. In the worst of circumstances, diseases such as toxoplasmosis may be transmitted to you and your family. Meat or fish which you have caught or been given by a friend should be thoroughly cooked before feeding it to your cat. This will kill any bacteria or parasites that may be present.

Some people recommend feeding a few ounces of raw liver once or twice a week. There is no evidence that this is either required or helpful for the cat. At worst, your cat may become ill with salmonellosis, toxoplasmosis, liver flukes, or a similar disease. Excess amounts of raw liver can lead to vitamin A toxicity (see Feed Components, above). If you give liver daily, the amount should be VERY small—no more than one-quarter ounce of liver per pound of the cat's body weight. Liver must be fed cooked to avoid the problems mentioned above.

MILK AND EGGS

Throughout nature, milk is a food for young animals, not for older ones, and cats are no exception. Milk causes diarrhea in many adult cats because as they mature, they lose the enzyme lactase, which enables them to digest lactose, the sugar in milk. If the lactose is not digested, it draws water into the digestive tract, resulting in a profuse watery diarrhea. Usually, milk should not be given to adult cats to drink, or used to moisten their food.

If you have given milk to the cat throughout its life, and it tolerates it well, by all means continue to do so. It can make food more palatable, and provide fat and protein. If you have been feeding milk to your cat and for some reason quit for a while, but want to reintroduce it, be sure to do so gradually to determine if the cat can still tolerate it. Gradually increase the amount each day until the cat reaches its limit. Cats that are fed ONLY milk may be deficient in niacin. If you have farm cats and a cow, cats that are fed milk from the time they are young may do fine on it. If they have diarrhea due to the milk, simply quit feeding it to them.

Cow's milk is a food for calves, not kittens. It can be used in an emergency, but should be replaced as soon as possible with a milk replacer specifically made for kittens, such as Pet-Ag's Esbilac®. You will save more kittens, more easily, and have fewer health problems.

Some people like to give eggs to cats. Raw egg whites (without the yolks) contain a protein, avidin, which ties up one of the B vitamins, biotin. This causes problems if the whites are fed alone in large quantities. When the white and yolk are fed together, the yolk contains enough biotin to compensate. Biotin is also synthesized by bacteria in the large intestine. If the gut is sterilized (as when the cat has been treated with oral antibiotics), raw egg whites should not be fed.

If you are feeding an adequate amount of a good quality cat food, eggs are an unnecessary addition to the diet. The cat will already have enough of the amino acids contained in eggs, and you will probably not notice any difference from feeding them. As with any table scrap or supplement, eggs should not, in any case, make up more than 10% of the cat's diet.

TREATS

Commercial cat treats or small, fat-free meat scraps are good treats when used IN MODERATION. Use them for rewards, or to let your cat know that you appreciate it. Cat snack or treat foods are not nutritionally complete foods, and should never be more than 10% of the cat's diet. When we give treats to our pets, we make ourselves feel good. However, we need to be sure we don't make ourselves feel so good (by giving too many treats) that our pet feels badly or becomes ill because of an unbalanced diet or obesity. Giving the cat ice cream and similar foods brings us to . . .

JUNK FOOD

Cats will eat many of the foods that humans eat, and they truly enjoy some of the same junk foods that give us problems. Excess sugar does not seem to cause tooth decay in cats, but it can easily lead to obesity when fed in excess. Foods such as meat scraps, which are high in fat, may also cause obesity, as can gravies and sauces.

Feeding junk food can also lead the cat to beg and try to persuade you that it much prefers your food. If you give in and feed human foods, you may displace good nutrition with empty calories. Two tablespoons of ice cream given to a cat are much like a human eating a pint. Little capacity would be left for good food. This is especially a problem with kittens because they are tiny and don't eat much. If you fill them with junk food, you may severely unbalance their diet. Continually feeding tidbits can also turn your cat into a constant beggar—a nuisance.

Your cat may choose not to eat a meal from time to time. This is much the same as it would do in nature, where the cat might not eat every day. If you give the cat tidbits to try to tempt it to eat, you are training the cat to be a picky eater.

To have a healthy cat, avoid feeding junk food. Stick to a well-balanced, nutritious cat food. Or, if you wish to make your veterinarian wealthy, feed LOTS of junk food . . .

Not all cats will chew bones. However, appropriately-sized bones such as those from a round steak, are great tooth-scrubbers for cats that will use them. They help keep the tartar scrubbed off the cat's teeth and massage the gums for better dental health. Never give poultry bones to a cat. It may break pieces off the bone and eat them, causing severe digestive upset, and perhaps a punctured stomach or intestine.

Cats rarely have a taste for liquor. Because of their small size, it would be very easy to kill a cat with even a tiny amount. Never give any liquor to your feline.

CATNIP AND OTHER HERBS

Catnip is an herb. Some cats will roll and may act as if in heat after smelling a scratching post or toy filled or scented with catnip. Other cats will nibble or even eat catnip, and may salivate profusely while doing so. The excitement may last about five to 15 minutes, followed by a period of an hour or more when the cat seems unable to become excited. Cats may return to catnip on a daily basis, and female cats may be especially attracted to the plant. Up to 50% of cats do not respond to catnip.

Your cat may enjoy it greatly if you start some catnip in a pot on your windowsill, or plant some outdoors in your yard. If you grow your own in the summer, it's easy to hang the stalks in a cool place to dry. After it is dry, remove the leaves and store them for the winter. Or, you can dry the leaves in a microwave or a moderate oven. In some areas, you may have to be careful, as it can grow so well that it will spread like a weed throughout your garden.

Cats may have a similar reaction to valerian plants. They may roll on the roots and urinate over them in their excitement. Papyrus plants and lime blossoms may be attractive to some cats. *Actinidia* species, including Chinese gooseberry, may be so attractive to some cats that they will stop eating when they smell the plant.

Some cats may appreciate a pot of parsley, oats, or a lawn grass mix as a treat. This may also help keep the cat from grazing on your house plants, some of which may be toxic. Wheat can also be grown to make wheat grass for your feline. Some cats enjoy alfalfa sprouts, cucumber (peel it first), or finely chopped celery. Some will enjoy a couple of green beans, lima beans, carrots, peas, or broccoli with their dinner (all cooked). In small amounts, these are fine additions to their diet. It is probably natural for cats to eat small amounts of grass and other plants which add fiber to their diets, even on a daily basis. Greens may also help the cat to remove hairballs from its stomach.

SUPPLEMENTS

If you are feeding a nutritionally complete commercial cat food, the manufacturer will have added all the vitamins and minerals needed by a normal cat. Additional vitamins and minerals are not necessary, but if used in recommended amounts, will not increase the overall quantity to harmful levels. Do not, however, think that if a little is good, a lot more is better. If you give more than the recommended amount, the cat's total intake may result in an excess of vitamins or a serious imbalance, causing illness. This may be dangerous, or in the worst case, fatal to your cat. If you do supplement, give only one product at a time, in the dosage given on the label or by your veterinarian.

Your veterinarian will prescribe a specific supplement if there is a need for it. Otherwise, supplementation is an unnecessary expense and bother. Never give human vitamins to your cat, no matter what your friend or health food guru says. Human dosages are usually huge overdoses for your cat.

WATER

A constant supply of clean water is essential for all cats and especially for those that are fed dry food. Without it, severe digestive problems may occur. Cats that eat canned food may drink less water than those that eat dry food. Because about 75% of the cat's body weight is water, your cat must be able to drink when it wishes in order to maintain this percentage. The availability of water is a matter of life or death in hot weather. A cat may quickly die in a place like Phoenix in the summer if it is without water for even part of a day. More water is also needed if the cat is on a high-salt diet, has a fever, or has water loss due to diarrhea or vomiting.

Metal or glass containers are best for both food and water. Plastic dishes may hold odors of previous meals or cleaning products, causing the cat to refuse to eat its food or drink its water. Some plastic dishes may cause an acne-like allergic rash on the chin where it touches the bowl. Because unglazed ceramic crockery and containers may contain lead, be sure the glaze is as lead-free as you would use yourself. The water dish should be heavy enough that it does not tip while the cat is drinking. It is important to wash and sanitize the cat's dishes frequently.

Some cats may refuse to drink stale water while others prefer water that has "settled" for a few hours. Some won't drink water that has been soiled by a slobbering dog drinking from it. Occasionally, a cat will refuse to drink water when it is "different," as when the cat travels or goes to the veterinary clinic or boarding kennel.

Do not let your cat drink from the toilet, or from water standing in the sink. A small kitten, or even an older cat, may try to get a drink, fall in, and drown. Cats of all ages may become ill from drinking waste-contaminated water. Keep the lid down to keep the cat from getting into the toilet, and have all family members close the lid. If your cat does take an occasional drink from the stool, never use a toilet bowl disinfectant.

Inadequate (or unpalatable) water may result in the formation of plugs or stones in the urinary tract, especially in male cats. If your cat has had urinary tract problems, your veterinarian may ask you to give the cat distilled or purified water. You can purchase it at the grocery store, or use a home purifier or reverse-osmosis unit. Do not use water that is labeled "drinking water," as this is often only tap water sold in gallon jugs.

Cats that are both indoors and out should have water in both places so they can always get to it. Outdoor cats in cold climates should have a dish of lukewarm water at least twice a day. Better yet, put out a heated water dish that never freezes. Outdoor cats that do not have enough water in winter will not utilize their food well, and may have digestive upsets, as well as forming plugs or stones in the urinary tract. These problems are easily prevented by supplying clean, ice-free water to your outdoor cats.

WHEN TO FEED

Feral cats eat small mammals, birds, insects, and occasionally reptiles such as lizards or snakes. Mice are a favorite meal, but it takes 10 to 15 adult mice to provide an adult cat's daily needs. Domestic cats are normally nibblers; they may eat 10 to 20 small meals each day. These may be evenly spaced around the clock. Most cats are happiest having food available at all times so they can eat whenever they are hungry.

Many cats do well when dry food is provided on a free-choice basis. The cat may go through a short initial period of overeating, after which it will regulate the quantity eaten. Cats that are free-feeding on dry food will eat a number of small meals, eight to 16 times in a 24-hour period. Just put out the amount of dry food the cat will eat in a day or two. Kitten foods are very dense in calories, and may cause obesity if fed free-choice to adult cats. When feeding any dry food, FRESH WATER MUST BE AVAILABLE AT ALL TIMES. It's fine to put the water dish next to the food bowl.

If you are feeding several cats, convenient feeders are available. These usually consist of some type of cylinder or box with a tray or hopper below. The tray refills as the dry food is eaten. Large numbers of barn cats are easily served with a hanging cylindrical chicken feeder, which may hold as much as 20 pounds of food at a time. Suspending the feeder a couple of inches above a workbench or similar raised surface will help keep out dogs and pest animals.

If you are feeding the cat a limited amount of dry food or a canned cat food, it can be fed either once or twice a day. If you are feeding a canned food, it should be given once or twice a day to make sure it does not spoil before it can be eaten. Cats that tend to be obese can be fed measured meals once or twice a day. Having one or two regular mealtimes each day is useful for outdoor cats, as it trains them to come home at certain hours, and makes it easier to catch them for veterinary visits or to check up on them.

If you feed the cat in the morning, it may get to the point where it awakens you very early. This is because most predators become active an hour or two before their meals, and house cats are no exception. When the cat annoys you early in the morning, change its feeding time to later. This will delay its high activity period. Be prepared for a fight; don't give in to its demands. If your cat is stubborn, it may take as much as two weeks to change its meal "timer."

If you feed your cats at dinner time and find they are ready to play around your bedtime, try feeding their last meal when you go to bed. Cats also may prefer to eat late in the day when the weather is hot because they and the house are cooler and more comfortable.

If a cat remains overweight after a trial period of three to four weeks, it is eating more than it needs. It may be necessary to feed a measured amount, once a day. Like some humans, some cats can't afford to eat all the food they would like to eat! For some cats, changing to a slightly less palatable food may be all that is needed to reduce the animal's intake and regulate its weight.

When going on vacation, some people take their cats to a kennel or boarding facility. Check with kennel personnel to see if you should bring food for them. If a cat is on a special diet (as for heart or kidney disease), it is important that the cat stays on the diet while in the kennel.

It is convenient to leave cats at home if you are gone for a brief period—two or three days. Put out a large dish of water and plenty of dry food, or a full dispenser, as well as a fresh, clean litter box. If you are going to be gone more than a couple of days, it is important to have a friend or neighbor check on the cat to make sure that it has the necessities of life and is healthy, and or to take it to the clinic if the cat should become ill. Many cats appreciate some petting and attention from the caretaker, too. Do NOT change a cat from canned food to dry food when you are going on vacation. The cat may not eat it, or it may not drink enough water to avoid urinary problems. Put the cat on dry food several weeks before you leave if that will be the cat's diet while you are gone.

Some cats gulp their food so rapidly that they vomit after eating. Sometimes this is due to excess hunger before being fed. These cats often benefit from twice-daily or free-choice feeding. If the cat has been without food for a couple of days for some reason, give it half its normal amount of food at first. Then, in a couple of hours, give the cat the rest of the meal.

WHERE TO FEED

Pick a feeding location that is out of the main traffic pattern in your house. It's hard for the cat to pay attention to its meal when it is in the middle of a hallway or the kitchen. Feed in the same place every time, with the food and water dishes in the same place. If you put them near the litter box, however, the cat may not eat well because of the odor.

Many cats prefer to eat alone. If you have several cats and there is fighting at the food dish, you may need to put several dishes in different places so that each cat can have a bit of privacy. If you have both cats and dogs, feed them separately, as neither one's food is good for the other. Feed the cats in a separate room or on a countertop so that they can eat in peace. When feeding measured meals, it usually works better when each cat has its own dish.

If you have one cat that drives the other from its food and eats both, you may end up with one fat cat and one thin cat. With a group of cats, feeding may occur by social pecking order, with dominant cats getting the lion's share. Young, elderly, or shy cats may not get their fair share if eating from a common dish. Kittens may race to the dish, gulp enough food to take the edge off their hunger, and then leave. They may get enough food to survive, but not enough to prosper. An older cat that has been a mother may have waited for her kittens to eat first. Even if she has since been spayed, this instinct may still have her waiting until younger cats have finished eating. This may also occur with a neutered male that has a mothering instinct. All these problems can be prevented by feeding the cats in separate rooms at the same time.

A cat dish with a wide, flat bottom will not tip and make a mess on the floor. It should have a smooth, easily cleaned surface, inside and out. Some cats prefer to eat out of a saucer or flat dish instead of a bowl, as they seem to be annoyed when their whiskers touch the sides. Keep the dish clean. If you are feeding canned food, the dish should be washed daily with soap and hot water and rinsed well.

Cats with long, luxuriant hair, such as Persians, may need some help with their meals. Experiment with different sizes and depths of dishes to help keep the fur out of the food. Raising the dish on a small platform or step may make it easier for the cat to reach. If the cat soils its fur while eating, wipe off the food with a damp cloth. This keeps the cat smelling sweet and avoids skin infections. Persians, especially, may not be able to adequately groom their face and neck areas.

HOW MUCH TO FEED

Cats eat to supply their energy needs and caloric requirements rather than eating a specific volume of food (Houpt, 1979). A normally active cat that weighs 7 to 9 pounds will need about 32 to 34 calories of food per pound of body weight each day. For most dry foods, this is around two-and-a-half to three ounces of dry food daily for an adult cat. Canned food, because of its water content, will require about two to three times that amount.

More than 90% of cats will regulate their own food intake and can be fed on a free-choice basis. Even a self-regulating cat may overeat when it is suddenly given canned food instead of its regular dry food, when it is given unusually appetizing food such as table scraps, or when it has gone without eating for longer than usual. This can happen when the cat is accidentally shut in a garage or room away from its food. In these situations, give the cat only a small amount of food, with further amounts in two to four more feedings over a period of several hours. Otherwise, the cat may overload and vomit. Or, it may make abrupt retching motions without vomiting. This is no cause for alarm, and will take care of itself as the cat either removes the overload by vomiting, or gradually digests it. As with many other species, including humans, studies have shown that cats are healthier, live longer, and more easily avoid chronic disease when they are slightly underweight rather than overweight.

When your cat becomes mature, it will need much less food than when it was growing. Be sure to cut back on the amount you are feeding. Do not encourage the cat to eat the same amount as previously, or it may rapidly become obese.

Use the recommendations on the cat food sack or can ONLY as a GUIDE for your particular cat. It is a starting point and no more. The individual cat's needs will differ depending on its metabolism, temperament, exercise, and the climate where it lives. If the cat is new to you, begin with the recommended amount, by volume (cups) or weight (ounces). Feed it daily for three weeks. Then, decide whether the cat is fatter or thinner than is healthy,

and whether it has changed. Adjust the amount being fed accordingly. Since the manufacturer is in business to sell cat food, the recommendations will usually be on the high side. Cat foods differ in bulk so that feeding a certain volume of food will result in widely varying calorie content from one brand to another. However, if the cat doesn't like its food, it won't eat it, and may become seriously thin. Change to a different food if necessary.

Some experts recommend removing any food that isn't eaten within 30 minutes, whether the cat is finished or not. This may not, however, satisfy the nibbler(s) in the bunch. Make sure the food doesn't spoil and is fresh two to four times a day if you are feeding canned or moistened dry food. Best of all, switch your nibblers to free-choice feeding of a dry food. It may work to feed some canned food twice a day, and leave dry food out at all times, if the cats do not become fat. Or, you may separately feed your thin cat some canned food, while keeping everyone on dry food.

A normal cat's food consumption will vary a bit from day to day, eating more one day and less on another. Unless there is a definite trend over several days, there is no need to worry. A cat that is very active, whether playing or hunting, will need more food than a couch-potato cat that lies around all day.

Outdoor cats' food requirements will vary with the time of year and outdoor temperature. An outdoor cat in a Wyoming winter needs far more food to maintain the same body condition than an Arizona cat in the middle of summer. Also, as fall comes on, many northern cats instinctively seem to eat more, putting on some extra fat to help them through the winter. Needs also vary according to how much they are supplementing their diet by hunting. When this is taken into consideration, cats in the winter may consume three to six times more cat food than they eat in the summer.

Outdoor cats in the city may eat varying amounts of food based on what other cats' feed dishes they are visiting in their rounds, and how many of your neighbors are feeding them. If your cat is gone several days at a time and comes back looking fit and fat, you're probably sharing it with another family!

Especially for a cat that is long-haired, it is important to FEEL the cat's condition every few weeks if you are not weighing it regularly. Some cats, such as Persians and Maine Coons, may look fat while they are extremely thin because their build and hair coat appear so bulky. With the cat standing on the floor or on a firm chair or table, stand behind it. Put your thumbs side by side, on the backbone, with fingers spread over the ribs. Ideally, you should be able to feel a thin layer of fat. If the ribs are visible or you can feel them, or if the backbone protrudes noticeably, the cat is too thin, and should be evaluated for health or feeding problems. If there is so much fat that the edges of the ribs are totally covered and the chest feels smooth and only slightly wavy, the cat is probably too fat. Outdoor cats should be checked often during the winter, when there are heavy caloric demands on their bodies, to make sure they do not become thin beneath their winter coats.

Incidentally, the average cat will eat about 66 pounds (30 kg) of dry food or 200 pounds (90 kg) of canned cat food per year. (Beaver, 1992, p. 181).

THE VEGETARIAN CAT?

Nature has made cats carnivores, in contrast to dogs that in nature can eat a certain amount of plant material or spoiled meat. In the wild, cats eat freshly killed animals or birds. In rare instances, they will eat meat which another animal has killed, but only if it is fresh, or they are desperate. Cats do not have the enzymes necessary to digest vegetable material, and cannot make some of the nutrients they need such as vitamin A and taurine. They require meat or meat by-products (including, of course, fish). You may be a vegetarian, but if you want a healthy cat, please don't expect it to live according to your lifestyle. The cat is not made that way.

Cats should have an acidic urine to prevent many urinary tract problems. This is difficult or impossible to achieve on a vegetarian diet.

FINICKY AS A CAT?

Cats are often considered to be finicky eaters. However, some of what is called finicky is because the owner has been trained to give the cat what the cat demands. What a cat will eat depends largely on what it is fed when it is young. A kitten that is fed a single food may be difficult to change to another food. As an adult, the cat may starve to death before it eats a new or different food, no matter how good it is for the cat, or how necessary for its health. A cat that is given a variety of different foods during its first few months of life can be switched to another food with relative ease. Changing foods often during this period is a good investment in the cat's future health.

Some experiments have shown that cats are sensitive to deficiencies of thiamine in their diets. After trying a food for a few days which is lacking this vitamin, they may refuse to eat it.

When cats are under stress, they tend to prefer foods with which they are familiar. This is important when the cat needs a prescription food because of a medical problem. Some of these special foods are not as palatable as we (or the cat) would like. For this reason, if the cat will not eat its new diet, it may be easier to mix the new food with the old, making the change over several weeks. Begin by adding one-fourth or less of the new food to the old diet. Feed this for up to two weeks until the cat accepts it well. Then, add another one-fourth and feed this for another couple of weeks. Keep doing this until the cat is completely converted to the new food. It may also help for the cat to be a bit hungry. However, starving the cat to force it to eat the new food does not work nearly as well with cats as it does with dogs. The cat may refuse to eat for several days, and get into severe metabolic problems requiring special veterinary care. Or, it may simply die without eating.

When you change a cat to a new diet, it may eat eagerly for two to three days and then refuse to eat any more. If it is necessary to change it to the new food (such as a prescription diet), it may be helpful to mix in table food for a few days. Use a small amount; the goal is to flavor the special diet, not replace it. Try pouring a little clam juice or shrimp broth on the cat food, or stir-fry it with a little butter. Check with your veterinarian to be sure what you are adding is appropriate. It would not be good to add cottage cheese to a low-protein diet, or chicken fat to a low-fat diet.

If you do end up adding some "people food," it should not make up more than 15% of its diet. And, it should be discontinued as soon as possible so that the cat will have the full benefit of the carefully balanced cat food. Also, continuing to add scraps or treats to its diet may encourage the cat to be a "finicky" eater.

Rarely, a cat may have a depraved appetite, called pica. It may lick at a rock or eat dirt or cat litter. This is not due to a lack of minerals or a craving for a particular mineral. The most common cause of pica is anemia, and one of the most common causes of anemia in cats is feline leukemia. Have the cat checked by your veterinarian.

A cat may have a poor appetite or completely quit eating with many diseases. This also may be due to anxiety, as when a cat is kept in a large group, is boarded, or is disturbed by traveling when it is unaccustomed to it. The cat may lack appetite because it is nauseated or not feeling well, or has a tumor. It may associate a particular food with having been ill or hospitalized. If the cat goes without eating for more than two to three days, it may have metabolic problems that need to be treated by your veterinarian.

It may be helpful to play with the cat before feeding. In the wild, the cat has to run and work as it catches its prey. This helps stimulate the appetites of some cats.

SPECIAL NEEDS

BREEDING AND PREGNANCY

As with any baby animal, feeding a kitten begins when it is conceived. The queen will nourish the kittens inside her uterus for nine weeks, and may need as much as two to four times as much food as does an inactive adult cat. The queen needs good nutrition during her pregnancy in order for the kittens to develop normally, and to be at a normal weight when they are born. It is also important to help her begin good milk production after the birth.

A good-quality, balanced, nutritionally complete commercial diet is adequate for reproduction. It should contain at least 1700 digestible calories per pound of food and have at least 30% high-quality, easily digestible protein (Purina, 1989). Dry cat foods made for prevention of obesity in adult cats are usually not adequate for pregnancy and nursing. This type of food may be supplemented by adding moderate amounts of a nutritionally complete canned cat food to her diet. Or, change her to another food.

Before she is bred, the queen should be at a normal body weight and in good physical condition. Shortly before breeding, she should be placed on the same diet that will be used throughout her pregnancy. This will avoid refusal of the food after she is bred. Also, it will put her on a high plane of nutrition, giving a greater chance that she will conceive.

Cats, like humans, may have wide hormonal swings during their reproductive cycle. A cat that is in heat may stop eating completely. If she resumes normal eating patterns after she is bred, there is no cause for concern. Pregnancy may cause the cat to overeat, undereat, or stop eating. Having her on a high-quality, palatable ration can help maintain normal eating patterns.

About three weeks into the pregnancy, many queens will have a reduced appetite for a short period, usually three to 10 days. The cat may lose a small amount of weight. If there are no signs of illness, this is normal. The cat's weight gain will resume when she starts eating normally again.

Many cat foods for inactive adult cats produce low-volume, firm stools. This is not good during pregnancy because the queen may become constipated and strain excessively while attempting to defecate. The food should have enough bulk to keep the cat's stool regular without constipation. It also should be concentrated enough to allow her to meet her body's needs without having to eat excessive amounts.

Between the fourth and sixth weeks of pregnancy, the queen will show a gradual increase in weight. Allow her to eat as much food as she wants, within reason. She should gain a healthy amount of weight, but do not let her become obese; this may make for a difficult delivery because fat narrows the birth canal. In the worst cases, a Caesarean section may be needed to deliver the kittens; they will be less likely to survive and thrive than those born normally.

The queen's body weight will increase even more rapidly during the last three weeks of her pregnancy, as she will be providing nutrition for the rapidly growing kittens. In addition, her body must manufacture the membranes that support them, the fluid that surrounds them, and her developing mammary glands. At this point, the cat may be allowed to become "slightly" overweight. She should either be fed several times a day, or fed free-choice, because the expanding kittens and uterus leave less room in her abdomen to hold food. The queen's appetite may decrease, and she will need frequent small meals to make up for her lack of digestive capacity. Toward the end of her pregnancy, the cat may be eating more frequently than she did before she became pregnant.

Water is extremely important for the pregnant cat. It carries nutrients into and wastes out of the developing kittens. It also helps the queen maintain a normal body temperature. This is especially critical if she is pregnant during the summer in a hot or humid climate. Carefully wash and rinse the water container and refill it frequently with fresh water to encourage her to drink.

A cat that is carrying a large number of kittens, or a few large kittens, may become very uncomfortable in the last couple of weeks of pregnancy. She may sit or lie around, avoiding exercise, and have a poor appetite. If you own a cattery, having the extra kittens may not be worth the extra trouble and risk. Some cattery owners remove

from their breeding programs cats that routinely have large litters.

During the ninth week of pregnancy, the queen may completely quit eating. With many cats, this is a sign that she will have kittens within 24 to 48 hours. Be sure to remove any uneaten food so it does not spoil. Offer a few tablespoons of fresh food three to four times a day so she will have food if she wants it, but don't be surprised if she doesn't eat. After the kittens are born, the queen will usually resume normal eating within 24 hours. If, either before or after the kittens' birth, the mother goes without eating for 48 hours, she should be examined by a veterinarian to make sure everything is normal and she is not ill.

Tom cats that are only occasionally used for breeding do not need a special diet. They can be kept on normal adult maintenance food, being careful they do not become fat. If the cat is used frequently for breeding, or is around females in heat (causing him to be upset), he may not eat his normal amount of food, and may become thin. Help him to stay in good body condition by feeding a diet high in nutrient density, as you would the pregnant female.

LACTATION

After the kittens are born, the queen should be kept on the same nutritious food she ate throughout her pregnancy. Some mother cats are reluctant to leave their litter to eat or drink, and some with large litters may not feel like eating the quantity necessary to support themselves and the kittens. Both these queens need extra encouragement to eat and drink. Otherwise, they may not produce enough milk to feed the kittens, resulting in stunted, malnourished offspring. However, a queen with only one or a few kittens will not need much extra food, and you may have to limit her food consumption so she does not produce too much milk, resulting in engorged, painful mammary glands.

As the kittens become larger, the queen's food intake usually increases. Peak milk production usually occurs three to four weeks after the kittens are born. At this time, she may eat (and need!) as much as two to four times what she ate before pregnancy. Be sure to divide it into three to four meals a day, with fresh food each time to tempt her to eat. Until they are able to eat solid food, kittens are totally dependent on their mother's milk for their nutritional needs.

Be careful not to overwhelm the queen's digestive system. If she has diarrhea or shows other signs of digestive problems, decrease the quantity (but not the quality) of the food. The intake of protein and fat should be maintained at fairly high levels. Feed less dry food and more canned or semi-moist food. Or, you can moisten the dry food, which may help her eat as much as 20% more than usual. Adding too much water will change the mouthfeel and may reduce food consumption. For this brief time in her life, you can add gravy, broth, or meat juice to the queen's food to tempt her to eat more.

In any case, do not add more than 10% table scraps to the food, or you risk unbalancing it. Do not add calcium supplements to the diet of a lactating cat. Excess calcium may decrease the level of parathyroid hormone in the cat's body, causing her body to react slowly to the rapidly increasing demand for calcium. Blood calcium levels may drop rapidly, causing metabolic problems for her.

Around three to four weeks of age you can begin supplementing the kittens' nursing with food (see below). This will reduce the load on their mother. At the same time, she will be less interested in nursing and more interested in spending time away from them.

By the time the kittens are weaned, the queen's food intake should be back to her normal maintenance level. If she has become very thin during pregnancy and nursing, carefully raise the amount of food to get her back to normal body condition. If she does not return to normal within a few weeks after the kittens are no longer nursing, or if she shows any signs of illness, have her examined by your veterinarian. Do not breed her (or allow her to become bred by running loose outdoors) until she is back to her normal weight.

Weaning occurs gradually as the kittens learn to eat or hunt and the mother spends less time with them. In the wild, the queen does not wean her young, but after they are 12 weeks old, her milk has little nutritional value (Beaver, 1992, p. 174). Meanwhile, the mother is bringing small dead prey to the kittens. Around five weeks of age, she will eat in their presence, and they will eat with her by about six weeks of age.

If you are weaning the kittens all at one time by removing them from the queen, she may be quite uncomfortable because her body does not yet know it needs to stop producing milk. You can reduce her misery by feeding her no food at all the day before you wean the kittens. Feed her one-fourth of the amount you have been giving on the first day after weaning; one-half on the second day; three-fourths on the third day; and then back to normal. This will help stop the flow of milk and make her much more comfortable.

KITTEN FEEDING

The first day after birth is the most significant time in the kitten's life. During the first one to three days after the kitten is born, the queen produces colostrum. This is a special form of milk which is high in water content and low in protein and fat content. Most important, it contains antibodies which protect the kitten from disease until its immune system is able to produce its own antibodies. A kitten that does not get colostrum is very susceptible to contagious diseases. In addition, colostrum tends to be laxative, and helps the kitten's digestive system begin functioning. As lactation progresses, the protein, fat, and mineral content of the milk gradually rises to meet the needs of the rapidly growing kitten. A normal kitten will gain almost a pound per month until it is close to its mature weight. Consider that your cat will grow as much, proportionately, in its first year of life as a human does in 18 years.

Kittens need more energy, protein, calcium and phosphorus than do adult cats. They may need as much as four times the energy per unit weight as does an adult cat.

Supplemental feeding of a normal litter of kittens nursing a normal queen can begin at three to four weeks of age. Giving food to the kittens helps reduce the load on the mother, especially if she has a large litter. If the mother is not well, or is severely drained by the kittens, begin feeding them around 14 to 16 days of age. The kittens will try to crawl into their mother's food if nothing else is offered. Some kittens learn faster than others, but all should be eating by the end of their seventh week of age.

Put a small amount of dry kitten chow moistened with water, or canned or soft-moist food in a very shallow pan or plate. Or, you can use a milk replacer especially made to mimic cat's milk, or a kitten weaning formula, both of which are available commercially. The edge of the pan should be no more than a half-inch high so that the kittens can make their teetering way into the food. Saucers tend to tip when the kittens wade in, and are not very successful. The consistency of the food should be that of gravy, but not quite soup. It is better to mix the food with milk replacer or water than with cow's milk. You may want to put the whole procedure on newspapers to help catch the mess, or feed them outside on the lawn. It is almost guaranteed that some of them will walk in it, and they will get food all over themselves. And just when you think they'll never get the hang of it, they start eating by themselves! As the kittens get older, decrease the amount of liquid mixed with the food until they are eating dry or canned food unmixed by the time they are weaned.

Whichever kind of food you use, make sure it is labeled as complete and balanced for all life stages. Or, use a food specifically made for kittens. Make small batches of food so it is fresh each time you offer it to the kittens, three to four times a day. Wash the container between feedings so there will not be any spoiled or contaminated food left to harm the kittens.

Take each kitten in turn, and gently dip the end of its snout into the food mixture, being careful not to get the food into its nostrils. The kitten will sputter and blow bubbles, but will lick it off its face. Or, you can moisten a finger in the food and offer it to the kitten to suck. Then, lead its head downward to the pan. By the second or third time you do this, most of the kittens will be eating. As the kittens get older, reduce the amount of liquid you mix with the food until it is offered in its regular consistency. Kittens should have access to fresh water at all times after solid food is added to their diet.

It is both expensive and time-consuming to make a homemade weaning formula. Leave that up to the cat food companies which have laboratories and entire staffs of nutritionists to do the job. Feed a good brand of kitten chow or cat food, and DO NOT supplement it with "a bit of yogurt and a dab of cereal" or any other of the random food mixtures that circulate among cat owners and breeders. Kittens should NOT be weaned onto human meat-type baby food, nor should it be fed to their mother. These foods are severely lacking in calcium. Remember, when a cat eats a mouse, it eats bones and all, and thus gets calcium. Human baby foods are entirely meat, making them high in phosphorus and badly lacking in calcium.

By the time the kittens are six weeks old, they should be weaned. Usually the mother cat does this, becoming less available and more grouchy when the kittens attempt to nurse. Some super-mother cats will allow offspring to nurse even when adults. It may be necessary to separate this queen from her kittens to allow her to dry up and quit producing milk. This will stop the continued drain on her bodily resources. It also gives her a better chance to conceive and carry a new litter if you want to rebreed her shortly.

Weaned kittens can be fed a good-quality kitten chow. One advantage of kitten chow is that the pieces are small and easier for the kitten to eat. Or, feed them any nutritionally balanced and complete food which is suitable for both them and their mother. When you are feeding this type of food, no extra nutritional supplementation is needed, either for the kittens or for the queen. Kittens make up for their increased need for vitamins and minerals simply by eating more food, which contains the necessary balance in every bite. Oversupplementation of vitamins and minerals can cause far more problems than it cures.

Most kittens can be given all the food they will eat up to the point where they start to become obese. If your kitten becomes overweight, switch it to an adult cat food as this is less calorie-rich and will act as a diet food. Avoid abrupt changes in diet which may cause digestive upsets such as diarrhea.

Judge the proper amount to feed by the look and feel of the kitten. The kitten should look trim, with only a slight layer of fat over the ribs. If the ribs cannot be felt with gentle pressure on the rib cage, the kitten is too fat. If you can easily see the ribs as the kitten moves, it is too thin. The abdomen should be nicely rounded but not tightly swollen. Diarrhea can indicate overfeeding or intolerance of the food. Excessive crying and a failure to gain weight can indicate underfeeding. Adjust its diet to keep the kitten in proper condition. Change the feed quantity weekly if needed.

Change the food you are giving the kitten from time to time. This will provide nutrition from a variety of sources, and will keep the kitten from becoming fixed on only one flavor. This way, if the kitten is ill or hospitalized later in life, it will be more willing to accept a new food.

If you are feeding measured meals rather than free-choice, kittens that are just weaned (about six weeks of age) do best if fed four meals a day, four to five hours apart. From three to six months of age, three meals a day are enough. Be sure to increase the quantity at each meal to balance having fewer of them. After six months of age, one or two meals a day are sufficient for most cats. Or, you can make life easy for yourself and the cat and encourage it to become accustomed to free-choice feeding. This can be done around 12 to 14 weeks of age. When changing from moistened dry food to feeding the same food dry, decrease the amount of water added to the food over seven to 10 days.

Cats reach their full size about nine months of age, but are not internally mature until about 12 months of age. You can switch your cat to an adult food around the time you have it neutered (five to six months of age), or you can keep it on kitten chow until the cat is a full year old. (For feeding orphaned kittens, see Reproduction Chapter).

THE ILL OR CONVALESCENT CAT

Nutrition is extremely important to a cat that is sick or recovering from an illness. Cats that are ill or seriously stressed are less likely to eat or drink on their own than are dogs in the same situation. If left without food long enough, the cat may reach a point where it has no appetite, and will not eat by itself no matter what food is offered. Do not assume that the sick cat will eat when it becomes hungry enough. It may not, and may actually starve to death. Most injured or ill cats, however, do well voluntarily eating high-quality foods that are highly digestible and relatively high in protein and fat.

A cat that is ill can lose strength and muscle mass twice as fast as a cat that is starving. The cat's body will use its own tissues for survival. First, its fat is burned for energy, then muscle mass is used to keep it alive. Within five days, skeletal muscle is lost. This may cause liver failure if it goes on long enough. Then, it proceeds to the smooth muscle of the digestive tract. If it goes further, it will paralyze the diaphragm, followed by cardiac arrest. This is especially a problem in fat cats that have become ill and stopped eating. It is critically important to provide them with adequate nutrition.

The loss of 10% of a cat's body weight is cause for concern. That's only 1 pound on a 10 pound cat! However, the change from 10 pounds to 9 pounds may not be obvious. The loss of 2 pounds on that same cat is a SERIOUS matter.

Fever increases the cat's need for energy. Ideally, the cat with a fever should have a palatable, bland, easily digested food that is rich in calories. It will, of course, need plenty of water. If the cat has diarrhea, foods high in fiber should be avoided.

Sick cats need especially high levels of some nutrients, and may be sorely lacking them if they do not eat for more than a few days. Supplementation with potassium may help the appetite. Zinc may be helpful, too (.5-1 mg/lb (1-2 mg/kg/day)). Also, vitamin B12 may be added to the diet (50-100 micrograms/day orally). Other water-soluble B vitamins may be helpful. Thiamine should be supplemented, especially if the cat is on (or has been on) intravenous fluids. If the cat is not eating, it may be necessary for your veterinarian to inject the vitamins for more rapid response.

Cats that are healthy normally require high levels of protein in their diet. A cat that is ill needs at least the same level of protein and often more. Food for a sick or recovering cat should contain 30-50% good quality, easily digested protein, and 35-60% percent fat. If a cat on a fat- or protein-restricted diet becomes ill, consult your veterinarian for a proper diet.

Healthy cats have almost no need for carbohydrates in their diets, and there is evidence that sick cats also do not need them. They need protein and fat far more than they need just "calories" supplied by carbohydrates. In other words, it's better to give the cat meat broth than sugar water! One exception to this rule is when you are feeding an extremely ill animal. Your veterinarian may have you feed a product high in carbohydrates, as well as containing many amino acids and vitamins. If the cat will eat by itself, feed a highly digestible, high-fat, calorie-dense food such as c/d (Hill's). Calories may also be added to the diet by putting a teaspoon or two of salad oil on the cat's food.

Because the odor of its food is so important to a cat, it is common for a cat with an upper respiratory infection to completely quit eating. Much the same thing is seen when a human has a "cold" in the nose. The difference is that humans know they need to eat, so they do it whether they can smell the food or not. A cat doesn't have this intellectual process to drive its food intake. If it can't smell food, it probably won't eat.

For a sick cat, it is often better to offer four to five small fresh meals during the day rather than to leave food setting out. Warming the food to body temperature will make it more attractive and will make the odor stronger. It also keeps the cat from having to use precious calories to heat food to body temperature. Cold food may also cause diarrhea or vomiting. Be sure to check the temperature before feeding it. Food at body temperature will feel just slightly warm when touched to the inside of your wrist. Check the temperature of the food and not that of the container. If any medication is to be added, do so after heating the food.

You can also tempt the cat with table foods. Try beef (well cooked, not raw), turkey, chicken, cheese, fish or shrimp. Some cats may eat strained meat baby foods, especially lamb, veal, beef, and chicken. These are NOT nutritionally balanced, and should not be fed for more than about three days. They do not contain the minerals or vitamins necessary for your pet. Milk may cause diarrhea in the adult cat; offer canned beef or chicken broth instead. It may also help to lightly sprinkle the food with onion or garlic powder (NOT onion or garlic SALT). Food with a strong odor may induce the cat to eat. This may be the time to feed sardine-flavor food, even if you can't stand the smell!

Provide a quiet, secure place for the cat to eat. A cat that is already ill may be reluctant to eat if surrounded by other cats, dogs, or noisy children. A cardboard box covered with a cloth makes an instant "dining room." It may also be helpful if you sit with the cat and feed it by hand, or pet or touch it as it eats.

It may be possible to stimulate the cat's appetite with diazepam, a drug given intravenously by your veterinarian. This acts rapidly to temporarily make the cat ravenously hungry. It does not work well orally, so is not helpful if you have the cat at home. If the cat is very ill, appetite stimulants may not work.

Force-feeding may be necessary. In some cases, the cat may swallow if you put food into the back of its mouth, thus stimulating the swallowing reflex. Try small pieces of cooked fish or beef. Bite-sized chunks of a regular or gourmet cat food or a meat-based baby food also can be used. This is better for the cat than giving it high-carbohydrate or sugar-based foods. It is difficult to force feed a cat for a long period of time, even using a well-balanced diet or supplement (see Viral Respiratory Infections for more information on specialized diets).

Or, your veterinarian can give you a high-calorie liquid diet that can be fed with a syringe. Strain the mixture before using it so it will flow smoothly. If you use a 12 cc syringe, it may require up to 16 to 18 filled syringes to sustain a 9 pound cat. This is a lot to get down, however, it can be a lifesaving measure for the cat that is treated at home.

For a critically ill cat, the veterinarian may place a tube (called a nasogastric tube) through the cat's nose into its stomach. Or, a tube may be placed through the back of the cat's mouth (the pharynx) into its stomach. Sometimes, it may be surgically placed into the stomach or intestine. The cat must be either sedated or anesthetized to insert these tubes. Once in place, the tube may be taped or sutured to the cat's neck or to a bandage to keep it in place. If necessary, the tube can be left in place three to four weeks until the cat is feeling better and eating on its own (the tube doesn't interfere with its eating). Tube-feeding is useful for a great number of ailments. You can feed the cat at home, greatly reducing the cost of care. Being able to easily feed your cat via this tube may make all the difference in its recovery.

The tube will allow you to feed the cat with a syringe, giving a tiny, fresh meal every two hours. A gruel can be made from cat food. Make sure the product you are using is "nutritionally complete" so the cat is getting all the nutrients it needs. Human baby foods, baby formulas, and dog foods are extremely lacking in the proper balance of nutrients, especially for the ailing cat.

Special liquid diets are often the easiest way to get nutrition into the sick cat. These foods contain all the essential nutrients in easily digested form. For this reason, much smaller quantities are needed than would be if you were using regular cat food. Enteral products (liquid foods) for humans are severely lacking in several amino acids needed by cats, and can cause severe deficiency if fed for more than a few days.

An emergency tube-feeding formula can be made by mixing 3 ounces strained chicken-flavor baby food or egg yolk baby food, 3 ounces water, 1 teaspoon cooking oil, and 1 teaspoon corn syrup. Give one ounce per pound of cat weight per day, divided into at least four feedings (Whitford, 1989).

Diarrhea and vomiting are the most common side effects of a liquid diet. It may be necessary to decrease the amount being given to the last amount the cat was able to handle, and remain at that level until it has been free of side effects for eight hours. Then the amount given can again be increased. Liquid foods usually contain some glucose. If they are given to a diabetic cat, urine and blood glucose levels should be monitored.

Liquid feeding will help keep the cat alive until its body can overcome the illness. If necessary, the cat can be restrained by having someone hold its front legs in one hand and hind legs in the other. When treating the cat by yourself, the cat's legs can be taped together in pairs with adhesive or masking tape, or it can be securely rolled in a towel.

Water must be added to most food slurries as they are mixed. Otherwise, the nutrients will draw water into the digestive tract from the cat's body, and the cat may become seriously (or even fatally) dehydrated. If the cat is not drinking, you may need to give "drinks" of water via the tube between feedings. Be sure to follow each feeding with a syringe partially full of clean, lukewarm water to help keep food from caking in the tube. Food and liquids are given in small amounts, 30 to 40 milliliters (2 or 3 tablespoons) at a time, frequently throughout the day. As the cat improves, mix the liquid diet with pureed canned cat food. This will add high-quality protein and help get the cat started on solid food.

Intravenous feeding may be needed in cases where the cat is vomiting uncontrollably, or where the animal should not be sedated or anesthetized for tube placement. For most cases, enteral tube feeding can completely eliminate the need for intravenous feeding. Your cat can go home from the hospital much sooner.

The cat that is fed special foods or a liquid diet may quickly gain weight. Since it was so far behind when the feeding was started, this does NOT mean it is "out of the woods" yet. Much of the early gain is fat and water, neither of which helps heal wounds or restore immune functions. It takes a longer period of good nutrition to replace protein that has been lost. Do NOT overfeed the cat, trying to make it gain weight. This may overload its digestive tract and metabolic systems. Giving the cat numerous small meals each day is important to speed its recovery without overwhelming its body's systems.

THE UNDERWEIGHT CAT

At with many conditions, there are degrees of being underweight. This may vary from the cat that is always a bit thinner than you'd like, to the cat that is malnourished or starving. Let's just discuss the thin cat.

Is the cat normal for its breed? An Abyssinian is naturally a much leaner cat than a plump, robust Maine Coon. And, by the way, is the Abby really thin? Feel through its hair to see whether its ribs are covered with fat. You should be able to feel the ribs but not dip your fingers deeply between them or see them sticking out through the skin.

Begin by making sure the cat is healthy. Take a stool sample to your veterinarian and have it checked for worms. If any are present, have the cat dewormed. Then, see whether it gains weight in two to three weeks. If not, or if the cat shows signs of physical illness, have it examined by your veterinarian.

To put weight on the cat by feeding, increase the amount of food, providing the cat will eat it. If the food is not palatable to the cat, try another brand. Some of the least expensive cat foods provide good nutrition, but have poor flavor, and some cats will not eat enough to maintain good condition.

If you are feeding a dry food, changing to a canned food may help the cat put on weight. You can also feed small amounts of fresh, lukewarm food so the odor will be stronger and more attractive.

A cat that is thin because it has been crowded or bullied away from the food dish by another cat should be fed by itself, preferably two to three times a day until it reaches a normal weight. Other thin cats are stimulated by competing for their "vittles."

A few very nervous cats, such as some Siamese, may be anorexic because of stress when visitors or strange animals come to their house, when they are taken to the veterinary clinic, or when there are too many animals in the household. Sometimes a cat like this will benefit from tranquilizers or by being able to eat by itself in a quiet dark place. Many feline diseases can cause the cat to lose its sense of smell and quit eating. This will correct itself when the cat is well. If the cat goes without eating for more than a few days, it may need intensive medical treatment and possibly tube-feeding to get it going again.

Extreme thinness is one of the few instances where, if lack of calories is the only problem, one might recommend feeding "people food." The fat also will increase palatability of the cat food. Start with a teaspoon or so of bacon grease or other pork fat on the cat's food, and work up to two to three teaspoons per day, depending on the size of the cat. You also can use corn oil, but other cooking oils do not work as well. If diarrhea occurs, reduce the amount of fat. A bonus with this program will be a good, shiny hair coat. Be sure to discontinue or reduce the fat feeding when the cat reaches its normal weight.

THE OVERWEIGHT CAT

Cats in the wild get plenty of exercise because they have to hunt down and kill or scavenge everything they eat. Overeating is not a problem. And, the cat that might overeat in the wild is automatically regulated because it will be too sluggish to chase anything until it goes without food for a few days. Under domestication, some cats overeat if they have the chance.

Most cats tend to regulate their eating quite well. Only about 10-20% of the cat population is obese. How do you determine if your cat is overweight? Many times it is obvious—the rolls of fat bulging between the last rib and the hip bone, ribs that can't be felt with your fingers, and the general look of the animal. Obesity is sometimes considered to be 25% more than the animal's normal weight. A few cats may be as much as 50-100% above normal weight. You should just be able to feel the ribs when you run your fingers across the side of a normal weight cat, but not dip in between them. With the possible exception of Maine Coon Cats, almost any cat that weighs more than 12 pounds (5.5 kg) is probably over-weight (Burkholder, 1995). How do you determine your cat's weight? Cats can easily be weighed on a baby scale if you have one. Or, the cat may stand on a bathroom scale by itself. If it won't, hold the cat in your arms and weigh both of you. Then, put the cat down and weigh yourself, alone. The difference is the cat's weight.

Some cats, especially older males, may have a large hanging flap under the belly. Some of this is sagging skin, and some of it is fat. This may be normal for the particular cat, so judge it by its ribs, not just by its flabby abdomen. If in doubt, consult your veterinarian, who will tell you if your cat is overweight, and give you a realistic goal for weight loss and condition. Some cats that are overweight remain fairly healthy. A few become diabetic (see Diabetes). Others that are extremely fat will have problems with dermatitis in the skin folds around the vulva or penis.

Cats that are slightly overweight may not be harmed by it, and it may not be critically important to reduce them if they do not have any other health problems. Small amounts of extra weight seem to be far less harmful to cats than they are to humans and dogs. It takes very little food to feed one of these "easy keeper" cats, and it's hard to feed it even less than the small amount it is already eating.

Why is your cat overweight? Cats today generally live indoors and are far less active than when they are out "catting" around. Cat foods today are far tastier than they were in past years, and many cats can't resist the temptation. Some cats can't handle being fed free-choice. They overeat instead of regulating their intake. Also, some people associate a plump cat with a healthy cat. This is not true!

As with humans, overfeeding a kitten can predispose it to being a fat adult, as it develops more fat cells than normal. If you allow the kitten to become overweight while it is growing, it may have problems with obesity throughout its life. Keep the cat at a normal weight as an investment in its future.

Severe obesity can be a serious health problem in cats. It can significantly shorten your cat's lifespan and make it miserable while alive. Cats that are overweight have more physical ailments than those of normal weight. Because the fat holds anesthetic agents, an overweight cat has greatly reduced chances of surviving surgery, especially emergency surgery due to an injury. Excess weight strains the heart and puts extra stress on ligaments and tendons. Locomotion problems increase. These may include herniated disks, ruptured ligaments, and arthritis. Cats that are overweight can even have their legs collapse so severely they must be euthanized because they cannot stand. Fat deposits may cause the skin to bulge into rolls which then rub against each other and produce skin irritation. The resulting skin disease can be difficult to cure. A cat that is overweight may have sanitation problems because it cannot reach around to groom itself as would a cat of normal proportions.

The overweight queen, if she can becomes pregnant, is more likely to have a complicated delivery. If she has to have a Caesarean section, she is less likely to survive than an animal of normal weight. An obese tom cat may have decreased semen quality and a poor libido. Layers of fat make it difficult for your veterinarian to give your cat an adequate examination. Wounds heal more slowly in fat cats, and they have less resistance to viral and bacterial infections. Cats that are overweight also are less resistant to the effects of heat, and some may be irritable because they are miserable. Cats that are overweight show a large increase in digestive problems, including constipation, diabetes, and gas. The bad effects of being overweight can begin when the cat is only 10-15% over its normal weight. That's only a pound or pound and a half on an average sized cat.

Some cats are more prone than others to put on weight because of their conformation and heredity. A cat with a chunky, stocky build is more likely to be overweight than is a long lean racing model Abyssinian.

The only legitimate excuses for weight gain are as a side effect of medication (such as corticosteroids), or a physical disorder causing the animal to put on fat. Both of these are very rare, however, compared to the "too much food" cats. If your cat is obese, the first step is to rule out a medical problem.

Obesity is easier to prevent than to cure. Don't let it get started. As with humans, obesity comes from too much food, food with excess calorie content, or inadequate exercise. The first step in taking weight off the cat is to stop feeding "people food." Food which is fattening for people is fattening for your cat. Also, the size difference between humans and cats must be taken into account. Allowing a small cat to lick an ice cream dish is like a human eating an entire bowl. Cut out all table foods and "treats."

Stick to the diet without exceptions. It is kinder to control the food than to let your pet suffer from the medical problems that obesity can cause. You are NOT showing love and proper care for your beloved pet by giving it treats and human foods that are high in calories. Ignore the meowing and soulful looks. Do you really want to "kill your cat with kindness?" I hope that by now you are convinced that a very fat cat is neither healthy nor happy. If you are paying attention to what your cat eats, it should never become obese. However, if you look at your cat and decide that it needs to go on a diet, here's what to do . . .

If you are feeding a very tasty, yummy food, switch to a less palatable food. A calorie-controlled food is the easiest, first step in dieting. For a cat that is only slightly overweight, or for the adult cat that simply needs fewer calories, grocery store brands such as Purina Cat Chow Mature® can be fed. Or, you can use prescription diets such as Science Diet Feline Maintenance Light® Formula (Hills Pet Products) or CNM Clinical Nutrition Management OM-Formula®.

For the severely overweight cat, Feline r/d® is one example of a low-calorie, high fiber food. The added fiber helps the cat feel full and less hungry so it eats less. It is important for a cat on a high-fiber diet to have an adequate caloric intake each day. Gradual reducing is important. Starvation diets are not healthy for cats. The cat may end up with a fatal case of hepatic lipidosis (fat accumulation in the liver) from it. Let your veterinarian know if the cat goes more than a day without eating. It is sometimes difficult to change the cat to a diet food, because these foods are deliberately less tasty than regular foods. When a cat is first placed on a diet higher in fiber, it may have intestinal gas, and will probably produce a greater volume of feces. The gas usually goes away after the cat is on the new food for several weeks. If it does not, try (or ask your veterinarian to recommend) another brand of low-calorie, high-fiber food.

Cut out all table scraps and people-food treats. Avoid giving semi-moist cat treats, as they are very high in sugars and your cat doesn't need the extra calories. The attention you give your pet is more important than the treat you give.

When first putting your cat on a diet, it may be helpful to put it outdoors or in another part of the house when you are eating meals or snacks. This keeps it away from the tempting odors and sounds of food preparation and consumption. It can't beg if it's not present—and many obese cats are skilled beggars. Do not feed an obese cat with other pets. It may be easier for the cat if you feed it before you or your other pets eat. Make sure it has plenty of fresh water, and keep your cat indoors so that it cannot hunt, scrounge in garbage cans, or beg from the neighbors.

Frequent small feedings, especially in the beginning, may make the new regimen easier for your cat to tolerate. With time, its stomach will shrink and it will become used to smaller meals and less food. Give your cat plenty of attention and emotional support to help compensate for the lack of groceries. Make sure children don't tease the cat with food and make the diet more difficult. Hand-feeding may help when you are starting the cat on the new diet. Free-choice feeding usually cannot be used with the obese cat—it just helps itself! Another alternative is to feed the cat measured meals of its regular food, but to leave out a bowl of a less palatable dry food such as Prescription Diet r/d®. This will allow the cat to crunch a few pieces when it becomes desperate.

It is vital that you have the cooperation of ALL family members. It does no good to limit the amount of food if the four-year old is pushing food off its plate, or grandmother is letting the cat lick the gravy pan. It is best not to give the cat anything but the diet food. Overall, it's better to get the obese pet out of the begging habit—it's better for its long-term health!

The average household cat is a rather sedate beast. It is rarely active for prolonged periods, and most of the energy that it expends is used in short bursts. Overweight tends to perpetuate itself. The cat doesn't feel like doing anything, so it moves even less, and reduces its expenditure of energy. Increased exercise will help reduce your cat's weight, but it can be difficult to get it to cooperate. You might try coaxing the cat to play, or encourage it to chase a toy on the end of a string. If you are thinking about getting another cat, a young cat or kitten may encourage (or harass) the older cat into more vigorous activity. For the most part, however, activity has little bearing on the weight of the normal house cat.

In extreme cases of obesity, it may be necessary to have your pet hospitalized until it has lost enough weight that it can go on a home-reducing program. Hospitalization can also be a last resort when a home program is not working.

Don't give up on the diet program. As with humans, weight reduction may be slow. An overweight cat may only lose a half pound per month, and it may take several months to reach your goal. Eventually, you will notice that your cat is feeling younger and more full of life. It will enjoy the remaining years of its life, and you will enjoy your cat!

THE ELDERLY CAT

The older cat's body becomes less efficient. It digests its food less easily, and since it is less active, it needs fewer calories. If you are lucky, your cat will adjust its intake to its activity level and eat less, keeping its weight normal. Unless the cat has kidney disease, it should be kept on a food containing high-quality protein because it is eating a smaller quantity of food. The older cat's sense of smell may not be as good, so be sure that the food is tempting and palatable. Fish-based foods have strong odors that may tempt the older cat to eat. Warming the food also may help it to eat more readily.

Chapter 6

THE DIGESTIVE SYSTEM

TEETH

Kittens, like humans, are born without teeth. Their 26 deciduous teeth, also called milk teeth, baby teeth, temporary teeth or kitten teeth, begin to show from the gums around three to four weeks of age. The permanent teeth begin to replace the baby teeth at three to five months of age. Adult cats have 30 teeth.

Up to about seven months of age, you can estimate the cat's age by its teeth. The kitten's first pair of incisors (the small front teeth in the center, between the fangs) come in between two and three weeks of age. These are its "two front teeth." The second and third pairs of front teeth come in between three and four weeks of age. The first two pairs of permanent incisors erupt between three-and-a-half and four months of age. The third pair of permanent incisors comes in between four and four-and-a-half months of age. The temporary incisors are thinner and more needle-like than the permanent ones. The incisors are the smallest teeth. They are meant to help cut food, although in the modern cat they are not very useful.

The canine teeth (fangs) are the large pointed ones at the front corners of the mouth. Yes, they're called "canines," even in cats. They allow the cat to securely grab its prey and kill it. Temporary canine teeth come in between three and four weeks of age. Permanent canine teeth erupt around five months of age. As with the incisors, permanent canines are thicker and broader at the base than are kitten teeth. The teeth further back in the cheek, behind the canine teeth, are the premolars. They shear food and let the cat chew through tough, fibrous material. Cats have six premolars in the upper jaw and four in the lower jaw. The rear cheek teeth are called molars. They work like scissors and slice food into bite-sized chunks. Cats have two molars in each jaw.

Normally the "baby" teeth are pushed out of the way by the incoming permanent teeth, and fall out unnoticed. Occasionally, a baby tooth refuses to fall out. In this situation, there are two canine teeth side-by-side. If the baby tooth stays, all the teeth may be permanently misaligned. Don't attempt to take the extra teeth out yourself. Ask your veterinarian to remove them (see Corrective Dentistry, below).

The cat's short jaw with few teeth is adapted to a hunting lifestyle. Cats eat small prey (such as mice) with very little chewing, or rip pieces from larger prey (such as a rat or gopher). They are unable to chew their food very effectively, and merely tear it into chunks which can be conveniently swallowed. The rest of the digestive system is made to compensate, and is capable of digesting food that has not been well chewed. The tongue is rough and scratchy, which helps the cat groom itself.

With most feline dental problems, there is a choice between repairing the tooth and removing it. The incisors, the tiny front teeth, are far more ornamental than useful in the cat. They are perhaps of importance only in cats which are being shown or bred, to prove that the conformation of the animal's mouth is normal. The back, shearing teeth (premolars and molars) are used very little in the average household cat that is fed either dry or moist food. Cats that have had all their teeth removed because of dental disease can still eat and digest food quite adequately if the pieces can be swallowed.

The canine teeth, the large, pointed fangs—two in the upper jaw and two in the lower jaw—are a different matter. The fangs are very important in maintaining the shape of the face and in keeping the tongue in place in the mouth. If at all possible, these teeth should be repaired and retained, even if all the other teeth must be removed.

CORRECTIVE DENTISTRY

Short-faced cats, such as Persians, usually have the same number of teeth crowded into a much shorter jaw. The lower canine teeth may be so cramped that they protrude outside the lips. Your veterinarian can put braces on the cat or refer you to someone who can. Orthodontic treatment will make the cat more attractive and comfortable. Correction should not be done on cats that are going to be shown, as it would lead to further breeding of cats with this hereditary defect. A cat that had braces should be spayed or neutered.

For most cats, braces which are firmly fixed to the teeth and periodically adjusted by the veterinarian or dentist doing the work are more successful than those you apply and care for yourself. Small movements of teeth may take as little as two to eight weeks. If the tooth must be moved a long distance, the time period will be much longer. If you don't want to have orthodontic work done, your veterinarian can anesthetize the cat and remove a few teeth, giving considerable relief.

Some cats may not shed their deciduous ("kitten") teeth when the permanent (adult) teeth are ready to erupt. If this occurs, they may end up with two canine teeth side-by-side. This can cause poor alignment of the lower permanent canines, making them strike the roof of the mouth and causing ulcers. For this reason, many veterinarians prefer to remove the offending kitten tooth as soon as it is apparent it is not coming out by itself. The cat must be anesthetized for the removal, but it is simple and can prevent many problems in the future. In some cases, it may be necessary to put braces on the lower canine teeth to spread them sideways until they clear the roof of the mouth.

A common cause of hard bony swellings on a cat's face is a tumor called squamous cell carcinoma. It may be seen on the face, in the cat's mouth, or under its tongue. By the time it is discovered, it is usually too late to successfully treat the tumor. Hard swellings may occasionally be seen because of tooth problems. In either case, the cat should be checked by your veterinarian.

Cervical line lesions are eroded areas on the tooth enamel at or below the gum line. They are also called feline neck lesions, external and internal root resorptions, external odontoclastic resorptive lesions (EOR), and cavities or caries. They look much like cavities in humans, but seem to have a different origin. Cervical line lesions are caused by malfunctioning cells which begin to remove tooth material, replacing it with fibrous material. The cause of this cellular malfunction is unknown. Bacterial action, calicivirus infections, metabolic imbalance, diet, or an immune deficiency may be involved. This makes prevention difficult. For some reason, these lesions are seen more often in modern cats than in cats that died before 1960 (Harvey, 1990).

Cervical line lesions may be found in as many as two-thirds of cats more than four years of age. The cat may have only one lesion, or several teeth may be affected. You may see a heavy accumulation of tartar-like material at the gum line, extending up onto the tooth. The gums may be swollen, reddened and bleeding and the cat may have trouble chewing. These areas may be very painful,

and just touching the spot with a cotton swab or toothpick may cause jaw spasms. Many cats do not show any clinical signs. Disease is discovered during a checkup or when the teeth are cleaned.

Cervical line lesions may eventually lead to loss of the tooth. A veterinarian experienced in dentistry can often clean, repair, and restore these teeth to near-normal function. Minor lesions can be treated with fluoride, applied every three months. The other alternative is to simply have them removed.

Badly diseased teeth, or teeth with abscessed roots can be removed. Teeth also may be broken, and will be very sensitive if the nerves are exposed. They may show up as a swollen cheek. In any case, the cat should be treated promptly. Otherwise, infection can spread to the jawbone and then throughout the cat's body via the bloodstream.

Some cats have continuing gum infection, even with tooth brushing and antiseptic treatment. It improves with antibiotic treatment, but promptly returns when medication is stopped. Removal of the offending tooth, and in worst cases, all teeth, will give the cat permanent relief from the pain, and will stop the infection from shedding bacteria to the rest of its body.

If an abscess occurs over the fourth premolar in the upper jaw, it may erode through the thin wall of bone that separates the tooth from the sinus, filling the maxillary sinus with pus. The cat's eye may swell partly shut, and a lumpy swelling or draining lesion filled with pus can be seen just below the eye. Most owners, however, do not notice the abscesses which occur over the roots of the other teeth. If the upper canines are involved, the root abscess can break out into the nasal cavity, and is not easily detected. Abscessed roots on other teeth sometimes drain to the outside, and may appear to be nonhealing abscesses on the face, or ones that heal, then recur. If you notice any of these signs, or discolored teeth, have your cat checked. If you do not wish to have root canal surgery performed, or cannot find a veterinarian to do it, or cannot afford it, simply have the tooth extracted.

The cat can do quite well without any teeth. It will raise its head and work food back into its mouth with its tongue. However, if one or both of the canine teeth are taken out, the tongue may loll out of the mouth and the face becomes misshapen. In some cases, root canal therapy (endodontic treatment) can save teeth that would otherwise be removed.

There are five steps to root canal therapy. The condition is diagnosed by dental exploration and X-rays. The cat is anesthetized and the veterinarian will go into the pulp chamber inside the tooth. The root canal is cleaned, using special instruments to remove dead tissue. Then, it is sealed with a surface restorative sealer. After surgery, the cat will be given antibiotics to help prevent infection. It should have soft food for the first week after surgery. Contact your veterinarian if there is excessive bleeding or swelling of the gums, or if the cat shows pain or is reluctant to eat after you bring it home. Many veterinarians X-ray the treated tooth six months later to make sure the procedure was successful.

TEETH CLEANING

A healthy mouth should have clean, white teeth with coral pink gum tissue tightly and evenly surrounding them. The breath should have an acceptable odor. Early signs of dental disease include yellowing of the teeth and bad breath. The gum tissue may be reddened, especially where it adjoins the teeth. As the gum disease progresses, the separation of the gum tissue from the tooth becomes irreversible. It is an indication of shrinking bone mass in the jaw, and loss of ligament support of the tooth. In the later stages of periodontal ("tooth-surrounding") disease, the teeth are very yellowed, and may be loose. The breath has a fetid or "rotten" odor. The gum tissue is swollen, with areas of ulceration; it is softening and may separate from the neck of the tooth. At this point the teeth may be loosened or fall out completely. The gums can be extremely sore, and the cat may refuse to eat. One hundred percent of older cats that are fed soft food will develop periodontal disease. Diseased teeth are nothing new—evidence of it has been found in cat skulls from Pharonic Egypt (Harvey and Alston, 1990).

Cats rarely get cavities, but they do develop tartar accumulations which can lead to periodontal disease. This is a lot worse than cavities, because it can cause kidney disease, heart infections, and other disease problems. Routine dental care is usually not necessary for a younger cat. Cats five or more years old should have their teeth checked frequently. Examine the cat's mouth once a month. Look for an accumulation of plaque or tartar around the gum area. Plaque is a colorless, yellow, gray, or greenish bacteria-filled scum or growth on the teeth around the gum line. Plaque can be scraped off with your fingernail or a soft object such as a wooden toothpick. Plaque forms rapidly and is basically unavoidable (Watson, 1994). If plaque stays on the teeth for a long time, it will accumulate bacteria and minerals, which harden it into tartar. This hard, rocklike substance is NOT easily removed with a fingernail. Tartar shows the same unhealthy colors. Both can be accompanied by a foul odor.

Either plaque or tartar can cause infection along the gum line. Neglected, infection will work its way along the tooth, under the gum line. In time, it will undermine the entire root of the tooth. At that point, bacteria contained within the infected mass can be picked up by the bloodstream and carried throughout the body, causing infection in the kidneys, heart valves, and elsewhere. In fact, periodontal disease is a leading cause of kidney disease in older cats. Routine dental maintenance is an inexpensive investment in continuing good health for your cat in its old age.

Periodontal disease causes perhaps 95% of bad breath in cats. Even some cases of vomiting and diarrhea may be due to gum disease. Painful teeth may cause the cat to be upset when its head or face are handled, and the cat may be irritable and grouchy. Occasionally, an abscess on the face may be due to an infected tooth.

Gingivitis and stomatitis are general terms used to describe infection of the gums and tongue. They also may extend to the cheeks and under the tongue, where painful sores or ulcers make it difficult or impossible for the cat to eat or groom. The inside of the mouth may be fiery red. The cat should have a complete laboratory exam to be sure there are no complicating diseases such as feline leukemia. Extensive periodontal care may be necessary, including removal of all the teeth. About 85% of cats have gum disease. Some of them are helped by antibiotics, while others may get relief from the use of steroids. Current thinking is that many of these unhealing gum infections are autoimmune reactions to some component in the cat's own teeth. For some cats, the only cure is removing all teeth.

Keep an eye on your cat's teeth to make sure they stay healthy throughout its lifetime. If the cat will chew on bones, give it the bone from a round steak. Do NOT give your cat poultry leg bones or the bones from pork chops, as it may splinter them and swallow the pieces. Chewing provides cleansing action for the teeth and exercise for the small ligamentous fibers which help hold the teeth in place. Many cats do not care to chew on bones and, for them, medical care may be needed.

Cats that have misaligned teeth often have trouble keeping their teeth clean and may need more frequent professional care by your veterinarian. Most cats lose incisors from time to time throughout their life. These front teeth are tiny, poorly attached, and unnecessary when eating. You probably won't even notice they're gone. The only time their loss is a problem is if you are showing the cat.

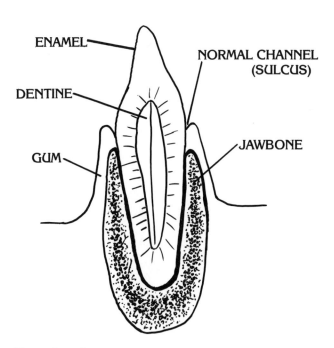

Normal tooth anatomy.

Why does periodontal disease occur? Where the gum meets the tooth, a narrow groove is formed. It is easily filled with soft food material. Mixed with saliva and bacteria normally found in the mouth, food builds up within the groove and sticks to the surface of the tooth. When plaque is first formed, it is soft and only slightly stuck to the teeth. It can easily be removed by brushing the cat's teeth, or by the cat as it chews dry food or bones. Gum disease will occur if the plaque is not promptly removed.

Plaque is the perfect place for bacteria to grow and prosper. The rotting food, along with the dead bacteria and waste products, causes huge quantities of white blood cells to invade the gums around the tooth. The gums become inflamed. Minerals seep from the inflamed gums into the plaque, settling out to form a material called calculus. Plaque and calculus together are sometimes called dental tartar. If the buildup of calculus is allowed to continue, the material accumulates along with the dead white blood cells, forming a pocket of pus around the root of the tooth. This pocket begins to separate the gum from the tooth, forming a larger channel between the gum and the tooth. Still more food material gets packed into the space, and the process accelerates. This debris eventually becomes so toxic that it kills the tissues surrounding the diseased tooth. The thin, bony walls that hold the tooth in place begin to erode, loosening the tooth.

If not treated, periodontal disease becomes progressively worse. The erosion process will eventually involve the whole bony socket holding the tooth. When it is no longer adequately attached, the tooth falls out. Now the hole is large enough that the cat can clean it out with its tongue. The food, debris, and pus disappear, the inflammation subsides, the hole fills with scar tissue, and the cat has one less tooth. However, the likelihood of having only one tooth involved is small. Chances are very good that the entire mouth and all of the teeth are undergoing the same process. If this is the case, it's only a matter of time before all the teeth fall out.

Cats' teeth are more likely to have problems with decay than dogs' teeth. This is perhaps because cats are less likely to chew on hard objects on a regular basis. It may also be because many owners are not aware that the cat's teeth need careful, regular attention.

Many factors may contribute to dental disease in the cat. Among them are feeding canned or semi-moist cat foods. High sugar levels in the soft-moist products may add to dental disease. Human sweets, such as ice cream, are as harmful to cats' teeth as they are to human teeth. A diet high in raw liver may increase gum inflammation in young cats (Seawright, 1974). Prepared and processed foods accumulate at the gum line due to the shape of feline teeth, which were originally meant to tear at meat. As the wild cat eats animals and birds, its teeth rip through the feathers and crunch at the small mousie bones, all of which act as natural toothbrushes and toothpicks. Advancing age seems to contribute to the development of tartar. Cats that chew and bite at their coats and eat large amounts of hair have more problems with tartar, as do cats with crowded or misaligned teeth.

Basically, any condition that contributes to dirty teeth is a potential cause of periodontal disease. Cats that are on soft diets are especially in need of frequent dental cleaning. When you begin to notice tartar or plaque accumulation, it is time to take action. Dental disease develops over a long period of time. If the process is interrupted often enough, the various factors will never accumulate to the point where they cause problems. If the factors can be interrupted every 24 hours or so, progress of the disease can be stopped. It is important to regularly inspect your cat's mouth to make sure there are no problem areas. It will also allow you to obtain prompt veterinary help when you find the teeth need cleaning or care.

It is best to brush the cat's teeth daily, or every other day at the latest, especially with older cats. Studies have shown that brushing even once or twice a week is helpful in reducing plaque and gum disease.

Soft tartar can be easily removed by gently brushing the cat's teeth. Brushing the cat's teeth may seem ridiculous, but taking care of the mouth isn't pampering—it is protection against serious health problems. It can greatly help the cat's comfort, as well as saving you a considerable amount on veterinary bills. Use a very soft child-sized or preschool toothbrush, or one especially made for cats, with a convenient size and angle. The latter are very soft (even softer than a child's toothbrush) to ensure the cat is

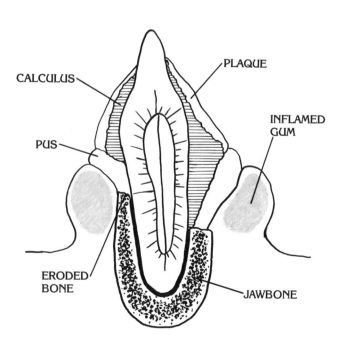

Gums recede as periodontal disease becomes worse.

not irritated by the brushing and will tolerate the process. A piece of damp cloth or gauze or the corner of a washcloth wrapped around the end of your finger can also be used. Brushes are made that are like a gauze glove which slips over your finger. Soft foam swabs are also available for cleaning cat's teeth, or you can use a cotton swab, either by itself or with a bit of gauze wrapped around it. A few cats, with some gentle coaxing, may tolerate a quiet battery-powered toothbrush.

It is a good idea to use a toothpaste made especially for cats. Some of them are even beef or malt flavored, which seem quite acceptable. Other cats prefer mint flavor. C.E.T.® Animal Prophypaste (Veterinary Prescription, St. JON Labs, Inc., Harbor City, CA 90710) is an example of a more abrasive toothpaste which will help remove moderate buildups of plaque and tartar. Most of these products do not need to be rinsed out of the mouth, which is very convenient. There are also powdered products that can be squirted into the cat's mouth to help reduce the quantity of tartar and bacteria present. Human toothpaste is not good to use on cats because it contains ingredients which cause excessive foaming in the mouth, and which can cause stomach problems or vomiting if they are swallowed. It's hard to teach a cat to spit! Baking soda and salt have been recommended for brushing cats' teeth. However, both have a high level of sodium and may cause problems with some cats, especially those with heart disease. Oral hygiene sprays are available which do not need to be rinsed from the cat's mouth, and can be used with a brush or gauze.

Train your cat to accept brushing from an early age. Begin to teach it about brushing by handling its mouth for several minutes each day. After several days, hold the mouth gently closed with one hand, lift the lip on one side of the mouth, and brush the outside surfaces of the teeth. A circular motion is most effective, although a back-and-forth motion can be used. Be sure to brush all three surfaces—the cheek side, the tongue side, and the biting surface. Brush a few more teeth each time, until your cat cooperates willingly with the procedure. You can hold the cat gently but firmly, either on its back, or upright, under your arm.

To clean the inside surfaces of the teeth, place your hand over the muzzle from the top. Gently squeeze and push the cheeks on one side between the back teeth. This will help keep the mouth open. At the same time, pull the head back gently but firmly so the mouth will remain open. Do not pull it back too far or the cat will struggle. Then brush the inside surface of the teeth on the opposite side. Repeat the process for the other side. When you and the pet have become accustomed to the procedure, it should only take one or two minutes. If you have a small cat that is not cooperating, wrap it completely in a towel or blanket, with just the head sticking out. Be careful not to brush too hard and injure the gums. Remember, you are brushing teeth about a tenth or twentieth of your size. The gums may bleed when you first start brushing. This indicates that some gum infection is present. It will stop in two to three weeks, when the teeth are well cleaned and the gums are beginning to heal and return to normal.

Brushing teeth should be a pleasant routine for the cat. It is good to pick a time when you are both relaxed, such as after the evening meal. Give the cat plenty of praise and attention for allowing you to brush its teeth, and occasionally give the cat a small, non-sugary treat. Start brushing the teeth with plain water or chicken or beef broth to get started. Or, save the juice from water-packed tuna, and mix a little bit of it with water to give a slight tuna taste. Some cats will tolerate a bit of garlic salt sprinkled on a moistened piece of gauze in the beginning and can be switched to a toothpaste or powder later.

Oral cleansing solutions are available for use in the cat's mouth if you are not inclined to brush its teeth. One, for example, contains chlorhexidine (Nolvadent Oral Cleansing Solution®, Fort Dodge, KS). This is a powerful disinfectant which helps kill plaque-forming bacteria. Using it is simple—place the spout inside the cat's mouth and squeeze a small amount between the teeth and the side of the mouth. Then massage the cheeks over the teeth to spread the liquid over the surface of the teeth. The product also helps eliminate bad breath, much like the mouthwash humans use. You also can use this type of product instead of toothpaste when brushing your cat's teeth. Cats with more advanced dental disease can benefit from the use of a spray or gel containing zinc ascorbate three or four times daily. Rinse the mouth with a chlorhexidine rinse afterward, using it twice daily for two weeks. After the two-week period of intensive treatment, a stannous fluoride gel can be used instead of the chlorhexidine product (Holmstrom, 1992). Oral cleansing is NOT a substitute for regular visits to your veterinarian.

Some biscuit-type products are recommended for keeping the cat's teeth clean. They are better than no oral hygiene, but many cats won't eat them. Whole turkey or chicken necks (cooked to prevent transmitting salmonellosis) make good chews for some cats. Others enjoy rabbit (also cooked). Give chews three or four times a week for best cleaning. Some cats are not inclined to chew on anything. For them, dry food is better than a softer diet. Regular brushing of your cat's teeth is the best form of dental hygiene. If your cat shows signs of aggression such as scratching or biting, stop trying to brush its teeth. Consult your veterinarian, who may be able to help you teach the cat to accept the process.

If the tartar has become hardened, its removal is a job for your veterinarian. Normally, teeth cleaning (dental prophylaxis, sometimes called a "prophy") is done under either a sedative or general anesthetic. This allows your veterinarian to get deep down under the gum line and remove accumulated plaque without causing the cat pain or having to wrestle to restrain it. Removal of deep plaque and tartar is crucial to continued good dental (and physical) health. If your cat is very old, your veterinarian will probably use gas anesthetic so there is minimal risk and the cat will awaken quickly.

Some groomers offer teeth cleaning as a part of their service. However, they are not allowed to administer anesthetic or sedatives. For this reason, the cleaning they perform is cosmetic only and does not adequately clean down into the groove between the teeth and gums. It should NOT be considered adequate dental hygiene for your valued pet. Have the cat's teeth thoroughly cleaned by your veterinarian with the cat adequately sedated so a good job can be done. Studies suggest that antibiotics are not necessary after routine tooth cleaning (Harai, 1991). However, they are probably a good idea if there is severe infection around the teeth.

If infection has already invaded below the gum line, it may have undermined the roots of the teeth and loosened one or more of them. If this has occurred, removal is necessary. Signs of dental problems include swollen, reddened, ulcerated, or bleeding gums. The cat may have bad breath or be reluctant to eat. It may hold food in its mouth, then spit it out and drool. There may be dark spots on the molars, or raised, orangish-red spots inside the mouth. Cats with dental disease may have sudden personality changes. They may become aggressive for no apparent reason, or may be droopy or less willing to play than usual.

Please DO NOT ask your veterinarian to try to "save" the teeth at this point. Chances are good that infection has invaded much of the surrounding tissue, and perhaps even the bone in the area. Removing the tooth is the best insurance against future kidney and heart problems. Tooth removal is also a good idea if the cat has infected teeth and you are unable to brush its teeth or otherwise care for them.

In severe cases of dental disease, a number of teeth may be pulled in one session. This is easier on the cat than anesthetizing it twice. If they're that bad, they needed to come out and probably were easily pulled. A cat CAN eat without any teeth. It will lap the food into its mouth with its tongue, and then lift the mouth upward (much like a chicken drinking) before swallowing it. If you think about it, cats rarely chew their food, anyway. Most veterinarians try to preserve the canine teeth (eyeteeth) if possible. However, if preservation is not possible, it is better to remove these teeth than leave them as a source of infection.

Other health problems may show up in the cat's mouth. A cat that is reluctant to eat and has an ulcerated mouth may have kidney disease or diabetes. Some tumors may show up as sores or swelling on the mucous membranes and tongue. If your cat has any of these signs, or if it has a sore in its mouth that does not heal, have the cat checked by your veterinarian as soon as possible.

TOOTHACHE

Your cat will not tell you it has a toothache! You might notice it is not chewing its food as much as it used to. The cat may mouth it and wallow it around with tongue and lips, or it may scratch or paw at the affected side, or rub it along the floor or ground. The cat may drool reddish or brownish saliva, and may have an extremely foul odor in its mouth, as well as being quite grouchy and resistant to having its head handled.

These also can be signs that the cat has a foreign object, such as a sliver of poultry bone, caught between its teeth or wedged across the roof of its mouth. Also, plant slivers, grass blades, or awns may be caught in the roof of the mouth or between the teeth. The gums may be reddened and bleeding. You may be able to remove the object with a fingernail or pair of needle-nosed pliers. Other problems can cause painful chewing, including abscesses behind the eye, abscessed tooth roots, or broken teeth or jawbones.

Before you examine the cat's mouth, think of rabies. Cats with rabies may drip saliva, and may appear unable to swallow. These symptoms may cause you to think the cat has something caught in its mouth. IF YOU HAVE ANY REASON TO BELIEVE YOUR CAT MAY HAVE RABIES, OR IF YOU LIVE IN AN AREA WHERE RABIES IS COMMON, DO NOT EXAMINE THE CAT'S MOUTH. TAKE IT TO A VETERINARIAN IMMEDIATELY. Rabies is especially high on the list of possibilities if the mouth problems are accompanied by a change in the animal's voice, behavior, or attitude. (For further information, see Rabies, in Vaccinations Chapter).

To examine the cat, have someone hold it securely. If the cat resists, roll it in a towel. If an object is visible, remove it, using a pair of forceps or clean needlenosed pliers. If the object has been there long enough to cause infection, the area may have a membrane of pus and debris built up over it. This should be gently removed with forceps or teased away from the surface with a cotton swab. All infected areas, as well as the place where the object was resting, can then be wiped with a cotton swab dipped in povidone-iodine solution. Swab the area once or twice a day until it is healed. Antibiotic treatment may be needed if the infection involves a large area, or the cat is not feeling well.

ULCERS IN THE MOUTH

Between three and five months of age, when the cat begins to get its permanent teeth, it may have red, painful gums. This condition is seen either before the teeth erupt from the gums, or while they are doing so. In some cats, the gum tissue keeps growing, to great excess, and may completely cover the teeth by the time the cat is a year old. Surgery may be necessary to remove the overgrown gums.

Cats fewer than nine months of age that were "sickly" as kittens, or had severe upper respiratory disease, may have gum disease. Their gums will be reddened, and may be receding. The teeth are covered with plaque and tartar that one would not expect to see until the cat is much older. These cats may need to have their teeth cleaned every two or three months until they are about two years old. Then, they may outgrow the problem and cleaning can be done on a more normal schedule, once or twice a year. The cat's mouth may have a very foul odor, and the cheeks may be ulcerated.

Thrush is an infection in the mouth caused by a yeast called *Candida albicans*. It may result in ulcers or white, raised plaques. It occurs when the animal's resistance is lowered. While thrush is a disease in itself, it is frequently a symptom of something worse, such as infection with feline leukemia or feline immunodeficiency virus. It may also occur when the animal has been given antibiotics or corticosteroids for a long period of time. If the cat does not recover quickly from the thrush, it should be thoroughly checked by your veterinarian.

A cat may burn its mouth by biting an electric or phone cord, especially a coiled one. This is a particular problem with some kittens that chew on almost anything. Or, the kitten may eat or lick a caustic chemical in solid, powder, or liquid form. If the problem is chemical, rinse the animal's mouth for five to 10 minutes with lukewarm water. The cat can be placed under a sink or bathtub faucet. If you know the chemical is acidic, neutralize it with baking soda. If it is alkaline, neutralize with vinegar or lemon juice. After rinsing and neutralizing, have your veterinarian check the animal. It is possible that some of the chemical was swallowed and damaged the esophagus.

If the cat was not observed biting the cord or drinking the chemical, the first signs may be a cat that does not eat or drink even though it appears hungry or thirsty. Consider rabies (see below, and Rabies section). You may see excessive salivation, and the cat may not want you to handle its mouth or head. The mouth will show reddened membranes.

Keep the cat on a soft or liquid diet until it is healed. Flush the mouth with a solution of 1 teaspoon of salt per pint of lukewarm water. Or, use povidone-iodine solution. In most cases, using ointments on the affected surfaces (unless *Candida* yeast is involved) is of little or no use. Oral or injectable antibiotics may be needed for several days to help prevent the infection from going deeper—consult your veterinarian. Electrical and chemical burns in a cat's mouth can be difficult to heal successfully.

A common house plant, diffenbachia, can cause severe irritation and ulceration in a cat's mouth. Poinsettias also have a sap which is irritating to the cat's mouth.

If the cat gets a strongly acid or alkaline substance on its hair, the cat's mouth can be severely irritated when it tries to lick the material off its coat. The residual material can be neutralized with baking soda or vinegar, depending on which is appropriate. If the cat's mouth is severely irritated, it may be necessary for your veterinarian to give the cat intravenous fluids, B vitamins, and possibly feed it via a stomach tube until it is healed enough to eat on its own.

Ulcers in the mouth may be associated with systemic diseases which reduce the animal's resistance. They can also be seen with kidney disease and diabetes as well as with foreign objects, and with damaged, fractured, irregular, or diseased teeth. Large accumulations of tartar may abrade the cheek or tongue and cause ulcers. The treatment of ulcers is the same as for foreign bodies between the teeth. Deal with any underlying diseases and apply local treatment to the lesions in the mouth.

ORAL TUMORS

Oral tumors sometimes occur in cats. These are often seen as a single ulcerated lesion with no other symptoms. Most of these are squamous cell carcinomas. Research on inoperable oral tumors is being done at the University of Florida College of Veterinary Medicine. New medication is being tried to extend the life of these cats and to improve its quality. Call them if your cat has this type of tumor.

These tumors are usually seen in older cats, and most of them are malignant. "Malignant" means the tumors will grow rapidly and spread to other parts of the body. The most common tumors are lymphomas (which are also the most common in other parts of the digestive tract). Perhaps the next most common are squamous cell carcinomas (SCC). These often cause hard, bony swellings on the face. In the mouth, SCCs may cause abnormal, irregular growths or swellings. Unfortunately, by the time they are discovered, they are far enough advanced that they are rapidly fatal. Gum disease may occasionally cause a hard, non-painful swelling.

Since "benign" tumors (ones that are slow-growing, and don't tend to invade the tissues or spread to other parts of the body) are uncommon, it is very important that any abnormal growth in your cat's mouth be examined as soon as possible, and probably removed at the earliest opportunity. All lumps should be considered malignant until proven otherwise. Cryosurgery (freezing) is often used for removal. It has a low risk to the animal and helps to conserve tissue in the mouth. In some cases, radiation therapy is useful when combined with surgical removal of as much of the tumor as possible.

Cats sometimes develop polyps in the nasal passages and the pharynx. Some of them may become large enough that they hinder swallowing or breathing. They also may cause sneezing. It may be necessary to X-ray the cat to diagnose this condition.

VOMITING

Vomiting begins when the cat becomes nauseated. Early signs include licking the lips, stretching the neck forward, restlessness, excessive salivation, and swallowing. The cat may breathe deeply and gasp, open and close its mouth, and finally vomit. The vomiting cat has strong abdominal contractions.

Vomiting should be distinguished from regurgitation, where the cat voluntarily empties its stomach contents. Regurgitation is fairly common in cats. Because of the structure of the stomach and esophagus and the type of muscle of which they are made, cats can regurgitate voluntarily and with little discomfort. Almost all cats regurgitate from time to time.

Vomiting can occur from causes which have nothing to do with digestive tract illness. Cats may vomit because they have become excited after eating (such as with vigorous play). Some cats can't tolerate semi-moist foods, and will immediately vomit them. They sometimes vomit if they become very thirsty or hungry, and then overdrink or overeat. The cat may be a glutton that gulps its food, stuffing the esophagus full more rapidly than it can empty into the stomach. So, the food comes back up.

Cats can also vomit to get rid of foods they do not like. Sudden changes in diet may cause vomiting. Cats also will vomit to get rid of garbage or food which has spoiled from being in the dish too long. They may vomit from eating pieces of bone or junk like aluminum foil and plastic. Cats vomit because they have eaten grass or because they have a hairball. Cats also may vomit because of motion sickness. So, occasional vomiting is not a cause for alarm, especially if you can see a reason for it. In these cases, the cat usually vomits once and then is normal. It is both unnecessary and unrealistic to examine every cat that vomits once.

Frequent vomiting, on the other hand, should be cause for concern, because it can be a sign of many diseases. Be sure to check a vomiting cat (or one with diarrhea) for dehydration. Pick up a pinch of skin over the cat's ribs between your thumb and forefinger. Pull it upward until it is snug, pinching it firmly together. Then release it and let it return. If the cat is normally hydrated, it will quickly flatten to normal. If the cat is dehydrated, it will stay puckered up, or return very slowly to normal.

If your cat has vomited for one of the above reasons, keep it off food and water for a couple of hours. During this period, you can give it ice cubes to lick, or just 1 or 2 tablespoons of water in the bottom of a dish so it cannot overload. Drugs such as Maalox®, Kaopectate®, and Pepto-Bismol® can be given to coat the stomach (see below for dosages). After a couple of hours, give water, about one-third cup at a time. The cat may WANT more than this, but if you overload it, the water will come back up again. And, repeated vomiting can irritate the stomach, leading to yet more vomiting. Give water every 10 minutes or so until you have satisfied the cat's thirst and can put out a dish of water. You also can offer salted meat broth. Wait two to three hours (or until the next routine meal) before giving the cat any more food. Resume regular feedings at the next meal if there is no more vomiting.

Spitting up small amounts of whitish or greenish phlegm may mean the stomach is empty at the time of vomiting, or that the cat has been eating grass. It may be due to an irritation in the stomach, or to an infection in the throat or tonsils. In any case, if it persists, have the cat checked by your veterinarian. Some cats eat grass when they have hairballs; it may help them vomit. Unless it happens frequently, don't worry. Vomiting large amounts of bile-laden greenish-yellow phlegm may mean that the cat has intestinal parasites, kidney disease, an infection in the uterus, an intestinal blockage, or an infection or foreign body in the stomach.

Vomiting blood IS a cause for alarm, and your cat should be examined as soon as possible. The vomit may be bright or dark red, brown (looking like coffee grounds), or black. Frequent vomiting is also a reason to have the cat examined, even if the amount of vomit is small in quantity. When accompanied by depression, listlessness, and fever, vomiting is often the sign of a systemic disease. The cat should be checked the same day, if at all possible. Disease of the pancreas will cause vomiting, as will liver disease and infectious diseases such as feline distemper. Vomiting can be an early sign of heart failure. It is one of the most frequent signs of inflammatory bowel disease (accompanied by diarrhea). It occurs with diseases such as kidney failure, diabetes, hyperthyroidism, and pyometra (uterine infection). With these diseases, the cat also may be drinking more water and urinating more than normal. Vomiting accompanied by weakness, depression, frequent (but unsuccessful) attempts to urinate, bloody stools, or severe abdominal pain are also indications for an immediate visit to your veterinarian.

Cats that vomit lose fluid, which can result in dehydration and electrolyte imbalance. Intravenous fluids may be necessary to rehydrate the animal. They may also lose sodium, chloride, and potassium. Loss of potassium may cause weakness and an irregular heartbeat. A cat that vomits more than a couple of times should be examined to find the reason.

Cats that have swallowed a foreign object (a toy, coin, yarn, etc.) will vomit, usually a short time after they have eaten. They may otherwise appear normal. Have the cat checked. X-rays may be needed to determine whether a foreign body in the stomach is the problem. Make sure that toys for your cat are too large to be swallowed. The cat should not be allowed to chew small pieces of childrens' toys, either. Other tests may be needed to determine why a cat continues to vomit. These include laboratory blood work, test diets, and abdominal ultrasound. Endoscopy, which uses a long, lighted tube to look directly into the cat's stomach, may be useful. In the worst cases, an exploratory laparotomy may be done. This is surgery to take a look into the abdominal cavity to see what is wrong, and may be needed if other tests do not give answers and vomiting continues.

Dosages of medications to help control vomiting and soothe the stomach are: Pepto-Bismol®—one-half teaspoon per 10 pounds (2.5 milliliters (ml) per 4.5 kilograms (kg)), Kaopectate®—2 teaspoons per 10 pounds (10 ml per 4.5 kg). Give either of these every four hours. Do not give more than 7 ml/kg of Pepto-Bismol per day, as it could possibly cause salicylate toxicity in the cat (Papich, 1987). If you are using Maalox®, give one-half teaspoon per 10 pounds (2.5 ml per 4.5 kg) every eight hours. If your cat is on any other medication, consult your veterinarian before giving any treatment. Why? 1) The medication may be causing the vomiting; and 2) The vomiting may prevent absorption of the drug, and it may be necessary to change to an injectable form until the vomiting is under control.

HAIRBALLS

Hairballs are wads of undigested hair that have reached the cat's stomach and not proceeded through the digestive system. Hairballs occur because cats groom themselves. The tiny, rough barbs on the tongue face backward, making it easier to swallow the fur which the cat has combed out of its coat than to spit it out.

Every cat continually sheds small amounts of hair. In addition, when hot weather arrives in the spring, a cat may shed much of its coat. Hairballs are as much of a problem for shorthaired cats as they are for the longhairs. Since the cat may spend one-third of its waking hours grooming, there is plenty of opportunity for hairballs.

When the cat swallows a small amount of fur, it passes harmlessly through its digestive tract (and probably acts as fiber in the diet, too). If the cat is eating large amounts of hair, it may form a wad or ball in the stomach, instead of passing on down the digestive tract. The cat may simply vomit up this mass, usually on your white carpet! If the cat is otherwise feeling fine, there is no problem. Sometimes, a cat with a hairball in its stomach will eat grass, then vomit the mass of grass and hair. Or, it may eat a large amount of dry food and then vomit both it and the hair. Rarely, a large ball of hair will accumulate in the stomach and stay there, or clump together elsewhere in the gut. This can be much more serious, as it may interfere with the cat's digestion or elimination. In the worst cases, an obstruction may form between the stomach and lower intestine, resulting in a fatal strangulation. This, fortunately, is rare.

A cat with hairballs may have a hacking cough and make retching motions, as if trying to vomit. It may vomit greenish-yellow fluid which includes some hair. Or, the cat may have trouble keeping meals down, vomiting soon after eating. In some cases, the cat may have a touch of intermittent diarrhea. It may be depressed and lose its appetite.

Most cats will vomit hair from time to time. This may be a small bit of hair in a bit of clear or greenish phlegm, or it may be a larger, tubular-shaped "hairball." Either this will cure the problem or further treatment may be needed. Hairballs are at best uncomfortable. At worst, more serious complications may follow. Some cats that are itching badly may groom excessively, and will vomit hairballs, or pass excessive hair in the feces.

The simplest cure is to use a commercial cat laxative (such as Laxatone, Kittymalt or Petromalt) to help move the hair on through the digestive tract. The laxative does not dissolve the hairball—it just passes it on through the system. These products come in a tube or pump dispenser and are flavored so that most cats eat them willingly. Some cats will lap the gel from the tube or your finger. For those that do not, simply mash the gooey paste into the fur of the cat's front leg, about an inch up from its paw. Do this in a bathroom or place where, if the cat shakes some off or rubs against furniture, it will not make a mess. The cat will lick the "offending" substance off its fur, taking it in as it does so. After a few days of feeding, most cats will willingly lick the substance from your finger or right from the tube. About an inch and a half of the laxative is sufficient for the average cat. Give it once a day, about an hour before mealtime. Feed the laxative daily for five to seven days, until symptoms disappear, or the worst of shedding season is over. Then, use it once or twice a week. The laxative should not be mixed with food or given with meals. Any hairball remedy should be given between meals.

Be sure to consult your veterinarian if the cat is not feeling well, if vomiting continues, or if the cat is not noticeably better after the five days of treatment.

The best long-term cure for hairballs is regular grooming, whether your cat has short or long hair. It is especially important for long-haired breeds such as Persians and Himalayans. It is even more necessary in the spring when the cat is shedding its winter coat. A little brushing every day or two can reduce, or even completely eliminate hairballs. Use a soft brush, a comb, a grooming mitt or rough cloth, or even your hands to remove loose hair before the cat can lick it off. Any grooming tool is helpful as long as it gently removes loose fur without hurting the cat. If you train the cat to accept it, you can even use your vacuum cleaner. A cat that is outdoors also can use a bit of grooming help—the wind and rough weeds are not always enough to get rid of dead hairs.

Some publications recommend home remedies such as mineral oil or butter. Mineral oil can be fatal to your cat because it cannot taste it. The oil may go down its windpipe into its lungs, causing a fatal pneumonia. Butter is usually digested before it can do much good. Either of these may cause diarrhea. If you are going to use a home remedy, use petroleum jelly, rubbing about a half-teaspoon of it into the fur on the cat's front leg and letting the cat lick it off. Hairballs are usually a sign that the cat needs more help with its grooming—brush the cat often and the problem will usually go away.

ESOPHAGEAL STRICTURES

Constriction of the esophagus is generally due to the presence of scar tissue. The scarring may be because the cat drank or ate a strong acid or alkali. It may occur after a foreign body, such as a bone or toy, has become lodged in the cat's esophagus. Or, it may occur when the cat is anesthetized and food mixed with acid flows backward into the esophagus. This is just one more good reason for a STRICT fast and an EMPTY stomach before your cat goes in for elective surgery. Because it takes some time for scar tissue to develop, strictures may occur weeks to months after the initial injury to the esophagus.

A cat with an esophageal stricture usually cannot eat solid food. The cat may vomit it, while keeping down liquids or gruels. Many of these cats have ravenous appetites, yet lose weight because the food doesn't make it to the stomach. They usually do not show any signs of pain or discomfort.

Your veterinarian will diagnose this problem by giving the cat liquid barium to drink, followed by an X-ray of the esophagus while it is coated by the barium.

Two treatments are available. One is surgery, which may have less than a 50% success rate. The other is to anesthetize the cat and gradually stretch the area to a more normal size by threading dilators through it. This should only be attempted by a veterinarian who is trained in and familiar with the procedure. If your veterinarian is not, ask for a referral to a university hospital or to a surgical specialist who is. Even in the most skilled hands, the procedure occasionally results in further injury and even more scarring.

FOREIGN BODIES IN STOMACH

A foreign body may be anything the cat swallows other than food, water, or medication. The cat may eat metal, wood, rubber, cloth, etc., or may swallow a splinter of bone while chewing on it. The cat may eat a wad of aluminum foil soaked with grease from a barbecue. A kitten may eat a rubber ball, or piece of a child's toy.

Signs associated with the ingestion of foreign bodies are quite variable. Some objects may remain in the stomach for long periods of time without causing illness. Others will cause serious illness almost immediately. The cat may vomit occasionally, especially after it has eaten solid food, and may gradually lose weight. A large, rough object, such as a bone with sharp points, may irritate the stomach severely. It may tear the stomach lining, causing the cat to vomit blood. On rare occasions, the object may completely perforate the stomach wall, causing peritonitis.

Surprisingly, cats are able to pass many odd items without damage. So, if you see your cat swallow something, do not try to get it to vomit. The anatomy of the stomach is such that it will probably not come back up. Wait and see if vomiting develops. Also, watch the stools for a few days to see whether the object passes. If the cat has swallowed string, cut off any that is still in its mouth or hanging out of it. Watch to make absolutely sure the rest of it is passed.

A history of swallowing various objects, or of intermittent vomiting after meals, is suggestive of a foreign body in the stomach. Your veterinarian will probably diagnose the foreign body by taking an X-ray. The object may be visible on a plain film, or it may be necessary to give barium, which will coat the object and make it visible.

Some small objects can be removed from the stomach by passing an endoscope and pulling the object through it. Larger objects may require abdominal surgery for removal. If surgery is necessary, have it done soon, while the cat is still in good condition. Don't let your cat go downhill until it is unable to tolerate the surgery.

DIARRHEA

Diarrhea is a common problem in small animals. In the cat, it is seen as abnormally frequent, watery bowel movements, which may be reddish-brown or brown in color. These may also contain mucus, blood, undigested food or worms. The cat may have a poor appetite or completely stop eating. Its bowel movements may be quite urgent, and it may not make it to the litter box in time, leaving watery feces on the floor. The cat may keep straining after it is finished defecating. If you notice straining, check the cat to be sure it does have either constipation or diarrhea. The straining may be due to a urinary tract blockage (especially in male cats), and failure to get prompt treatment can lead to serious kidney damage, or even death (see Urinary Tract Chapter).

Most often, diarrhea is a temporary problem caused by dietary factors. For example, raw eggs can cause diarrhea in some cats. Milk or rich gravies may cause diarrhea when they are added to the cat's food, or fed along with it. Removal of the offending food will usually stop this type of diarrhea. Excessive quantities of fats or oils in the diet also may cause diarrhea. If you are feeding fats or oil to deal with coat dryness or to provide extra calories, be sure to add it to the diet gradually, increasing to the amount you wish to feed over a two-week period. If diarrhea occurs, reduce the quantity given to the point where diarrhea stops.

A change in food can cause diarrhea, especially if the change is made suddenly. Eating garbage or spoiled food may cause diarrhea as well. Are you or your neighbors feeding your cat inappropriate foods? Some purebred cats have delicate digestive systems and are easily upset by even minor changes in diet, resulting in vomiting and/or diarrhea. Table foods, especially if they are spicy, cause problems for some cats. Other cats have diarrhea when given foods to which they are allergic. A change of water or routine while traveling may cause diarrhea, as can fright or nervousness from being in unfamiliar surroundings.

Treatment with antibiotics may kill bacteria in the intestine or change the kind and quantity. This may cause diarrhea. If your cat is on medication and develops diarrhea, check with your veterinarian, who may be able to prescribe a different drug.

Some types of worms and other intestinal parasites can cause diarrhea. It may be a chronic, continuous diarrhea, or it may come and go between periods of normal stools. Diarrhea caused by internal parasites may be bloody and should be checked by your veterinarian. Some parasites which cause diarrhea in cats (and dogs) are contagious to humans. For this reason, it is important to determine whether parasites are causing a cat's diarrhea, especially if it comes and goes, or does not clear up with home treatment.

Viruses and bacteria can cause diarrhea, and some of them are contagious from one cat to another. A profuse bloody diarrhea is one of the most prominent symptoms of feline distemper (panleukopenia) infection, which occurs most commonly in young unvaccinated cats. Distemper requires aggressive treatment, often including intravenous fluids. In some cases, diarrhea may accompany respiratory disease. Chemical poisonings can cause diarrhea, but, fortunately, they are quite rare because cats are generally finicky eaters. Colitis (an inflammation of the large intestine) is also a relatively common cause of diarrhea.

If the diarrhea is mild and the cat has no other symptoms, keep it off food for the rest of the day. Give a medication such as Pepto-Bismol® or Kaopectate® in the same dosages used to control vomiting (see above). If the diarrhea persists, is bloody, or if the cat otherwise shows illness, have it examined by your veterinarian.

Medium-sized and adult cats with diarrhea should be taken off food for 12 hours. They can be given clear broth after five to six hours, but no solid food until the next day. Then they should have frequent small meals of a highly digestible food. Kittens have very few reserves to protect them against the weakness and dehydration that can accompany diarrhea. They should be given small amounts of food at regular intervals and their condition should be closely watched. Both kittens and adult cats must have water available at all times to help avoid dehydration.

After 12 hours, start the cat back on four to five small meals a day of its regular food, gradually working up to normal feeding quantities and times. Or, for a couple of days, you can use a food which is specially made for digestive tract problems. This type of food will contain only a small percentage of fiber, often less than 1%. If your cat has colitis, a diet high in fiber may be needed instead.

Carbohydrates in the diet should be easily digested, as from dextrose or rice. Also, the diet should provide a moderate amount of highly digestible protein, and should be low in fat. Do not give any food which contains bran, wheat middlings, other cereal by-products or lactose (milk sugar). Avoid all table scraps and snacks until the cat is well. These foods may complicate diarrhea and prolong healing. During the recovery period, feed frequent small amounts of fresh food, three to six times a day.

Contact your veterinarian if diarrhea lasts more than 48 hours or if the cat shows signs of general systemic illness, such as vomiting, listlessness, depression, fever, etc. Do NOT deprive a cat of food for more than two days.

Some cats with severe dehydration will need intravenous fluids to stabilize their condition before the cause of the diarrhea can be determined. Check the cat for dehydration by picking up a pinch of the skin over the ribs between your thumb and forefinger. Pull it upward about an inch, hold it there for a few seconds, and let it go. In the normal cat, it should spring back fairly quickly and stretch itself flat. In the dehydrated cat, the little ridge of skin will just stand there, or it may take five to 10 seconds to flatten back to normal.

If the diarrhea goes on for a long period of time, your veterinarian may wish to take a biopsy of the intestine. This procedure is done under sedation or general anesthetic. A tiny section of tissue will be removed through a small surgical opening made in the abdominal wall. Only a stitch or two will be needed to close the opening.

Chronic diarrhea is often seen in young cats, especially those from pet shops or shelters or, occasionally, from breeders. They may have eaten spoiled food or have worms. Home treatment can sometimes lead to chronic diarrhea. If someone gives the cat a course of broad-spectrum antibiotics, which changes the water flow inside the intestine, it appears to "cure" the diarrhea. However, when the treatment is complete, the cat still has diarrhea so perhaps the person changes the diet (or the antibiotic). This might happen three or four times. By this time, the normal bacteria in the cat's intestine have been killed and unusual varieties of bacteria have taken over the gut. For some kittens, all that is necessary is to give their intestinal bacteria time to return to normal. Giving the cat lactobacillus from your health food store may help. In some cases, it may be necessary for your veterinarian to treat the cat with metronidazole. If the cat is on dry food, try switching to canned food.

Diets with large quantities of modified food starch sometimes cause diarrhea. Cats with intestinal problems do best on high-fat diets. Science Diet® and Iams® foods work well for many cats. Cats with diarrhea should be taken off high-sugar content soft-moist foods.

Treatment with oral antibiotics for routine diarrhea may not help the diarrhea. At worst, it may allow the overgrowth of salmonella bacteria, causing salmonellosis. Only 2-4% of diarrhea has been proven to be caused by bacteria. For this reason, it's not a good idea to throw antibiotics at every cat with diarrhea. Neomycin, one of the most commonly used oral antibiotics, may also be the one that causes the most continuing problems. It has been shown to actually cause diarrhea, at least in humans, by killing the normal bacteria. Other antibiotics such as gentamicin, erythromycin, and amoxicillin may also help continue the diarrhea or make it worse. Changing the cat to a diet with a different protein, such as lamb and rice, cures many cats (Burrows, 1989). Some cats may be helped by giving them a small amount of a fiber product such as Metamucil.

Because cats with diarrhea may lack vitamins that have been flushed from the body, it is always a good idea to give them extra vitamins. It may be necessary for your veterinarian to give an injection of fat-soluble vitamins; water-soluble ones can usually be given orally.

Diarrhea in an adult cat which does not improve within a few days may be due to inflammatory bowel disease. This may occur with or without vomiting. It may be due to disease of the pancreas or liver. Or, it may be due to a serious disease such as lymphoma. Have your cat checked by your veterinarian.

SALMONELLOSIS

This disease can sometimes infect cats. It has been reported in the northeastern states as "songbird fever." It occurs when the cat eats a bird that is infected with *Salmonella* bacteria. The disease occurs suddenly, five to seven days after the cat eats the bird. It can also be seen when large numbers of cats are kept closely confined with poor sanitation. Under these conditions, adult cats may not show any obvious signs of disease, but kittens may become ill.

The cat will have a fever, as much as 104 to 105 degrees F (40-40.5 C). A few cats may go as high as 108 F (42.1 C). The fever lasts from two to seven days. Because of both the fever and the infection, the cat may be severely depressed, and may completely lose its appetite. Some cats may vomit, and diarrhea is common with severe cases. The symptoms may make this look much like feline distemper (panleukopenia). Cats with severe acute infections may die suddenly. For this reason, cats with acute salmonellosis should be hospitalized and treated aggressively if they are to survive. Milder cases have fever with nonspecific signs of illness. These cats recover in three to five days.

Some types of salmonella spread easily to humans and may cause serious illness. If your cat has this disease, keep it confined to an area that you can easily clean. Wash and disinfect the litter box frequently until the cat is completely well, and then for three to four months more, as the cat may still shed the bacteria from its intestine even though there are no obvious disease symptoms. Be sure to wash your hands after each time you handle the cat, and especially before you eat, drink, or smoke. These precautions are a good idea when dealing with any pet with diarrhea. While a considerable number of cats carry salmonella in their intestinal tracts, human infections from them are uncommon. When infection of both cats and humans occurs in the household at the same time, they may both have come from a common source, such as contaminated, inadequately cooked meat.

This disease can be prevented by keeping the cat from eating birds (another reason to have an indoor cat!). Keep it away from areas around bird feeders if the disease is a problem in your part of the country. Thoroughly clean and disinfect bird baths and feeders every few days with a diluted solution of chlorine bleach. One part bleach to 32 parts water works well. Maintain good sanitation in groups of cats.

CAMPYLOBACTERIOSIS

Campylobacter species are bacteria which cause diarrhea in many species of animals. Until a few years ago, this disease was called vibriosis. It is sometimes a problem in young kittens, but is uncommon in adult cats. The kitten may have a poor appetite, and lack the energy to move around or play. Worms may be found on the fecal examination, and be considered the cause of the problem. If after worming, the kitten doesn't get well and still has diarrhea, take your pet back to your veterinarian to be reexamined. It may be necessary to perform laboratory tests on a fresh sample of the soft feces in order to find the bacteria. The diarrhea may last up to a week, but the feces may be soft for another two to four weeks.

The disease is most often seen in kittens six- to 12-weeks-old that have just been weaned. The diarrhea is usually soft and covered with mucus. Occasionally it is thin and watery, and may quickly kill the kitten by dehydration. The kitten usually does not have a fever.

Campylobacteriosis is especially common in kittens and cats from animal shelters, catteries, or other areas where large numbers of cats and dogs are gathered. Some animals, while appearing healthy, may carry the bacteria in the intestinal tract, infecting others with whom they come in contact. Stress lowers the animal's resistance, allowing the disease to start and spread. The infection passes from one animal to another by the oral route, from feces from animals that have the disease, and via contaminated water, unpasteurized milk, and raw or undercooked meat or poultry. The bacterium is normally found in the digestive tracts of many animals, where it causes little or no problem until it contaminates meat or milk. Pasteurization of milk and cooking of meat will kill the organism and prevent its spread. This disease is usually treated with erythromycin or another suitable antibiotic.

One of the biggest problems with campylobacter infection is that it is also contagious to humans, although transmission is uncommon. If your cat has it, the safest course of action is to hospitalize it until the infection is well under control. If you can't do this, keep the cat confined to the smallest area possible, preferably one that is easy to clean. Thoroughly wash and disinfect all containers and materials that come in contact with the cat. Be sure to wash and disinfect your hands after you have handled the cat, or anything that comes into contact with it. Keep children from handling the cat (even petting!) until it is well.

In humans, the disease is more severe in young children, for the same reason it is more dangerous for kittens than adult cats—lack of physical reserves. It causes vomiting, sharp stomach pains, and diarrhea, which may contain mucus (Williams, 1988). It is more commonly spread to humans by contaminated milk, meat, or water than from pet animals. Anyone who has diarrhea after handling a kitten with a similar illness should see a physician.

PROTOZOAL DIARRHEA

Diarrhea caused by protozoan parasites such as *Coccidia* (called coccidiosis), Trichomonas or Giardia is contagious from one cat to another. These organisms are normally present in the digestive tract in very small numbers. They multiply if the cat is stressed or sick, or its digestive tract is irritated by worms or a viral infection. Diarrhea caused by these parasites cannot be treated with wormers, nor are they touched by antibiotics. Some home remedies may help temporarily, but the disease will inevitably return.

These diseases spread from one cat to another by contact with feces from an infected cat. A healthy cat may lick its feet after having walked where a cat with the disease has defecated, becoming infected. It can be spread by contact with contaminated water or food dishes left in pens where sick animals have been held. Protozoal diarrhea is a particular problem where numbers of young kittens are brought together, such as pet shops and kennels.

Cats with protozoal diarrhea have a watery or "mushy" diarrhea (often with much mucus), loss of appetite, and weight loss. Vomiting is sometimes seen. The disease is much more severe in weakened or young animals. It, in turn, can weaken the animal still further, making it susceptible to other diseases.

Your veterinarian will diagnose the disease by examining a fecal sample under the microscope. In some cats, several samples may be needed over a period of a few days, as it can be difficult to find the organisms on a single sample. The organisms tend to occur in waves and aren't present all the time. The cat will be treated with a drug which is specific for protozoan parasites.

Good nursing care will be needed to bring the pet through the disease, especially for a young kitten or very small cat. Keep the cat's cage or yard and its bedding dry, clean, and free of bowel movements because reinfection from it own feces can occur. Feed a high-quality, balanced diet and make sure the cat eats! Encourage the cat to drink, as diarrhea can quickly cause dehydration. Replacement of the lost fluids helps prevent dehydration. Isolate new cats until you are sure they are free from infection. Isolate the affected pet to keep it from spreading the disease. If you have more than one cat, keep the sick one in a cage or kennel so it cannot contaminate the yard, or another cat's food or water dishes. Disinfect runs and kennels with chlorine bleach (diluted 1:32 in water). Give vitamins as needed to help increase the cat's appetite and keep up its strength. Return the cat to your veterinarian for a recheck if it quits eating or drinking, becomes weaker, vomits more than occasionally, or if the diarrhea continues for more than two days without improvement after treatment has been started.

COLITIS

Colitis is a condition in which the large bowel (the colon) becomes inflamed and irritated. It may strike suddenly, or come on gradually over a long period of time. If the problem develops rapidly, it may respond to less than a month of therapy, and heal well. If it has come on gradually, it may be more chronic, lasting for years, or even for the rest of the cat's life.

The inflammation of the colon causes the intestine to be less effective than normal at absorbing water back from the material in the digestive tract. Because of excess water being present, the main sign of colitis is diarrhea. The loose stool may be streaked with blood or mucus. The diarrhea may be continuous, or it may come and go. The bowel movements may be more frequent and more urgent than normal. The cat may otherwise look healthy and act normal. In some cases, the cat may be depressed, have a fever, show abdominal pain and weight loss, and have a dull and dry coat.

There are many possible causes of colitis. A fecal sample should be checked to determine if the cat has any parasites; if any are present, the cat should be treated.

Colitis can be caused by various agents, including bacteria, viruses, parasites, tumors, food allergies, dietary changes, or the ingestion of a foreign body. Colitis should be suspected when your cat does not respond to standard treatment for diarrhea, and if the diarrhea persists for a period of time.

Your veterinarian may need to run an entire battery of tests, including bacterial cultures, fecal exam for intestinal parasites, X-rays (possibly with barium to show irregularities and defects in the intestinal lining), and colonoscopy (visually inspecting the colon with a lighted fiber optic tube inserted into the anus). Biopsy of the colon and exploratory surgery to examine the abdominal organs may be needed. Additional tests may be required throughout the course of the treatment to monitor the cat's progress.

The majority of cases of colitis, especially the chronic ones, cannot be cured. They can, however, in most cases, be managed well enough that the cat can live a nearly normal life.

Two approaches are commonly used to treat colitis. The first approach is to increase the amount of fiber in the animal's diet. Fiber can be, and often is, used to treat constipation. It can also be used to treat the diarrhea of colitis. The fiber stabilizes and lengthens the amount of time material takes to move through the intestine. This allows more water to be absorbed from the food material, and less to be lost in the stool.

The second approach is to feed a hypoallergenic diet to avoid food allergies which may be at the root of the problem. With some cats, it may be necessary to try both diets (high fiber diet and hypoallergenic diet) for a period of time, and then use the one which works the best. A trial of two to six weeks may be needed on each diet in order to give them a fair evaluation. The diarrhea may become worse for several days before the cat's digestive tract stabilizes and adjusts to the new food. Be patient and give it some time. Whatever you are feeding, feed only the prescribed food. Do not feed ANY treats, bones, or anything else. Do not give ANY "people food" at all, or the cat may go back to where it started, a miserable situation for the cat and an expensive proposition for you. Drugs may be used to help control the diarrhea and relieve the inflammation and pain. Azulfidine and metronidazole are sometimes used to treat colitis for which there is no obvious cause and for which no other treatments work. In some cases, antibiotics will be given to control related infections.

INTESTINAL OBSTRUCTION

Intestinal obstruction is occasionally seen in young kittens, and diarrhea may be one of the signs. Any cat with a diarrheal problem which does not clear up rapidly with home treatment, or is accompanied by other signs of illness should be examined by your veterinarian. Laboratory blood and fecal examinations, X-rays (possibly with barium), and other tests may be needed to determine the cause.

Do not let your cat play with string or yarn, as they may cause a fatal intestinal obstruction when swallowed. The most dangerous situation is when the cat eats a piece or wad of thread with the needle still attached. The needle catches in the stomach or upper part of the digestive tract, while the string continues on through the gut. Then the peristaltic action causes the thread to act like a saw, cutting through the intestinal loops. If this isn't diagnosed in time, the cat dies a miserable death. If the cause is found, surgery may possibly save its life. In some cases, the thread may be looped around the base of the tongue. If discovered early enough, it may be possible to cut the loop. In some cases, the wad (and the needle) may then pass through the digestive tract without further harm.

If you find a piece of thread or string looped around the base of the cat's tongue or caught on a tooth, do NOT pull on it, because you could cause severe damage to its digestive tract. Cut the thread VERY carefully, and watch the cat closely. If you are lucky, the cat may pass the material and be fine. If the cat shows ANY signs of illness, including depression, lack of appetite, vomiting, diarrhea, or constipation, have your veterinarian check it as soon as possible. Make it a rule to keep ALL thread, yarn, buttons, sequins, beads, and other sewing materials stored safely away from your cats. Keep wood screws, tacks, small nails, and other building or craft materials put safely away after they are used.

CONSTIPATION

Constipation is a condition where the cat has infrequent stools or strains to pass feces. The bowel movements which are passed may be small, hard, and dry. With constipation, the feces remain in the colon and rectum for an abnormally long time. The walls of the large intestine absorb water to conserve it for the body. So much fluid is absorbed that the feces become very dry. Do not worry if your cat does not have a bowel movement every day. Normal cats, especially if not eating much and not getting much exercise, may only have bowel movements every two to three days. Constipation also should be considered to be a decreased frequency of bowel movements. This may or may not be accompanied by straining. Make sure the straining is not due to diarrhea.

A cat with constipation will pass little or no stool. The cat may be depressed, and may vomit or pass foul-smelling, blood-streaked stools. They may be dry, coated with mucus, or filled with hair. They may be less frequent, and larger or smaller than normal. The cat may have no appetite, and may be depressed. Its abdomen may be bloated and it may feel hard.

EMERGENCY NOTE: It is critically important to determine that your cat (especially if it is a male) is not straining because of a urinary tract blockage. If it is trying to urinate and cannot do so because its urinary tract is plugged by a stone, giving laxative will only cause you to delay getting treatment. This may be fatal to your cat. If the cat is dribbling small amounts of urine, with or without blood, the cat still has a urinary tract problem and should be examined by a veterinarian (see Urinary Chapter).

Constipation is more often related to dietary problems than to any other cause. An irregular or imbalanced diet may cause constipation, and an inadequate water supply is sure to cause it sooner or later, especially if you are feeding a dry food. Remember that the cat's body is 75% water. But, the water doesn't stay put. It keeps coming out the back end so you have to keep it going in the front end. If you are using an automatic or lick-type waterer for outdoor cats, check it every couple of days to make sure that it is functioning normally. Check it once a day in a hot climate, or the cat may die before it has a chance to develop constipation. Or, the cat may drown while trying to get into a bucket, stock tank, or swimming pool as it tries to get a drink.

Pieces of bone, foil, or plastic eaten by the cat may also cause constipation, as will hair or other foreign materials. Long-haired cats should be brushed daily to remove hair which they might otherwise swallow, causing constipation. A cat with a fractured, healed pelvis may have a narrowed opening through which the rectum passes. This may cause the animal problems with constipation, and it may need frequent doses of cat laxative for the rest of its life. Tumors, foreign bodies in the abdomen, and damage to the hind part of the spinal cord also may cause chronic constipation. In an older cat, even a minor dietary change may cause constipation. Low taurine levels may cause constipation because the smooth muscle in the intestinal wall does not contract efficiently. Correcting the taurine deficiency will correct the constipation.

The mere fact that our pet cats are housebroken may be a major contributor to constipation. The better housebroken the animal is, the more it is conditioned to wait for the appropriate place to defecate. If the cat needs to be hospitalized or boarded, it may simply wait. When you take your cat home after a week at the kennel, it may be unable to have a bowel movement because the material in the colon has solidified. When the cat does try, the large, hard, dry stool in the colon is hard to pass. The resulting pain causes reluctance to try to defecate. Sometimes liquid

feces may dribble around the retained stool, resulting in an otherwise constipated cat that has diarrhea. A cat that has recovered from diarrhea may not have a bowel movement for several days, ending up constipated.

Older cats often have trouble with constipation simply because their digestive system is less active. Older cats may exercise less, as well. Changing to a diet with more bulk may be helpful. Prostate disease, nervous disorders of the large intestine, endocrine disorders, and metabolic problems may cause constipation in the older cat, as can tumors in the intestine, colon, rectum or prostate. Have the cat checked by your veterinarian if the problem persists. Dehydration, extreme malnutrition, and debilitation can lead to constipation.

Cats that have had pelvic injuries with subsequent nerve damage or a crushed pelvis which narrows the pelvic opening may also have constipation. These animals may need stool-softening foods or medication for the rest of their lives. This will allow the softened feces to pass more easily through the narrowed opening. Surgery (symphysiectomy) can also be done to enlarge the pelvic opening, allowing the cat to defecate easily. Cats with spinal cord injuries also may have chronic constipation and will need similar treatment.

Long-haired cats may have fecal material caked onto the hair under their tails until they can no longer defecate. This is a horrible, foul-smelling mess, and the only way to fix it is to cut it off. Use clippers or scissors to cut off all the hair at the skin level until the entire mass is removed. Hair may have to be cut from the underside of the tail as well as the hind legs. Then, gently wash the whole area, using povidone-iodine or chlorhexidine solution. Afterward, a soothing cream may be applied. If sores are present, the cat may need injectable or oral antibiotics in addition to the local treatment of the area. Keep the hair in the area clipped to avoid the problem in the future.

Mild cases of constipation may be treated by adding Metamucil® to the food. Give 2 teaspoons per 10 pounds body weight up to a maximum of 2 teaspoons (10 ml per 4.5 kg up to 10 ml maximum). Metamucil® should NOT be used if your cat has kidney disease. Laxative products made for pets are also available. One of these is Laxatone® (Evsco). It comes either in a squeeze tube like toothpaste, or in a pump dispenser. These products are flavored especially for pets, and most cats take them readily. Many cats will lick the medication directly from the tube as you squeeze it out for them. One of my cats licked the laxative off the end of the tube and actually begged for more! One or two teaspoons of canned pumpkin can be mixed with the cat's food as a laxative. It adds insoluble fiber to its diet, and most cats find it quite palatable. You can add bran to the cat's food (one to two tablespoons per can). Petroleum jelly works for many cats—put half a teaspoon of it on the top of the cat's front leg; the cat will lick it off.

Products such as those containing cascara, senna, or castor oil, if given often, may cause the colon to fail to function, permanently. Agents which add bulk to the cat's stool, such as celluloses, gums, and colloids, can safely be given on a long term basis.

DO NOT try to pour mineral oil down your cat's mouth for a laxative. The cat cannot taste it, and instead of swallowing it, may inhale the oil into its lungs. The resulting pneumonia can kill the cat. Another problem with mineral oil is that if given over a period of several days, it will tie up vitamins in the cat's body, and may eventually result in a vitamin deficiency. It is FAR safer to use a pet laxative.

Cats that are straining to pass small quantities of blood-streaked feces may be given a gentle warm water enema with plain tap water, using two to five milliliters per pound of body weight (1-2.5 ml/kg). This can be repeated in 20 to 30 minutes, but not more than twice. There is no advantage in adding soap, as it may irritate the mucosa lining the bowel. Try this no more than twice. If it does not produce results and relief, consult your veterinarian. Commercial phosphate enemas such as Fleet® enemas may be toxic to cats and SHOULD NOT be used.

A cat food containing a higher quantity of fiber will help compensate for a less active digestive tract in the older cat, much as it does in humans. The bulk helps stimulate the walls of the digestive tract, aiding the movement of food materials through the intestine. The fiber also helps hold water in the intestine, softening the stool and making it easier for the cat to have a bowel movement. Don't feed your cat snacks if it is prone to constipation. Finally, the only thing your cat should ever eat, whether it is prone to constipation or not, is clean, wholesome, nutritious food and treats. Keep your cat away from and don't let it chew on, eat, or swallow anything else. Splintering bones, string, yarn, garbage, foil, paper—the list of foreign materials is endless—can all, at one time or another, cause problems.

Last but not least, make sure the cat has a fresh, clean litter box, filled with a material that it finds suitable. Many feline cases of constipation occur when the box is unacceptably dirty, and the cat waits beyond the time at which it would normally defecate. The cat's body absorbs much of the water from the fecal material in the colon, leaving it so hard that the cat cannot easily push it out.

Megacolon is a disorder which occurs mainly in older male cats that are overweight and sedentary. It is seen in cats that have been frequently constipated for months or even years. Failure to defecate leaves the colon distended with feces. When this goes on for a long time, the muscle is stretched to the point where it no longer returns to normal. This stretched, feces-filled colon is called megacolon. In some cases, the constipation may start with dysfunctional nerves to the muscles of the colon. Treatment to keep the cat's stools softened so that they are more easily passed is helpful to these cats. Psyllium laxatives or enemas work for some animals. Drugs such as cisapride are helpful to some cats.

When drug therapy is not successful, surgery to remove 90-95% of the colon may be a safe cure. This leaves the cat with a watery diarrhea for a short time. With time (within one to 12 weeks), the cat's fecal consistency will stabilize, and it will pass soft, frequent stools. This may be much easier and more acceptable than attempting to manage a chronically constipated, chronically miserable cat.

RECTAL PROLAPSE

Rectal prolapse occurs when continued straining pushes one or more layers of the rectal lining out of the anal opening, where they are visible. The straining is usually due to either intestinal problems such as diarrhea, or to a urinary problem.

Young cats are especially susceptible to rectal prolapse. It can occur because the cat has worms which cause a loss of protein from the blood. This is added to vitamin loss, continuing diarrhea, and non-stop straining to defecate. Rectal prolapse can occur with any severe diarrhea for these reasons. Other causes are tumors of the colon or rectum, bladder or kidney stones, bladder infection, and diseases of the prostate gland. A queen that is straining excessively to have kittens may push the rectal lining out.

Rectal prolapse is diagnosed when you see a reddish, wrinkled mass of tissue sticking out from where there should normally be an anal opening. It may be small and rounded, or it may be large and long, resembling a sausage. The large protrusion may be more than just a simple prolapse. It may be one piece of intestine which has telescoped inside another piece. If it has been out for some time, it may be dried, crusty, and blackened.

A rectal prolapse may not be a simple thing to repair. It is best to take the cat to your veterinarian for examination, diagnosis, and treatment. Keep the exposed tissue from drying out by moistening it with lukewarm water with a small pinch of salt added per cupful of water or a povidone-iodine solution (see below). Treatment usually includes surgery. If the portion of intestine sticking out has died, it may be necessary to amputate it. Understand in advance that this repair may be quite expensive, and that the results are not always satisfactory. If it's in a young kitten, are you willing to spend the money?

After the prolapse is replaced, it may be necessary to feed a special diet, or keep the animal on a stool softener until it has healed, or perhaps, for the rest of its life. If the original cause was diarrhea or a urinary problem, that, of course, must be treated or the prolapse will recur.

If you do not have access to a veterinarian, you can attempt to replace the prolapse yourself. This may or may not work, but if you have no other help and want to try to save the cat's life, it's worth a try. If the prolapse has dried, moisten it very gently with lukewarm water. Add enough povidone-iodine to the water so that it is the color of weak tea. Gently wash the tissue with a soft cloth and the iodine solution. If the prolapse is severely swollen, pack powdered sugar onto it, patting it gently, all the way around. This will help soften it and draw out some of the fluid which is the cause of the swelling. Alternate the sugar and water treatment for half an hour. After it has softened, locate the opening in the middle. Begin to gently tuck the edges into the middle, as though you are rolling a sock. Continue until all of it is back in the cat. Insert a little finger into the rectum and gently push the lining forward, flattening and straightening it as much as possible. The cat will need antibiotic treatment for a week or so. If the prolapse has been caused by diarrhea, this must be treated. The cat must be kept on a soft diet for one to two weeks until the prolapse is healed.

Keep a close eye on the cat for those two weeks. It is not unusual for the prolapse to recur.

Hemorrhoids are a small version of a rectal prolapse in which just a small portion of the rectal lining pushes out through the anal opening. These seem to be especially common in Siamese cats, and may occur from the time the animal is a kitten. Hemorrhoids look like one or more bright pink or red lumps or nodules protruding from the anus. These can be helped when they begin to develop by gently using a finger to replace them inside the cat. Make sure your fingernail is clipped short, and lubricate it with a bit of sterile lubricant (such as KY Jelly®) or petroleum jelly. Gently massage the lump, easing it back into the anal opening. Hemorrhoids often recur. If they are a continuing problem, your veterinarian can surgically remove them. As with rectal prolapse, if diarrhea or worms are starting the problem, they also must be treated to prevent recurrence.

PANCREATITIS

The term pancreatitis refers to an inflammation of the pancreas. It is uncommon, but occasionally seen in cats. The pancreas, an organ on the upper part of the small intestine, provides enzymes to the digestive tract. It also produces insulin to regulate the animal's blood sugar levels. Pancreatic insufficiency, in contrast to pancreatitis, is a deficiency of the products of this gland, whether digestive enzymes or insulin. Pancreatitis may be associated with feline infectious peritonitis, and fluke infestations (Stewart, 1994). The most common cause of feline pancreatitis may be toxoplasmosis.

Acute pancreatitis can come on suddenly. The cat may have severe abdominal pain, and may have a fever. It will show depression and vomiting, and may have greasy, loose or diarrheic bowel movements, which may be grayish in color. Signs of diabetes may also be seen because the inflamed pancreas is not producing enough insulin. Complications are common.

Pancreatitis can be VERY difficult to diagnose. Your veterinarian will use a combination of clinical signs and laboratory tests, often accompanied by a lucky guess, to make the diagnosis. You can help by giving the veterinarian a good history of your observations of the cat.

Some cases of acute pancreatitis improve within a day or two without treatment. The digestive organs get a rest because the cat will not eat. This period of inactivity gives the body a chance to repair the damage. However, some cats won't eat or drink for many days. Don't let this go more than a day. Eventually, if the problem is not diagnosed, the cat may have to be euthanized because it is starving to death and no cause is found to treat.

In cases of chronic pancreatitis, enough of the pancreas may have been destroyed that slowly, over time, the cat will have difficulty digesting food. It may have chronic or intermittent diarrhea, and lose weight or stay very thin, even though it eats normal quantities of good food. The cat may have large quantities of grayish, foamy stools. Some cats will have a greasy, soiled coat.

While the pancreas will never return to normal, the cat can have a normal life by supplementation with pancreatic enzymes to help digest food, and insulin to control diabetes (if it is present). Cats that are lacking in digestive enzymes may, in some cases, be helped by adding a teaspoon of meat tenderizer containing papain to each feeding. Your veterinarian can advise you, or, perhaps, prescribe a pharmaceutical preparation containing the necessary enzymes. With treatment, the diarrhea will usually stop, allowing the cat to be a comfortable and acceptable pet. Some cats will never maintain a normal weight.

PERITONITIS

Peritonitis is not strictly a disease of the digestive tract. It is an inflammation or infection of the peritoneum, the membrane which lines the abdomen. Peritonitis may be due to trauma such as a penetrating abdominal wound, whether from a tree branch, a bullet, an arrow, or some other object. It may be due to the rupture of some part of the digestive tract allowing intestinal contents to drain into the abdominal cavity. Or, it may be a more localized infection due to rupture of an abscessed lymph node.

Signs of early peritonitis may be as vague and nonspecific as lack of appetite, vomiting, and fever. Or, a case which is rapidly becoming critical may show severe signs within a few hours. These may include a high fever and fluid in the abdomen. The cat will show a lot of pain, standing with a humped back, being reluctant to move, or not wanting anyone to touch its abdomen. If your cat is acting like this, get care IMMEDIATELY. You have a possible emergency on your hands. A similar human condition is acute appendicitis. The cat may rapidly go into shock. Laboratory tests may give conflicting answers, suggesting several different diagnoses. In some cases, it may be necessary for your veterinarian to tap the abdomen with a needle to see what kind of fluid is present. This may enable the veterinarian to make a positive diagnosis. In some cases, it may be necessary to do exploratory surgery to confirm it. Don't hesitate if surgery is recommended. It may be your cat's only chance!

Without prompt and intensive treatment, the cat with severe peritonitis nearly always dies. With treatment, the chances are much better. In most cases, it will be necessary for your veterinarian to give large amounts of intravenous fluids to counteract the shock and replace the fluid which was lost into the abdominal cavity. Oxygen therapy may be needed to counteract the respiratory depression that occurs. Electrolyte imbalances will have to be corrected. Antibiotic therapy will be needed. Corticosteroids will be needed to treat the shock. It may take several days to a week or more of hospitalization before you will know if the cat will live or die. Be prepared for the veterinarian's bill—a full-blown case of peritonitis is expensive to treat.

Acute pancreatitis may follow a case of peritonitis. This is because the digestive juices and enzymes which spilled from the damaged intestine have partially digested and damaged the pancreas. The cat may end up being deficient in pancreatic enzymes or become diabetic. Even with these possible problems, many of the cats that have peritonitis can be saved, and will have long, useful lives after recovery. Prompt and aggressive treatment is the key.

Chapter 7

REPRODUCTION

TO BREED OR NOT TO BREED

Do you really want to breed your cat? Why? Is there a market for the kittens you would produce? The "market" includes not only being able to sell the kittens, but to find homes for those you plan to give away. Please remember that there are always more cats available than there are homes. A queen can easily produce four to six kittens twice a year. Currently, 16 to 18 million cats and dogs pass through the nation's animal shelters each year. About 13 million of these animals are eventually put to sleep (euthanized) because homes are not available. This includes young, healthy pets as well as older, unhealthy animals that no one wants. If the numbers don't shock you, visualize heaps and tons of dead pets in a crematorium or city dump. This fate may await the kittens you produce. Now, do you REALLY want to breed your queen?

Is your cat a purebred or a "mutt"? If she is a mixed breed or "Heinz 57," there may not be homes for the kittens. You might end up taking them to the pound, or giving them to less than desirable homes. If you give the kitten to someone and in a month or six it ends up in the pound, the result is the same as if you had taken the kitten there yourself. Is that what you really want? Kittens are cute, but sometimes people don't want them when they become "cats."

If your cat is a purebred, registered animal, is there a good chance that you can sell the kittens? Do you know other people who have had the same breed of cat and are successfully selling kittens? Just because you saw a breed for sale in the classified ads for "$800 each" does not mean that is what the breeder actually got for them, or that all the kittens the queen produced were sold. Do your homework. Call and check how many kittens the breeder has. Call back in a couple of weeks to see if there are any left. Ask what is the least the breeder will take for a kitten. If they are 14 to 16 weeks old, you can be sure they are NOT selling like hotcakes!

If you have a purebred, do you have one with a desirable bloodline? Often in show cats, certain lines become popular and sell for much more than cats of comparable quality from less-known heritage. Whether male or female, the cat to be bred should be a reasonably good example of its breed so it will produce quality offspring. The cat should be free from hereditary defects.

There are definite reasons for high selling prices in some breeds. Some breeds are known for reproductive problems, beginning with hormonal upsets that keep them from coming into heat. One of my clients bought a pair of Abyssinian females, hoping to produce enough kittens to pay for her pets as well as make a profit. One of the females stayed in heat ALL the time, rolling all over the floor, rubbing and howling. The owner finally got tired of this and spayed her. After a LOT of hormonal evaluations and therapy, the other cat finally came into heat. The Abby male wouldn't even look at her—something was not right about her hormone balance. In desperation, the owner tried to breed the cat to a friend's tabby, hoping that if the cat would get pregnant, it would settle her hormonal state and she could be bred to an Abby the next time around. Even the alley cat wouldn't look at her. Eventually, this cat was spayed, too. The result was two lovely pets, but not the cat-breeding empire originally planned. Find out if there are similar problems in the breed you hope will make you rich.

In general, there are two types of cat breeders who seem to make money: those to whom the purebred cat is a pet and hobby, and any monetary gain is incidental and welcome; or serious breeders with professional, long-term catteries. Breeders who make money usually breed for show-quality cats. They stay in it through thick and thin, through high prices and low. With luck, they make a small living which rewards them for devotion to their particular breed or type of cat. Very few people have become wealthy from cat breeding.

There is an old wives' tale which says that the female will be a better (or more settled, calmer, etc.) cat if she is allowed to have a litter of kittens before she is spayed. Most veterinarians do NOT believe this is true. All it does is produce more unwanted kittens to be killed. If you want to have the cat spayed, it will be far more convenient (and less expensive!) to have it done before the first heat. Her maturity and final form will in no way be affected by your decision. This also saves you the bother of putting up with having her in heat, keeping her indoors and having all the males cluster around your house, fighting for a chance to get at her.

Some people feel their cats will become fat and lazy if neutered. The animal may be less active because he or she is not out "catting around." If you don't overfeed the cat after surgery, it will not be overweight.

Some people want to breed the cat so their children can see her having kittens, and witness the "miracle of birth." Animals have some ability to control the time at which they have their offspring. The chance of your children seeing kittens born is perhaps one in 10. They are much more likely to arrive in the middle of the night or when the kids are at school than when there are spectators. This is NOT a good reason to breed a cat. Go to your library and borrow a video for the kids to watch if you want them to see the birth process. Having another pet "just like Fluffy" is also not a good reason to breed your cat. If you breed two purebred cats, there is only a remote chance of getting a pet exactly like the one you already have. With mixed breed animals, the chance is nearly zero.

What about breeding your tom cat? There is no physiological need for him to reproduce. While the male cat seems to take pleasure from the coital process, it is not necessary for his well-being. If toms are not specifically being kept for breeding, nearly all of them make better pets if neutered. They are less prone to run away from home looking for a female, and get hit by a car, poisoned, attacked by another cat, or even shot. If the male is out running around and fighting, there is a high chance that he will have abscesses. He also has a much greater chance of catching diseases, from upper respiratory problems to feline leukemia or feline infectious peritonitis. Your veterinary bills will be much cheaper if he is neutered! Also, neutered males are less prone to urine spraying to mark their territory indoors. All in all, they make far better pets when neutered.

The male cat, by the way, usually reaches puberty several weeks later than a female of the same litter. Sexual maturity usually occurs soon after he reaches his adult weight, around eight to 12 months of age (up to 18 months for feral males). The female reaches puberty between five and 12 months of age. A few individuals may come into heat as early as three-and-a-half months of age. Feral females and Persians may not reach puberty until they are a year and a half old.

BREEDING SOUNDNESS EXAM, FEMALE

There are two ways to approach breeding the female cat. The first is to put her with the male and see if you get kittens a couple of months later. This is cheap, easy, and usually works best when you don't want kittens. The second way is to go about it with science and deliberation, starting with a veterinary examination. This may include a complete health history. If the cat is receiving drugs that may harm the kittens or affect her pregnancy, she may be taken off them. Some drugs, especially corticosteroids or hormones, may affect her current ability to reproduce. Tell the veterinarian how old she was when she first came into heat, how often she comes into heat, and any breeding behavior you have observed. Let the veterinarian know whether she has had kittens before, and how many were in the litters. The veterinarian also will need to know if she was bred naturally or by artificial insemination.

Have your veterinarian go over the cat's nutritional program to make sure it is adequate for breeding, as well as how she should be fed during pregnancy. The queen

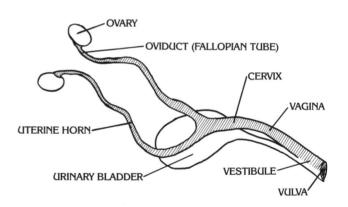

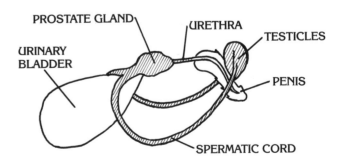

Reproductive tracts, female and male.

should be in good condition—neither too fat nor too thin, and have good muscle tone.

If the queen is more than seven years old, it may be a good idea to run a CBC (complete blood count), urinalysis and blood chemical profile to make sure she does not have any health problems which might affect her or her kittens.

Booster vaccinations should be scheduled a bit more than 30 days before breeding, so the vaccine will not interfere with early growth of the embryos. Otherwise, it may cause early abortion, resorption of the embryos or abnormal development of the kittens. Boosters will ensure that her colostrum (the first milk she produces) is full of antibodies to protect the kittens against disease until they are old enough for their immune systems to produce their own antibodies. When you take her to the veterinarian, take a fresh fecal sample to be checked for worms. Any worming that is needed can be done well before breeding. A female that is infected with ascarids may pass them to her kittens while they are in the uterus. Begin a control program for external parasites such as fleas. Dental care or other surgery requiring anesthesia (other than that of an emergency nature) should be done at least six weeks before breeding.

BREEDING SOUNDNESS EXAM, MALE

Tom cats are fertile year-round. Fertility may decrease with age, but the tom cat usually retains male behavior, including spraying and breeding females as long as he lives. Aggression between males can be lessened if tom cats cannot hear or see each other or females in heat. Very few males are seen in the calico or tortoiseshell colors. While most males in those colors are sterile, a few will be fertile. Blue-eyed white cats may or may not be sterile.

The male also should be examined for breeding soundness. A physical examination by your veterinarian will determine if he is in good health, normal, free of worms and blood parasites, and fit to breed. It should also include a semen examination to show that the cat is fertile and can be expected to impregnate a normal female. Both testicles should be in the scrotum, and the penis should be checked to make sure that it is normal and will extend fully from the prepuce (sheath). The tom cat's penis has tiny, rough projections on it. These induce the queen to ovulate when he breeds her.

The tom cat that is heavily used for breeding may not groom himself normally. He will benefit from being brushed daily and bathed as needed. If you do not give this care, skin and coat problems may occur, especially if he is long-haired. If you don't want to bother with caring for him, the cure is simple: Have him neutered.

Occasionally a male will mount females persistently, thrusting for long periods of time without actually finishing the act. This may be due to irritation from a ring of hair around the base of the cat's penis. The abnormal behavior will go away when it is removed.

The other extreme may occur with a male that grows up in a household with a dominant male. He may be psychologically castrated, and won't spray or show other male behaviors. He may not breed females that are presented to him. This cat may become a normal stud if he is taken to a home where he can be the only cat. Give him time and start him by presenting him with experienced females that are fully in heat. It may take a year or more for him to come into his own.

Rarely, a male will show an abnormal interest in a stuffed toy, pillow, or your leg. Sometimes this behavior can be suppressed by squirting the cat with a spray bottle. Other toms may be cured with female hormones. If neither treatment works, you may let him have the pillow or toy in a location where it does not bother you, such as behind the sofa. If he is already neutered, the only other cure is to get rid of him.

BASICS OF BREEDING

The queen should be physically mature before she is bred. It is usually best to wait until the second heat, or around one year of age, whichever comes later.

The age of the female also has a bearing on kitten survival. Queens more than two years of age usually wean more healthy kittens than those that are younger when they give birth. Aged females will generally have less reproductive success, although some keep shelling out kittens until they die. What is too old? If the older queen is in good physical and mental condition and gets around normally, there is no reason why she should not be bred. She will need careful feeding and care. It is especially important that she not become overweight. In general, older queens are more prone to having a prolonged labor.

If you are taking the queen to a tom and she is not accustomed to travel or has to be shipped, do so early in her heat cycle. This will give her time to recover from the trip and get acquainted with her new location. In any case, the female should be taken to the male. Tom cats are extremely territorial, and may not breed if taken to an unfamiliar place.

Queens often show definite preferences for one tom over another. For this reason, a queen may refuse to allow the tom of her owner's choice to breed her. She also may refuse to accept a tom cat that is brought to her home or yard. Leaving them together for some time, or introducing them gradually, often will allow a successful breeding. Tranquilization may also help.

A queen that has never before mated, or is shy or timid, may go completely out of heat when placed with a tom she does not know. Upon arrival at the male's location, she should be exposed to him for 15 to 30 minutes, two to three times a day. Put her where she can see, smell, and hear him. A cage where she is separated from him by wire, so she still feels safe, often works well. This will help bring her completely into heat, and allow her to become gradually acquainted with him. Another possibility is to put her with a group of breeding queens. They often synchronize heat cycles with each other. Conversely, some timid queens will come into heat if kept away from other cats.

When she is ready to be bred, the queen will crouch on her elbows with her hind end thrust upward. She will pull her tail to one side. She may tread with her hind feet, making tiny steps and going nowhere, signaling that she is ready to be bred.

The tom cat usually approaches the female, attracted by her calling or scent. He usually sniffs her genital area, curling his upper lip (called flehmen) in response to the odor. A tom that is frequently used for breeding may run directly to and mount any female brought to the breeding area. The tom cat usually grips the neck of the female in his teeth, especially on their first mating. He straddles her first with his front legs and then with his hind legs. He makes treading movements, stepping from side to side, which may help him arch his back. The entire mating process takes only one to four minutes. After breeding, the tom jumps out of striking distance of the queen. Because a single mating may not be enough to induce ovulation, the queen should be bred several times, at least three times per day, until she goes out of heat.

Outdoor males may fight violently over a female in heat. After their initial battles, tom cats do not usually fight when they meet again. More than one male may breed the queen before she goes out of heat. Thus, a litter of feral cats may have more than one father.

In a cattery, one male can usually breed about 20 females. Only about one out of three males will become a reliable breeding tomcat. Testosterone therapy will not usually make a breeder out of an uninterested male.

It is important to locate the tom to which you want to breed your female before the onset of her heat period. That will give you time to find one whose conformation and bloodlines you like. If the male is registered, you will want to make sure his registration is in order so the breeding will be valid and recognized by the appropriate cat fancier's club. Two of the largest cat registries are: The Cat Fancier's Association (CFA), 1309 Allaire Ave., Ocean, NJ, 07712, (201) 531-2390, and the American Cat Fancier's Association, Box 203, Point Lookout, MO 65726, (417) 334-5430. Smaller registries can be located through pet magazines such as Cat Fancy, the public library, or your veterinarian.

THE REPRODUCTIVE CYCLE

Puberty in the female occurs between five and 12 months of age. She may be fertile at her first heat cycle and may accept the male, become pregnant, and produce kittens. Queens are seasonally polyestrous, coming into heat from spring through fall. They are out of heat in the winter, usually from September until late December or January. In the northern hemisphere, the peaks of breeding activity are between mid-January and early March and between May and June. (Beaver, 1992, p. 142).

Signs of estrus (full heat) in the queen include unusual meowing, crying, or even howling. Some females, especially Siamese, may yowl endlessly. The cat may rub her neck and head against objects or against you, appearing more friendly than usual. She will roll on the floor or ground, twisting and pushing herself along the floor. Others may climb the curtains and try to escape from the house. Meanwhile, males are clustering around your house, fighting in your yard, screaming at all hours, and spraying on the doors, walls, windowsills, and bushes.

Cats are induced ovulators. This means that they do not ovulate unless they are bred. When the female is bred, she goes out of heat within 24 hours. If the female is not bred, she will come into heat at 14- to 19-day intervals from spring until fall. She will be receptive to the male for between one and four days each time. Having to put up with a cat in heat for half the year may make you believe in spaying! Females that are not in heat will usually claw and hiss at a male that is so impolite as to approach them.

An especially fertile female may have two or even three litters in a particular year. A queen may have 50 to 160 kittens in 10 or more years of production. This is why it is very important to spay your queen if you don't want her to keep shelling out kittens like a kitty machine.

Gestation: 56 to 68 days (average 63-66 days)
Litter size: 1 to 8 kittens
Rarely, up to 12 or 13 kittens

BREEDING THE QUEEN

As the cat goes fully into heat, she accepts the male as he tries to mount. She crouches on the floor and pulls her tail to the side. There may be a little bloody discharge on her vulva. Breeding takes less than five minutes. Cats may mate eight to 10 times per hour if left together or outdoors.

The tom cat also may let out a howl, often called a caterwaul. He may give a softer version of the call before mating, advertising his readiness to mate with the queen. After she is bred, the queen may let out a loud cry. She will twist away from the male and continue to roll on the ground.

Once the female has been bred to the male you have selected, keep her away from all other males. You may get undesirable kittens if another male breeds her while she is still in heat.

When a sterile mating occurs, the queen may experience a pseudopregnancy. This false pregnancy will last about 40 to 45 days. The cat may mother a stuffed toy, another queen's kittens or another baby animal. Some queens experiencing false pregnancy may have mammary gland development and produce milk. Treatment is usually not needed—it will go away, given time.

If the queen fails to conceive after she has been bred, both the male and female should be evaluated for infertility. If the male has sired other litters of kittens during the time he bred this female, it is not necessary to check him, as he has proven himself fertile. Otherwise, a semen sample can be checked to make sure the male has adequate numbers of sperm cells.

Several types of bacterial infections can cause infertility in the queen. Viral diseases such as feline leukemia, feline distemper, feline infectious peritonitis, and feline rhinotracheitis have been linked to abortion in cats. In some of these, the cat may simply absorb the fetuses while they are in the uterus, then come into heat again later in the season.

Genetic abnormalities and imbalances in endocrine hormones can cause the queen to fail to come into estrus. Or, the cat may have normal heat cycles, but the signs may be so slight that they go unnoticed. This is called "silent heat," and may lead you to think she is not coming into heat. Older queens can have irregular and less frequent estrus cycles, coming into heat fewer times per year, even when no abnormalities can be found.

Cystic ovaries can cause variations in the estrus cycle, including a shortened time between heat cycles. They can also cause the queen to be continuously in heat. One of these can REALLY make you believe in spaying! Severe liver disease or congenital abnormalities of the liver can result in decreased metabolism (destruction) of reproductive hormones. This can also lead to the queen staying in estrus for a prolonged period or continuously.

MISMATING

A mismating is when the female is bred to the wrong male, or is bred when she was not supposed to be bred. First, let's clear up an important misconception. The male to whom the female is bred for one litter has NO influence on future litters. In other words, the queen is not "contaminated," as some people would lead you to believe. If your purebred queen is accidentally bred to a common alley tom, this litter (if you allow her to have it) will be crossbred kittens. But there will be NO influence at all on future litters. In most cases, it is safer to go ahead and allow her to have the kittens than to abort her and try again. Aborting the litter may injure the queen, reducing her ability to conceive and give birth in the future.

Injections of hormones may be given by your veterinarian to produce an abortion in a female if you do not care about her future reproductive abilities. One type should be given as soon as possible (within a day or so) after the mismating has occurred. Another (dexamethasone) may be given as late as 45 days into the pregnancy. The problem with these injections is that they cause a high incidence of pyometra ("pus in the uterus," uterine infection). This infection often necessitates spaying the queen to save her life. The injections also may cause bone marrow suppression, a sometimes fatal condition. It is easier (and safer!) to allow her to begin the pregnancy, then have her spayed as soon as she is out of heat if you don't want to keep her as a breeding animal. While you are waiting for her to go out of heat, it is necessary to keep her from being bred again if you do not want her to have kittens. The more times she is bred, the higher the probability that the matings will result in a pregnancy.

The same recommendations hold true when you want the queen to have kittens, but not at this time. If she is bred by accident, it is usually better to let her go through the pregnancy and have the kittens. If you do not want the kittens, most veterinarians will euthanize them for you as soon as they are born. If the kittens never have a chance to nurse, the queen will not start a milk flow, will not bond to them, and will have minimal side effects from the pregnancy. Then you can breed her at her next heat, if you desire—to the male of YOUR choice. Pregnancy has less likelihood of permanent damage to her reproductive system than an abortion does.

Vaginal douches after mating are of little or no use in preventing pregnancy in the cat and their use may cause injury or infection in the female. This technique should not be considered.

If you wish to use your queen for future breeding, it is far easier to keep her from getting pregnant by careful confinement than it is to try to fix the problem later. And, just because your female wouldn't think of climbing out of your yard doesn't mean that an enterprising and athletic tom cat won't climb in. They can and do! Otherwise, it's easier to have her spayed and not worry about the problem any more.

ABORTION

In the section on mismating, deliberate abortions to end an unwanted pregnancy were discussed. This section deals with spontaneous or unwanted abortion. Bacterial infections of the uterus (metritis, endometritis) may cause spontaneous abortion or prevent pregnancy. The only way to diagnose them is for your veterinarian to check a culture from the vagina or uterus, or take a biopsy sample from the uterus. In this examination, a small piece of tissue is taken from the lining of the uterus and examined for normal cellular structure and/or the presence of bacteria. Bacterial uterine infections may necessitate treatment with systemic antibiotics for a prolonged period of time (three to four weeks).

If you don't wish to breed the queen again, spaying is the easy cure. Your veterinarian will perform the surgery after the queen's infection has cleared up as much as possible and she is healthy enough to withstand the surgery. In some cases where the uterus is not draining, emergency surgery may be done to save the cat's life. If you DO wish to breed her again, bacterial cultures, blood tests, urinalysis and possibly a thyroid hormone evaluation may be needed before you attempt to mate her.

Taurine deficiency in the queen's diet (or the inability to utilize dietary taurine because of some types of liver disease) may cause abortion around 20 days of pregnancy. Make sure that the queen's diet contains adequate taurine, or add a taurine supplement to her diet.

INFERTILITY

Hormonal imbalances or deficiencies may cause either infertility or abortion. One of the most common causes is hypothyroidism, in which the thyroid gland is not producing enough hormones for normal ovarian function. The queen may not come into heat, or may have abnormal, irregular cycles. Males that are hypothyroid have little or no interest in breeding. Or, they may have such low sperm counts that they can not impregnate females, even if they are interested. Your veterinarian can run tests to check if your cat is hypothyroid. The problem can at least be partially corrected with hormone therapy.

Cysts or tumors on the ovaries also may keep the queen from coming into heat. In most cases, the only sure diagnosis is an exploratory laparotomy—surgery in which your veterinarian opens the abdominal cavity and "takes a look" at the ovaries. If only one ovary is affected, it may be removed. The other ovary may still be functional. In some cases, hormones from one ovary will suppress function of the other to the point that it never returns to normal. If the cat is very valuable as a breeding animal, it may be worth removing the abnormal ovary (especially if the problem is a cyst) and waiting to see what happens. If you do not want the cat for breeding, complete ovariohysterectomy will cure the problem permanently.

Some cysts or tumors may produce an excess of hormones, keeping the female in heat continuously. Hormone injections may be used in an attempt to resolve the cyst. If injections do not work, surgery may done to collapse the cyst(s) within the abdomen, or to remove the abnormal ovary if only one is involved. If a tumor is causing the queen to stay in heat, the affected ovary should, of course, be removed.

Malnutrition or extreme parasitism may cause abortion, but these problems are usually so severe they are obvious. If you have a number of related queens, you may have unintentionally kept cats with inherited infertility. In nature, longer days trigger heat cycles. Cats that are kept indoors may be in heat year-round.

Males that have tumors in the testicles are generally infertile. If only one testicle is involved and is removed, the other may regain reproductive function. However, in many cases, hormones from the affected side have destroyed the function of the other testicle. Don't get your hopes up that you will have a fertile male after surgery is done.

Extremely high environmental temperatures may cause either temporary or permanent low sperm count in the male. Breeding males should be kept cool in the summer if you wish to maintain their reproductive ability.

Occasionally, a young tom will not be inclined to breed a female. This is a real problem if he is your choice for stud-cat to breed to your purebred female. Young male cats may be intimidated by older, more aggressive female cats. A hostile environment, such as the presence of aggressive toms, may also inhibit the shy male from breeding. Less than half of all toms will mate in a group situation. Take the cat to a neutral area with no other cats except a young submissive female in heat. This may help him get the idea and realize breeding is permitted.

Some females do not show strong signs of estrus. Your veterinarian can do a microscopic examination of vaginal smears from the queen to determine when she is fertile. They may need to be done on several consecutive days so that a trend can be seen.

PREGNANCY DETERMINATION

Most normal, healthy queens become pregnant when bred to a normal, healthy male. Most of the time, nature works as intended (or as the owner didn't intend!). The most obvious sign is the end to the cat's heat cycle. She will suddenly stop her "calling," rolling on the floor, and other signs associated with heat. She will seem much more mellow and calm. Keep an eye on her eating habits. A loss of appetite for more than two days may be a sign of trouble. Cats are creatures of habit and do not take kindly to change.

The queen will have an increased appetite and may begin to gain weight. There are few signs during the first couple of weeks of the pregnancy. The cat's nipples gradually get much larger and more pink. Around the twenty-first day of pregnancy, if the cat is not overweight, your veterinarian may be able to palpate the tiny kittens as a string of lumps in the uterus, assuming that the queen cooperates and will relax. Around the thirtieth day of pregnancy, the lumps in the uterus are no longer individually distinct. Late in the pregnancy, after about 50 days, it is usually possible to feel individual kittens. If the cat is X-rayed, bones can be seen in the fetuses after about 38 days of gestation. Some clinics have ultrasound machines, which can make a determination of pregnancy around days 21 to 35.

If the queen has a two-pound weight gain within a month, she is probably pregnant. The cat that started out at a normal weight will not gain weight all over her body. She will look more like she has swallowed a grapefruit. Most of the weight gain occurs in the second half of pregnancy when the kittens are growing rapidly.

If you are fairly certain the cat is pregnant, positive veterinary diagnosis may not be necessary. This diagnosis, however, is important where a small female has only one or two kittens. They may each become so large that they will not easily come out through the birth canal, and you may need to be prepared for a Caesarean delivery. If she has a larger number of kittens, chances are good that they will individually be small enough that she can give birth normally. At any rate, it is better to anticipate the problem than to deal with an emergency. Exposure to X-rays late in pregnancy will NOT cause problems for the kittens; they are too far along in their development to be affected by the low dosages used. There are currently no chemical or biological tests which can determine feline pregnancy.

CARE OF THE PREGNANT CAT

The gestation period in cats may range from 56 to 68 days, with an average around 63 to 66 days days. In other words, be prepared from the fifty-first day on, counted from the day the female accepts the male. The length of gestation varies slightly from one cat to another, however, a queen will usually carry her kittens about the same number of days from one litter to another.

Around 50 days of pregnancy, the breasts will begin to enlarge in many queens. This does not occur in all of them—some do not show breast enlargement until after the kittens are born. Kittens born earlier than 60 days may be considered premature, and some of them may be born dead or die shortly after birth.

Adequate (but not excess) nutrition is necessary for the queen during pregnancy. Malnutrition may cause her to have kittens that are too small to survive after they are born. Also, a malnourished mother may not care for the kittens properly, and may not provide adequate milk for them after they are born (see Feline Gourmet Chapter). During pregnancy, she will need a larger quantity of food to give more calories. The daily ration should be divided into three to four smaller feedings. There will be less room left in the digestive tract for food as the kittens take up more of the abdomen. Taurine deficiency may cause reproductive problems in the queen, including absorption of the kittens, abortions, and stillborn or poor-growing kittens. The cat will have a greater need for water—make sure she has a fresh supply available at all times.

Normal exercise, especially during the first half of pregnancy, will help keep the queen from becoming overweight. It also will keep her in good muscle tone to help make her delivery easier. On the other hand, don't allow her to run free without supervision. Later in the pregnancy, she will restrict her own activity as she becomes less comfortable with exercising—but don't let her get fat and lazy. The queen that is nearing term will be awkward and may find it difficult to get out of the way of a vehicle or a dog or other animal that may chase her. For this reason, it is a good idea to keep her indoors after her seventh week of pregnancy. Keep her from any strenuous exercise for the last three days before her anticipated delivery date.

Drugs given during pregnancy may be hazardous to the fetuses. No medication should be given except on the advice of your veterinarian. If you have to take the queen to a veterinarian for an injury or illness, be sure to point out that she might be pregnant. In some cases, it may be necessary to treat the queen and risk the kittens in order to save her life. The antibiotic tetracycline may cause liver failure in pregnant queens. Other antibiotics must be used carefully, if at all. Drugs such as corticosteroids and griseofulvin are known to cause deformities in kittens. Some drugs may require higher concentrations in the pregnant queen, while only half as much of others may be needed. Many wormers cannot be given to the pregnant queen. It is best, if possible, to have all worming and other necessary treatments done before the queen is bred, as a part of getting her ready for breeding and pregnancy.

DELIVERY

Fifty days have passed since your queen was bred to the male. You are expecting kittens around 63 days, but it doesn't hurt to be prepared a bit early. A normal litter is four or five kittens. A small cat such as an Abyssinian may have only one or two kittens. A larger cat—a Siamese or Siamese mix—may have as many as eight or nine kittens at a time, and may carry them a few days longer.

It's good to have a box for the queen to use while giving birth. Otherwise she will certainly pick your laundry basket, closet, or drawer. Most queens prefer a dark, quiet hiding place. Try putting the box in her favorite hiding place or where she normally sleeps. If you let the cat "find" the box by herself, she is more likely to use it than if you stuff her into it. The box should be long enough that the mother can stretch out at full length. It should be low enough that she can step comfortably in and out, yet high enough to keep the kittens from crawling out. Prepare the box at least a week before the expected birth so the cat can begin to sleep in it. This will saturate it with her odor, allowing her to relax in its security. Some cats may prefer to be around people when the birth occurs. A social cat may prefer to have

her box near your bed. She may even end up giving birth in bed with you—something you might want to avoid.

A cardboard box can work nicely for the cat, and is easily discarded if it becomes wet or soiled. Line the bottom with layers of newspaper. Cover them with clean towels, rags, mattress pads, or carpet. Be sure that whatever you use goes completely to the edge of the box so the kittens cannot crawl underneath the padding and smother. The same guidelines apply to loose strings or holes in which the kittens could become tangled. Hay and sawdust are too dusty to be good bedding. Farm cats can be born on straw, if it is VERY clean and dust-free. Whatever you use, the area should be clean, dry, free of drafts, and attractive to the queen. The prettiest box in the world isn't much good if she won't stay in it.

If you can keep the birthing box at a temperature around 80 degrees F (26.7 C), more kittens will live. Chilling is one of the commonest causes of death of newborn kittens. They cannot regulate their own temperature for as much as two weeks after they are born. The box can be placed near a radiator or electric heater, a heating pad can be used under about half the box IF your female is not prone to cord chewing. Put the pad and a thermometer in place several days before the kittens are due; check the thermometer frequently to see that the proper temperature is being maintained. If it is too hot, the queen will not use the box. If it is too cold, it won't do any good. Remove the thermometer after you have the temperature adjusted to around 80 degrees.

If the queen has long hair on her belly (such as a Persian or Himalayan), clip it quite close with a pair of clippers (or have your groomer do this) about a week before she is due; otherwise, kittens may begin sucking on a lock of hair because they can't tell it from the nipples. It's not very nutritious! If she has long hair under her tail and around her vulva, this should be clipped at the same time. The female can more easily be kept clean and fresh with the long hair gone from the area. Clipping the mother's belly also allows the kittens to have direct contact with her skin, which gives them more warmth than if her skin is insulated by the hair. A bare tummy may make females with heavy hair more aware of the cold, so they will more readily snuggle with their kittens.

Within two to three days of the time she is due, wash the queen's belly and vaginal area with a good pet shampoo and lukewarm water. Then, rinse it a half-dozen times to make sure that ALL soap is off the skin and hair. Any soap left on her skin may be ingested by the kittens as they nurse and may make them ill. Dry her off with a towel and keep her in a warm place until she is completely dry.

Delivery of a litter may occur quite rapidly, within three to four hours after the queen goes into hard labor. Or delivery could take as long as 18 to 24 hours. The queen may be able to delay the birth for up to 24 hours if she is upset or stressed—which is why she may not have the kittens when your kids are watching. No drugs are available at the current time to safely induce delivery at a time that is convenient to humans. We have to take potluck and watch to see when she is going to have kittens.

How do you know that birthing is near? Two or three days before the event, the queen may become restless and nervous. She may pace and meow, and lose her appetite. She may urinate and defecate frequently because of the decreasing space within her abdomen. Nesting behavior is usually seen within 12 to 24 hours before the kittens are born. The queen may dig and turn around in her nest box (or chosen nest site). The muscles of the pelvis and abdomen will relax and look loose or sagging.

At this point, the queen may go into the first stage of labor, when contractions of the uterus begin. Shortly before kittens are born, she may repeatedly scratch at the carpet or bedding. There may be a dark greenish discharge from the vulva several hours before the birth of the first kitten, as well as throughout the birthing process. This is normal. It is stale blood breakdown products being released as the membranes separate from the uterus.

The queen may have droplets of milk oozing from the nipples. This may occur a week or two, or just a few hours, before she has kittens. Some queens do not show any mammary development until the kittens arrive and try to nurse. This depends a lot on the queen, and is perhaps more common with those having their first litter.

As labor approaches, the cat may pace the floor, dart aimlessly around, or circle. The kittens will be moving inside her, and this changing pressure may confuse her. She may cry, much as she did when she was in heat. She may lick her vaginal region, and squat in the litter box without eliminating. Some of these signs may occur as many as 24 hours before delivery begins. On rare occasion, the female may become hysterical. If so, call your veterinarian, as she may need tranquilization.

When the cat goes into labor, move the birthing box to her and try to coax her into it. If she doesn't want to go, don't force her. Allow her to pick the birth spot and remove any fragile items from the area. Try to get bedding under her which you can throw away.

The queen may experience labor pains from time to time within a day or two before she gives birth. As long as they are occurring one or two at a time and she is not settling down, they are just "practice runs." When the queen lies down and has rhythmic contractions, labor has begun in earnest. She will voluntarily push with her abdominal muscles during the contractions, and she may stretch and turn. From the time that this occurs it should not be more than two hours until the first kitten is born.

It may take as many as two to three hours between the first and second kittens if the contractions are weak, or as few as 15 to 30 minutes if they are strong. Intervals between the remainder of the kittens should be shorter. During intervals between kittens, the female will continue to strain if there are more kittens to come. If it is longer than about three hours between kittens, or if the cat strains for more than four to five hours without producing the first kitten, she may be having problems or be getting tired. Consult your veterinarian. Also, if she strains hard and constantly for more than an hour without producing a kitten, she should be examined as soon as possible.

An emergency situation may have developed. Delivery of the entire litter is usually completed within six hours. However, in some cases it may be spread over twenty-four hours without problems. A litter may range from a single kitten to about eight.

When birthing starts, it is a good idea to have the queen in the birthing box. She won't want to be moved until all the kittens are born. Children should either be VERY quiet or out of the room. Keep noise to a minimum. Maintain enough light so that you can see what is happening, but not so much that it is harsh, glaring or distracting for the mother. No strangers should be around a birthing queen if it can be avoided. This may upset her so much that she will not pay attention to giving birth and taking care of the kittens. If the female is distracted or frightened, labor may be prolonged, and she may have less milk than she would otherwise. She may accidentally roll over one or more of the kittens and smother them.

Don't overdo attention to the mother cat. A very young queen, five to 10 months of age, may not have a good idea of what is happening. An affectionate cat may want to be near you during delivery. She may follow you around the house rather than staying in her box, and you may have to sit with her when she starts into labor. A dependent, nervous cat may also need more attention than usual. The queen that is giving birth to kittens is not a circus performer—be quiet and unobtrusive.

Everything which touches the mother's birth canal or the kittens should be either sterile or as clean as possible. Be sure to wash your hands before touching her. Scrub well with soap and plenty of water. Brush under your fingernails with a brush to remove any dirt that is caught there. Dry your hands with a clean cloth or paper towel. If you have a disinfectant available, rinse your hands with it. Povidone-iodine mixed with water until it looks like weak tea works well.

When the kittens appear, they may come feet first or head first. It doesn't matter which—they are usually rather sausage shaped, and either way is normal. The queen will tear open the sac and lick the fluids from the kitten's head. The kitten should start breathing when the membranes are removed.

When the kitten begins to emerge from the birth canal, give the mother time to push it out, which will usually happen within a dozen or so contractions. If it isn't out by then, you can GENTLY help. If you do help, keep your movements slow and quiet so you don't disturb the queen from her work. Grasp the kitten with a clean rag or paper towel. Pull only on the kitten's legs, grasping as near the body as you can. Don't pull on the head if you can avoid it. Work with the mother. Pull when the mother pushes, and relax when she does. Don't pull the kitten straight out of her, but curve the kitten downward as if you are pulling it toward her heels. It may be helpful to have someone hold the mother on her back. If the kitten comes head first, you can tear open the membranes covering its face as soon as you can see it. It should not take more than three to four pushes to remove the kitten from the mother. Some kittens may not be covered with a sac, or the mother may pass one kitten, and then a couple of sacs within five or 10 minutes, and then another kitten or two. This is also normal. There is one set of membranes per kitten.

If the cat is having the kittens easily, and you just want to watch, that's fine. If she does not remove the membranes from the kitten's head within a minute, gently pull it off yourself or the kitten may suffocate. She will usually lick the membranes off the kitten's head, then vigorously lick it to stimulate its breathing. She will chew at the umbilical cord to separate it from the membranes. At times, this action may be vigorous enough to tear the kitten's abdomen open, exposing the intestines. Or, it may cause an umbilical hernia. These accidents are rare, but watch her carefully. Be prepared to intercede if the mother seems excessively rough with her kittens.

If you are helping with the delivery, remove all membranes from the kitten's body. Tie off the umbilical cord about an inch from the kitten's body, using string which you have soaked in alcohol. Now dip the end of the umbilical cord into tincture of iodine or tamed iodine. Dab off the excess iodine with a cloth or paper towel. Using scissors that have been dipped in alcohol, cut the cord on the side AWAY from the kitten, leaving the string on the part attached to it. Dip the end of the cord into the iodine again. Do these steps quickly in order to go onto the next procedure:

Wrap a single layer of cloth or paper towel around the end of your finger. Use this to clean out the kitten's mouth, removing mucus and fluid. If the kitten is not breathing, cradle it between your two hands, head downhill. Swing the kitten GENTLY in a long, wide arc, using the whole length of your arms. If you use too much force, you may lose your grip and fling the kitten to the floor. You are helping mucus to flow out of its lungs. If you do this too vigorously, you may rupture the diaphragm or cause other internal damage. Having the kitten supported by your full hand will keep the head from swinging from side to side, which may cause injury. Sway the kitten from one side to another six to eight times. Repeat the mouthwiping. If the kitten is still not breathing, blow a tiny amount of air GENTLY into the kitten's nose until the chest expands. Too much force will rupture its lungs. Squeeze its chest VERY GENTLY with two fingers to help it exhale, and repeat the artificial respiration. Efforts to get a kitten breathing may continue up to 20 to 30 minutes if you really want to save it.

Now take the kitten in your hands and rub it vigorously but very gently with a paper towel or a soft rag. This will remove mucus from its hair and help stimulate breathing. By this time, the kitten should be gasping nicely. If it does not, repeat the gentle swinging. If you are taking the kittens away from the mother, they can be placed in a box held at 90 degrees F (32.2 C). Otherwise, the kitten can be placed at the mother's breast for nourishment and warmth. Allow it to find the nipple by itself if it can. The struggles and crying help to strengthen the kitten and get its lungs open and working properly.

Chilling is one of the main causes of kitten loss. The kitten wanders away from its mother while it is still damp and becomes cold. If you come to the box and find that the mother has had a kitten, has not cared for it, and it is chilled, take it to the sink and run lukewarm water (NOT HOT!) gently over it, holding it with the head straight down. Then, dry and rub it as above. Some people try to warm the kittens with a hot water bottle. One disadvantage is that this will cool off during the night, and it may also leak and further chill the kitten. A heating pad may help keep the kitten warm.

Breeders who have large numbers of queens and raise valuable kittens may wish to invest in a heated kitten warmer, or an incubator with oxygen capabilities. These are available from Thermocare Inc., P.O. Drawer YY, Incline Village, Nevada, 89450. Digitally controlled models are sold by Lyon Electric Co., Chula Vista, CA. The ideal temperature for newborns is 80 to 85 degrees F (26-29.5 C).

If all is going well, you should have a kitten which is warm, partly dry and breathing with a normal rhythm. If the queen is having another kitten, pass this one to a family member and help her with the next. As soon as the queen is through having kittens (if they are coming close together), you can put all the little ones up to her to nurse. If she is going a long time between kittens, or lying quietly between births, kittens should be given to her to nurse and cuddle as soon as they are dried off and breathing normally. The sooner they eat, the better chance they have to live.

The queen may reach around and take the placenta (membranes or afterbirth), either picking it up after it is passed, or actually pulling it out of her body. She may eat it, even before it is fully out of her body. This is normal—let her do it if she wants to. The placenta is laxative, and may also help start the flow of milk. It has considerable nutritional value when her appetite is otherwise depressed, and eating it helps keep the nest area clean. The cleaning process also seems to help the queen bond to the kittens. Allow her to eat at least one set of membranes if she wants to do so. You may remove the rest of them if you are squeamish. Make sure she has access to a convenient litter box because of the laxative effect. The queen may also want to eat kittens which are born dead. You can remove these and dispose of them, although there is no harm if she does eat them.

There may be just a few minutes between kittens, or the birth process may take seven to eight hours. This is still normal. If actual labor lasts more than eight hours, or if the cat cries constantly or seems exhausted, check with your veterinarian.

When the queen is through having kittens, she will stop straining and relax. She will start licking them and paying attention to them. At this point, you can wash her off with a warm, damp rag if she is soiled. Do not make a big production out of this, or take her away from her kittens. Just get the big pieces and leave the rest for her to clean up herself, or for you to deal with in a day or two. Put clean bedding in the litter box if it is soiled with birth fluids. Make sure that everything is warm and cozy, and then LEAVE HER ALONE. She needs time and quiet to bond to the kittens. If you pay too much attention to her, she may think she is supposed to be with you and leave her kittens at this critical time, which would likely be fatal to them. She is a mother now, with a mother's responsibilities. Don't distract her, or make her choose between you and the kittens. Keep children away.

Make sure each kitten is warm and has had a drink of milk. Occasionally a cat will push one of her kittens to the edge or out of the nest, or may even pick it up and remove it. You must take action quickly. Make sure the kitten is warm—being cool is one reason the mother may have rejected it. You can hold the kitten next to your skin to warm it. When the rest of the kittens are nursing, mix the rejected kitten in with them. If the mother continues to reject the kitten, you may have to raise it yourself using a commercial milk replacer. Some kittens are rejected because they do not remain as warm as the rest. In other cases, the mother truly knows best, and the rejected kitten, after being carefully hand-raised, turns out to have a serious congenital defect and is never normal. A first-time mother may be confused by the birthing process, and may try to harm her kittens. Watch her for several hours to make sure she cleans the kittens and allows them to nurse.

The kitten's umbilical cords will separate nearer to the body than you have cut them off initially. This is a natural separation point, and is normal. The remnant of the cord usually falls off in two to three days.

Most of the time the wonderful and amazing process of birth goes without a hitch for a healthy mother cat. However, things can go wrong . . .

BIRTHING PROBLEMS

Call your veterinarian immediately if you have a kitten stuck in the birth canal and you cannot gently pull it out within several minutes. The veterinarian may be able to give you helpful suggestions over the phone, or may ask you to bring her in immediately. A stuck kitten IS an emergency.

If more than two hours pass between kittens, or if the queen quits straining and you suspect there are more kittens, have her examined as soon as possible by your veterinarian. Likewise, if she is still straining, but appears to be doing so only weakly, have her checked. If she is still very enlarged, or she is a cat that normally has a large litter, or if she has been X-rayed and the required number of kittens have not come out, get her to a veterinarian as soon as possible. A Caesarean section may be required to deliver the remainder of the kittens and save the queen's life.

Occasionally the mother will quit trying to have kittens during delivery. This can occur if she is stressed, as when many people, or people whom she doesn't know, are present. This is especially a problem with a cat that is overly dependent on humans, such as one that was orphaned or weaned early. The cat may labor for a day or more, stopping for many hours between kittens. When a kitten begins to come out of the vulva, she may stop straining. She will not remove the membranes after the kitten is born. Consult your veterinarian, who may want to give you a mild tranquilizer to give her at home rather than have you bring her to the veterinary clinic.

In the worst-case scenario, all but the last one or two kittens are passed before the mother's uterus completely quits trying, and a Caesarean section has to be done to deliver the remainder of them. When one of these cases is finished, you may wonder why you didn't have the surgery done at the beginning. Even so, it is often better if the kitten can be born naturally, so it's worth trying.

Other factors may affect the queen so she has difficulty giving birth. One of these is a previously fractured pelvis which narrows the birth canal. If your cat has had a fracture which has not healed well, it is worth having her spayed so she will not become pregnant—unless you really want kittens and are willing to consider a Caesarean section each time she becomes pregnant.

Difficult births may also be due to problems with the kittens. One or more kittens may be deformed, or extremely large. Dead kittens may hamper the birth process. Sometimes a kitten gets stuck crosswise at the fork of the uterus. The uterus has two horns and is "Y" shaped. Imagine a kitten lying crosswise across where the two horns come together. Not only can it not get out but none of the others can, either. Sometimes when a small queen has only one or two kittens, all the nutrition goes into growing HUGE kittens, and they cannot pass through the birth canal. This is especially true if she has been bred to a much larger male. All of these situations may require a Caesarean section to save the queen and/or her unborn kittens.

CAESAREAN SECTION

If you are planning on a Caesarean section, you will be taking the queen to the veterinarian when the calculated days of gestation suggest she is very close to giving birth.

In performing this surgery, an incision is made down the midline of the abdomen and the kittens are removed from the uterus. Depending on the anesthetic used and how well the surgery progresses, you may or may not be able to take the queen home immediately after the surgery. She should be able to nurse the kittens soon after the surgery is completed, even if she is groggy. Stitches will need to come out in 10 to 14 days.

If you are planning to have the cat spayed, ask your veterinarian about it before surgery begins. If conditions are favorable, it may be possible to do it at the same time. Also let the veterinarian know if you do not want the kittens. That way, the staff will not be tied up in heroic efforts to save them. If you do not want the kittens, they will be painlessly euthanized shortly after they are removed from the uterus.

Before the veterinarian does the Caesarean section, you should make a decision as to whether the mother or her kittens are more important to you. Tell the veterinarian. That way, if there are complications and the veterinarian must choose to save either the queen or the kittens but not both, your choice is known and the veterinarian can act accordingly.

THE NORMAL NEWBORN

If any of the kittens is dirty, wipe it gently with a clean, damp, warm washcloth. When the kittens are all cleaned, check each one to see if there are any defects or injuries from the birth process. The skin should be intact, with no bruises or tears. The coat should be shiny and clean. The umbilical cord should be dry and clean. If a hernia is present, it will look like a bulging area or small knob where the cord attaches to the kitten. The membranes of the mouth should be pink. Check to make sure the kitten does not have a cleft palate (split in the roof of the mouth).

Newborn kittens should be rounded and plump. They will usually breathe between 15 and 35 times per minute. The heart rate is more than 200 beats per minute until they are a couple of weeks old. The rectal temperature is usually around 96 to 97 degrees F (35.6-36.1 C). The rectal temperature will gradually increase to 100 degrees F (37.8 C) by one week of age. If you have a chilled kitten that is less than a week of age, it should not be warmed any higher than 97 to 100 degrees F (36.5 to 37.8 C).

A normal newborn kitten should be able to crawl and turn itself right side up. It should be able to nurse shortly after birth, although some newborn kittens may not nurse well the first day. By the second day it should have the hang of it and suckle eagerly. The kitten will mostly sleep and eat for the first week.

CARE AFTER BIRTH

The queen should pass one set of membranes per kitten. Keep count to see that she has done so. Retained membranes may lead to uterine infection. However, if you haven't been watching her all the time, she may have passed and eaten some of the membranes. In that case, don't worry right away. Just watch for odorous drainage or passage of membrane fragments from the vagina.

The day after the queen has given birth, take her to your veterinarian, who will palpate the abdomen to see that all kittens have been born. The veterinarian may give her an injection of the hormone oxytocin, which helps shrink the uterus and expels fluids and any membranes that are left inside. It also stimulates milk production. If you see anything abnormal about the kittens, have them examined by your veterinarian at this time. Put them in a SMALL box (just big enough for them all to sleep in a single layer), and cover them with a towel or piece of cloth. Be sure you are not smothering them, but keeping them snug and warm. If you need to take one kitten to be examined, take them all.

It is a good idea to take the queen's temperature twice a day for 10 to 14 days after birth. If it goes over 103.5 degrees F (39.7 C), she may have an infection of the uterus (metritis) or of the mammary glands (mastitis). Have her checked by your veterinarian as soon as possible.

It is also a good idea to squeeze a couple of drops from each of the mammary glands once a day. Colostrum, the milk produced for the first two to three days, is slightly thick and may be straw-colored or yellowish. After about the third day, normal milk is bluish-white. It should not be off-colored, bloody, sticky, or odorous. If any of these conditions occur, have her checked. Meanwhile, take the kittens away from her and put them on milk replacer until your veterinarian has examined her. Milk from a queen with mastitis can make the kittens very ill.

You can offer food to the queen soon after she has finished giving birth. If she has eaten the placentas, she may not be hungry yet. It is normal if the cat does not eat for a day or two after she has kittens. Have food and water available close to the box in case she wants them. If she is an indoor cat, you may want to move her litter box within the same room as the birthing box, but not too close to the food and water. If she is an outdoor or in/out cat, you can let her outdoors for a few minutes. Try to avoid handling the kittens while she is gone. The mother may be disturbed by any change in the odor of the box that happened while she was away.

The queen may have a black, watery diarrhea for 24 to 36 hours after giving birth if she eats the placentas. This diarrhea is normal and is not a problem unless it continues.

Keep a close eye on the queen's vulva for a couple of weeks after birth has occurred. A small amount of drainage may be seen for up to two to three weeks after the births. Odd colors are normal—it may be greenish, blackish, or reddish but should NOT show fresh blood. The drainage should not have a foul odor, nor should there be much of it. If fresh blood, a yellow or white discharge, foul odor and/or a large amount of drainage are present, the queen may have a a uterine infection. Weakness, vomiting, drinking excessive amounts of water, or vomiting after drinking also may be signs of pyometra (a uterine infection). Consult your veterinarian immediately.

For the first three days, other than the visit to the veterinarian, leave the new mother alone with her kittens as much as possible. Do NOT let children handle the kittens. Keep a close eye on the kittens for signs of illness. Remember, "A Quiet Kitten is a Happy Kitten." Healthy kittens are well fed, warm, comfortable and plump. It is normal for them to whimper for a few minutes when they wake up or when their mother gets in and out of the box. But there should not be any loud, continuous crying. The kitten may cry if it gets caught in the bedding and cannot get to its mother. Or it can occur if the kitten is not feeling well, or is cold or hungry. If ALL the kittens are crying much of the time, the mother may not have enough milk (or any at all), or she may have an infection in the breasts (mastitis) so that the milk there is not good. If the problem is only with one kitten, take it to your veterinarian to be checked. If all of them seem to have a problem, take the mother as well as the kittens.

Kittens are so small and have so few reserves that diseases easily can be fatal. Take them to your veterinarian at the first sign of a problem if you want to save them. If you are not interested in saving every kitten at any price you may want to make your best guess as to the problem and treat it as best you can with home treatment and nursing. This may be the most realistic course if they are mixed breed and you are uncertain about finding homes for them. Be careful, however. Some problems in kittens may reflect a serious problem in their mother. You may want to consult with your veterinarian anyway.

For the first few days, most queens want to be with their kittens almost all the time, and will only get out of the box to urinate, defecate, or eat. Some will stay so close to their kittens that they become constipated, or have urine retention. The queen should be taken outside her box for a short break several times a day so she will urinate and have a bowel movement.

Some queens may be very protective of the kittens and may not want you to handle them. Limit the number of visitors and strangers for the first three days. After that, it is good to have your entire family handle the kittens frequently so they will be socialized to humans at an early age. After their eyes open, baby kittens do not see very well for a few weeks. They may not see the shapes of adults and children as being the same sort of animal, so it is important for the kitten to be handled by both.

Socialization to the world of cats also is important. It is good to find feline companionship for kittens that have been orphaned so they will be comfortable in the feline world when they are grown. This is especially important if they will be used as breeding stock. Otherwise, they may be so bonded to humans that they will not breed normally. This is not a problem if the kittens are going to be pets. Exposure to dogs or exotic pets during this period will help the kitten accept them without question in the future.

The kittens will soil their nesting box. On the third day, when their mother is outside taking care of her needs, change the bedding. Once a day, wash her breasts and belly with a washcloth and clear, warm water. DO NOT USE SOAP OR DISINFECTANT PRODUCTS.

The colostrum that the queen produces for the first 24 hours is thicker and more yellowish than milk produced later in lactation and contains antibodies against diseases such as panleukopenia. In humans, much of the baby's early immunity is transferred from the mother through the placenta, before the baby is born. In cats, only about 10% of the antibodies responsible for the kitten's immunity comes to it through the uterus. The other 90% comes to it in the colostrum after it is born. That is why adequate early nursing is essential to protect the tiny kitten until its body is capable of producing antibodies against disease when it is vaccinated.

The queen's appearance and milk production are the best way to know if you are feeding her enough (see Feline Gourmet Chapter). Cats with large litters that are producing large quantities of milk may need extra vitamins and calcium. Consult your veterinarian for products and dosages. It is very important that the female have clean water available at ALL times. Without it, she cannot produce enough milk.

If you have a small, sensitive scale (how about a postage scale?), weigh the kittens soon after birth. Ten to 14 days later they should have nearly doubled their birth weight if they are growing normally.

Kittens' eyes will open between five and 16 days of age. At first they only open slightly, but by the seventeenth day, every kitten's eyes should be fully open. From that point on you will notice rapid mental and physical growth. It is normal for the cornea to be slightly cloudy for the first two or three weeks the eyes are open, but the surface should be shining and perfect. When the eyes first open, the iris is usually blue or bluish-gray. It will change to its normal adult color around three to six weeks of age. Before this time, the kittens' vision is poor, and their ability to see is still developing. The eyes may be cross-eyed or staring until the cat is about eight weeks old. The ear canals open around 11 to 17 days of age, a day or two after the eyes open.

Newborn kittens cannot stand. They move by making "swimming" motions with their legs and sliding along on their bellies. Kittens may have occasional muscle twitches. This is normal. They can shiver by about one week of age. They will begin walking around 14 to 23 days of age. They are very curious and interested in the world around them, and easily become lost. For this reason, it is good to keep them confined in their birthing box, a bathroom, or other simple environment where they won't become trapped behind or under objects. Kittens need the queen's licking to stimulate their urination and defecation for about two-and-a-half weeks.

As the kittens grow larger, the mother will spend less time with them and have less patience with them. Their sharp toenails may scratch her breasts, and their teeth are sharp when they nurse. The queen will usually growl and move away from the kittens, or swat them on the nose with a paw if they bite her too hard. You can trim the kitten's nails, which will help for a time, but this is nature's way of making sure their mother weans them. If the kitten chews on you, use the same gentle thump on the end of the nose, combined with a firm "no!".

Mother cats that give birth to litters around the same time may share kittens, letting each others' babies nurse without distinguishing between them. In some cases, the more dominant female may steal kittens from the shy queen. Shortly after birth, the queen may take other animals into her litter, such as baby squirrels, puppies, or rabbits. You've seen pictures of them in the newspapers.

Most kittens tend to nurse from the same nipple at each feeding, and unused mammary glands dry up if they are not nursed for 3 to 4 days. You can tell how many kittens the queen has by counting the active teats. If you are feeding orphans, use the same bottle and nipple from one feeding to the next, and try to keep your hands smelling the same. The kittens might not like it if you've just finished peeling onions! Kittens knead the mother's belly with their front paws as they suckle. Also called the "milk tread," this movement may stimulate milk flow.

If you have a queen that dies or has no milk, you may be able to graft her kittens onto another female. This is most successful during the first week after they are born. The substitute mother may ignore or kill the extra kittens if there is a great difference in size between them and her litter.

You can begin feeding the kittens around 16 to 18 days of age, and the entire litter should be eating a kitten-food gruel by 21 days of age. Put food in a shallow pan or small cookie sheet. It is normal for the kittens to walk through the food, sit in it, fall over in it, even romp in it for a few days until they get the hang of eating. If you are using dry kitten chow, soak it in water until thoroughly moistened before feeding. This may help prevent the kittens from becoming bloated after feeding. Puppy or dog food is not properly balanced for kittens and should not be fed to them.

A kitten that stumbles out of the nest will usually let out loud cries. The queen comes running and carries it home by the skin of its neck. A first-time mother may grab a kitten by the leg or tail. A nervous mother may haul them from place to place. I had one scatterbrained farm cat that would often move her young kittens, leaving them strewn along the way to her new home. She would forget to come back and get them. Retracing her path, I would gather crying kittens and take them to the new nest.

COMPLICATIONS AFTER BIRTH

Retained kittens, as well as retained membranes, may be discovered on the day-after-birth visit to your veterinarian. At any time, if the queen is not feeling well, she should be examined as soon as possible.

If the kittens are not getting any milk or not getting enough, you will notice that they all whimper and cry much of the time. They settle into a restless sleep for brief periods, then wake and cry again. They are hungry. Have the queen checked immediately. Your veterinarian may give her an injection of oxytocin to stimulate milk production. If it works, you're in business, provided there is no infection in the breasts. If it doesn't work, you get to feed the kittens by hand (see Orphan Kittens, below). This situation may also happen after the first day or so—the queen may stop producing milk.

Mastitis is an infection of the breasts (mammary glands). It may result from bacteria invading through the nipples, especially if sanitation is poor. Infection also may occur because the gland has been injured, or because bacteria have been carried there via the blood from an infection elsewhere in the body. If mastitis develops, the kittens act hungry: restless and crying. In mild cases, the breasts (one or more of them) may be swollen, reddened, bluish or purple, hot (or in some cases, much colder than the others) and painful. The affected gland (or glands) may feel hard or have lumpy areas in them. Normal mammary glands should be soft and pliable. You may not be able to squeeze out any milk, or if you can, it may be grayish, reddish or off-colored instead of the normal whitish to slightly bluish color. It may contain clumps, clots, or stringy pieces and may be sticky.

In severe cases of mastitis, the queen may be droopy, have an elevated temperature, drink more water than normal and generally look ill. She may ignore her kittens. This is more serious—take her to your veterinarian,

quickly! Watch the kittens closely to see that they do not become ill from ingesting the spoiled milk.

Whether the mastitis is mild or severe, the queen will need treatment with antibiotics for seven to 10 days. You will need to milk out the infected gland(s). Warm packs will help resolve the infection and relieve her pain. If only one or two glands are affected, you may be able to cover the nipples with Band-aids® and let the kittens nurse from the rest of them. After several days of antibiotic treatment, the kittens can be allowed to nurse all the glands as usual. If the infection has progressed to gangrene or localized into abscesses, the kittens cannot be allowed to suckle and will have to be raised as orphans.

The mammary glands sometimes become swollen and hard with milk. This condition may be hard to differentiate from mastitis. You should have your veterinarian check the queen. The swelling may be so painful that she will not allow the kittens to nurse. Covering her breasts with towels soaked in warm (not too hot) water will help relieve the swelling and pain, as well as stimulating circulation in the area. Gently milk out the glands, and help the kittens to nurse. Reduce the queen's food to lower her milk production. If overproduction and swelling are continuing problems, get the kittens onto solid food as soon as possible (any time after about 16 days of age), and wean them when they are eating well. If the breasts become engorged with milk during weaning, use the warm compresses, but do NOT milk her out or massage her breasts, as this will stimulate continued milk production. You want production to stop.

Occasionally, a queen may seem to have no milk at all. If you squeeze the nipples, nothing comes out, and the kittens are continually restless and crying. This can happen if the queen is on a poor diet, especially one with low-quality protein, and may occur when a Caesarean section is done. Keep track of her temperature to make sure she does not have an infection. Encourage the kittens to suck, as the suckling action may help her to produce milk. In some cases, oxytocin may be given, as above, to bring about milk letdown. There is no drug that will stimulate milk production if the queen is not making any at all. Make sure the queen has adequate food (and is eating enough of it) and drinking enough water to produce milk.

Metritis, an infection of the uterus, may occur when the queen does not pass all the afterbirth (membranes) at the time the kittens are born. It can also occur if she has retained one or more dead kittens in the uterus. A few cases are seen after apparently normal births with nothing retained. Most cases develop within one to three days after birth. The queen may have a foul-smelling fluid draining from the vulva. She may have a fever, be depressed, stop eating, stop producing milk, and drink more water than usual. She may have little or no interest in her kittens. Get her to a veterinarian as soon as possible.

Blood tests and X-rays may be needed for your veterinarian to confirm the presence of metritis. If you do not want future litters, the simplest solution is to have an ovariohysterectomy (spay) performed immediately. If you wish to keep the queen for future litters, the veterinarian may treat her with antibiotics placed in the uterus, antibiotic injections or oral antibiotics, perhaps for three to four weeks. She may be given oxytocin, or other hormone injections, to try to eject the infected material from the uterus. There is a risk with hormone treatment in that the uterine wall, which has been weakened by the infection, may rupture, causing a fatal peritonitis. Or infection may spread throughout her system, again with fatal results. If the cat lives through the treatment, the uterine lining may be damaged enough that she will never carry another litter to term.

For some queens, the safest course of treatment for metritis is spaying, performed as soon as possible. Be aware that doing surgery on an infected uterus carries much more risk than a "routine" spay for a healthy animal. In some cases, the queen may not live through the surgery, or will die soon afterward. Queens with severe metritis are toxic, generally in borderline shock and very ill. They are very poor surgical risks, but there is little other choice.

The mother may ignore one or more of the kittens. If she is ignoring all of them, have your veterinarian check her immediately. She may have an illness or infection. No infection, no illness? Then, look for social causes. Is she so much a member of your family that she is not "acting like a cat?" You may pay for having excessively spoiled her by getting to play mother to her litter! It may help to move the kittens into an area of the house where you are. For example, if you are fixing dinner, move the box into the kitchen. Pay attention to her when she is in it, and ignore her when she is not. This will help to reinforce the idea that you want her to stay with the kittens. You may have to spend some time sitting by the box and petting her and telling her that this is where you want her to be. When you go to bed, take her and her kittens to the bedroom. When she jumps up to sleep with you, put her back in the box.

On the other hand, you may not be guilty of having excessively socialized the queen to you. She may have been removed from her own litter at a very early age, or she may have been raised by hand. Either way, she would not have an "example" of mothering skills from HER mother. Or she may simply lack the skills for genetic reasons. Some females in all species (including humans!) are not good mothers. You may either have to help her raise the kittens or raise them yourself as if they were orphans. Think long and hard about whether you want to raise another litter out of this female or one of her offspring and, perhaps, perpetuate the problem through the next generation.

NEWBORN KITTEN PROBLEMS

A rough, dry hair coat on a kitten is either a sign of illness, or of the mother neglecting it. A kitten that has decreased muscle tone and looks "flat" is probably seriously ill; saving it may not be possible. Have it checked by your veterinarian as soon as possible. Bluish color and labored breathing are also problem signs, possibly of a congenital heart defect.

Kittens that are widely separated from each other may be too hot, as may kittens that are panting and have reddened gums. A litter of kittens will pile together if they are cold.

Hypothermia is a common cause of death in newborn kittens. Until the kitten is several weeks old, its system is not capable of regulating its body temperature. If it is not getting (or eating) enough food, is in a cold environment or is neglected by its mother, the kitten may become chilled. At this point, the queen may decide she doesn't want the kitten. This is a natural reaction on her part. However, it may be fatal for the kitten when it is pushed away from its only source of warmth and food. Kittens cry constantly when they first become chilled. Later, they will stop crying and stop moving. The queen may push the cold kitten out of the nest as if it had died.

Feeling the kitten is not an adequate test of its temperature. A kitten that feels warm may still be cold enough to be dying. If the kitten's rectal temperature drops below 93-94 degrees F (33.9-34.4 C), it may not be able to nurse effectively. Chilled kittens cry pitifully and weakly. If not rewarmed, they may die within a few hours.

Take its temperature, and if necessary, warm it until the rectal thermometer registers between 96.8 and 99 degrees F (36 to 37.2 C), and NO higher.

Gently warm the kitten by wrapping it in a towel and placing it on a hot water bottle filled with lukewarm water. Electric blankets or heating pads may cause the kitten to become too warm and should not be used. You can tuck the kitten inside clothing next to your skin to warm it. If you are wearing a bra and are not squeamish, this is an excellent place to warm a cold kitten. Do not warm the kitten so fast or so hot that the skin is burned, or that you overheat it and raise its body temperature too high. Too-rapid heating raises the oxygen needs in the outer tissues, while the heart and breathing rates are still too slow to adequately oxygenate them. You are trying to bring the kitten back up to normal, not parboil it. Rewarming may take one to three hours, depending on how badly the kitten is chilled.

In many cases, when you have warmed the kitten, the queen will take it back. If it does not begin to warm up within an hour or two, it is unlikely to do so, and will probably die. Hypothermia also may cause hypoglycemia by slowing the action of the digestive enzymes. A sugar-water solution (2:1), diluted honey, or corn syrup can be used to treat it. This allows energy-giving sugars to be absorbed directly from the stomach without needing digestion. Use a medicine dropper to place a few drops at a time in the kitten's mouth. If it swallows, you've probably succeeded. After the kitten is warm and has been fed, it can be allowed to nurse normally.

Cleft palate, a split in the roof of the mouth, is a defect sometimes seen in newborn kittens. Much of the time it is hereditary. A few cases of cleft palate are thought to be caused by factors affecting the mother during pregnancy while the kitten was developing, such as nutritional deficiencies, drug or chemical exposure, or stress. If the kitten has a harelip (split upper lip), check the roof of its mouth to see whether it is cleft, as the two problems are often found together. If no harelip is present, the first sign of cleft palate may be milk dripping from the kitten's nostrils as it tries to nurse. Pneumonia is common because the kitten inhales milk while trying to drink.

Kittens with cleft palate that are not treated usually die either of pneumonia as they inhale milk while nursing or of starvation because they cannot produce enough vacuum in their mouths to suck milk out of the nipple. In general, correcting cleft palate is difficult surgery because the patient is so tiny. Most veterinarians like to have the kitten about three months old before attempting corrective surgery. At this age, the kitten has a better chance of surviving the anesthesia. Meanwhile, you will have to try to keep the kitten alive for that long, which usually means feeding it by hand with a stomach tube to avoid getting milk and food into its lungs.

Cleft palate and harelip occur because the kitten did not quite grow together in the middle as it was being formed in the uterus. If the defects are large enough, the kindest course of action is to euthanize the kitten. Kittens which are successfully raised and treated should not be used as breeding stock because of the high probability of passing on the defect. Frankly, since the kitten could only be a pet, the bother and expense hardly seem worth it.

Umbilical hernia is another hereditary defect common in cats. You may notice a small bulge where the umbilical cord was attached to the kitten. Feel the swelling. If it is hot, it may be an abscess—have the kitten checked as there may be infection in the stump of the umbilical cord. If the swelling is of normal temperature, it is likely an umbilical hernia. If small, it will probably go away with time. What happens is that the kitten grows, but the hernia stays its original size. So, a "quarter-inch" hernia, which is large in a kitten, is negligible in an adult cat.

The biggest problem with an umbilical hernia is that a piece of intestine may crawl out through the defect (a hole) in the abdominal wall and become strangulated. It is pinched off by the edge of the defect and blood flow stops. The piece of intestine may die, endangering the life of the kitten if not promptly treated. If the umbilical hernia is large, feel it gently a couple of times a day, carefully pushing its contents back into the abdominal cavity. If you are suddenly unable to push the contents back in, take the kitten to your veterinarian immediately.

Umbilical hernias can easily be corrected surgically. Most veterinarians prefer to wait until the kitten is at least three months old so that it can better tolerate anesthesia. If the hernia is not giving the kitten any trouble, you may even wish to wait until you spay or neuter it around six months of age. Many times the hernia repair can be done as part of the other surgery, under the same anesthetic. It's a lot less expensive than having it repaired separately, and there's risk from anesthesia only once, not twice. If contents of the abdomen are not pushing into the pouch, there is no harm in waiting.

Atresia ani is the condition when the newborn kitten does not have an anal opening. It may be noticed as you check the sex of the kitten. The skin below the tail may bulge slightly where the opening should be. In some cases, the only problem is that the skin itself has not opened. Your veterinarian can quickly remedy this by puncturing the skin and making the opening that should have been there. In other kittens, part of the digestive tract may be missing. These kittens should be humanely euthanized.

Diarrhea can be a problem in newborn kittens, especially if they are orphans that are being hand-fed. Good sanitation will help prevent it. Overfeeding may also cause it—avoid giving them too much formula, or giving a few large meals instead of more frequent smaller ones. As with human babies, dehydration can quickly kill kittens because of their lack of bodily reserves. Cow's milk formulas can cause diarrhea when used for prolonged periods to feed some kittens. Switch to a feline milk replacer as soon as possible.

If the kitten that has diarrhea is valuable, take it to your veterinarian as soon as possible. If you wish to try home treatment, first look into the feeding problems mentioned above: sanitation, overfeeding, cow's milk. Then give the kitten one-half to one teaspoon (2-5 ml) of Kaopectate® or a similar product. Give this with an eyedropper or dribble it into its mouth with a spoon. Keep the kitten's head level. Repeat this every two to three hours. Keep the kitten hydrated by giving it feline milk replacer or, at least, water from a bottle if the kitten will take it.

Trauma is a common cause of kitten death. The cat may roll over and crush the kitten, or she may deliberately eat one. Some females may accidentally bite the kitten hard enough puncture its body, or squeeze it hard enough to cause an umbilical hernia while carrying the kitten around. These events are most often seen with queens that are frightened or nervous. Limiting the number of visitors (and strangers) around the mother for the first few days after the kittens are born will help prevent these injuries. Providing a stable, stress-free environment may keep the rest of the litter from being killed or "worn out" from too much motherly attention. If the queen shows this kind of behavior for more than one litter, remove her from the breeding program. This type of behavior can be inherited, and you may be breeding it into your cats by keeping her. Tranquilizing the queen may be helpful, but providing a quiet, stable environment from the beginning may be better.

Tom cats frequently kill kittens. Perhaps, like lions, they kill kittens sired by another male. The female promptly comes back into heat, and he may have a chance to impregnate her. Unless you are sure of his intentions, keep a tom cat (or any other adult cat) away from the kittens until they are several weeks old. This is also helpful in preventing transfer of disease to the babies. On the other extreme, a few males, especially Siamese, may sleep with and help to groom the kittens. Be sure you monitor him when he is with the kittens.

CAUSES OF KITTEN DEATHS

A certain amount of kitten loss cannot be avoided. Under average cattery conditions, as many as one in four kittens will die before three weeks of age. Even under very good cattery conditions, losses may be one in 10. Under home conditions, losses may be more or less, depending on both care and luck.

Malnutrition in the queen during pregnancy and afterward is a major cause of kitten loss. This may be because she is not given (or does not eat) enough food, or because she is unable to absorb certain necessary nutrients. It may be because her food is of low digestibility, her diet is unbalanced, or needed ingredients are lacking. As with human babies, low birth weight is a major factor in kitten loss.

The kitten may suffer malnutrition because it is too weak, small, quiet, or cool to nurse, or does not nurse effectively. The kitten simply may not drink enough milk to maintain itself or to grow. It may be oversupplemented so that its diet is unbalanced, or it may be unable to digest milk. Kittens that do not nurse well may quickly become hypoglycemic and die. The supplementation of these kittens with milk replacer with a small amount of corn syrup added may give them enough energy that they can recover and nurse on their own. Some kittens that die soon after birth are simply not developed enough to make it out in the world.

It is important for the newborn kitten to take a good, strong first gasp. This helps to open up and inflate its lungs. If they are not fully expanded and opened up, this will have to occur gradually over the next three days. During this time, the kitten may be weak, and it may be in doubt whether it will survive. Don't despair—many of them make it. Kittens that are not breathing adequately will not nurse well.

Some large kittens will have the umbilical cord pinched off by pressure as they pass through the birth canal. Or, the placenta may separate too soon, and the lack of oxygen from these situations may make the kitten try to breathe while it is still immersed in birth fluids. It may inhale some of these fluids, leading to its being born with lungs filled with liquid rather than empty and waiting to be filled with air. Removing as much fluid from the kitten's mouth and throat right after it is born is helpful. So is gentle swinging with its head held downward. Placing the kitten in an incubator which has a gentle flow of oxygen added to its atmosphere can be helpful.

Unhumidified oxygen should not be used for more than about four hours, or you risk drying out the lining of the lungs and causing even more problems. The atmosphere in the incubator should be enriched with oxygen, NOT 100% pure oxygen! A kitten that has fluid in its lungs also may be gently taped to a board. The board is then propped at a 45 degree angle, with the head downhill, in an incubator. The kitten will begin to cry, and this crying will help to open up the lung passages. The head-down position will help drain fluid out of the lungs. Do not leave the kitten on the board for more than half an hour to an hour.

Kittens that die within one to three days after birth, with signs of weakness and rapid decline, should be examined for signs of hemorrhage. You may see blood clots on the lips or tongue. All kittens are born with a marginally effective clotting mechanism. This may be due to a vitamin K deficiency and treatment with vitamin K may allow their survival. In some cases, hemorrhages may occur because a kitten was rewarmed too rapidly or subjected to temperatures above 103 degrees F (39.4 C). It may be necessary for your veterinarian to combine history, examination of the kittens, and laboratory tests to find the reason for the hemorrhages.

In some cases of hemorrhage, the queen may bite the umbilical cord off too close to the kitten's body, or pull too hard on the stump. The blood vessels pull back into the kitten's abdomen and it bleeds to death internally. These kittens will have blood or blood clots in the abdomen.

A few queens will eat their kittens. Sometimes, the kitten that is eaten is ill or defective. The queen may be high-strung or nervous. A cannibal queen that eats kittens in more than one litter should be spayed and placed as a pet as she will probably continue to do it. It is natural for the queen to eat kittens that are aborted or born dead. In the wild, this would keep from attracting predators to the nest. A queen that is starved may eat her kittens. As mentioned elsewhere, tom cats will often kill kittens. Queens that do not have kittens at the same time may also kill and eat young kittens. This may be because they are about the same size as many prey species.

A queen may carry streptococcal bacteria in her reproductive tract. Kittens are infected when they are born, either from fluids or when the mother bites through the umbilical cord, especially if she chews it apart exactly at the belly wall. Strep-infected kittens usually "fade," becoming progressively weaker and less active, and dying within the first week of life. The whole litter may die. However, future litters from this queen are less likely to die. In a group of cats where kittens have been lost to strep, the queen can be given benzathine penicillin. A single dose at birth often prevents kitten loss. Treatment of all cats in the group may stop further kitten loss, but sanitation and quarantine must be used to reduce contamination of the premises. Cats should be caged and fed separately during an outbreak.

Kittens which are four to 14 days old and are crying and bloated should be examined for red and swollen rectums. This may be a sign of "toxic milk" syndrome. Their mother looks healthy and normal. This distinguishes the problem from acute mastitis, where the queen will be sick. The kittens should be removed from their mother and placed where the temperature is 85-92 degrees F (29.4-33.3 C). Feed them a 1:20 mixture of corn syrup in lukewarm water until they are no longer bloated. When the bloat is gone, you can feed them a normal kitten milk replacer product for the remainder of the day. Meanwhile, take the queen to your veterinarian for examination. What has happened is that her uterus (or part of it) did not drain out completely after the kittens were born, or there is an early infection in it. Your veterinarian will treat the queen with a combination of antibiotics to control the infection and drugs to drain the uterus. In many cases, the kittens can be returned to their mother within one to two days.

Kitten septicemia may occur anytime from shortly after birth to six or seven weeks of age. Many of the cases occur within one to two days after birth. The very young kittens become hypoglycemic, chilled, and dehydrated—signs much like many of the other kitten diseases. Many will die within 10 to 12 hours after the illness begins. Older kittens breathe rapidly, have swollen abdomens, cry from time to time and die within 12 to 18 hours. At first, only one kitten may be affected. Soon others become ill, until most or all of the litter is sick. Few, if any, of the kittens in the litter will survive the first week.

Many bacteria are involved in kitten septicemia. In some cases, the exact species which is causing the problem can be determined only by laboratory cultures. Septicemia is especially a problem in cattery situations, and is more common in queens having their first litter. Kittens that do not get enough colostrum shortly after birth are more susceptible than those that nurse adequately from the beginning.

These are only a few of the problems which can befall newborn kittens. If you have kittens that are ill or are not doing well, and want to save them, gather them up and take them to your veterinarian for diagnosis and treatment. Even then, don't be too disappointed if all of them don't survive. A seriously ill kitten is a challenge to diagnose and treat under the best of circumstances.

ORPHANED KITTENS

Kittens need their mother's care and milk until they are nearly six weeks old. If at all possible, kittens should receive milk from the queen for at least the first two days of life. Her colostrum gives extra nutrition and a laxative effect to help start the digestive tract moving. It also transfers antibodies to the kitten.

Kittens whose mother cannot or will not take care of them are as much orphans as kittens whose mother is ill or has died. A queen may not have enough milk to feed a very large litter. The easiest solution, but one that is rarely available, is to graft some of the kittens onto another lactating cat.

Raising orphaned kittens can be a major task. It takes a great deal of time, and can be frustrating. It also can be heartbreaking when the babies, after a great investment of effort and emotion, die. Before you start, consider the consequences. If you do not want the kittens, or do not want the responsibility of finding homes for them, do the kindest thing. Have your veterinarian euthanize the kittens right now, and save yourself time, trouble, and heartache. Most veterinarians give a special rate for whole-litter euthanasia. You are in all likelihood saving the animals from the street or euthanasia in an animal shelter at a later date. Don't try to drown a batch of kittens—it really isn't humane. Their brains can tolerate 20 minutes and more of oxygen deprivation with little or no damage—a slow and terrible death.

Orphaned kittens that are younger than three to four weeks should be fed a kitten milk replacer product. They will not be as robust, or grow as rapidly as those kittens that have a good mother. However, with special care, they can become healthy, normally-socialized animals by the time they are several months old. In the end, most of them will catch up in size and development with similar non-orphaned kittens.

A cow or goat is NOT the best mother for a kitten. Cow's milk has most of its' calories in the form of lactose (milk sugar). In contrast, a large part of the calories in cats' milk are from protein. Use a milk replacer which has protein, fat, and milk sugar levels specifically made to mimic cat milk. KMR® (Pet-Ag, Inc., 39W432 Rt. 20, Elgin, IL 60120) is one well-known brand, and Nuturall™ is another. This product will keep up to two years on the shelf. If you live on a farm, and have nothing else available, cow's or goat's milk can be used. When using milk replacer, follow directions on the label.

In an emergency, cow's milk will do until you can get some milk replacer. An emergency formula can be made with one-half cup whole cow's milk plus one hard boiled egg plus 1 teaspoon calcium carbonate powder (limestone, from your health food store or drugstore). Add liquid cat vitamins according to package directions. Mix this together in a blender. Give about one-half tablespoon per ounce of kitten body weight per day, divided into several feedings. Another home-made formula is: 3 ounces condensed milk, 3 ounces water, 4 ounces plain yogurt, and 4 small or 3 large egg yolks (Wills, 1993).

The first two to three weeks are the most critical period in the orphan's life. Kittens that are orphaned at birth are especially delicate, as they did not receive colostrum and are much more susceptible to disease. Do not allow adult cats near them until they have received their first vaccinations. Do not go to a place where someone has had a sick cat if you can avoid it. Do not handle other people's cats. A respiratory virus which would give an adult cat a case of the sniffles can be fatal to a delicate baby kitten that has not received protective antibodies from its mother.

For the first hand-feeding, allow three to four hours to pass between the last nursing (if any) and the time that you start feeding milk replacer. If the kitten has had a chance to nurse, it will allow time for antibodies to be absorbed. It also will allow the orphan to become hungry, making it more likely that it will start to drink milk replacer.

Give kittens that weigh 3 to 5 ounces (90 to 150 grams) one teaspoon (5 cc) of milk replacer for the first feeding. If you are feeding the kittens with a bottle, they will usually stop sucking when they are full. If you are using a feeding tube, it is important to avoid overfeeding them. A tiny kitten's stomach capacity is around four teaspoons per pound of body weight (50 cc per kg). A kitten that weighs a fraction of a pound has a VERY small stomach! Kittens that are orphaned in the first week of life may drink less than 10% of their body weight per day.

Feed the kittens through the night for the first several days if they are crying and awake. Otherwise, you can let them sleep through the night, if they will, and feed them during the hours you are up and around. Waking sleeping kittens to feed them is stressful and unnecessary. If they're not crying, let them (and yourself) sleep. Let sleeping orphans lie! It is normal for the kittens' legs to twitch during sleep. This muscular activity helps prepare them to walk in a few days. A normal litter of kittens will huddle together, especially when they are sleeping. Kittens that constantly cry or stay away from the rest of the litter should be suspected of having problems. Be sure they are warm (also see Nursing Chapter).

Feed milk replacer at room temperature or very slightly warmed. As with baby formula, you can put one or two drops of the kitten formula on the inside of your wrist to judge its temperature.

In an emergency, you can feed kittens with a medicine dropper. If you don't have one handy, steal one from a bottle of nose drops or children's vitamins. Be sure to wash and rinse it well before use. An eyedropper is also useful for kittens that are extremely small or weak. If you have one handy, you can use a small syringe in place of an eyedropper, squeezing out one drop at a time. For emergency use, try a doll-sized baby bottle. Most doll nipples, however, do not work very well for feeding kittens. Pet stores or veterinarians have special pet nursers with nipples which fit the kitten's mouth and are of the right shape and softness so the kitten can nurse easily. If you have litters of kittens often, it is a good idea to keep nipples, bottles, and other supplies on hand.

Wash all utensils, bottles, and nipples thoroughly after each use with hot, soapy water. Rinse well to remove ALL soap. Formula can be mixed every two or three days and kept in the refrigerator. Shake well before you measure the amount needed for feeding. Once opened, liquid milk replacer should NOT be left in the can. Put it in a glass jar or bottle and refrigerate. Cleanliness is not only next to godliness, it will help prevent serious illness in your kittens.

Be sure when feeding the kitten that you hold it nearly level with its head slightly upward. Squeeze one drop at a time when using a medicine dropper. If you feed the kitten too fast, or hold its head too high, you may force liquid into its lungs and the kitten will get pneumonia and die. If milk comes out the kitten's nose while nursing, you are feeding it too fast (or it may have a cleft palate). When using the nipple and bottle, put the nipple in its mouth, and pull it up and away slightly. This helps the kitten raise its head and will encourage vigorous sucking. Try to avoid getting air from the bottle into the kitten.

Warm the formula to around 100 degrees F (37.8 C). The kitten, especially at first, may not open its mouth and nurse automatically. In that case, place the kitten on its stomach and open its mouth with your finger. Put the nipple on top of the tongue. The kitten should start nursing. If it does not, squeeze the bottle to let out a drop or two of milk so the kitten can get the taste of it. If it still won't nurse, feed a drop or two at a time until it gets enough. When you are finished, the kitten's belly should be nicely rounded but not tight or bloated looking. Burp the kitten much as you would a human baby, placing it on your shoulder and patting its back. Remember to use a towel on your shoulder!

The proper amount of a balanced formula to feed is around 60 to 70 calories per pound of body weight per day (28-32 calories/kg). Less should be given to kittens that are orphaned during the first week of life, and for the first few feedings to kittens that are orphaned at an older age. You can weigh the kittens on a postage scale to see how they are doing, and to help determine how much to feed. Follow the instructions on the milk replacer product that you are using. In general, when in doubt, it is both safer and healthier to feed a bit less rather than giving too much. In addition, it is good to give the kittens water each day. Use about two-and-a-half to three ounces (70-85 ml) of water per pound of kitten per day.

When you increase the amount of formula you are giving, the kitten may have diarrhea. If this occurs, return to the previous level of feeding for several feedings before trying to increase it again. Diarrhea may upset the bacterial balance in the kitten's system. Supplementing the formula with an oral product containing normal digestive bacteria may be helpful. One product is Bene Bac® (Pet-Ag, Inc., Elgin, IL., 60120). It also may be helpful to give plain water instead of milk replacer for one feeding, followed by diluted milk replacer or a smaller amount of it. A small amount (one-quarter to one-half teaspoon (1-2 cc)) of Kaopectate® also can be given. If diarrhea persists, or the kitten becomes weakened or is otherwise ill, consult your veterinarian. Tiny kittens have very few reserves, and can quickly die.

Feeding is only part of your job. In addition to nourishment, the queen provides warmth, security, and socialization. Her licking cleans the kittens, and helps provide moisture in their environment. It is also a massage which stimulates the circulatory and sensory systems, and stimulates the digestive tract to help the kittens' elimination. So YOU have to lick the kittens, right? No, not really. Here's what you do:

After you have fed them, take a washcloth or rag dampened with warm water and wipe their skin. Work from head to tail, first down one side and then the other, then down the back and down the belly. This also helps to clean the milk mess off the kitten's face and the other mess off the other end. Now take a dry rag and stroke a few more times to help dry the kitten. A reasonable amount of gentle petting will also help things along—you can let your children stroke the kittens for a few minutes four or five times a day (after you have done the washcloth scrubbing). Normal bowel movements will be yellowish and have some shape to them.

If you have access to a commercial incubator, this is perhaps the ideal environment for orphan kittens. If not, prepare an appropriate-sized incubator box for them. It is important to provide good ventilation, but keep drafts away from the kittens. For very small, delicate kittens, you can use a clear plastic cover with holes in it, or even clear plastic wrap safely secured to the box so that it will not fall and suffocate the kittens. Poke air holes in the plastic wrap.

The kittens must be kept warm to compensate for the absence of their mother. When they are born, the temperature should be around 90-92 degrees F (33 C). By the end of the first week, you can drop it to 88 degrees F (31 C). Between 8 and 14 days of age, the temperature can be gradually reduced from 85 degrees F (29.4 C) to 80 degrees (26.6 C). The temperature can be kept at 80 degrees F (26.6 C) through the end of their first month of life. By five weeks of age, the temperature can be dropped to 75 degrees F

(23.9 C). After the kittens are about six weeks old, temperatures of 70 degrees F (21 C) are fine. Smaller kittens generally need higher temperatures than do larger ones, but not much higher. Set the box halfway on a heating pad.

If the box is very thick, you can put the heating pad inside at one end, wrapped securely in a towel so the kittens cannot burrow under it. Begin by turning it to low, and check the temperature in the box every hour for five or six hours until you are sure the temperature has stabilized. Use a thermometer, placed at kitten level. The bedding at the end with the heating pad should be near the desired temperature. If not, adjust it and check it again.

Having heat at only one end of the box will allow the kittens to crawl to the other end if they feel too warm. Whatever heat source you use, make sure it will not burn the kittens or cause a fire hazard in your house. A bit of humidity is important to keep the kittens' membranes moist. A humidifier in the room, or a pan of water near the box, will add moisture to the air. Placing an old-fashioned, wind-up alarm clock with a loud tick in the box may help keep the kittens calm and quiet.

As the kittens' eyes open and they become more active, they will want more food, and will be able to cope with eating more. You can continue to feed them by hand. Or, you can make a small rack to hold the nursing bottles at a height and angle that is convenient for the kittens. Place the kitten near the nipple, in its normal feeding position, and squeeze some milk out of the nipple. If it doesn't get the idea or loses interest, finish hand-feeding the first couple of meals. After that, you can leave the bottle, with the remaining milk, in the rack. Be sure to check the nipple frequently to be sure it is not clogged or open and flowing freely. Once the kittens get the hang of eating from the bottle in the rack, they will gain weight faster and be more content than when hand-fed specific meals. Milk replacer will become sour in the bottle, and should be changed at least three times a day to keep it fresh and safe. After the kitten is lapping food from the pan, discontinue feeding from the bottle over a period of two or three days. Eliminate one bottle feeding per day as you wean them. (See Feeding Chapter for further information on feeding kittens.)

WEANING

Kittens should be walking by the time they are a week old. By 16 days of age, their eyes should be open. By three to four weeks of age, they can begin to eat soft canned food or dry kitten food moistened to a soupy consistency with water. Handle young kittens as much as possible from the time they are a couple of weeks old. Some people feel that frequent handling results in friendlier cats later in life. The time from when their eyes open until about seven weeks of age is critical to their socialization. The kittens should be gently exposed to a wide range of experiences. This is an investment in having a normal adult cat later in life.

Normal, healthy kittens can be weaned any time between six and eight weeks of age, assuming they have started eating cat food. At this point, they can safely be taken from their mother and can go to their new homes. Kittens that are taken away from their mother and littermates before six weeks of age can have behavioral problems, including abnormal sucking. A normal kitten will usually weigh eight ounces (500 mg) or more by six weeks of age. Kittens that are smaller or sickly may benefit from another couple of weeks of nursing their mother, if she is healthy and has not become thin from nursing. Kittens may be fed canned or dry cat food with water (not milk) added to make a thin gruel. Or, you can use a product such as Kitten Weaning Formula® (Pet-Ag Inc., Elgin, IL 60120) as a transition from mothers' milk to solid food. (See Feline Gourmet Chapter.)

It is easy for kittens to be malnourished when they are depending on their mother for all their needs. Affected kittens are smaller and lighter in weight and may appear to be "runts." They may nurse poorly and make sucking motions. They may either cry continuously or be abnormally inactive. The kittens may feel rubbery or limp and weak when you handle them. Supplementing them as above and feeding the weaker individuals by hand may remedy this problem. Make sure the kitten is warm enough—its temperature should be 95 degrees F (35 C) or higher. If the kitten is colder, warm it up and make sure it is sucking and swallowing normally before you feed it.

It is easiest on the queen to take one or two kittens off her every one or two days until they are all gone. This may be easy if you are selling them or giving them away. Getting the little ones eating supplemental food before weaning serves two purposes. It helps get them ready to live on their own without mother, and it helps reduce the burden on her for their nutritional support.

A queen that comes into heat before the kittens are weaned should not be bred. Wait until after they are off her and she has had a bit of time to relax and recover before starting the work of producing a new litter.

If both the mother and father of the litter are purebred and registered, you can register the kittens. This makes them eligible to compete in cat shows, and they may sell for considerably more than "alley cats." Make sure the papers are in order, and that you have the necessary forms to give to each kitten buyer.

SPAYING

Why spay? Spaying (called an ovariohysterectomy) prevents pregnancy and the birth of unwanted kittens. It avoids the need to confine the queen during her heat period. It is even more useful in cats than dogs. Dogs only come into heat two or three times a year, while queens stay in heat most of the year if they do not become pregnant. The spayed cat does not attract males that urinate on everything, fight, scream, and howl at all hours, and generally make nuisances of themselves. If your cat lives outdoors, it keeps her from roaming because she is in heat and looking for a mate. If she is an indoor cat, you will not have to put up with her howling, rolling on the floor, climbing the curtains, and tearing the screens in an attempt to escape. Spaying also avoids reproductive problems such as pyometra and false pregnancy. Tumors of the reproductive system are eliminated, and the incidence of mammary tumors is greatly reduced.

When to spay? In general, most veterinarians do not like to spay cats before they are five to six months old. The more nearly mature the cat is before she is spayed, the better she is able to withstand the stress of anesthesia and surgery. Spaying at this age will catch most females before they come into their first heat (estrus) period. There is no need to let the cat have a heat period before she is spayed. You can avoid the problems associated with estrus by spaying her before it occurs. There is evidence that the hormone estrogen, which is secreted by the ovaries when she comes into heat, may sensitize the breast tissue to later tumor development. Over 95% of mammary tumors are malignant and life-threatening, and early spaying helps prevent them. It completely removes the chance that the cat will ever have uterine or ovarian cancer or pyometra (a potentially fatal infection in the uterus).

It also is not necessary to let the female have a litter before she is spayed. There is no evidence that it changes her disposition, or makes her "calmer" or "more settled." Spaying does not slow or change her physical or mental development, nor does it alter her personality. It does not change the cat's activity level (except to remove the fact that she might normally have gone roaming, looking for a male when in heat). Cats that get fat after they are spayed do so because they get too little exercise and too many groceries, NOT because they were spayed.

What about spaying the older cat? A cat that is not in heat or pregnant can be spayed at any time. Cats that are in heat can be spayed, but there is slightly more risk because the hormones keep the blood from clotting normally. This may increase bleeding during surgery. When the cat is in heat or pregnant, many veterinarians charge more because the cat bleeds more easily and the surgery takes more time and is more difficult. Cats can be easily spayed during the first month of pregnancy. If your cat is in heat, she may stay in and out of heat for several months. You may prefer to let her get with a male, because she will go out of heat as soon as she is bred. Then, you can take her in to be spayed a few days later. A cat that is spayed within 45 days after a mating, whether sterile or fertile, may produce milk within three or four days after surgery (Johnston, 1991). This minor sign of false pregnancy will go away in a few days.

If the cat has just had a litter, wait until milk production has completely stopped, but have her spayed before she gets pregnant again. A good time for the operation is usually between two and four weeks after the kittens are weaned. If you have a queen that you have been breeding and no longer wish to breed, it is strongly urged that you consider spaying her to prevent the same problems which can occur in all unspayed females.

What is a "spay?" The word "spaying" brings visions of a simple piece of surgery. The technical name, ovariohysterectomy, gives a better view of the operation. It is removal of the entire reproductive tract—uterus, Fallopian tubes, ovaries, and part of the ligaments that hold these organs.

A spay is major abdominal surgery, but is routine to veterinarians because they do a large number of them.

PREPARATION FOR SURGERY

For a "routine" spay, the cat should be in good condition, preferably not overweight or in heat or pregnant. Her immunizations should be current. Call several days in advance to make an appointment for her surgery. Most veterinarians schedule a limited number of spays per day, and will not accept any more than that in order to have time for any emergency cases which must receive care. A few veterinarians like to have the cat brought to the clinic the night before surgery is to be performed. Most of them, however, want her to come in the morning of surgery.

The cat should be kept off food and water before surgery. Do not give any food after her evening meal, and no water after midnight. That means closing the toilet and shutting off the dripping faucet so she can't sneak a drink. DO NOT try to be "nice" to the cat and feed or water her after these times. This is one time you could kill her with kindness! If she has anything in her stomach, she may vomit when she is given the anesthetic, or even after the surgery is completed. If she inhales this material, it will likely cause pneumonia and death. The food material and the bacteria on it cannot be removed from the lungs.

Incidentally, this preparation holds true for most surgery on cats—adult or old, male or female. One important exception is surgery on very young (six to 14 week-old) animals (see below).

THE OPERATION

Spaying is done under general anesthetic, which means the cat is completely unconscious during surgery and does not feel any pain. The front leg may be shaved to install an intravenous catheter. If a gas anesthetic is used, a tube may be placed in the cat's trachea. Some veterinarians use an intravenous anesthetic agent instead of, or addition to, gas anesthetic.

After the cat is anesthetized, she will be placed on a surgery table and sterile-draped just like a human surgical patient. The veterinarian will make an incision into her belly and remove her uterus, ovaries, Fallopian tubes, associated ligaments, and blood vessels. For a normal cat, the incision may be as little as an inch long. When surgery is over, the cat is taken to a recovery area.

Especially at some low-cost spay clinics, the cat may be sent home while still groggy. Put the cat in a warm, dark place (a cage or airline crate works well) and leave her alone! It may take the rest of the day and through the night for her to sleep it off. Check her every half hour or so to make sure she is comfortable. If you have the cat out around your family, she will try to walk and follow you and will be very upset that she cannot. It is much kinder to have her confined. The cat will "go up and down," alternating between being more and less conscious. DO NOT give her any water until she is able to walk without staggering and acts like she knows where she is. Then give her a couple of sips every half hour. Do not give her food until the next day.

AFTERCARE

The cat's throat may be sore from the tracheal tube. She may have a dry cough for a day or so. If it lasts longer, have her checked by your veterinarian. Restrain the cat from excessive activity for two to three weeks after surgery. Do not allow her to jump onto the sofa, bed, or windowsill. The stretching may tear open the incision.

Check the incision twice a day. A little swelling on each side is normal for a few days. If it is reddened, very swollen, hot, or if pus oozes from the area, contact your veterinarian within a day. DO NOT bathe the cat or allow her in the bathtub or shower or outdoors in wet grass until the incision is completely healed. If the cat needs to be cleaned, wipe her off with a lightly dampened washcloth. The cat should feel well and eat and drink normally.

If the cat licks or chews excessively at the stitches, it may be necessary to put an Elizabethan collar on her. It may help to put Bitter Apple or Variton Creme on each side of her stitch line. Some veterinarians close the skin with stainless steel sutures. The stiff, prickly ends keep some cats from licking them. If the cat pulls out one or more stitches within four or five days after surgery, have her checked. The suture line may be weakened enough that it might open. It's better to take her back for an extra visit than wait and have the incision rip open.

The stitches may be hidden, with no removal required. Visible stitches should generally be removed in 10 to 14 days. You can take them out with a pair of fingernail scissors. Clip about one-sixteenth inch (1 mm) to one side of the knot. Take your fingernails or a pair of tweezers and pull out each stitch. Or, you can take the cat back to your veterinarian for removal—the price is usually included in the spay cost (ask!).

If the cat is fat, pregnant, or difficult to spay, the incision may be long. Sometimes it is very hard to tell if a cat is already spayed without going inside and looking, surgically. Don't laugh—this can easily happen if you take in a stray or get a cat from a shelter. A long incision should not have any more trouble healing than a short one. As is said in the veterinary world, "incisions heal from side to side, not from end to end." However, with a long incision, it is even more important to limit her activity.

If the cat has a weak abdominal wall or is overweight, she may come home with a wide bandage around her belly. This may also be the case if the cat has suffered excessive bleeding (usually due to her hormone status rather than to any fault of the veterinarian). Carefully follow recommendations for aftercare.

The most serious problem which can occur after a spay is for the abdominal incision to tear open, allowing the intestines to fall out through the hole. This usually occurs either from excessive activity or due to infection of the surgical site. THIS IS AN EMERGENCY. Your immediate care may make the difference between life and death for your cat. Soak a towel or strip of bedsheet with lukewarm water. Wrap it around the cat's belly to keep the intestines moist and clean. Get the cat to the nearest clinic. This is a VERY rare consequence of surgery, but it is good to know what to do if it occurs. It is important to limit a cat's activity after ANY abdominal surgery until the incision is healed.

If the cat was in heat or starting to call to males when spayed, keep her away from toms for a few days after she gets home. Hormones still in her body may make her attractive to males. One of them may injure her while attempting to breed her, or their rough play may help to tear open the incision.

A farm cat or one that lives outdoors or goes in and out should be confined until she is completely healed and the stitches have been removed. Otherwise, if she becomes ill or infected, she may hide. You may not find her in time to get treatment for her and she may die.

SPAYING THE VERY YOUNG CAT

Some humane societies and veterinarians are spaying kittens (and puppies) as young as six to 14 weeks. They find this avoids the situation where 70% of the adopted animals are never neutered. Studies have shown that most kittens are produced by female cats between one and three years of age. Early spaying helps stop this production, and thus stop the tragic numbers of cats going from womb-to-tomb as they are euthanized en masse at shelters and humane societies. No problems later in the animals' life have been observed from early spaying or neutering. However, for my own animal, I would wait until around five to six months of age, depending on the size and maturity of the cat, because the animal is sturdier and better able to withstand anesthesia.

The young cats should be carefully screened for anemia due to parasites and for other illnesses such as diarrhea, dehydration, and hypoglycemia. One advantage of the early surgery is that the very young animals do not yet have a well-developed blood supply to the reproductive tract, making surgery easier and safer. The bad news is that if there is any excess bleeding, the animal is so small that it has very little "extra" blood to provide a margin of safety.

Procedures for surgery are different for the very young cat. These little animals have a poor glucose storage mechanism. In general, they should be given a small meal one to two hours before surgery and fed again within an hour after they wake up from the anesthetic to help keep their blood sugar levels normal. It also is important to keep the kitten warm after surgery. Be sure to discuss this with your veterinarian if you are having ANY surgery done on a very young cat.

ALTERNATIVES TO SPAYING

The easiest and safest alternative is to keep the cat confined when she is in heat—the abstinence method of birth control. This is simple with a cat that lives indoors all the time. Just be extra alert when you or others are going through the door, as she might try to escape when her hormones urge her to go forth and find a male.

Some drugs which do not involve permanent sterilization have been tried to keep the queen from coming into heat. They are not safe for long-term birth control.

Drugs used to keep dogs from coming into heat have serious (or even fatal) side effects when used in cats. Side effects may include the development of diabetes or adrenal gland suppression.

Megestrol acetate (Ovaban, Schering Corp., Kenilworth, NJ) has been used in Europe for preventing pregnancy in cats. It is not approved for use in cats in the United States. It should not be used in cats with liver or uterine disease, diabetes mellitus, or tumors in the mammary glands.

Mibolerone (Cheque Drops, Upjohn Co., Kalamazoo, MI) has been used to keep female dogs from coming into heat. It is not approved for cats in the United States. Don't even think of using this product on your feline. Side effects include masculinization, which is not reversed if administration of the drug is stopped. It may also cause thyroid and liver problems, even in small doses. Larger doses may kill the cat.

A very few veterinarians offer tubal ligation as a method of birth control. Their theory is that it allows the ovaries to function, retains the uterus within the cat's body and keeps her "natural." It still allows her to come into heat and be serviced by a male, although kittens will not result. This surgery, in the opinion of the majority of veterinarians, has all the disadvantages of having an intact female: coming into heat, males hanging around and breeding her, a uterus which can become infected, ovaries which can have tumors, mammary tumors, and the nuisance of caring for a cat in heat. It has none of the advantages of spaying (removal of the organs so heat periods and diseases do not occur).

Research goes on to produce a vaccine which will induce sterility in cats (and dogs), keeping the animals from coming into heat. When available, an injection should be a quick and easy (and hopefully, inexpensive!) alternative to surgical spaying.

NEUTERING

The term "neutering" applies to the removal of the reproductive organs of both male and female cats. It is also called "altering." However, the word is more commonly associated with the removal of the testicles and epididymis of the male (castration). This surgery renders the male unable to reproduce, and has many advantages if you do not specifically want him for breeding. It reduces roaming, especially if performed before the cat becomes sexually mature and establishes a territory. While roaming, the tom cat has a greater chance of getting hit by a car, getting into a fight with another tom cat (and developing an abscess), being attacked by a dog, becoming lost, or contracting a contagious disease from another cat. Neutering reduces the tom's tendency to urinate to mark his territory, especially in the house and yard. It does not usually change a cat's position or cause loss of status in the social order in large groups of cats.

Neutering stops fighting and roaming behavior in about 90% of male cats that have the surgery, regardless of their age or breeding experience. In general, the neu-

tered tom cat is simply a better, more pleasant pet. In some areas, the neutered male and spayed female have the advantage of much cheaper licensing fees.

When should the tom cat be neutered? Much like spaying the female, it is preferable to have the surgery done before the cat is sexually mature—around five to six months of age. At this point, you may notice him spraying to mark his territory. This is different from normal voiding of the urine. A tom cat that is urinating to relieve itself will squat toward the litter box or carpet. One that is marking will back up, stiff-legged, toward an object, with his tail raised rigidly over his back. He will urinate on the object level with his body, without squatting. He may howl or growl as he does so. As sexual maturity approaches, the cat may also roam and fight.

Preparation for surgery is the same as for spaying (see above). The cat is put under general anesthesia. An incision is made over the scrotum, and the testicles and epididymis are removed. Most veterinarians do not suture the incisions closed; this is normal procedure. The cat will lick the incision to keep it cleaned and open, and for cats, that is acceptable.

Complications can occur if the incisions close prematurely. The scrotum may be swollen and reddish or purple. If you see this, if the cat is not feeling well, or if there is pus, blood, or a foul-smelling discharge, return the cat to your veterinarian to be checked. Otherwise, there is no aftercare other than keeping an eye on the cat and checking the incision daily. If the scrotum has been sutured, the sutures may need to be removed in seven to 10 days. Or, absorbable sutures may have been used, with no need for removal.

Male kittens can be neutered at a very young age, in the same manner as spaying female kittens; the same pre-operative conditions apply (see Spaying the Very Young Cat, above). For early neutering, both testicles must be in the scrotum. If they are not, surgery should be put off until the kitten is around six months old.

Occasionally, a neutered male cat will appear to mate with a female cat that is in heat. He does not have any sperm, so he cannot make her pregnant. This sterile mating will usually cause the female to ovulate and go out of heat. Approximately 10% of male cats that are neutered will still exhibit male behavior such as fighting and urine spraying, regardless of the age at which the castration is done. This can be suppressed by the administration of hormones. They can sometimes be given for a short time and then withdrawn gradually. The hormones can cause side effects if given for long periods of time.

A vasectomy could be done on the tom cat to keep him from reproducing. He will still have all of the annoying characteristics of an intact male which make neutering so desirable. A vasectomy really serves no useful purpose.

The normal kitten's testicles develop inside the abdomen when he is in the uterus. They descend into the scrotum at birth or shortly afterward. If they are going to descend into the scrotum, they will ALWAYS do so before six months of age. If one or both testicles are not in the scrotum, the cat is said to be a cryptorchid (meaning "hidden testicle"). This is an uncommon problem in cats, but is occasionally seen, especially in Persians. It is hereditary and cats with this defect should not be bred. For this reason, surgery done to pull the testicle(s) into the scrotum is considered by most veterinarians to be unethical. There is no medical treatment which will make the testicle(s) descend into the scrotum.

Neutering a cryptorchid is more like spaying a female than neutering a normal male, and a cat with one descended and one retained testicle will probably have two incisions when he is neutered—one over the scrotum where a standard castration would be performed, and one more nearly like a spay incision. Surgery on a cryptorchid cat is much more complicated, as well as more expensive, than normal neutering.

Cryptorchid cats that have only the external testicle removed will still show tom cat behavior. An undescended testicle will still produce male hormones, and may be more likely to develop a tumor than a normal testicle. For this reason, a cryptorchid cat should always be neutered. Neutering also removes any chance of passing on this genetic defect.

REPRODUCTIVE PROBLEMS

Prolapse of the uterus is occasionally seen in cats. This usually happens shortly after the queen gives birth. It will show up as a reddish, meaty-looking mass of tissue pushing out of the vulva. This can vary from a swelling that just shows through the opening, or a mass which sticks out several inches behind the cat. Keep the tissue moist and take the animal to your veterinarian.

Some Persians may be late or slow breeders, and you should take this into account if they are your favorites.

Pyometra is an infection in which the uterus becomes filled with pus due to a bacterial infection of the lining. Estrogen injections, sometimes given for "mismating," may contribute to the occurrence of pyometra, as can some drugs used to produce abortion, prevent pregnancy or treat some skin diseases and behavioral problems. A hormone imbalance within the queen's body may also initiate a case of pyometra. Pyometra is most commonly seen in middle-aged cats, around seven to 10 years of age. When hormones are used to produce abortion, the disease can be seen in queens less than a year of age.

Endometritis, an inflammation or infection of the lining of the uterus, can occur before a full-blown case of pyometra. It may be diagnosed by a uterine biopsy and treated with hormones and antibiotics which may be needed for several weeks. With intensive treatment, the queen may (or may not) be salvaged for breeding. It is best to allow her to go through one heat cycle before breeding her, to make sure she is over the infection. Females that have had endometritis must not be treated with progestagens, as they may cause it to recur. If you do not want kittens, the cure is simple. Spay her and be done with it.

Signs of pyometra vary, depending on whether the cervix is open or closed. If it is open, a bloody or cream-colored pus-like discharge may be seen dripping from the vulva. It may stain the hind legs and cake the hair, and often has a foul odor. If the cat cleans herself well, the only thing you may notice is a tiny droplet of pus on the vulva between her cleanings. Pyometra often occurs one to eight weeks after the queen goes out of heat. The cat may be depressed, vomit, and quit eating. She may drink more water than usual, and may urinate more frequently. If the uterus is closed, depression, vomiting, and lack of appetite may be the only signs—drainage will not be seen. The abdomen may be swollen. If not PROMPTLY treated, non-draining pyometra can quickly result in shock, dehydration, coma, and death. THIS IS AN EMERGENCY, even if it's the middle of the night. If drainage is still present, she should be checked within 24 hours.

Pyometra is sometimes difficult to diagnose. Your veterinarian may need to run blood tests, and possibly take an X-ray to confirm the diagnosis. Spaying the cat immediately is the best treatment, even though the risk from anesthesia is higher than in a healthy cat.

If you wish to salvage the queen for breeding AND she is not too ill, a more conservative treatment using hormones and antibiotics may be tried. In some cases, prostaglandins have been used to drain pus out of the uterus and attempt to save the cat's reproductive capability. If the cervix is still open and draining, this is often successful, and the cat may later become pregnant and deliver a normal litter. You may wish to try this if a valuable breeding queen is involved (Davidson, 1992). However, overall, spaying seems to save more animals than do more "conservative" treatments. This is because the bacteria present in the uterus are spreading infection throughout the body. It's like having a balloon filled with pus inside the abdomen. The blood supply to the uterus is less than adequate, making it difficult to get antibiotics into the uterus to treat the condition.

Spaying a cat with pyometra is a delicate piece of surgery. The uterine wall is thin and tears easily. It's much like trying to remove a pus-filled balloon. The cat is already ill and has less physical reserves than a cat being spayed under normal conditions. She also will have less tolerance to anesthetic than she would otherwise have. For these reasons, there is significantly more risk than with a normal spay (but less risk than if the surgery is NOT performed). Also, it's more expensive surgery because of the complications. Intensive care, including large quantities of intravenous fluids, may be necessary to save the animal's life. After surgery is performed, the queen will be kept on antibiotics for about seven to 10 days to get rid of the bacteria in her body. If you and your veterinarian try conservative treatment and are successful, it is highly likely the problem will recur at later heat cycles. The cat should be bred at each heat cycle until you no longer wish to breed her, and then she should be spayed. Pregnancy sometimes prevents conditions from developing in the uterus which lead to pyometra. Mammary tumors are sometimes seen in cats (see Tumors Chapter).

Finding the cause of male infertility begins with a complete physical examination, including a medical and breeding history. Some males may be rendered temporarily sterile by the administration of drugs. Be sure to tell your veterinarian if the cat has been given any medication within the last six months.

Chapter 8

THE IMPORTANCE OF NURSING

THE IMPORTANCE OF NURSING

*". . . grant me the serenity
To accept the things I cannot change,
Courage to change the things I can,
And wisdom to know the difference."*

These words by Rheinhold Niebuhr seem particularly applicable to the field of veterinary medicine. There are problems veterinarians CAN change, such as suturing a wound, splinting a broken leg, giving the proper antibiotics to help control infection-causing bacteria, or helping your cat give birth to her kittens.

The difficulty comes with problems that cannot be directly relieved—those that leave the veterinarian and cat owner feeling helpless. If you are cursing your veterinarian's inability to cure panleukopenia (caused by a virus) in your beloved cat, stop and consider how little human medicine can do for the common cold! Medicine cannot yet influence, much less cure, most viral diseases. Diseases such as panleukopenia and rabies can be prevented by immunizing your cat against them, but little can be done if it catches the disease. A cat with one of these problems leaves all of us feeling helpless. Only good nursing care can aid an animal with many diseases.

It is with diseases such as panleukopenia that you can influence the outcome of the disease through careful and diligent nursing care. Veterinarians can only give the animal the best conditions possible, hoping its immune system and bodily defenses are strong enough to overcome the disease. The day-to-day nursing care that you supply can make the difference between life and death. Even when dealing with diseases where a veterinarian can do something, nursing care often helps the cat heal faster and more completely. Let's discuss nursing the sick cat:

1) Shelter. The seriously ill cat must have moderate temperatures. If it lives indoors with you, this is usually adequate. However, a temperature which is comfortable for you may be too cool for a sick cat. Move the cat's bed to a warm, draft-free corner, out of the main traffic pattern but close enough that you can watch it. If it is still too cold for the cat, put a heating pad under one end of the sleeping area so that the cat can choose extra warmth if it wishes. Place at least two or three layers of blanket or towel between heating pad and cat. Otherwise, the pad may overheat and burn the cat before it realizes it is too hot. Hard plastic heating pads are the safest (such as Lectro-Kennel™, Pet Heating Products, P.O. Box 1674, Loveland, CO 80539-1674). If the cat sleeps quietly at night, you might want to cover it with a lightweight blanket.

If the cat normally lives outdoors and is sick in winter, bringing it inside may save its life. If the cat has diarrhea or a similar problem and you cannot bring it in, make a small, warm corner in a shed or garage, boxing it off with a couple of pieces of scrap plywood. Or, get a box to make a temporary house. Put a heating pad, turned on low, under one half of the box, as above.

You can use burlap bags, old blankets, or carpet for bedding, which should be soft so the cat will not develop sores from lying on it. The items can be washed or thrown away when soiled. The cat should be turned from one side to the other a half-dozen times a day to keep it from getting pressure sores ("bedsores").

If it is summer and hot outside, bring the cat indoors so it will not get too hot. And, the cat won't be disturbed by flies, mosquitoes, and other insects. The cat doesn't need heat stroke added to its problems!

If your home is hot, a fan will move air and make the cat more comfortable. If the cat is outdoors and you can't move it, shade the cat as best you can. Sponge the cat with cool (not cold!) water to help keep its temperature down to normal.

2) Nutrition. Your cat should have easily digested, high quality food. It should have adequate nutritional content to heal damaged or diseased tissues. The animal that is ill may not eat as much as normal; thus, it is important that the food provide as many nutrients as possible in a small quantity. However, avoid sudden changes to rich food that can compound the illness with digestive problems. Ask your veterinarian any questions regarding feeding your sick cat. In the worst cases, your veterinarian may place a feeding tube through the nose or into the stomach until the animal has improved. This makes it easy to give food and fluids.

A sick cat may need two to three times the National Research Council (NRC) requirements for nutrients. Give four to 12 tiny meals a day. The first weight gained after illness is mostly fat and water rather than protein. For that reason, initial weight gain should not be taken as a sign that the cat is out of danger.

3) Water. Water is very important—VITAL—to maintaining the fluid balance within the body to aid healing. Your doctor often advises, "drink lots of fluids." Especially with virus diseases, it is important that the body not become dehydrated. The water should be fresh and clean and changed frequently. Try to keep it cool, but not cold, in summer. If the cat will not drink, it may lick ice cubes—it's worth a try. A light chicken or beef broth might entice the cat to drink. Keep the salt content low unless your veterinarian advises otherwise. In winter, if the cat is outdoors, offer tepid water several times a day.

4) Freedom from insects. If your cat is indoors, this should not be a problem. Can you imagine lying in bed with a cold and having flies buzzing all over your body? Your sick cat surely can't enjoy it either. If the cat is outdoors, spray the area lightly with an insecticide that is safe for use around cats. Cover the cat with fly netting or put it in a screened area. Insect repellent can be used ON the cat—IF the label says it is safe for use on cats. Before you use a new repellent, try a small spot on the cat's neck skin and check for reaction 12 hours later. Testing a small patch will let you know if the cat is allergic to the product. Poisoned baits may help reduce fly numbers in the area—make sure they are safely outside the cat's reach.

5) Grooming. Don't overdo it, but a sick cat should be brushed to remove dirt, stimulate circulation in the skin, and generally help the animal feel better. Sponge drainage from the eyes and nose with a dampened cloth, or wipe it away with a tissue, to make the cat feel better and reduce the number of insects attracted to its face. Wipe mucus from inside its nostrils with a cotton swab, then coat them with petroleum jelly to keep them from drying and cracking. The cat's sense of smell is extremely important to its appetite, and cleaning the nose will help the cat to be more interested in eating, which, in turn, will help keep up its strength.

If the cat is an outdoor cat, it may be helpful if it is able to go outdoors to have a bowel movement and/or to urinate. When you bring the cat back in, be sure the cat is clean so it does not soil the bed. Wipe the cat clean with a damp rag if necessary. Don't let the cat lie down with damp hair, as this may cause an infection on the skin, and flies may lay eggs, which hatch into maggots. The cat may use a cardboard litter box with sides an inch or two high, so it can get into it easily.

You can make a diaper by pulling a soft piece of cloth up between the cat's hind legs and around the tail. It doesn't need to be pinned in place, especially if the cat is lying down. When it becomes soiled, wipe the cat gently with a cloth moistened in warm water. Dry the cat with a soft towel or rag, and dust the area with a light coating of cornstarch. This process will help prevent skin irritation and reduce odors. On a long-haired cat, it is helpful to clip all the hair off the hind end and underside of the tail so the area can be more easily kept clean. Be careful not to irritate the skin with the clippers.

6) Exercise or rest? The decision to exercise or rest your cat depends on the illness and your veterinarian's instructions. If you don't understand or agree, ask the veterinarian why rest or exercise is recommended. Also, be sure you understand how much, when, and what kind of exercise to allow the cat, if any. After surgery or with some diseases, "cage rest" is essential. This means confining the cat to a small area so it cannot move around and injure itself. Restriction of movement is particularly important with fractures of the legs and pelvis.

7) Medication. Pills or injections should be given as close to the prescribed times as possible. The veterinarian may tell you to give a pill every 12 hours because the drug only stays in the blood for 14 hours. If you go much beyond the prescribed interval, you might give bacteria a chance to start growing again. Bandages should be changed or wounds cleaned according to the veterinarian's instructions.

Painkillers may not be given to the cat after surgery. Cats often show pain by moving very little or refusing to move, and by becoming grouchy. Pain is nature's way of limiting the animal's activity so it does not overexert itself and end up with even worse damage. Also, there are almost no painkillers which are both safe and effective in cats. If the cat does not eat because of its pain, check with your veterinarian.

If you have any questions about treatment or progress, don't hesitate to call your veterinarian. Most would rather get an extra call or two than have an owner treat the animal in a way that would be harmful or delay healing. Regular medication or bandage changes will give faster healing than treatment in "fits and starts." Do what you are supposed to do and when you are supposed to do it, and you will save time and money on medications, bandaging materials, and extra veterinary visits.

8) Miscellaneous. Some cats do best with a companion around, while others should not be fussed over and pushed around by their normal housemates. Separation may be the only way for the animal to get some rest and relaxation. And, speaking of rest—don't worry your cat to death by hovering over it. Take care of the cat so it is comfortable, but don't fuss all day long. That's why hospitals have visiting hours—so that sick people can get some rest!

Strangers may be upsetting to a sick cat—think of that before you have all your friends over. It's definitely NOT a good time for the kids to have a slumber party at YOUR house! When you are home, your cat may appreciate it if you sit nearby from time to time, perhaps just touching the cat with your hand or foot as you read the newspaper or watch TV. Knowing that you care can make a real difference in your cat's recovery.

No matter how difficult it is, hang in there. Many problems can be cured if you keep after them long enough and give the animal a chance to heal itself.

9) Medications in general. The medication meant for your pet has been specifically chosen by your veterinarian for its needs. Unless directed otherwise, give ALL the medication until it is gone. Perhaps the most common cause of a cat not recovering completely, or having the disease return, is that the owner does not give all the pills as directed because the cat was "getting better." Stopping too soon allows the bacteria to come back, as it may not have been completely controlled at that point. And, if it does come back, you have only the resistant bacteria. It is always more difficult to treat recurrent infections. If you think your cat is having a reaction or side effect to medication, let your veterinarian know immediately. Be sure to consult him or her about the dosage and safety of over-the-counter medicines in cats. Cats have some unique sensitivities, and a drug such as aspirin can easily be fatal.

Be sure you understand how to give the medication. Your veterinarian will be glad either to write out instructions, or show you what to do.

Give all medication with as little fuss as possible. Keep an eye on your cat for signs of excitement, such as panting and weakness. If you have any questions, stop your attempt and consult your veterinarian before continuing. Better to miss one dose than to fight with the cat and cause a relapse.

10) Restraint. Safe restraint is important when handling or medicating cats. Most cats can be talked into many unpleasant things, including injections, with gentle handling and petting. It is no fun, and may even be a hazard, if the cat is hostile about being handled. Both cat bites and scratches can become infected. Some cats are easily handled by putting them on a table or counter about waist high. Don't use a counter where the cat is not normally allowed, because it will be upset by being in a place that is "off limits." One person can scratch the cat's ears and the top of its head while gently restraining it.

If persuasion doesn't work, give up and roll the cat in a large bath towel. Leave its head sticking out if you are giving medication. If you are giving injections, you can roll the towel over its head, too, as long as the cat can breathe easily. Then, pull out a hind leg and give the injection. If you are treating the cat by yourself, wrap it in a towel and place the bundle on the floor, holding it snugly (but not too tightly!) between your legs. Then you can give the medication or put ointment in the eyes or ears. For oral medication, pull a pillowcase snugly around the cat's body and pin it at the neck, leaving the cat's head sticking out. This will keep the feet from getting into trouble.

A folded blanket can be used to corral an antisocial cat that is cowering and hissing in the bottom of a closet or behind the sofa. Fold the blanket into quarters and use it to completely cover the cat, gently pressing the cat against the wall. Then, fold the blanket over the cat and scoop it up.

If you are catching feral cats, don't attempt to handle them. They are best caught and transported in a live trap. If you are taking the cat to a shelter or veterinary clinic, be sure to tell the staff the cat is wild, even if it looks calm at the moment. This will keep someone from getting seriously clawed or bitten when reaching into the cage. If you have one of these cats cornered, don't push it too hard as it may attack you, or run up one side of you and down the other while trying to get away. A fish net may be used to capture the cat until it can be wrapped in a blanket or placed in a carrier. Next, let's cover some treatment methods which you may be using:

ORAL MEDICATIONS

LIQUID MEDICATIONS

Liquid medications are sometimes given to cats. Your veterinarian may prescribe a human pediatric liquid medication, especially for an antibiotic or other drug which is not easily available in veterinary dosage or form. Liquid human anti-diarrheal drugs are often given to cats. They are convenient, safe, and most people have them handy. Cough syrups also can be used, especially pediatric formulas.

Liquids should be measured as closely as possible. You can use a measuring spoon from your kitchen. You can ask your veterinarian for a syringe, or you might be able to acquire one at the feed store. Use it without the needle, of course. You also can buy a small measure at the drugstore which has a calibrated cylinder and a spoon-like top. Pour the liquid in it up to the amount needed, and then use it to pour the medication into the cat's lip. You can also use a bead-tipped plastic eyedropper. Insert the dropper between the cheek and teeth. Tilt the cat's chin just above level and slowly squeeze the medicine into the cat's mouth.

Approximate measures are: 20 drops = 1 ml (cc), 1 teaspoon = 5 ml, 1 Tablespoon = 15 ml, and 1 cup = 250 ml = 8 oz.

If you are by yourself, you can either put the cat on a counter at a comfortable height (see Restraint, Emergency Chapter) or on a towel on your lap if you are seated. If you are right-handed, tuck the cat under your left arm. If the cat is grouchy, have someone else hold the cat's legs or wrap the cat securely in a towel. Hold your left hand on top of its head, hooking your fingers under the bone just below its eyes; then, gently raise this upward to open the mouth. Or, you can pull out the flap of the cheek outside, and place the liquid in it. Do not put in more than a teaspoon at a time. Hold the cat's head SLIGHTLY above level, but NO more than that. If you hold it too high, you risk the cat inhaling some of the medication. Wait until the cat swallows before you put more into the pouch.

Maybe the cat won't swallow. What do you do? Stroke its throat gently, in a downward direction, from the base of its tongue part way down the neck. Sometimes you can put a small drop of the medication on the end of its nose. When the cat licks it off, it will end up swallowing the rest of it. When the cat's tongue pokes out through its teeth, you will know it has swallowed. You also can tell the cat has swallowed by watching its throat bob as the medication goes down. If the cat gags or coughs, stop immediately, allowing time for swallowing and relaxing. Then, gently give the medicine again.

Continue until you have given the entire dosage of medication. Wipe the cat's face with a dampened washcloth or paper towel, as medication left there may cause the hair to fall out. At the very least, it may become smelly and spoiled, causing discomfort to both you and the cat.

Coat supplements and some worming medications can be given by mixing them with the cat's food. Try a bit of the medication with just a little food in the bowl, however, before you give the cat the rest of its "spiked" dinner. Otherwise, the cat may smell the different odor, and leave the medicated portion in the bowl. It is often helpful if the cat is a little hungrier than usual before giving medicated food. Important medications, such as antibiotics, should not be given in the cat's food because they might not be eaten. It is often easier to give the cat its medicine before dinner. In this way, dinner becomes a reward for taking the medicine. Some oral medications are irritating to an empty stomach; feeding immediately afterward may help. Ask your veterinarian about feeding along with, before, or after giving the medication.

PILLS AND TABLETS

Pills and tablets are handy, and many common medications come in a variety of dosage sizes to accommodate cats from kittens to adult size. Your veterinarian also may prescribe human drugs, as this allows administration of modern antibiotics which are not yet available in veterinary form, as well as drugs which are rarely used for animals. It may help to coat the pill with butter or salad oil before giving it.

Give a pill to a cat by placing one hand over the top of its head. It is easiest for many right-handed people to use the left hand to open the cat's mouth and the right hand to give the medication. Press the cheek into the space behind the canine teeth, and gently but firmly open the cat's mouth, pressing inward and upward. Pull the upper jaw upward and backward, toward the cat's back. Do not pull it too far back, or the cat will fight you. However, pulling it a little way back will make it easier to hold. Do not count on keeping its mouth open by wrapping its cheek over its teeth with your fingers. The cat may bite through both the cheek and your skin. It is helpful if you are clearly dominant over your cat, so that when you speak sharply, it will stop struggling immediately.

Next, using your other hand, pull the lower jaw down, and place or drop the pill as far back on the tongue as possible, in the middle of it. Close the cat's mouth, and hold it gently shut until the pill has been swallowed. Stroking the throat will help some cats swallow. Other cats respond if the skin of the throat is pulled outward. This helps open the throat and lets the pill slide down.

You also can use a "pill gun" which holds the pill, allowing you to place it far back into the cat's throat. The good ones have a soft rubber tip. You then squeeze the plunger (much like a syringe), which pushes the pill out onto the cat's tongue. Be careful! You can injure the throat area if you go too far back into it with the instrument or handle it too roughly. These are available from

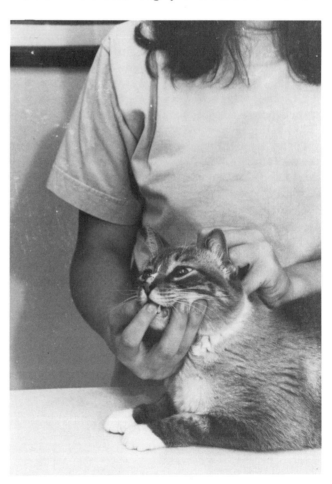

Drop the pill onto the back of the cat's tongue, pushing it back with your finger.

many veterinarians. A pill gun also can be made by cutting the end out of a small syringe (2 or 3 cc) and rounding the edges with a fingernail file. Leave the plunger in place to "shoot" the pill into the cat's mouth.

If the cat tries to claw you with its front feet, have someone hold them or wrap them in a towel. Some cats are easily pilled by gathering up the skin across the back of the head below the ears (just above the scruff of the neck). Pull it snugly together, pulling the cat's head slightly upward and back. The cat's face will pull into an open-mouthed grimace which looks horrible but works well. Cats don't seem to be bothered by this restraint. It may be like the grip the queen uses to carry her kittens, or resemble the mating bite of the tom cat. Whichever method you use, be sure to praise the cat lavishly after you are finished treating it.

It may be helpful to take the cat into a different room, such as the bathroom. The cat may be surprised by being handled in this manner and you can pill the cat before it is aware of what is happening. Another trick is to stick the cat on a window or door screen. When the cat is hanging on with all four claws, it can't hang onto you, and can easily be given the pill. The "screen method" is not good for liquid medication because it would be possible for the cat to inhale it.

Sometimes you can feed the cat pills by disguising them in any food which is "legal" for its diet. Putting the

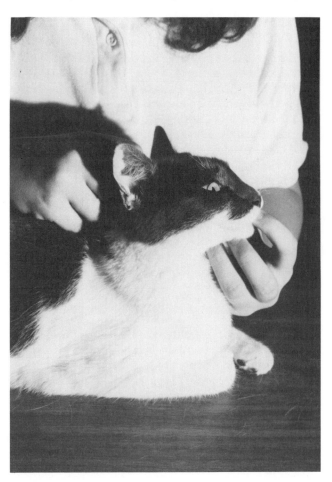

If necessary, hold the cat by the scruff of its neck to give medication.

pill in a piece of cheese, hot dog, or meat works well with some cats. Don't use salty meat for a cat on a salt-restricted diet. Some cats will learn to take the pill if you give them a (legal!) treat afterward. Try a couple of the treats without pills, followed by the one with the pill. If you are going to be giving the cat pills for a long period of time, it is well worth the effort to train the cat to take them easily; this makes it easy on BOTH of you. Some cats will take the pill if you coat it with butter. Margarine works with some cats and not with others. You can use sugar pills, harmless vitamins, or small cat treats as trial pills to see which, if any, of these methods will work for your cat. Some pills can be crushed, mixed with a tiny bit of water, and given with an eyedropper or syringe. Other cats will take the tablet if it is crushed up and mixed with something sticky like Nutri-Cal, Petromalt, or butter. This can be pushed firmly into the fur on the cat's front leg. Most cats can't stand anything sticky on them, so they will lick it off, medicating themselves in the process.

Capsules are occasionally used for cats. They may be used to give drugs too bitter or distasteful for the cat to take as a powder or a liquid. If you are giving a capsule, you may have trouble with it sticking to the cat's tongue. Then, the cat spits it out. This can be avoided by lubricating the capsule with salad oil before popping it onto the cat's tongue. It will slide down without sticking.

Whatever method you use, watch the cat carefully for several minutes after you have given the pill or capsule, to be sure it has been swallowed. If the cat spits it out, try again until it goes down. If you have tried everything and still can't get the cat to take the pill, ask your veterinarian for help. He or she may be able to think of something you haven't tried, or furnish a liquid or injectable form of the drug. Or, you may need to bring the cat to the clinic for daily treatment. It's cheaper and more convenient to train your cat to take pills.

OTHER ORAL MEDICATIONS

Paste medications are sometimes used, especially vitamins, laxatives and high-calorie supplements. They come in tubes much like toothpaste, and the dosage is usually measured in inches of material squeezed out of the tube. The paste easily can be squeezed onto the cat's tongue, and it will usually swallow. To get your cat started taking the paste, squeeze a half-inch or so onto the fur of its front leg, just above the paw. Mash it well into the fur as you put it on. Then, of course, the cat has to wash it off. These products are made with liver extracts and other good flavors, and most cats accept them eagerly. Nutri-cal® (Evsco Pharmaceuticals) is an example of a nutritional supplement which comes either in a tube or in a pump-type dispenser.

Powdered supplements or medications are occasionally used. Sometimes they can be mixed with gravy or with one of the tasty paste products mentioned above. Or, they can be put into empty gelatin capsules and given.

TOPICAL MEDICATIONS

Fresh wounds should not be cleaned or medicated if they are sizeable or deep. Cover the wound with a clean bandage or wrap and take the cat to your veterinarian. Small wounds can be treated with topical medications, directly on the skin or into the damaged area.

Minor wounds can be flushed with chlorhexidine (Nolvasan, Fort Dodge Laboratories, Fort Dodge, IA). This is one of the most effective disinfectants, and has a residual action against bacteria. It should not be used in wounds which may open into joints. Tamed iodine (povidone iodine) should not be used in wounds, even if diluted. It can increase wound infection and retard healing. Hydrogen peroxide has almost no value as a disinfectant, despite the impressive appearance as it bubbles and foams. It can even be damaging to tissues (Swaim, 1987). Don't bother using it.

Antibiotic ointment containing the combination of neomycin, bacitracin, and polymyxin is effective against many different bacteria, and is helpful to healing. Gentamicin is another good topical antibiotic. It is useful for wounds that do not respond to the neomycin-bacitracin-polymyxin treatment. Treatment with gentamicin solution seems to be more effective than gentamicin ointment (Swaim, 1987).

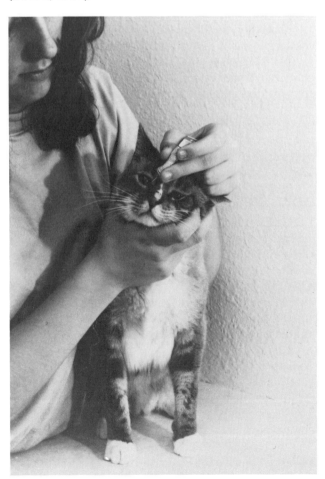

Squeeze ointment into inner corner of the cat's eye.

EYE MEDICATIONS

To put any medication into the eye, it is often easiest to have the cat in a sitting position, with its head extended upward. Placing the cat on a table or counter gives you better control of the cat and a better working angle. Use the thumb of the hand holding the cat's head to pull the upper eyelid upward, as well as to keep its mouth shut so it cannot bite. Rest the hand holding the medication against the side of the cat's face so that if it moves you can move with the cat and avoid jabbing it in the eye.

After putting the drops or ointment in the cat's eye, distract its attention for a minute or two by playing or feeding. This will keep the cat from rubbing its eye and injuring it or removing the medication.

Eye medications occasionally cause sudden allergic reactions or irritation, resulting in an itching, weeping, reddened eye. These are individual reactions to the particular medication being used, and are more annoying than serious. However, if a reaction occurs, discontinue treatment immediately and consult your veterinarian as soon as possible. He or she may wish to change your cat to a different medication, or the same medication in a different base.

These medications, as is true of all drugs, should be kept out of the reach of children. Wash your hands after treating your cat's eye. This can keep you from getting an infection if the cat has one, as well as keep you from getting any of the medication into your eyes or mouth by accident.

EYE DROPS

Eye drops are a common form of medication. Putting drops into your cat's eyes is easy. Hold its head slightly above level. Rest the hand which is holding the dropper or dropper bottle on the bridge of its nose. Then drip the drop onto the surface of the eyeball, or drop it onto the white area just inside the skin at the inner corner of the eye. To avoid contamination of the dropper, do not touch the tip to the eye. Just get close and allow the drop to fall. The biggest mistake is to hold the dropper too far away from the cat's eye, because when the drop falls on the eye, it is uncomfortable.

Many eye drops need to be put in the eye four to five times a day, or even more often. The cat's blinking washes them off the surface of the eye and flushes them away with tears. Let your veterinarian know if you cannot follow this schedule.

EYE OINTMENTS

Eye ointments are often used because they have a longer duration of action than drops. The greasy film holds the medication in place and keeps it from being washed away by the cat's tears. They are used in other cases because the oiliness provides good lubrication for the corneal surface. Eye ointments are used to carry the same drugs as drops: corticosteroids, antibiotics, and others.

Eye ointments are even easier to use than drops. Again, hold the head with one hand and steady the other (holding the tube of ointment) against the cat's forehead. The cat will normally close its eye when you get near it with the end of the tube. Pull the lower lid down, and squeeze a small amount of ointment into the pouch that is formed, using a steady, gentle pressure. Try not to touch the tip to the eye, to avoid contaminating it and to avoid scratching the surface of the cornea. In most cases, you will want to squeeze out about one-half inch (1.3 cm). When you are through, pull the tube gently away from the eye and stop squeezing. Sometimes a small dab of ointment will be left on the eyelashes. Use a tissue to wipe it gently away as your cat closes its eye again. The most common mistake with ointments is using too much at one time and wasting the drug. This can be very expensive with some ointments!

Some eye ointments are very stiff when cold. Warm the tube in your hand or in warm water before using it.

If you are using chloramphenicol ointment, be careful. Chloramphenicol is a good antibiotic, and seems to be safe for your cat. It can, in rare cases, however, cause blood problems in humans. Wash your hands well, with soap, to remove any traces after using it, or wear rubber gloves when applying it.

If your cat's eye is injured and you use an ointment with a corticosteroid in it, you may cause the loss of the eye. If in doubt, use an ointment containing only an antibiotic (the names of corticosteroids often end in "-sone"). Your veterinarian or pharmacist can quickly tell you if the ointment contains a corticosteroid. If the cat's cornea has been cut or torn (such as from a branch on a bush or tree limb), DO NOT put ANY ointment in it if you can get the cat to a veterinarian within an hour or so. An oily ointment may prevent successful suturing of the laceration.

OTHER EYE TREATMENTS

Any cat can occasionally have a bit of matter or discharge in the corner of its eye. Remove this quickly and easily with a cotton ball moistened in warm water. Avoid scratching the eyeball. Wipe gently in the same direction as the fur lies.

Eye powders are sometimes used in animals such as cattle, but must not to be used in cats' eyes. They are coarse and irritating, and the cat may claw violently at its eye, causing even more damage.

In some cases, as with a prolapsed eye, it may be necessary to suture the cat's eyelids shut. This is an extremely safe and secure treatment, especially with cats such as Persians, whose heads are hard to bandage without choking them. It's a lot like bandaging a bowling ball with eyes and a mouth. The sutured eyelids will act as a bandage, allowing the eye to heal. The stitches are usually removed in one to two weeks, depending on the problem. In some instances, you will need to put eye ointment into the corner of the eye, under the sutured lids, to help healing. This is a simple and very effective process. Ask your veterinarian to show you how to put ointment in the sutured eye.

EAR MEDICATIONS

Ear drops and washes often are used on cats. Ear drops work well to spread medication evenly over the inner surface of the ear. Washes contain products to dissolve wax in the ear, helping to liquefy and remove it.

To put either drops or washes into the cat's ear, hold its head steady (or have someone else hold the cat if it is actively trying to move around). Steady the ear flap with one hand and drop in the medication with the other, using the prescribed number of drops or amount on the dropper. Let go of the ear flap and massage the ear canal below the opening with your thumb and forefinger, rubbing firmly. This spreads the liquid around the ear surface, and works it into the nooks and crannies. It also helps loosen debris so the cat can shake it out. Last but not least, you are "scratching" the cat's ear, which often makes it feel better. When all this has been done, get out of the way. Many cats will naturally shake their heads vigorously, but will not shake out very much of the medicine. Because of this shaking, ear treatment is best done outdoors or in the shower, and NOT while wearing good clothing! Or, hold a towel or rag loosely over the cat's head until it quits shaking.

Ear ointments are used much like drops. Squeeze the recommended amount (for example, one-half inch) into the ear and massage the ear canal. Warm the ointment tube in your hand or in warm water before you use it and it will squeeze out easily. Do not use powders in a cat's ears. They stay in the ear and cause more problems.

COLD THERAPY

Cold therapy is a valuable treatment for injuries, such as bruises, sprains, muscular strains, and similar problems which have JUST occurred. Cold helps relieve pain. Cold therapy is also good for cats that have just been burned.

Cold helps reduce the inflammation which is occurring in the FRESHLY injured tissues. It can reduce swelling, and reduce the amount of fluid which leaves the blood and lymph vessels and pools in the damaged tissues. It also can help stop bleeding by constricting capillaries in the area. The less blood that escapes from the blood vessels into the tissues, the less there is to be removed in the healing process. Think back to the times when you have had a severe, large, purple bruise—and remember how long it took for it to heal! If you can avoid some of this blood oozing out, the wound will heal more quickly and easily. For all these reasons, prompt application of ice or cold water may significantly reduce healing time by reducing damage from the injury.

Cold is most valuable when used during the first 24 to 48 hours after the injury has occurred. After this time, it is of little or no value. By slowing circulation, it may even hinder recovery.

If available, ice may be used to chill an injured area. Ice cubes can be placed in an ice bag or plastic sack, and then wrapped in a towel or rag, which may be held over the injury by a loosely applied elastic bandage. This procedure works best if you can hold the cat, or sit beside it so it remains still. The refreezable, artificial-ice bags are convenient, and often stay frozen longer than ice made with water. They can be molded around a box of frozen vegetables or package of meat and then frozen so they approximate the curve of the cat's leg. If you use ice or cooling material, be sure to wrap it in a towel or other material to avoid freezing the skin.

Cold water may be run directly onto the area with a garden hose or under a faucet if the skin is not cut or damaged. Put it ONLY on the affected area, NOT all over the leg or cat. Don't keep the cat in the cold water for more than about 20 minutes, or you may drive it into hypothermia.

If you are using cold water on a cat that has been burned, do not use it for an excessive length of time as it may contribute to the shock that the cat is experiencing. In general, if the animal is in shock, large amounts of cold water or ice should not be used. Treatment with cold water also should not be used if infection is present.

When water is put on an open wound (this includes third degree burns where open tissues are present), the cat's tissues tend to absorb it. This may carry infection into the cut, and swell the tissues, slowing the healing process. For this reason, cold running water should not be used on open wounds—use an ice bag instead. Again, be careful using ice so you don't freeze the skin, as that will severely retard healing. The injured cat doesn't need frostbite in addition to a cut!

Cold should not be used for more than 20 to 30 minutes at a time. Around that time, it may cause blood vessels to open up and increase circulation to the area—the opposite of the desired effect. Using cold in addition to a compression bandage will help prevent this. Place the cold material over the bandage.

Heat and cold may be used alternately in some problems, such as sprains and similar injuries, after 24 to 48 hours have passed. Temperature therapy can be a tricky business, although it is a valuable adjunct to treatment. If you aren't sure how to do it, ask your veterinarian for advice.

HEAT THERAPY

Heat may be used to warm a cat in certain situations, such as a very ill outdoor cat in a cold climate, a kitten born in a snowbank, a kitten that has wandered into the rain and is suffering from exposure, or a kitten suffering from hypothermia from any cause. Fill plastic gallon jugs or similar containers with warm water, and use them as hot water bottles to help warm the cat. If you put very hot water in the bottles, wrap them with a thick cloth or towel to avoid burning the cat's skin. A chilled cat may be warmed in a tub of lukewarm (NOT HOT) water. It should then be carefully dried. A good way to do this is to wipe the kitten with towels or other cloths, and then finish the job with a hair dryer. Warm the cat slowly, as too-rapid warming can cause shock. A kitten can be returned to its mother after it is warmed and dry. For newborns, your body is a very good heat source—just put the kitten under your shirt next to your body as you go about your activities. Your movement will help stimulate its circulation.

Infrared lamps can be used to heat kittens in a garage or in a horse stall. Make sure they have plenty of bedding. Be very careful with these lights, as they can burn the cats if they are too close. They also present considerable fire danger if they are near bedding or other flammable materials. The queen (or another animal) may accidentally knock the bulb down and break it, injuring herself or the kittens. A minimum bulb-to-skin distance is 18 inches for a 125-watt bulb and 24 inches for 250-watt bulbs. Lay a thermometer next to the cat—its temperature should not exceed 103 degrees F (39.5 C). One disadvantage is that lamps disrupt the normal day-night cycle. With a bit of ingenuity you may be able to find a substitute method for providing heat which is at least as effective as an infrared lamp—and much safer.

Hard plastic kennel heaters are available which can keep the mother and kittens nicely warm—and safe, too. (One source of kennel heaters is R.C. Steele, 15 Turner Drive, Spencerport, N.Y., 14559). Whatever method of heating you use, the cat's enclosure or box should enable the animal to move to the other end if it is too warm and wishes to be cooler. This can be accomplished by using a box (with heat at one end) or by placing the box halfway over the heat source.

Heat is often used on injuries after 24 to 48 hours have passed. At this point, heat helps to stimulate circulation. This aids the body in removing blood and toxic products and speeds healing by bringing fresh oxygen to the cells. This in turn reduces the swelling, allowing the cells to return to normal.

Heat should not be used if infection is present in an area—or even suspected! It can cause the infection to spread. Heat also can cause problems because of increased absorption of infection-related toxins into the body. Increased circulation in the area may lead to severe edema and swelling, which may further complicate the infected injury. If heat is used on a fresh injury, it may make the problem worse than it would have been without it. For this reason, DO NOT use heat on a fresh injury, nor any time within 24 to 48 hours after the injury.

Hot water can be applied with moist cloths, as when a queen has edema in her mammary glands. Make sure the cloths are not so hot that they scald the animal or she may become rapidly worse instead of better. Second degree burns are severe problems all by themselves. Begin with lukewarm water and gradually make it hotter as the animal becomes accustomed to it. If the cloths are too hot for you to handle with comfort, they are too hot to put on the cat.

If she will cooperate, the cat may be put into the bathtub or a dishpan and given a heat treatment. Begin with lukewarm water, and gradually heat it up as the cat becomes used to it. Again, if it is uncomfortable to you, it will be uncomfortable to the cat. This type of therapy is used, for example, for cats with disk disease.

Deep heat and diathermy have been used to produce heat below the surface tissues. These should be used only under the direct supervision of your veterinarian, as severe damage to bones and other tissues can occur with improper usage. Like other forms of heat, deep heat techniques should not be used for at least 24 to 48 hours after an injury has occurred; likewise, they should be NOT used when ANY infection is present.

Infrared light has occasionally been recommended as a way of producing heat in tissues. It is not a good idea because of the very great danger of skin burns. Like a sunburn, these burns may not show up until some time after the treatment which caused them.

SOAKING SOLUTIONS

Epsom salts (magnesium sulfate) are sometimes used to help draw swelling and fluid out of an injured area. One or two cups of epsom salts are used per gallon of water. Use warm or cold water, depending on how fresh the injury is. Commercial soaking solutions are available. They are mainly based on epsom salts, with menthol and other aromatic substances added. The aromatic substances are generally oily and become stuck in the cat's hair and make a mess. Plain magnesium sulfate is probably better, and also cheaper.

Epsom salts are usually available from a drug store. Before you use a soak of epsom salts on your cat, carefully check for cuts, scrapes, or other breaks in the skin. Do not soak an area that has anything but intact skin.

MASSAGE

Massage is often used in addition to heat treatments to help heal sprains and similar problems. Massage often helps to lessen swelling and reduce pain. Many people like to use liniments, "braces," and other products, rubbing them into the skin over an injury. In general, liniments don't help much, and make a real mess in the cat's hair. They may produce some reddening and irritation in the skin over the injury, but don't do anything for the underlying tissues. A strong liniment may even cause a chemical burn on the cat's sensitive skin. It also may get into its eyes as it tries to wash itself, or could be harmful when the cat licks the material off its coat and swallows it. A dry gentle massage with the fingers is beneficial and a liniment isn't needed.

For best effect, massage should be repeated three or four times a day. Massage often helps to keep scar tissue from forming adhesions between the skin and the underlying tissues.

REST

Rest is often used to help keep leg problems from becoming worse. It also helps with disk problems in the back and pelvic fractures. Some leg injuries will become much worse if the cat continues to move around and use the leg: more fluid and blood may leak from the injured area, causing more swelling and pain, and lengthening the time needed for healing.

Make sure you know what your veterinarian recommends in the way of rest for your cat. He or she may want the cat totally confined to a small space. My favorite area for total confinement is a playpen. It keeps the cat from exercising, while allowing it to see and be a part of what is going on in the household. It is large enough that you can put a small litter box at one end and still have room for the cat's bed, food, and water. You can cover the top with mesh, netting, or lightweight plywood if the cat wants to get out.

Perhaps the best location for the cat is one that is out of the main traffic pattern, but close enough that its "humans" are visible. After all, your cat is still a member of the family, and not in isolation. Your veterinarian may want the cat to have a small amount of exercise, or recommend that the cat be completely confined. If it is an outdoor cat, the exercise may be limited to going outside a couple of times a day to urinate and defecate. Be sure you know what the veterinarian has in mind, and follow his or her instructions. Don't feel sorry for your cat because it was "cooped up all day." You could set progress back considerably—or even cause permanent damage by letting your cat out to exercise and play.

EXERCISE

Exercise may be used to help your cat lose weight. It can also be used to build up the cat's muscles and tendons after prolonged confinement. In either case, it is VERY important to start gradually. With a very fat cat, walking once or twice around the living room may be all that it can do as a beginning. Give the cat lots of encouragement, and don't carry the cat if you can avoid it. It is better for the cat to get halfway down the hallway and back by itself than to get accustomed to being carried. You can't do the exercise for your cat! Match your pace to the cat's, at least while it's getting in better shape. A toy on a string or flexible pole will let you exercise the cat a bit while you are watching television or relaxing. It is often difficult to encourage sedentary cats to exercise.

Be careful about turning your cat out to play with another cat, dog, or other pet if it is recuperating from surgery or injury. The cat may forget that it has a problem, and reinjure the area or tear something loose if they start to play vigorously.

ACUPUNCTURE

Acupuncture has been touted as a cure-all for anything and everything that ails. It also has been debunked as being total quackery. Like many disputes, the truth probably lies somewhere in between. No one knows for sure HOW it works. However, there are definitely times when it DOES work. It often can help relieve pain, as from arthritis. If you've tried everything else, and an acupuncturist who is familiar with cats is available, why not give it a try? This author will be the first to encourage any treatment which works.

Acupressure (kiatsu or shiatsu) is often helpful, especially with bruises and fresh bleeding under the skin. You can press your thumb firmly into the area, and hold it there for six to eight seconds. Release the pressure SLOWLY, gradually removing your thumb from the area. This action presses blood and stale fluids out of the area, allowing fresh lymphatic fluids to seep into the area. If you can do this three or four times a day, it can make a difference in how fast the bruise will heal.

INHALANT TREATMENTS

A humidifier may help your cat breathe more comfortably if it has an upper respiratory disease, or a vaporizer may be used to raise the humidity of the air. Check with your veterinarian whether to use one that puts out cold moisture or steam.

Your veterinarian may treat certain diseases and lung conditions by putting your cat in a cage with a nebulizer. It creates a small fog of medicated droplets so the medication is inhaled directly into the lungs. Nebulization is not usually a treatment used at home. As a hospital therapy, it can sometimes be a lifesaver.

INJECTIONS

"Injection" is the general name given to the process of putting a vaccine or medication into the animal's body with a syringe and needle. Injections placed under the skin are known as subcutaneous (S/C or Sub-Q for short) injections. Injections into the muscle are called, logically, intramuscular injections. Other specialized injections may be used by your veterinarian. Some drugs are given intravenously (in the vein). Intraarticular injections are those made into joints. Intradermal injections go into the upper layer of the skin. This route is tricky and used more for diagnosis than treatment. You are not likely to find a veterinarian willing to teach you these techniques—too many things can go wrong that would endanger your cat.

There are advantages to giving your own routine injections. Depending on the availability of quality vaccine, you may be able to save substantial amounts of money, especially if you have several cats. It can be much more convenient to bring vaccine home than taking cats to a clinic, especially if you have a "herd" of them. You may be more likely to keep vaccinations current if you can vaccinate at your convenience, giving your cat better protection. If your pet requires a prolonged course of antibiotic injections and you live a long way from nowhere, your veterinarian may PREFER that you give these "shots" yourself.

Make sure the vaccine comes from a reliable source. It must be refrigerated throughout the distribution chain. If it sits in the back of the feed store for a week until it is unpacked, it will not be any good, even if it is then refrigerated. You will be falsely relying on it for protection. Freezing and light are even more damaging to vaccines than heat. When you buy vaccine, take a cooler and ice pack to chill it on the trip home. Then, refrigerate it until used. Vaccine which has passed its expiration date may no longer give protection and should be discarded.

Do not use syringes which have been cleaned with chemical disinfectants or alcohol. These products do not kill some contaminants, which may later cause disease in the cat. And they do not kill all blood-borne parasites which can be transmitted from one cat to another. However, they CAN kill modified-live vaccines, rendering them useless. Use only new, sterile, disposable needles and syringes, one for each cat.

Before exploring the common types of injections and how to give them, it is important to discuss a few problems and liabilities involved in giving injections to your animals. Any injection has some small risk of reaction, which you should consider before deciding to give your own injections. If you are uncomfortable living with this risk, spend the money and take the cat to your veterinarian for immunizations. Anaphylactic shock is rare in cats but could happen—and it could kill the cat. If you give an injection to your own animal, you are obviously assuming the risk of doing so.

Some veterinarians, when accepting a cat as a new patient or for boarding or hospitalization, insist that your pet have a veterinary certificate of current vaccination, which is proof of immunization with an effective vaccine. The veterinarian is concerned about his or her liability if the cat is hospitalized and later contracts a disease against which it should have been protected.

Some veterinarians worry about children finding used needles and syringes, or about improper disposal of medical waste. They are concerned that you may be bitten while trying to vaccinate your pet. They worry that you may give the vaccine to a pet that is ill, when it may be completely ineffective. They worry you will not get an annual medical checkup for the cat. A veterinarian with this policy will insist on revaccinating the animal before he will admit it to the hospital. This can be both expensive and redundant if you have properly vaccinated your own cat. Find out in advance, BEFORE your cat needs hospitalization, if this is your clinic's policy. If it is, it will be a waste of money and effort to vaccinate your own cat. If you don't like this policy, look around until you find a veterinarian that will accept you vaccinating your own animals. Keeping GOOD records of vaccine products, routes of administration, and dates will alleviate some veterinarians' concerns.

NOTE: If the cat is insured, the insurance company may REQUIRE that any immunizations or injections be given by a veterinarian, and the policy may be voided if you treat the animal yourself—be sure to check with your insurance agent or read the policy before giving the animal ANY medication. You will be taking the responsibility for any reactions that may occur. Reactions are of two types: local and systemic. Systemic reactions are the most serious and life-threatening. Fortunately, they are also extremely rare.

ANAPHYLACTIC SHOCK

Anaphylactic shock is a very acute, powerful allergic reaction. It may follow an injection of vaccine, antibiotics, or products for desensitization to allergies. Normally, it does not occur the first time the animal is given a drug (although it can in exceptional cases). The body usually requires previous exposure to the substance to become allergic, so it follows the second or later exposures to a substance. Anaphylactic shock can occur when the cat is stung by a large number of bees, fire ants, or yellow jacket wasps. Very rarely, it can occur because of allergy to something the cat has eaten.

Anaphylactic shock occurs from within a few minutes to four or five hours after the offending material has been injected. Signs include pale, cool mucous membranes, increased heart rate, and difficulty in breathing. The cat may have sudden, acute, explosive diarrhea and vomiting, and both may be bloody. It may have hives, or a generalized swelling as its skin fills with fluid. Collapse and death can follow, due to complete failure of the circulatory system.

If the problem is not treated promptly, the cat can quickly DIE. If the cat survives long enough to call a veterinarian or get to a clinic, it will probably make it anyway. It will be important for the veterinarian to know that you gave an injection (and what you gave) within the preceding minutes or hours.

Treatment for anaphylactic shock must be immediate and sure. Epinephrine (also called adrenalin) is used at a dosage of about .005 cc per pound (.01 ml per kg) of a 1:1000 solution. Check the vial to make sure of the dosage and method of administration BEFORE you need it. Chances are good you will never have to use it. But, if you do, there will be NO TIME to read the label. Give it intramuscularly or subcutaneously, according to the label. A small spot of white hair regrowth may occur at the site of local epinephrine placement. Don't give it in a visible area on a dark-colored show cat.

A bottle of epinephrine and suitable syringe and needle (a 3-cc syringe and 20-gauge, 1-inch needle) should be handy WHENEVER you give an injection. It should never be more than a few yards away in your medicine kit. Tape a sterile syringe and needle (still in its plastic case) to the vial of epinephrine so they are always convenient—and so you are never tempted to use them when short of supplies. Don't cover the label. If epinephrine is not available, prompt administration of an antihistamine tablet or solution according to the directions on the label may save the cat's life. Have the cat checked by a veterinarian as soon as possible to be sure it is all right.

Occasionally, hives (also called urticaria) may be seen as a milder systemic reaction following an injection. See your veterinarian if they are numerous or do not go down within 12 to 24 hours.

LOCAL REACTIONS

Reactions may occur at the injection site. They may not show up immediately, but occur from a few hours to a week later. Swelling is the main sign, and may range from a small bump to a large blob. Pain may accompany the swelling. It will go down in several days (with or without treatment).

The swelling may be due to an infection. This can happen when bacteria are carried into the tissues by the needle when the injection is given. Or bacteria may be brought by the bloodstream to tissues which are damaged or weakened by an injection. Abscesses tend to form in the swelling, and feel hotter to the touch than the surrounding area. After several days, the abscess may come to a "point," forming a soft area at the highest part of the swelling. The presence of the point indicates that it should be drained (see Skin Care Chapter).

An abscess may affect the cat's well-being, causing it to go off feed and appear "droopy." An abscess on the neck may cause the cat to turn stiffly. Because the cat may be sore after an injection (even if it does not develop an abscess), it is not a good idea to vaccinate right before the cat is to travel or compete in a show.

The possibility of an abscess makes it important to utilize injection sites that will drain well if an abscess occurs. This is why intramuscular injections are often made in the lower part of the hind leg.

The animal may get a hematoma at the injection site. This is a blood clot which occurs because a small (or large) blood vessel has been punctured while giving the injection. It is impossible to prevent an occasional hematoma. But, by utilizing good injection techniques and giving injections in the proper sites, the possibility of getting one can be minimized. It would be a good idea to ask your veterinarian to coach you in both injection site selection and proper technique. If he or she refuses, and you are determined to give injections to your cat(s), find one who WILL help you.

As sometimes happens after a human "flu" shot, the vaccine itself can make the cat feel ill for a day or two. Don't worry if your cat is droopy for up to two days after an injection, as long as it does not show other signs of illness.

LEGAL COMPLICATIONS

In some cities and states, vaccine is available through the feed store, drugstore, or veterinarian, so you can purchase and give it yourself. In other areas, it is illegal to even possess a syringe or needle. Make sure that "doing-it-yourself" is legal where you live.

If you are treating your own animal, you are accepting the risk of anything that might happen. The cat is your property, and—short of cruelty—you can do almost anything you want with it. It becomes another matter entirely if you are treating a cat belonging to a friend or neighbor. Several things happen if a reaction occurs, whether it causes the animal's death, or "merely" an abscess or other "minor" complication. First, you feel horrible and will probably lose a friend. The second reaction is even worse. There is a good possibility that the owner may sue you for the loss of his or her animal—his or her property—and stand a good chance of winning.

Finally, YOU may be charged with practicing veterinary medicine without a license, which is a serious crime in some states—enough to get a stiff fine or even a jail sentence. It usually doesn't matter whether the other person is paying you. What does seem to matter is that you were illegally practicing medicine on someone else's animal.

How do you avoid this problem? Easy. Don't work on other people's animals. Period. If someone wants you to help and you know how to give injections, that's fine. Show the person how to give the injections (and make darned sure you're right or that could be another possible liability). Even better, suggest the person ask his or her veterinarian to demonstrate how to give an injection, or tell the person to get a copy of *The Cat Repair Book*.

Some veterinarians are reluctant to show clients how to give injections because of the problems which may occur. However, if you offer to pay for the time it takes to teach you, it will be money well spent, and may change resistance to cooperation. This is because veterinarians get tired of being milked for free information by clients, who then misunderstand or misuse it. We get a little gunshy about freely dispensing it. If, however, you can show your veterinarian that you are aware of the dangers, and that, despite the risk, you would like to learn to give injections properly, he or she may have a change of mind. Some veterinarians don't want you to give your own injections in any situation.

Now that the advantages and dangers of giving your own cat injections have been discussed, let's talk about technique.

ROUTE OF INJECTION

It is very important that injectable drugs be given in the manner prescribed on the label. A drug which is meant for intravenous injection but given in the muscle may cause the cat severe pain. A large chunk of muscle may die. If a drug meant for intramuscular use is injected into the cat's vein, carriers and other agents in the medication may cause a severe reaction and/or death. If there is ANY doubt as to how a vaccine should be given, read the label or the package insert and do only what it says. The cat you save may be your own.

PROCEDURE FOR GIVING INJECTIONS

What do you need in order to give an injection? You need the vaccine or medication which is to be injected. Check whether it is labeled for intramuscular or subcutaneous use. You need alcohol or other disinfectant for the skin. Apply it with a cotton ball or just spray or flood it onto the skin. If the cat has long hair, part it and inject into the "valley" you have formed. If the animal is very dirty (muddy or bloody), comb the dirt from the fur before beginning the injection. In warm weather, wash or hose the area first. This is unnecessary when the cat is reasonably clean; alcohol will cleanse the skin adequately.

Syringe sizes should closely match the injection being given. Too large a syringe is awkward with a small amount of liquid. Syringes are sized in cubic centimeters, also called cc's. A cubic centimeter is the same as a milliliter (ml). A 3-cc syringe is adequate for most vaccines, as well as dosages of antibiotics and other drugs for cats. In most cases, you will not inject more than one or two ml in any one site intramuscularly. This is because larger amounts cause considerable pressure and pain, and slow absorption, as compared to dividing the same dosage into smaller amounts and giving it in a couple of places.

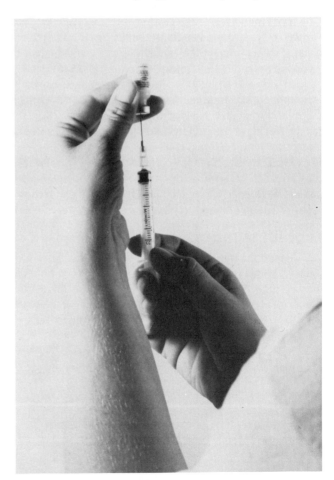

1) Draw air into the syringe.

2) Inject air into the bottle with liquid.

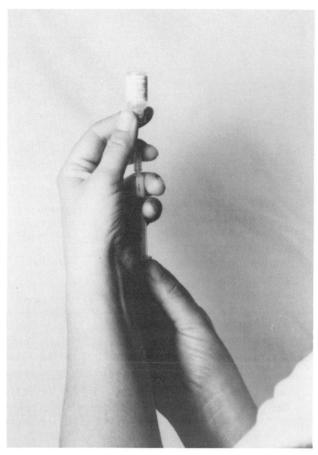

3) Draw liquid vaccine out of the bottle. Inject it into the bottle with dried vaccine if it comes in two bottles.

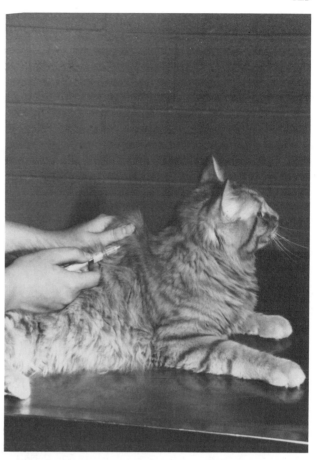

5) Subcutaneous injection. Insert needle at base of skin. Pull back on plunger to check for blood.

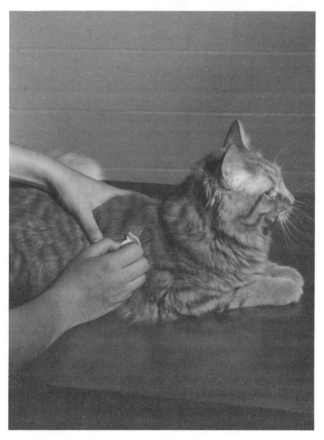

4) Cleanse injection site with alcohol.

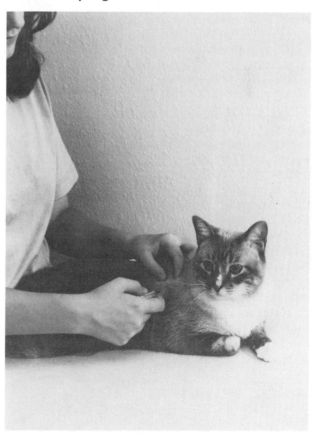

6) Hold skin firmly down while pulling out needle.

Syringes come with two different types of tips. Luer-lock syringes have a threaded end which must be screwed onto the needle. Luer-slip ends, which slide into the end of the needle with a snug fit, are also available. Either one is suitable for cats. If you have both cats and horses, you may wish to keep only syringes with Luer-slip ends on hand, as they are handy for both species. Syringes have the business end either centered or offset to one side. For most injections, it doesn't matter which you use.

The size of the needle depends on the material you are injecting. Most vaccines, for example, are placed under the skin. They are generally given in small doses and are usually liquid enough to flow easily through a needle. A small-bore needle can be used, causing the animal less discomfort. My preference is a 20-or 21-gauge needle, 1 inch long, for both intramuscular and subcutaneous injections. These needles also will handle penicillin and similar small-quantity antibiotics which are given to cats. If you are giving vaccine to a VERY small cat or to a kitten (under two pounds), you may wish to use a smaller, 22-gauge or 23-gauge, 3/4-inch needle.

Needles and syringes may be purchased individually in sterile plastic containers. Some veterinarians prefer needles and syringes made by Monoject (Monoject Division, Sherwood Medical Industries, St. Louis, MO, 63103). Others are made which are less expensive, but some brands are not consistently sharp and are more subject to breakage and leakage.

There is no excuse today for using anything but new, sharp, disposable needles and new, disposable syringes for cats. Old-fashioned needles could be sharpened, but it seems no one ever bothered to do so. Using a dull needle on a cat can cause considerable pain. Soon, you have a wrestling match each time you give an injection.

No method of cold sterilization (such as soaking in alcohol) will kill some virus diseases, or all the parasites which may be transmitted through the blood from one cat to another. Boiling the needles and syringes also does not always kill these organisms. The ONLY sterilization method which kills viruses and parasites is sterilization with live steam under pressure. Your veterinarian uses an autoclave to prepare instruments for surgery with live, pressurized steam. Most cat owners do not give enough injections to bother with such sophisticated methods. Besides, disposable syringes and needles are very inexpensive. Don't try to save a few cents and maybe lose a cat by using syringes and needles which are not sterile. Use a separate, new, sterile needle and syringe for each cat.

If you are treating the same cat day after day with a medication such as penicillin, you can put the syringe, with needle still attached (after you have used it) in the refrigerator along with the penicillin bottle. This will keep the penicillin in the syringe from spoiling. Then, take the syringe out when it is time for injection, put a new needle on it and give the injection. You can use the same syringe for three or four days in this manner if you have NOT drawn any blood into it in the process of injection. If you do draw blood, start with a new syringe for the next injection.

Now it's time to fill the syringe with the medication or vaccine. Let's assume that you are starting with a new bottle of the product, such as penicillin. Use the tip of a fingernail or sharp knife and remove the small, protective flap of metal covering the center of the bottle cap. It will usually have one or more raised edges which make it easy to remove. Lift off the metal cover if there is one. Place the needle on the syringe, remove the protective sheath, and draw air into the syringe, in an amount equal to the amount of drug you are going to remove from the bottle. For example, 2 cc of drug will need about 2 cc of air to replace it in the bottle. This need not be an exact measurement. Shake the bottle well. Wipe the center of the rubber cap with a cotton ball moistened in alcohol. Rubbing alcohol from the drugstore is fine for this and for wiping the cat's skin.

Hold the bottle of medicine upside down and insert the needle (attached to the syringe with air in it) into the center of the rubber cap. Push the air from the syringe into the bottle. This equalizes the pressure and prevents a vacuum from forming in the bottle, allowing you to remove the medicine more easily. Draw out the amount of drug which you need. If there is a bubble of air in the top of the syringe or hub of the needle, merely inject it back into the bottle and draw out enough product to fill the syringe to the required amount. Measure to the top of the black plunger in the syringe (with the needle upward), not the bottom of

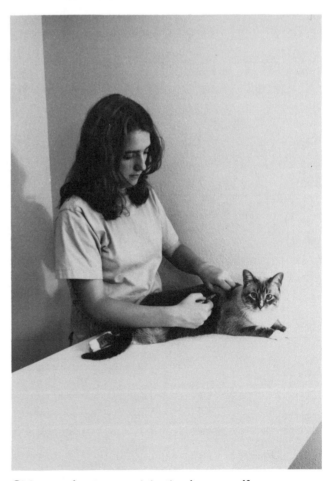

Giving a subcutaneous injection by yourself.

it. Now you're ready to give the injection. Proceed according to the instructions given below for subcutaneous or intramuscular injections, depending on which one the drug label tells you to use.

Perhaps the single biggest cause of problems while giving injections is the owner's attitude. If you are upset or anxious about having to give your cat a shot, you may communicate it to the animal. It will then become upset and will squirm and protest. One thing that helps is to have your assistant (the one who is holding the cat's head with one hand) rub the cat's head FAIRLY HARD while talking to it. It sometimes also helps to have the helper blow in the cat's nostrils. But he or she should keep his or her face safely out of reach of a front foot so as to not get scratched. These actions take the cat's mind off what you are doing. If necessary, wrap the cat in a towel.

If it bothers you too badly to give an injection, it's probably best to have your veterinarian do the dirty work. But if you are determined to do it, get your own mind under control before you approach the cat. Take a deep breath, slowly let it out, and RELAX! You're just giving your cat a shot to help it, not facing a firing squad! Now that you are calm, cool, and collected, approach the cat.

Pick the site where you are going to place the needle. Cleanse a spot two or three inches in diameter with disinfectant. Having a large area disinfected allows you some leeway. If you don't hit the exact spot you have in mind, you can still hit within the cleansed area.

Be sure to safely dispose of your needles and syringes so they cannot be used by children or addicts. They are tools, not toys. When you are finished using it, you can disable a needle by bending it over before you throw it away. Bend it against a hard surface while holding the syringe. DON'T use your finger to bend it. Put the syringe on a firm surface and step on it with a hard shoe heel, cracking it so that it cannot be reused. Watch that you do not put the needle in the trash and reach in and scratch or stick yourself on it. If you drop it in a soup can or milk carton, it won't be a hazard for the sanitation engineer who picks up your trash.

SUBCUTANEOUS INJECTIONS

The most commonly used site for injecting vaccines into cats is the loose tissue right under the skin. "Subcutaneous" means "under the skin." This is also a convenient site to give large quantities of fluids, and is sometimes used for cats with severe diarrhea. It is currently recommended that rabies vaccines designed for subcutaneous administration should be given as low as possible in the right rear leg. Vaccines containing leukemia vaccine should be given in a similar location in the left rear leg. This will make surgery easier if

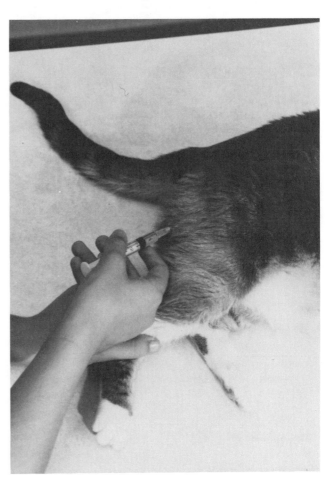

Giving an injection with a helper. Be sure not to give the injection TO the helper!

Intramuscular injection. Be sure to pull back on plunger before injecting here, too.

any reaction occurs at the site (Rude, 1995). Remember, "rabies-right, leukemia-left."

Safe restraint of the cat is important. If the cat is not carefully held, it may turn and bite you when you give the injection. Have someone hold the cat for you at a convenient height. The cat can be placed on a counter, a table or a bench, or it can be held on the floor. Have everything ready before you restrain the cat. Most of them resent being restrained more than they dislike the injection!

Many cats can be given subcutaneous injections of vaccine by one person alone. Put the cat on a slick surface at a level that is comfortable for you. Gently press the cat down onto it, so that it is lying comfortably upright on its sternum, facing away from you. You can raise the skin on the scruff of the neck with one hand while injecting the vaccine under the skin of the neck with the other. Try the gentle approach before you escalate the level of restraint.

A cat that is less cooperative can be held by an assistant with the left hand under the cat's jaw, holding the muzzle slightly above level. The right hand holds the two front legs above the elbows, with one finger between the legs. The right elbow clasps the cat gently to the assistant's side. This assumes that the helper is standing on the cat's left side. Reverse the position if the helper is on the cat's right side. If the cat is antisocial or nasty, it can be rolled in a towel. Adjust it to allow you to expose the upper part of the rib area for a subcutaneous injection or to pull a

hind leg out for an intramuscular injection. Just make SURE your helper has a firm grip and is strong enough to hold the cat. If you don't feel you have safe, adequate restraint, don't attempt to vaccinate the cat.

For subcutaneous injections, let's assume that you are right-handed (reverse the directions if you are left-handed). You are on the cat's right side, with its head to your right. Two convenient sites are over the shoulder, and over the ribs just behind the shoulder blade and an inch or two below the backbone. Pick up a fold of skin with your left hand, between thumb and forefinger. With the syringe in your right hand, insert the needle just through the skin. Don't thrust the needle as if it were a dart. Push it firmly through the skin as if you were sewing heavy canvas, holding it nearly parallel to the skin. A new, sharp needle will encounter almost no resistance. Be extra careful not to stick the needle clear through the fold of skin and into your thumb or finger! It is better to insert the needle below your finger at the base of the fold rather than directly into the fold itself.

When the needle is under the skin, pull back gently on the plunger to make sure you are not in a blood vessel. If you get blood back into the hub of the syringe, you have hit a blood vessel. Withdraw the needle and insert it at another nearby spot. If no blood appears in the syringe, go ahead and gently inject the contents of the syringe. The liquid should flow in smoothly. If it does not, you may have the needle within the skin itself rather than under it. If this happens, withdraw the needle and reinsert it, holding it at a slightly greater angle in relation to the skin. In most cats, you will be going about one-fourth to one-half inch deep for a subcutaneous injection.

Your veterinarian may give fluids subcutaneously. He or she might put a hundred or more milliliters (three ounces or more) of fluid under the cat's skin to treat an illness. Several days after fluid has been given in this manner, you may notice large amounts of fluid hanging in pouches of skin under the cat's belly. Gravity has pulled the fluid down into the area because it has not yet been absorbed. This is fairly common in cats because the skin over their chests is quite loose, and it is easy for the fluid to migrate from the area up high where it was originally placed. If the pockets of fluid are cool and soft, there is no problem. If they become hot and more firm, consult your veterinarian immediately about possibly draining them, and the cat's possible need for antibiotic treatment, as an abscess may be forming from an infection.

INTRAMUSCULAR INJECTIONS

Some vaccines can be given to cats ONLY by the intramuscular route. Certain brands of rabies vaccine are the most important of these. Read and follow the manufacturer's instructions.

There are several reasons for using the intramuscular route. A large cat has large hind leg muscles which provide plenty of space for injecting materials. Many antibiotics are specially formulated to be injected intramuscularly. The muscles have a good blood supply,

SUBCUTANEOUS INJECTIONS

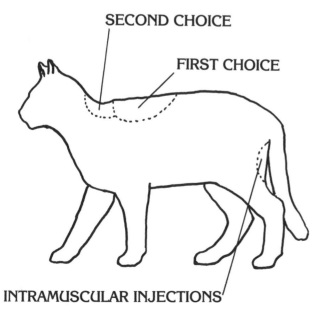

SECOND CHOICE

FIRST CHOICE

INTRAMUSCULAR INJECTIONS

Injection sites, in order of preference.

giving a rapid absorption of medication into the blood, which will then spread it throughout the body. For many people, intramuscular injections are more difficult to give than are subcutaneous ones. For many cats, intramuscular injections may be somewhat more painful than subcutaneous injections. This is especially true of tiny kittens. They have little muscle mass and have more of a tendency to tense their muscles.

When should medication be given intramuscularly? Vaccines should be given intramuscularly when so directed by the labeling or package flyer. This is especially important with rabies vaccine. If you have a choice of giving a rabies vaccine either subcutaneously or intramuscularly, put it in the muscle, as this seems to give a longer acting, more durable immunity. If the vaccine says it SHOULD be given intramuscularly, be SURE to do so, as in some cases the vaccine may actually CAUSE rabies if given subcutaneously or more likely, fail to produce immunity.

Just because you have been giving a drug in a certain manner, don't forget to read the label occasionally for good measure. Manufacturers sometimes change formulas (and recommendations for administration) in midstream. Do NOT automatically assume that since you gave the medication subcutaneously a year ago, that a new bottle is still the same. Read the label to make sure. Any medication that your veterinarian prescribes to give in the muscle should be given according to his or her directions and dosage.

Sites for injection into the muscles should be chosen with an eye to avoiding bones, main blood vessels, nerves, and areas where the absorption of the material would be poor. The site should cause the animal as little discomfort as possible. It should be in an area which will allow good drainage if the worst possible side effect, an abscess, should follow the injection.

The site for intramuscular injection in the cat is the large muscle on the back side of the hind leg. In kittens or small cats, this is the ONLY sizeable muscle in their bodies! Also, it has good drainage if anything should go wrong and an abscess develops. The shoulder muscles of a cat are not large enough, and they are too close to critical bones and nerves to be used as sites for intramuscular injections.

The cat should be restrained by a helper, as described for subcutaneous injections. With a cooperative cat, you can have someone gently steady its head, cupping it in their hands from behind, while rubbing the cat's ears and side of its face. You grasp the hind leg and give the injection. With a grouchy cat, roll it in a blanket or hang it on a window screen as previously described.

Disinfect the skin and proceed. If you are right-handed, hold the needle and syringe in your right hand. If the cat is facing to your left, hold its hind leg from the front side with your left hand, stabilizing the muscle on the back of the thigh with your fingers on one side and thumb on the other side. Insert the needle into the center of the muscle with your right hand. Push the needle gently but firmly through the skin, perpendicular to it, with the needle

attached to the syringe. Place the needle halfway through the large muscle on the back of the leg, or about one-half inch (1.3 cm) deep. Be sure not to stick it in so far that you go clear through the leg and into your hand!

Pull gently outward on the syringe plunger to see if there is any blood. At first, it is helpful to hold the syringe with one hand and pull on the plunger with the other. As you become more experienced, you can pull out on the plunger while steadying the syringe barrel with the same hand. This procedure is done to make sure that you are in the muscle and NOT in a blood vessel. If you do get blood, don't panic. Pull the needle out and place it a half inch or so away from the first site. It is not a good idea to just push the needle deeper or to pull it out to a shallower position along the same track. Reactions or infections are more common when drugs are placed in an area where bleeding has already occurred, especially if vaccines or oily solutions are used. Pull the plunger back at the second site and check again for blood. There will be a little in the hub of the needle from the last puncture, but that is not a problem. No more blood should rush into the syringe. If you do not get blood the second time, go ahead and inject. It does not hurt to inject the small amount of blood which is in the syringe. It's going back into the same animal. Don't reuse the syringe.

You can inject small quantities of medication as fast as you can comfortably push on the plunger. It does not seem to be any more painful than doing it very slowly. The longer you take, the more chance there is that the cat may move its leg and pull the needle out, forcing you to start over and stick it again.

Some people find it easier to hold the hub of the needle with one hand and inject with the other. This helps keep the needle and syringe coordinated together. Occasionally, if you do not do this, the needle will pop off the syringe and medicine will spray all over you. If this happens, estimate how much medicine you have lost, draw that amount from the bottle, and give it in another location (except insulin: see Endocrine Chapter).

When you are finished, don't be in a hurry to get free. Place the fingers of your left hand against the skin at the base of the needle and hold it toward the cat as you withdraw the needle and syringe. This helps avoid pulling the skin away from the underlying tissues as you remove the needle. Otherwise, air may be sucked into the tissues. Remove the needle smoothly—don't jerk it out. After you have removed the needle, don't forget to praise the cat. Pet the cat and tell it that it was good. Any goodwill you can create will make it easier the next time you need to give a shot, whether it is tomorrow or next year. It doesn't hurt to give the cat a treat, such as some special canned cat food, provided it's a "legal" treat and fits its diet. If you have any doubt about being able to give injections by yourself, wait until you have adequate assistance.

If you have to give injections for several days in a row, alternate sides from day to day. Give it in the right hind leg or ribs one day, and the left one the next. Also try to alternate between sites on the same leg. Give it higher up on the right leg the first day, and perhaps a half-inch or inch lower on the third day.

When you are repeating injections of a drug such as penicillin into a muscular area, you will sometimes hit a pocket of the drug which was previously given. When you pull back on the syringe plunger, you might get penicillin instead of blood or nothing. No problem—just pull the needle out and move it to another site. This happens because the body has not absorbed all the previous dosage. Just be aware that it occasionally happens.

Chapter 9

EMERGENCY CARE

RESTRAINT AND SAFETY

Before you can treat your cat, you must restrain it safely so that neither of you will be hurt in the process. No matter how much you trust your cat, it will be in pain, and may bite or claw you. This is an instinctive reaction, not a desire to hurt you. You must protect yourself.

Use the least restraint possible to do what is necessary. Many times, soothing words and gentle movements will work to talk a cat into taking a pill or injection, especially if the cat is accustomed to being handled with love and respect. Hold the cat firmly but not tightly. Picking a fight with a cat or using excessive restraint when it is not needed usually ends up with an upset, stressed, unhappy animal (and owner).

When you pick up a kitten, support it securely and comfortably. Tiny kittens may be picked up by cradling one

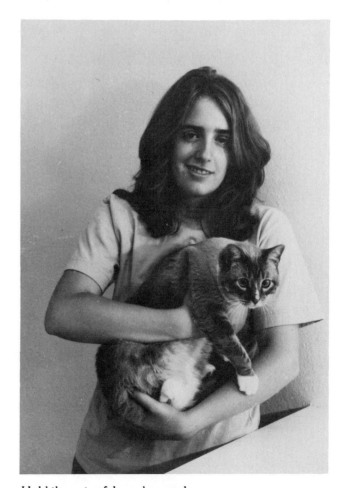

Hold the cat safely and securely.

adult hand (or two child-sized hands) around them. As it grows, two hands are needed to make sure the cat will not fall, and to keep it feeling comfortable and secure. It is easy to carry an adult cat by cradling its front feet or the underside of its chest with one hand, and supporting the hind feet or rump with the other hand.

Children often grab a cat around the chest, leaving its hind half dangling and unsupported. This is miserable for the cat, and may lead to the child being scratched or bitten by the uncomfortable animal. Teach the child to carry the cat properly or leave it on the floor. Do not pick up a cat by the scruff of the neck, whether it is young or adult.

Some cats simply do not like to be picked up and held. You can teach your cat to accept handling by gently restraining it. Hold the cat with the fingers of one hand above its elbows, with a finger or two between the legs, cradling the chest in the palm of your hand. This will allow you to securely restrain the front legs. Hold the hind feet together with your other hand. The cat should be held gently but firmly. Do not put the cat down until it has stopped struggling and is relaxed. After a few dozen times of holding the cat, it will learn that it has to relax in order to be put down, and will allow you to hold it. With a little bit of luck (and a little time), the cat will even learn to enjoy it!

A cat that is injured can easily be picked up with a blanket folded in quarters or a large towel folded in half. Press the cloth firmly over the cat, being especially careful to cover its head until you have picked it up, but not hard enough to smother the cat. Keep the blanket between you and the cat until you have it in a safe place and can evaluate whether or not it is hurt. The blanket can be used like a stretcher. If the cat is struggling and fighting, you can simply roll it up in the cloth like a jelly roll. This will keep the cat safe, as well as protecting the people around it. If you are outdoors, it is best to take the cat into a building or vehicle before you unwrap it. Otherwise, the cat may jump up, and in its pain and upset, flee the scene of the accident. You can immobilize the cat's head with the blanket and examine its legs and the rest of the body before opening the blanket fully. An injured cat is in pain, frightened, and very likely to bite.

An upset cat that has retreated into a corner or closet can be corralled by taking the same sort of heavily folded cloth and flattening the cat to the wall with it. Wrap the cloth around the cat and move it or place it in a carrier or box. You also can wear heavy leather gloves, such as welder's gloves to handle the cat. Remember that the cat might try to climb upward, toward your head; wear a heavy jacket if necessary. Turn your face away from the cat as you are handling it to avoid being clawed or bitten. Stay calm and speak in a soothing voice before you try to move the cat.

If you frequently handle nasty cats, a device called "Small Animal Control" (Robert Schilling Veterinary Products, Glendale, CA) may be useful. It is a netting-covered

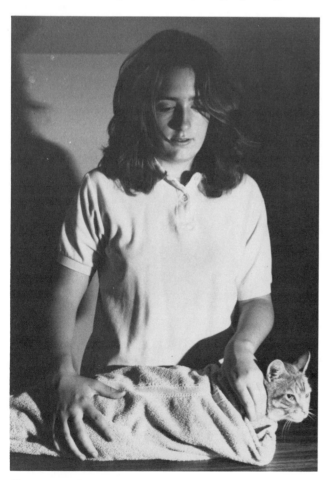

Cat wrapped in towel for restraint.

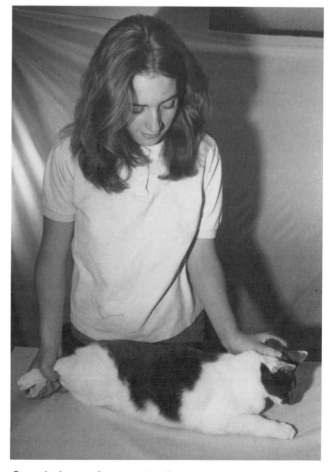

Stretch the cat for restraint if necessary.

frame, hinged like the cover of a book and clasped over the cat. The animal, now securely enclosed, usually settles down, and can be treated or transported.

A cat that is taken in a vehicle should be safely restrained. Otherwise, it may careen madly around the car, even if you think it is too badly injured to do so, and cause an accident. The cat can be placed in a cardboard box or airline crate. Or, you can put it in a pillowcase or laundry bag and tie it shut with string or wire, or a torn strip of cloth. Place the cat on the floor of your vehicle. If you put the cat on the seat, it may move around enough to topple onto the floor, adding insult to injury. Make sure you have not put the cat over the catalytic converter (under the floor of the back seat) or in the sun—it may get hot enough in either location to cause heatstroke or death. Be sure the temperature is comfortable for it—neither too cold nor too hot, and that the cat has plenty of fresh air.

It is very difficult to muzzle a cat. Muzzles are made, but most of them do not work very well. You can restrain a cat safely on its side by standing at its back (if the cat is on a table) and holding the front feet in one hand and the hind feet in the other. Gently rest one wrist across the neck to keep the cat's head snugly pinned to the table or floor so that it can't bite you. If the cat is too unruly, stretch it out flat with one hand holding the hind legs and the other holding the skin at the nape of its neck. Never use this method to pick up a cat (or even a kitten!), as you can cause injury. How would you like someone picking up your entire weight by the skin on the scruff of YOUR neck? This method should only be used to keep the cat down or stretched on a flat surface. Holding a cat by the scruff of its neck may also be difficult with an older tom cat, whose neck skin may be quite thickened.

When you are holding a very unhappy cat with either of these methods and want to let go, let go with BOTH hands at one time. Otherwise, the cat will often attack whichever hand is still holding it. If you let go all at once, the cat is usually startled, and will sit or stand up. At this point, you can pick the cat up in a more normal grasp. When two people are holding a nasty cat, both should let go at the same time to avoid injury. If the cat cannot be restrained by these methods, get help from your veterinarian.

If you are trying to handle a truly vicious cat, such as a feral cat that is rummaging in your garage, you may need to use a stick four to six feet long with a sliding loop on the end of it. Or, you can make a sliding loop in the end of a thin rope and lasso the cat. When you tighten the noose, the cat may struggle violently. Have someone standing by with a box or crate, slide the cat into it, and either release the noose, or toss it in with the cat and allow the cat to remove it itself. This is a desperation measure, but it beats being bitten or clawed by an injured cat, or leaving it in the middle of a road where it may be killed.

If the cat's injury has left it unable to move and it is angry, slide the cat onto a piece of cardboard or the edge of a box, or gently pick up the cat with a shovel and place it in a box or on a blanket. Roll or box the cat for transport. It also can be useful to toss a shirt or towel over the cat's head; a cat that can't see what's happening often calms down.

If you need to trap a cat that has escaped, or a feral cat that you wish to have neutered or disposed of, contact your local animal shelter. Some of them have live traps (Havahart or similar box traps) that can be borrowed or rented. When they work, they are both convenient and humane. Sometimes they are available from veterinary clinics, too. A squeeze-sided trap or cage also may be available, allowing easy treatment. Canned tuna makes a good bait.

CARDIOPULMONARY RESUSCITATION (CPR)

CPR may be needed if your cat has almost drowned or was hit by a car and does not have a heartbeat or is not breathing. In a few cases of injury or accident, prompt attention may make the difference between life and death. If after 20 minutes, there has been no sign of recovery, there probably never will be, and CPR can be stopped. If the cat has bitten an electrical cord, or otherwise tried to electrocute itself, prompt CPR may get the heart going again and save the cat's life. BE SURE TO SHUT OFF THE ELECTRICITY BEFORE YOU TOUCH THE CAT. Cats may come close to drowning in their attempts to get out of a swimming pool. They also may need CPR if they have heatstroke. Unfortunately, most cats whose hearts stop cannot be resuscitated. Of those that are resuscitated, many will have enough damage to their tissues that they will later die. It's still worth a try.

The seriousness of the problem must be recognized and treatment begun immediately. The cat may be unconscious and unresponsive. If you touch the eyelid, the cat may not blink. The cat probably will not be breathing, or if it is, it will be gasping deeply and irregularly. There may be no heartbeat. The membranes of the gums and eyes can be blue or grayish, pale pink, white, or even normal in color.

You can determine if the cat is breathing by watching the rise and fall of its chest. Check the heartbeat by gently putting your fingers around the bottom of the chest just behind the elbows, with your thumb on the other side. You should be able to feel a rhythmic thumping against your fingertips. It may be difficult to feel on a cat that has very long hair, that is overweight, or that has a weak heartbeat. If there is no breathing, or the cat does not have a palpable heartbeat, begin CPR immediately, without moving the cat. Of course, if the cat is in the middle of the road, move it to a safe place such as the sidewalk.

Remember the letters ABC when doing CPR. They stand for:

Airway

Breathing

Circulation

As a rule of thumb, use 120 to 150 compressions per minute and 8 to 12 breaths per minute.

Airway. Make sure the cat has an open airway. If there is any question, gently pull the lower jaw upward and backward, so that the head is above the level of the back. The cat should be lying on its side. An animal does not "swallow" its tongue, but it may fall back into the throat, blocking the airway. Grasp the tip of the tongue and pull outward. In some cases, this will stimulate the cat to breathe. If it does not, it still helps to open the airway. If there is any mucus or blood in the mouth, remove it with your finger or a piece of paper towel or cloth. Be careful the cat does not bite you.

Breathing. If you have an oxygen tank and face mask available, it can be used with a gentle flow of oxygen, (up to 20 to 40 pounds per square inch (psi) pressure) if the tank has a gauge. Oxygen from a welding tank can be used if medical oxygen is not available. If no oxygen is available, you can breathe for the cat, using your cupped hands around its nose, or using your mouth over its nostrils, forming an airtight seal. Hold the cat's mouth shut while doing this. For a cat, use only a small part of each of your breaths. Watch the chest and do not expand it more than it would if the cat were breathing for itself. Otherwise, you could force too much air into the lungs and rupture them. Use eight to 12 breaths per minute (one breath every five to seven seconds). After each breath, take your mouth away, and allow the cat's body to exhale by itself.

Circulation. External compression is used to stimulate the heart and circulate blood throughout the body. If you have someone to help you, ask that person to hold his or her hand on the femoral artery (see Pulse, Knowing Your Cat Chapter). Put your strongest hand around the bottom of the chest, just behind the cat's elbow. Squeeze your thumb and fingers toward each other. Stabilize the cat with your other hand behind its back. The cat can be lying on either side. The important thing is that you BEGIN CPR

IMMEDIATELY. At its best, external cardiac massage will only produce 20-40% of normal blood pressure—but even that is better than 0%!

Research has shown that if you can get 120 to 150 beats per minute going, with a strong pulse quality, many cats regain consciousness. The most successful techniques seem to use a brief duration of compression, done with moderate force, at a high rate of speed. If you have two people, one should do the cardiac compression while the other breathes for the cat in between periods of cardiac compression and monitors the pulse quality. Pulse can be checked by holding the fingers of one hand in the groove inside the hind leg where the femoral artery runs. Use whatever technique gives the strongest pulse in this artery.

Adjust the force of your resuscitation efforts to the small size of the cat. Pushing too hard can tear the liver, causing the cat to bleed to death. Or, it can break ribs, which puncture the lung or heart and cause death. Squeeze strongly, but not TOO strongly. Regardless of which method of artificial respiration is used, after you have inflated the lungs for each breath, remove ALL pressure completely. Allow the lungs to empty by themselves before you add the next breath. If you don't, the body cannot get rid of the carbon dioxide that has accumulated between breaths. The basic pattern is: breathe—compress heart five times—breathe—until the cat recovers or you quit.

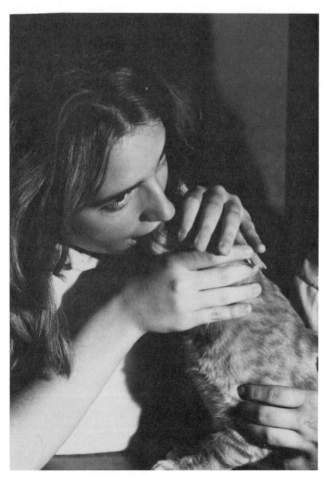

Mouth-to-nose resuscitation.

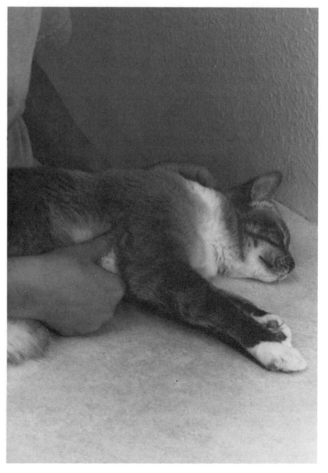

External cardiac massage just behind cat's elbow.

If you have epinephrine, a small quantity can be given—intravenously if possible. Otherwise give it subcutaneously or in the muscle. Use about 2/10 ml of 1:1000 concentration. The cat may die anyway, but it is worth a try if you cannot get to a veterinarian. Whatever you do, get the cat to a veterinarian as soon as possible, even if the cat begins breathing and its heart starts beating. If the cat has had enough damage to stop its heart or breathing, it will need serious supportive care to live. And the veterinarian will have to deal with the problem which caused the stoppage in the first place.

BREATHING DIFFICULTIES

Early signs of respiratory distress include stretching the head upward toward the back and an anxious expression. The cat may breathe with its mouth open, pulling the corners of the mouth backward as it inhales. The heart rate will be increased. The cat might hold its elbows outward, and have little or no interest in what is going on around it. Later, if the condition worsens, the cat will gasp and strain for air. These signs occur with an obstruction in the airway. They also may be seen with advanced cases of pneumonia. If the cause is pneumonia, the difficult breathing will be accompanied by fever and general signs of illness.

If a foreign object is lodged in the throat or trachea, hold the cat by its hind legs. Shake it vigorously (and watch that you don't get scratched). Slap the cat gently on the sides of the rib cage, alternating blows on one side and then the other. Remember that a cat is a small animal, so don't thump it too hard or you may break ribs or damage the lungs. Also try applying pressure up into its abdomen (similar to the Heimlich Maneuver for humans). If these actions are not successful within two or three minutes, quickly take the cat to the nearest veterinarian. He or she can do a tracheotomy (cut a hole in the trachea on the underside of the cat's neck), if necessary, to bypass the blockage.

If you are absolutely certain that a foreign object is causing the cat's distress, you are unable to get it out, and you are a long way from a veterinarian, you can try a desperate first-aid measure. DO NOT do this if you can get the cat to a veterinarian quickly. Lay the cat on its back, with one person holding the front legs and head and another holding the hind legs. Locate the trachea where it lies near the skin surface. This is about halfway between where the head joins the neck and the neck joins the chest. You can feel the trachea as a firm, bumpy tube, much like a small bumpy garden hose. Disinfect an area about two by four inches with alcohol or other disinfectant. Stabilize the trachea between the fingers of one hand. Feel for a space between two of the rings. With the other hand, pop a large, new, sterile hypodermic needle through the space between the rings. Use a 16- or 18-gauge needle, one inch long. Go straight in, perpendicular to the skin. You will need to end up with the needle in the lumen (open cavity of the trachea). When inserting the needle, it will only be necessary to barely go through the skin and about one-quarter inch deeper. If you use a longer needle, be sure not to push it in too far and go completely through the airway. When you are in the right place, you will hear air whistling in and out of the needle. This small amount of air should give the cat a bit of relief, and may buy you enough time to get it to your veterinarian. Leave the needle in place while you transport the cat. Have one or two people hold the cat and the needle so that it does not come out. This technique would not be of any help with pleural effusion.

Pleural effusion is an accumulation of fluid in the chest cavity. The fluid is present outside the lungs, between them and the chest wall. The fluid may be blood from being hit by a car or from a penetrating wound. Or it may be lymph from a ruptured lymphatic vessel. It can be pus from an infection, or exudate from a tumor. It can be the fluid that is seen with feline infectious peritonitis (FIP). Whatever the fluid, if enough of it is present it will cause breathing difficulties because it takes up space into which the lungs would normally expand as the cat breathes. It will be necessary for your veterinarian to drain as much of the fluid as possible, as quickly as possible. The cause for it must be found and corrected. If the cause is an infection or a tumor, the prognosis is poor at best.

Respiratory arrest is just that—the cat stops breathing. It must be corrected IMMEDIATELY. If it goes on more than three to five minutes, the cat will have heart failure and die. As a rule of thumb, more than four minutes without air will cause irreversible brain damage. Newborn kittens, however, can tolerate up to about 10 minutes without harm. Efforts at resuscitation should continue more than 20 minutes if oxygen has been given, or if the animal is colder than normal (the cat has been in cold water or exposed to cold temperatures). Either of these conditions will tend to prolong the time before brain damage occurs.

Respiratory arrest can occur from diseases such as chronic heart disease, blood clots in the lung, and chronic lung disease of any kind. It may result from depression of the centers within the brain which control breathing (caused by brain injuries), lack of oxygen to the brain, infection, or increased pressure within the cranial cavity. Overdosages of depressant drugs can cause the cat to stop breathing. These drugs include tranquilizers, narcotics and barbiturates. Paralysis of the respiratory muscles is sometimes the problem, as from poisoning by organophosphate insecticides or fractures of the spinal column.

Signs of respiratory arrest include slow, irregular, labored breathing. The chest stops moving and the cat's membranes turn blue.

Treatment is similar to the treatment for shock: Make sure the cat has an open airway and begin artificial respiration. Use mouth-to-nose respiration if necessary. Give oxygen if it is available. Remove the cause of the problem if you can determine what it is and correct it. Get the cat to a veterinarian IMMEDIATELY. In most cases, you won't be able to find the cause, and if you do, you won't be able to correct it. DO NOT waste a lot of time trying.

OXYGEN USE

Precautions: Before you use oxygen, be sure you understand and use appropriate safety measures. A steel tank pressurized to 2,000 or 3,000 psi is dangerous. Also, oxygen facilitates burning. No combustibles or open flame should be anywhere near the oxygen.

Any oxygen tank used to treat an animal (or human) MUST have a regulator attached before the main tank valve is opened. Otherwise, the pressure can be so strong that the tank may travel like a rocket. Open the valve gradually and gently. Be sure the tank is solidly held so that it will not fall over or roll around. The hose coming off an oxygen tank can be used to give oxygen to the animal by running it into the corner of a plastic bag. Place the open end of the plastic bag over the cat's head. Leave it loosely open so the exhaled carbon dioxide can escape. You are not trying to replace the air the cat is breathing with pure oxygen—you are only trying to enrich it with oxygen.

Oxygen must be kept away from cigarettes and other smoking materials, open flames (what about the pilot light on your cook stove or water heater?) and electrical connections. It is explosive in combination with grease or oil, and should be kept away from them—or a serious fire or explosion can result. If you are not absolutely sure about the safety of using oxygen, don't use it. It won't help you or your cat if you destroy your home in the process.

It is a good idea to give oxygen whenever the cat is not breathing normally. It can be given to a weak newborn kitten. It also is helpful with respiratory distress, such as the result of heatstroke, and for helping cats that are in shock.

Pure (100%) oxygen without any air should NOT be given to animals. It can cause permanent eye damage in kittens fewer than three weeks old if present in excess concentrations for more than a brief period of time. Pure oxygen also decreases blood flow through the lungs, drying up the mucus which helps protect the lungs against infection. There is no treatment for oxygen toxicity—and too much oxygen is toxic.

CONVULSIONS

A convulsion or seizure may be due to epilepsy. If this is the case, it will be over in a few minutes. The cat will awaken dazed and tired. Convulsions may be due to poisoning by lead, strychnine, organophosphate, or another toxic substance. Liver or kidney disease, brain tumors, injury to the head, and infection with bacteria or viruses also may cause convulsions. With almost all non-epileptic causes, seizures continue until the cat is treated or dies.

What do you do for a cat that has a seizure? Stay calm. Move any sharp objects out of its way. Keep your hands out of its mouth; you cannot help and you easily can be bitten. Cats do not swallow their tongues. Prevent the cat from falling off a porch or down stairs. If the convulsions do not stop within five minutes, get the cat to a clinic immediately. Unfortunately, if poisoning is the cause, the cat may die if the trip is more than a few minutes.

CONCUSSION

The cat's brain can be damaged by being hit by a vehicle, a blow from a blunt object, a fall from a height, a bite wound, and other traumatic encounters with the environment.

If you did not see the cat become injured, you may notice a skull fracture—one area of the skull may be caved

in. The scalp may be torn, and the cat may have a nosebleed. It may not be aware of who you are or where it is. The pupil of one eye may be enlarged; the other will be smaller than normal. The difference in size of the pupils is the most prominent sign of concussion. The cat may be uncoordinated, staggering, or falling. In cases of severe damage, the cat may be unconscious. It may make involuntary noises and might circle or tilt its head to one side.

Treat the cat for shock. If the cat becomes nearly normal within a few minutes, observe it closely for 24 hours. Take the cat to a veterinarian immediately if it does not return to normal within one to two hours, if it is obviously severely injured, or if its condition becomes worse. If you take the cat to a veterinarian, keep its head slightly elevated to help reduce bleeding which may be occurring in the cranial cavity—even though the cat might be in shock.

FRACTURES AND LIMB INJURIES

Cats' bones can be broken by a number of causes. Perhaps the most common cause is being hit or run over by an automobile. Fractures also occur from falls, being kicked by a horse or other animal, bite wounds (such as a dog attacking the cat), gunshot wounds, and blows from blunt instruments (such as a boot!). Nutritional deficiencies or imbalances and bone tumors can weaken the bone, making it prone to fracture.

Life-threatening fractures include those of the skull, which damage the brain; rib fractures, which prevent proper breathing or inflict damage on the lung; fractures of the jawbone and larynx, which obstruct breathing; and injuries of the vertebral column, which threaten the spinal cord. IF YOUR CAT HAS ANY ONE OF THESE, GET TREATMENT IMMEDIATELY. Other fractures (limbs or pelvis, for example) may cause severe pain, but with proper treatment most will heal and your cat will regain normal function.

Fractures and dislocations of the jaw are common in cats. Most are due to being hit by a car. Others are due to kicks by humans or large animals, falls, gunshot wounds, and fights with other animals. There may not be any bleeding, but the cat's lower jaw may appear crooked or lopsided, and its teeth may not mesh. Some jaw injuries may not need treatment while others will need to be stabilized with splints or pins or by wiring the teeth together. Damaged teeth may have to be removed. The cat may need a liquid diet or pureed cat food until it is healed. These fractures usually heal well. Have the cat checked by your veterinarian.

A cat with fractured ribs may appear to have a caved-in chest. Pick the cat up very carefully to avoid punching a broken rib into a lung, which could result in the cat bleeding to death internally.

Fractures may be closed or open (where the bone has pierced the skin from the inside to the outside). Fractures where the skin has been pierced from the outside, with an object penetrating the bone, are also considered "open." This type of open fracture may occur with a gunshot wound, for example. An open (also called compound) fracture should be kept clean. Do NOT put anything in the wound; put clean gauze or a Telfa® pad and pressure bandage over it and take the cat to the clinic.

It often is difficult to differentiate sprains and other injuries to the ligaments and muscles from broken bones. The injured area will be swollen and tender, much like a fracture. If you can take the cat to a veterinarian, have it examined. If you cannot obtain veterinary care fairly quickly, apply ice for 20 to 30 minutes. Then give the cat a night's rest to see how it feels. Sprains and other soft-tissue injuries generally heal well with time and rest.

Cats that show sudden pain or swelling on a limb may be suffering from an abscess. This swelling may be particularly warm and may feel as if it is filled with fluid. Or, it may already have opened and be draining a blood-tinged fluid. The cat may limp, or hold up its leg. This must be distinguished from a broken leg (see Abscess, Skin Diseases Chapter).

Joint luxations and subluxations are known as dislocations. Dislocations often occur when the joint is hit by an external force (such as by a car) or when the cat lands awkwardly on a leg, such as from jumping off a refrigerator or roof or out of a tree. The weight of the cat's body may tear the ligaments loose, allowing the joint to pop out of place or hang loosely. Dislocations are common in the toe, jaw, knee, and hip joint. The cat may hold the injured joint or limb at an abnormal angle. Do not attempt to replace the dislocation. Put an ice pack on it and take the cat to your veterinarian. In most cases, anesthesia will be needed to allow replacement with as little pain as possible. The sooner the joint is reset, the better the chance for normal and complete healing. Anesthesia also has the advantage of relaxing the cat's muscles, preventing further damage as the joint is maneuvered back into place. If left more than a day or so without resetting, it may be impossible to replace without surgery. If you leave it for several weeks, the cat may be permanently crippled.

Avulsions are injuries occurring when part of a limb is torn part way off, usually by a hard blow during an accident. The same kind of injury can occur when a tail is caught in a door or otherwise hurt.

How do you tell if your cat has a broken bone? It may be suddenly lame, carrying a leg completely off the ground or putting weight on it only reluctantly. If the cat has a neck or back injury, it may be uncoordinated, or unable to rise or walk. A cat with a broken leg probably will show abnormal movement, such as part of a leg moving sideways; however, a reduced range of motion of one leg may be the only sign. The cat may show pain and swelling of the limb. When the leg is examined, a grating sensation can sometimes be felt. Damage to the skin and muscle may be seen, with bleeding, bruising, and torn skin.

If the cat is lying down, or has just been hit, your first priority is to ensure that the airway is open. Deal with any life-threatening injuries first. Minor bleeding can be ignored until the cat's primary needs are met. Remember ABC: Airway, Breathing, Circulation.

Whether you see your cat hit by a car or it comes home limping, your first move MUST be to safely restrain it. The cat will be in pain and could accidentally bite you (see above). If there is bone sticking out through the skin, or

obvious angulation of the limb, there is no need to check the cat further. Take the cat to your veterinarian immediately.

Skeletal fractures, other than those few mentioned above, are obvious, painful, and dramatic, but rarely life-threatening. Do NOT give any painkillers or sedatives. These drugs can depress the cat's blood pressure and put it into shock. They also tend to mask signs of head injury or nerve damage, and complicate recovery from heart and lung involvement. Do not give your cat ANYTHING to eat. If the cat is thirsty, give it a sip or two of water—just enough to moisten its mouth, until you and/or your veterinarian determine the extent of its injuries.

If no broken bone is obvious, examine the cat. If possible, ask someone to hold the cat's head so it cannot bite, or hold the cat behind the head with one hand while checking it with the other. Feel the head and neck, checking for lumps, bumps, or rough edges. Gently feel down each leg, one at a time, looking for swelling, grating, or lumps. Move each joint in turn through its normal range of motion. If this causes pain, do not force it to move. If you find a possible broken bone, leave the cat wrapped loosely in the towel, and take it to a veterinarian. If nothing appears broken, unwrap the cat and encourage it to move a little. Watch how the cat moves across the room or yard. Is it favoring one leg? Dragging a toe, or not properly moving a leg through its normal arc, could mean there is nerve damage or a fracture that is not apparent.

Use direct pressure to stop any bleeding. For instance, if blood is spurting from an artery, put a sterile gauze compress over it. If you don't have sterile gauze handy, use a clean handkerchief or paper towel. Sanitary napkins are also good, especially for large open wounds. If the wound is deep, put the sterile gauze or clean material directly on the wound surface. If the material does not come up to the level of the surrounding skin, fill in the space with anything you have handy. Crumpled paper, or a rolled-up sock or rag, can be placed on top of the first layer. Then wrap a bandage around the entire area. The filler will help put pressure on the bleeding area deep in the cut. The bandage should be snug but not too tight. In most cases, this is much better than using a tourniquet, because you will not have to worry as much about cutting off the circulation below the bandage.

DO NOT put cotton batting or cotton balls on a wound. The cotton or polyester fibers will come loose in the clotting blood and be nearly impossible to remove later; their presence will delay healing.

DO NOT worry about splinting or setting a fracture if you can get the cat to a veterinarian within a reasonable length of time. This is true even if you have to drive three or four hours to a suitable clinic. It IS important that you keep the cat confined so that it cannot move around and cause further injury to it. If you live in the middle of nowhere, you will have to splint the leg.

Veterinary care for the injured cat usually will start with an evaluation of the patient to inventory its injuries. The veterinarian then will treat the cat for shock, and administer antibiotics to prevent infection. Open cuts may be sutured. If there are fractures, many veterinarians do not treat them until the next day. Do not feel that your cat is being neglected. A night in a cage (with four boring walls to help the cat rest quietly) will help your cat be a better candidate for successful surgery in the morning. It will allow the cat's body to stabilize and give the medication a chance to take effect. The veterinarian can then safely cast, splint, or pin the leg. The delay also gives the swelling around the fracture a chance to go down. Then, if a cast is applied, it will fit better and do a better job of holding the leg.

If the cat has suffered a dislocation, your veterinarian may need to suture ligaments and tendons, depending on what has been torn. A dislocated hip will be put back into place with the cat under anesthesia. It will either be pinned or bandaged to hold it in place, depending on the direction it has dislocated and the direction of force needed to hold it while it heals. Consult with your veterinarian to learn what will be required and what it will cost. If the cat's tail has been torn apart (an avulsion), the torn end will usually be amputated. The tail does not have a very good blood supply, and is extremely difficult to splint successfully.

Pelvic fractures are common in cats, usually from being hit by a car. There are two ways of handling these injuries. Your veterinarian can use multiple bone pins to put all of Humpty Dumpty's pieces back together. This surgery can cost $800 to $1,000 or more. As an alternative, you can confine the cat to a small space—about the size of a child's playpen. Pad it with fairly firm material such as carpet scraps or a small mattress, cut to fit the area. Firm material will enable the cat to turn around without getting tangled in the bedding. Put a litter box with shallow edges on one side and food and water on the other side.

Confinement will be necessary for about four weeks minimum, and perhaps as much as six weeks. Some cats will be more at ease in the kitchen or living room, in sight of much of the family's normal activity. Give the cat plenty of quiet attention. Do not let children induce the cat to play or become excited. The key to success is for the cat to use its rear legs as little as possible.

The cat may heal with some limping and may no longer win races, but this course of action is worth considering if you do not have the money for expensive corrections. This assumes, of course, that the cat does not have any complications affecting the urinary system or bowel. You can tell whether this is the case by watching to see if the cat is urinating and defecating normally. Feed the cat less than the normal amount of food. If the cat cannot defecate easily, feed a high-fiber diet or use a laxative. Enemas may be needed from time to time. Because the bone pieces from a pelvic fracture tend to reduce the size of the pelvic canal, a female should not be allowed to become pregnant unless you are prepared to pay for a Caesarean section. It is a good idea to have her spayed after her pelvis has completely healed.

With any fracture, rest and restricted movement are essential. Splints, casts, or bandages MUST fit properly. Be sure to feel the paw or foot below the splint to make sure it is still warm and has good blood circulation.

What do you do if you live in the middle of nowhere and your cat has been hit by a car or similarly injured? Or, if you cannot get to a veterinarian or do not have the money to do so? Give first aid for any open cuts. Administer CPR if needed. Check the cat for concussion. Then put the cat in a warm, QUIET place. Use a playpen if you have one, or a box which is just slightly larger than the cat. A travel crate works well, but be sure to shut the cat in. Otherwise, the cat will try to follow you around as it normally does, and may severely aggravate the injuries. Let the cat rest quietly overnight. Most veterinarians do this with many of their accident patients after checking them over. Go away and leave the cat alone. In the morning, you will be able to evaluate the cat's condition and the problems that are still troublesome. You can splint a leg as best you can, or apply other treatment. Please note that this treatment is to be used ONLY when you CANNOT do anything else—you could easily return in the morning to a dead cat if its injuries were severe. Yet, if you can do nothing else, this may enable your animal to survive.

CUTS

Skin cuts can occur when a cat is hit by a car or ripped by fighting with another cat or a dog. Farm cats sometimes are torn from charging through barbed-wire fences.

Cut arteries may bleed severely and, if not stopped, can be life-threatening. The end of the nose and the nasal cartilages are richly supplied with blood vessels and bleed profusely. Cuts on the tongue, ear flaps, tail, feet, penis, and mammary glands may bleed excessively from arteries. Pressure must be used to control arterial bleeding, and the cat should be taken to a veterinarian as soon as possible. Cats that have eaten warfarin or brodifacoum (rodent poisons such as D-Con®), or that have hemophilia or other clotting disorders, can bleed excessively from even minor cuts. If the bleeding is severe, or has continued for some time, the cat may have to be treated for shock. An ice pack may be used to help slow bleeding, but do not use it for longer than 15 to 20 minutes.

Blood which is coming from an artery is bright red and will flow irregularly, sometimes spurting in time with the heartbeat. Blood from a vein is darker in color and flows evenly.

DO NOT use "clotting" powders which are made for livestock or dogs. They can cause severe burning and pain in cats. And, it will be nearly impossible to suture the wound and have it heal if one of these products has been used. The only clotting products which are useful for cats are silver nitrate sticks, epinephrine, or styptic pencil. These can be used when you are clipping toenails and bleeding is caused by cutting one a bit short. None of these products is useful for open wounds. A pressure bandage is the only good way to control open-wound bleeding, whether arterial or venous. DO NOT use petroleum jelly in any open wound. It may keep the wound from healing if it is to be sutured, and it slows the healing of open wounds.

Your veterinarian will repair the laceration in somewhat the following manner: If the cut is large, he or she will completely anesthetize the cat. If it is small and the cat is calm, he or she may sedate the cat or have a capable assistant hold it. The veterinarian then will wash the cut with a mild disinfectant solution. Gauze sponges soaked with this solution will be put in the wound to keep it clean while the hair is clipped from around the edges of the wound. The dampened hair will be clipped from the edges at least one-half inch (1.3 cm) all the way around. This keeps the hair from getting into the wound, and from irritating it as it heals. It also will keep the area cleaner.

The veterinarian will anesthetize the skin edges by injecting small amounts of a local anesthetic, such as xylocaine, around the periphery of the wound, using a syringe and a very fine needle (about 25-gauge, 5/8 inch). The anesthetic will be injected about half an inch under the skin edge (away from the hole), in spots about a half-inch apart, in order to deaden the skin all the way around the wound. Following the use of the anesthetic, he or she will finish cleansing the wound, removing any hair, grass, dirt, or other foreign material. Any hanging shreds of arteries, tendons, or tattered muscle will be cut out. The veterinarian then will trim around the edge if the cut is more than a couple of hours old, or has a ragged edge, removing as little tissue as possible. In some cases, the veterinarian will take off only about one-sixteenth of an inch (1 mm)—the least amount that can be trimmed. If the wound surface is dried, it may be trimmed, again taking off the very thinnest layer possible. Trimming the wound in this fashion will give a fresh, clean surface which will heal well. Some veterinarians like to flood the wound with penicillin at this point, using 1-5 ml, depending on the size of the wound.

The veterinarian will use a surgical needle with a very sharp point to suture the skin; it is shaped like a half-circle. It is pushed through the skin with a pair of forceps which has a special gripping edge to hold the needle securely, called needle holders. The veterinarian will use a pair of "tissue forceps" with the other hand. Tissue forceps look like a large pair of tweezers with a toothed edge. The needle is pushed through the skin, first on one side and then the other, coming through about one-eighth to one-quarter inch (3-6 mm) back from the skin edge, depending on the location of the cut and thickness of the cat's skin. After the veterinarian has passed the needle and suture through both sides of the wound, a square knot is tied to complete a simple stitch. The stitches are barely pulled snug. Because the skin will swell, if they are put in too tightly, they will cut through the skin and pull out.

Many veterinarians like to begin suturing in the middle of a wound so they come out with the same amount of skin at both ends, with no wrinkles or puckers. The suture is often a nylon product similar to nylon fishing line, although a fine stainless steel suture is sometimes used. The stainless steel has sharp points on the knots which help keep the cat from chewing out the stitches. After the suturing job is finished, the veterinarian may apply a protective dressing spray along the stitch line. This helps dry any discharges which drain from the wound area, as well as kill any bacteria in the immediate area.

Some veterinarians use skin staples (the same kind used in human hospitals) instead of sutures. Whether staples or sutures are used, they usually will be removed in about 10 days.

Keep an eye on the stitch line. It should continue to be clean and free from pus, blood, or drainage. If the sutured wound becomes filled with pus because of infection, or swollen with serum or other fluid, it will need to be drained. Return the cat to your veterinarian. He or she will open the incision by removing one or two stitches at the lowest point of the pocket, and then push the blunt end of a pair of forceps into the pocket to open it so the fluid will drain out through the hole. This will take the pressure off the suture line and allow the rest of the wound to continue to heal. You will then need to swab out the pocket twice daily using a product such as tincture of iodine and long cotton swabs (available at the drugstore) (see Abscesses for Iodine Use). Do not be afraid to press gently with the swabs—you will not damage any tissues which have already healed. You are just cleaning out dead and infected material that is coming off the damaged tissue surfaces. Do not let the drain hole seal over all at once, or the pocket will fill up with pus again. It should get smaller day by day as it heals from the inside out. Each day you should notice that the depth to which you reach with the swab becomes more and more shallow. The condition and its treatment are very much like an abscess.

SHOCK

Shock is a condition in which the cat's blood pressure is lowered, causing inadequate blood flow through the tissues. It can result from severe blood loss, whether from a bleeding cut or from a ruptured spleen, liver or internal blood vessel. Acute heart failure results in shock, and shock may occur from fluid loss from diarrhea or severe vomiting or the plasma loss that occurs with burns involving large amounts of skin. Shock also results from massive crushing injuries, such as when the cat is hit by a car, leading to severe internal bleeding. Shock may occur when injury to the heart or heart disease results in lessened blood output, causing blood pressure throughout the body to drop. Severe stress, whether psychological or physical, can cause shock. Infections with some kinds of bacteria cause shock. The bacteria produce toxins which affect the blood vessels, causing blood to "pool" in the internal organs; a deadly drop in blood pressure occurs. Lack of hormones from the adrenal gland may leave the cat's system unable to maintain normal circulation and blood pressure.

Anaphylactic shock occurs when drugs or toxic substances trigger a severe allergic reaction within the body. In cats, the first sign may be intense itching, as the cat scratches its face and head. The cat may have difficulty in breathing. Other signs may include diarrhea, salivation, vomiting, and collapse. Anaphylactic shock is extremely rare in cats, but may occur because of reaction to antibiotics, foods, or stings from insects such as wasps, fire ants, hornets, bees, and yellowjackets. Take the cat to a veterinarian promptly, as treatment with epinephrine and other intensive medication, as well as intravenous fluids, may be required. If there is no way to take the cat to a clinic, antihistamines may be helpful.

Psychogenic shock can occur when the cat is subjected to severe mental stress. This can come from something as mild as preparation for surgery, stress from natural disasters, or the noise of war. It can occur from conflict with a human, dog, or other cat. One of my cats suffered this type of shock when a nasty tom cat ripped a screen and viciously attacked her inside our porch. He chased her into a screen door, which opened, allowing both of them to escape. After a half-hour search, I found her cowering near a neighbor's garage, unhurt but badly shaken. She huddled in a corner oblivious to the outside world. She was depressed, unresponsive, salivating, and had no appetite. This went on for more than a day. Then, she gradually returned to normal. This type of shock is an evolutionary survival mechanism that probably allows the cat to save its energy to recover from an assault. It can be treated by your veterinarian as any other shock. If you cannot get to a clinic, put the cat in a comfortable, quiet, warm place such as an airline crate or cardboard box. This alone may be enough to allow the animal to recover.

Whatever the initial cause of the shock, the events that follow are much the same. Some events decrease cardiac output, lowering the blood pressure. The adrenal gland and sympathetic nervous system cause arteries and capillaries in the skin and limbs to shut down. The spleen contracts and blood is shunted away from the intestines. The kidneys retain sodium and water. The entire process leads to complete circulatory collapse, ending with heart failure.

Signs of shock. Signs of shock include a rapid heartbeat and weak pulse. The cat will be breathing rapidly and shallowly, or may be panting. The cat will have a poor capillary refill, which can be checked by pushing your finger firmly into a pinkish portion of the cat's gums. When you release your finger, the color should return within one to two seconds. If it takes longer than two seconds to return, the cat's circulatory system is not doing well. The cat's temperature may be below normal, and it probably will be weak, depressed and restless. The eyes could have a "glassy" stare, and the gums will become pale, dry, and cool. If the shock continues to progress, the cat will go into collapse and coma, and the pupils will become dilated.

Treatment of shock. Support the cat's respiration. Make sure that the airway is clear by opening the mouth and checking it to be sure the cat can breathe. Be careful—you can be bitten if the cat is unconscious. If the cat is unconscious, pull outward on the end of its tongue, and tilt the head backward to open the back of the throat. If you have oxygen available, use it if you can do so safely. If there is visible bleeding, control it as soon as possible, preferably by direct pressure or bandaging. Keep the cat's head slightly lower than the rest of its body to increase blood flow to the brain (the same principle as raising the feet and legs of a human in shock). This

also will help drain any fluid out of the lungs. Be sure the cat is breathing before worrying about stopping the bleeding.

If the weather is cool, keep the cat covered with a coat or blanket until you move it. In hot weather, get the cat into shade. Keep the cat quiet, and avoid any noise that may make it attempt to move. Do not move the cat any more than necessary. Do not give painkillers or sedatives. Delirium or restlessness may be due more to a lack of oxygen to the brain than to pain. Painkillers can mask severe symptoms, and depressant drugs will further compound the shock.

If there is no visible bleeding, but you think the cat is bleeding internally into its abdomen, wrap a long piece of cloth snugly around its abdomen as a binder. A strip of bedsheet works well. Do not wrap the cloth around the chest area as this can restrict the cat's breathing. The membranes may be pale grayish in color, and the cat will be weak or prostrate.

At this point, your cat needs more help than you can give. Take the cat to the nearest veterinarian as soon as possible. It will be necessary, in most cases, to give intravenous fluids, and possibly a blood transfusion, as well as intensive drug therapy, to save the animal. Emergency surgery also could be required. Keep the oxygen on the cat while you are driving it to the clinic, if you can. DO NOT TO ALLOW ANYONE TO SMOKE AROUND THE OXYGEN!

PUNCTURE WOUNDS

DO NOT TRY TO MUZZLE A CAT THAT HAS A PENETRATING CHEST WOUND. It may interfere with the cat's breathing. Be sure the cat has a clear airway, and remove blood, mucus, or vomited material. Handle the cat carefully so it does not bite you.

The presence of air within the chest cavity is called pneumothorax. A pneumothorax is somewhat comparable to a sucking chest wound in a human. The difference is that in a cat, BOTH lungs are likely to collapse, while in a human, there is a good chance of one lung remaining partially functional. Pneumothorax in the cat is an EMERGENCY and must be cared for promptly.

Pneumothorax may occur because some of the air sacs of the lungs are ruptured. The ruptured sacs leak air into the chest cavity from the inside. Or, pneumothorax may occur with an open chest wound. This can happen when an object penetrates the chest cavity from the outside. These wounds are generally obvious. Penetration may occur in cats that are bitten by large dogs. If the penetrating object is still in place and is small, DO NOT REMOVE IT. This would apply, for example, to a small tree branch or archery arrow which had pierced the cat's chest. Just bandage it in place, while keeping it from penetrating any deeper. As long as it is there, it acts as a cork, plugging the hole. Take the cat to your veterinarian as soon as possible.

A large or immovable object (one you can't take along with the cat) will have to be removed before transport. It is important to bandage the cat securely, sealing the hole to prevent air from entering the chest cavity. Use a piece of plastic (a plastic bag will do in an emergency) to seal the hole—this helps keep the lung from collapsing. Put as many gauze sponges over the area as needed to cover the hole or bleeding area. Then put a large pad over them, to apply direct pressure. You can use a small folded towel or piece of clothing or rag. Finally, bandage around the whole chest. Bandage snugly so that the materials will not fall off, but not so snugly that the cat cannot breathe. Give oxygen if you have it safely available. Get the cat to a veterinarian as soon as possible.

Penetrating wounds of the abdomen are treated the same as chest wounds with respect to removing or leaving the penetrating object and bandaging. If the intestines have been pulled out or are dangling out of the wound, take a deep breath and get control of yourself—it's not pretty. Ask someone to hold the cat so that it cannot walk and drag the intestines in the dirt or step on them. Dampen a long, clean rag or towel with lukewarm water and wrap it around the cat's abdomen and up over its back, around and around to gently support the intestines in a sort of hammock. Do not attempt to replace them in the abdomen. Let the veterinarian do that so he or she can inspect them for damage and clean them. These wounds look grisly but, surprisingly, some cats survive the injury. Get the cat to a veterinarian as soon as possible.

The most common cause of puncture wounds is a cat or dog bite. These wounds are small at the skin surface, but are deep and become infected quite easily. Clip the hair away from the wound opening. If there is some doubt as to where the punctures are, it is better to clip away too much hair than too little. Cleanse the area with chlorhexidine or a similar mild disinfectant. If the puncture wounds are large enough, swab down into each one with a cotton swab and tincture of iodine solution. If the puncture seems to go into the chest or abdomen, don't swab—handle as above. If the bites are extensive, or if your cat becomes infected easily, it would be wise to take the cat to your veterinarian for an antibiotic injection. This will help prevent the possibility of tetanus, even though it is remote. Antibiotics also will help prevent an abscess from forming. The cat may need oral antibiotics for seven to 10 days to prevent infection.

HEAT STROKE

The most significant sign of heat stroke is an elevated body temperature. The cat may have a rectal temperature of 105 to 110 degrees F (40.6-43.3 C). Life-threatening complications may quickly follow. These include edema (fluid accumulation) within the brain, acid-base imbalances, and coagulation of the blood within the blood vessels.

Heat stroke usually occurs when the air temperature is high. It may occur when it is as low as 90 degrees F (32.2 C), however, most commonly, it occurs at temperatures between 100 and 115 degrees F (37.7-46.1 C). Most cats that are unconfined will not stay in conditions which will raise their body temperature to the point of heat stroke. For this reason, it is usually seen in cats that are confined, especially in places with poor ventilation,

or that are directly in the sun. A good example is a vehicle on a hot day, especially if the windows are rolled up. A cat in a transport crate is an even better candidate for heat stroke. If the cat has been in a fight or is otherwise excited so that its temperature is already raised, it is especially vulnerable.

High humidity can contribute to heat stroke because the cat is unable to evaporate as much moisture as usual through the membranes of its nose and mouth, even though it is panting as hard as it can. Young kittens and elderly cats have less heat tolerance and are more prone to heat stroke. Cats of short-faced breeds also are less tolerant of heat. Lack of water also can contribute to heat stroke. Fat cats have more trouble with heat than do thin cats.

One family took its cat on a 30 mile trip with the car windows open. The cat had been lying in the sun on this hot afternoon. Despite adequate ventilation, the cat's core temperature became hot enough to cause heat stroke and the cat died. Be sure to provide shade, even if you are driving with the windows open.

The first sign of impending heat stroke is hard and fast panting. The heart rate is above normal, the cat's mucous membranes are bright red, and the body temperature is above normal. As the condition progresses, the cat goes into a stupor, the legs and feet are hot to the touch, and the bright red membranes of the mouth become pale. The cat may have a watery diarrhea, which it cannot control. If it becomes bloody, or if hemorrhages are present on the mucous membranes, clotting may be occurring within the blood vessels. Coma and respiratory collapse occur unless the cat is treated. Take the cat to the nearest clinic. If you cannot get to a veterinarian, proceed as follows:

Treatment begins by lowering the cat's body temperature. Get the cat out of the sun or enclosed area, into shade or an air conditioned building. Immerse the legs and trunk in a tub of cold or iced water. Take the cat's rectal temperature at least every 10 minutes. Stop the cooling when the body temperature reaches 103 degrees F (39.4 C). The temperature will continue to drop, and it is easy for the cat to become too cold and develop hypothermia. After you stop bathing the cat, continue to take the temperature every 10 minutes to be sure it does not return to an elevated temperature. Ice water enemas have been recommended as a method of treating heat stroke. The disadvantage is that they interfere with the only way you have of monitoring the cat's progress and making sure the cat is not becoming too cold—the rectal temperature. Evaporative cooling methods which work to cool humans do not work well on cats because of their hair coats.

As soon as the cat is cooled and its temperature has stabilized below 103 degrees F (39.4 C), take the cat to a veterinarian for follow-up treatment. He or she may give corticosteroids, mannitol, or other drugs to help reduce edema in the brain. If the blood is starting to clot in the blood vessels, the veterinarian may administer intravenous fluids to dilute the blood and stabilize the cat's circulatory system. Antibiotics may be given to help prevent infection due to the cat's weakened condition.

The best treatment for heat stroke is prevention. If it's hot for you, it's probably miserable for your cat. It cannot sweat and cannot remove its coat. If there's the least doubt, leave the cat home, where it will be alive when you return, rather than taking the cat with you and finding it dying or dead. In many jurisdictions, you could be charged with animal cruelty for leaving a dog or cat in a vehicle on a hot day. It also may be legal for a passerby to break your window to relieve the animal's suffering, whether real or imagined.

DROWNING

Most cats can swim fairly well, if introduced to it gradually. Cats may drown when they have never learned to swim and are suddenly thrown or fall into the water, such as diving out of a boat in the middle of a lake. They may drown when they try to swim across a lake or large river, or are trapped during a flood and become exhausted. A tragedy often occurs when is a cat gets into a steep-sided swimming pool, pond, or irrigation canal, and finds it cannot get out. If rescue is necessary, be sure that you or the person who makes the rescue attempt, can swim well. Do not compound one tragedy with a second. You can drop a rope around the cat's neck and tow it to dry ground to avoid the cat trying to climb on top of you. Drowning cats act like drowning people. Don't leave a sink or bathtub filled with water, and keep the toilet lid closed.

When the cat is back on dry ground, hold it up by the hind legs with its head hanging clear of the ground. Hold the cat for 10 to 20 seconds while slapping it gently on alternate sides of the chest wall. Begin CPR on the cat. If you still hear gurgling noises, stop every couple of minutes to hold the cat up again to drain water out of the lungs. If possible, it also is helpful to have the cat lying with its head downward while doing CPR. As long as you can feel a heartbeat, there is hope that the cat will start breathing. Keep the cat warm. When it regains consciousness, take the cat to a veterinarian for examination if it has been unconscious for more than a couple of minutes, has swallowed water, or otherwise looks ill.

In some cases of cold water drowning, your veterinarian may wish to put the cat into a barbiturate-induced coma to reduce metabolism within the brain, thereby reducing damage to brain cells. This may give the cat its best chance of recovery.

POISONINGS

When we say "poisoned," the first thing that comes to mind is some vicious person deliberately trying to kill a cat. Luckily, these cases are quite rare. More often, the cat accidentally poisons itself by getting into insecticides, or herbicides, or chewing on a convenient poisonous plant because it is bored. Cats can be poisoned when tick or flea dip is mixed incorrectly and is too strong. If you suspect your cat has been poisoned, bring the container with you when you take the cat to the veterinarian. This will help the veterinarian determine what the problem is and how to treat it.

Cats are three to four times less likely to be poisoned than dogs. They are more finicky about what they eat. They are less likely to chew and worry at items that a dog would enjoy. They are less likely to roam and be exposed to dangers. Conversely, cats are much more vulnerable than humans (or even dogs) to most toxic substances. This is because they do not have the liver enzymes which break down many toxic substances.

Pesticides are chemicals used to kill insects and other pests in and around the house and garden, as well as on your pet. Their use is based on the principle that they are more poisonous to the pest than to you or your cat. Most of these are safe WHEN USED IN RECOMMENDED DOSAGES and at appropriate intervals. However, they all can be deadly when used in excessive amounts, or accidentally misused.

Organophosphate and **carbamate** poisonings will be discussed together because they are similar. These poisonings can occur from home and garden insecticides and related products. The cat can ingest a toxic dose if it eats (rare because cats are picky eaters) or walks on freshly treated foliage, such as a yard that has just been sprayed. If your cat is allowed outdoors, it may be poisoned while strolling through a yard a block or two from your house. Organophosphates may cause toxicity when the cat is dipped in an overly strong solution of flea or tick dip which is absorbed through the skin. It may inhale an overdose when the household is treated by an exterminator. Reactions to flea collars and pet wormers containing these products also can occur.

Pets can be poisoned when these compounds are incorrectly mixed or when the animal is treated at the same time with the same chemical for both internal and external parasites. Very small amounts, even the quantity left in an "empty" container, can cause death. Store these materials out of the reach of your cat (and other animals or children!). Dispose of the empty containers promptly and properly.

Common organophosphates include dichlorvos, DDVP, vapona, malathion, fenthion, parathion, trichlorfon, chlorpyrifos, prolate (Phosmet), Ruelene® (commonly used for cattle grubs) and Diazinon, to name but a few. Malathion is one of the safest of these compounds, while parathion is one of the most toxic. Names of organophosphates often contain "phosphoro." Carbamate insecticides cause the same symptoms. If one of these products is applied as a powder to the cat's coat, it will take it in as it licks while grooming. Some of the carbamates are carbaryl (Sevin®), aldicarb, some formulations of Golden Malrin (Zoecon®), and propoxur (Baygon®). More than 100 of these products are currently manufactured under many different names. Carbamates are also the main ingredient in some ant traps, such as Raid® Ant Trap (S.C. Johnson & Son) and Black Flag® Ant Trap (Boyle-Midway). Cats can chew them open and become poisoned. Be sure to place ant traps where pets can't get them (Hornfeldt, 1987).

Signs of organophosphate poisoning may occur within as little as five minutes after the cat has been exposed to the product. Most reactions occur within 12 hours after exposure. The cat may have a garlic odor on its breath or coat. The pupils of the eyes are constricted—this is one of the most consistent signs. The cat may be restless and confused. It will salivate, and have tears running from its eyes. Fluid is pouring into its lungs. As the cat breathes, this fluid will come out the nose and mouth as frothy bubbles. The cat will gasp and strain to breathe, and may turn blue because the fluid keeps the lungs from exchanging air. Breathing difficulties can be due to irregular muscular contractions, as well as fluid production in the lungs. The muscles of the face and tongue begin to twitch, followed by twitching of all the muscles in small, short convulsions. The cat might show muscular tremors, incoordination, stiffness, cramps, and vomiting. It may urinate and defecate (this may be a watery diarrhea). The cat may show muscular weakness along with the twitching, which can progress to convulsions and paralysis. If severe enough, the cat will go into a coma, followed by death. Death may occur within a few minutes, or the cat may live several days before dying.

ORGANOPHOSPHATE POISONING IS AN EMERGENCY. Take the cat to a veterinarian as soon as possible. The cat will be treated with drugs to specifically counteract the toxicity. Give oxygen if it is safely available. Artificial respiration may save the cat if it goes into respiratory failure—if you have someone to administer it while you are driving to the clinic. Even with prompt treatment, some cats cannot be saved. If the cat lives through the initial crisis, it has a good chance of returning to normal.

If there is no way you can take the cat to a veterinarian, do the best you can. Remove the cat's flea collar. If an insecticide or dip has caused the problem, give the cat a bath, using hypoallergenic shampoo if you have it. Otherwise, use liquid dish detergent and water, rinsing thoroughly. Wear rubber gloves so that there are not two victims! Towel dry the cat. Give hydrogen peroxide, 1 cc per pound of body weight (2 cc per kg), as an emetic to induce the cat to vomit. This can be repeated once. Or, you can give Syrup of Ipecac, 1 1/2 cc per pound (3 cc per kg), diluted half-and-half with water, and given once. After giving the emetic and allowing the cat time to vomit (it may not), give activated charcoal if it is on hand and can be given rapidly. Use 1 gram (gm) of activated charcoal per pound of cat (2 gm/kg). Do not give charcoal or anything else if the cat is in convulsions, or is having so much trouble breathing that it cannot swallow adequately. Repeat the activated charcoal at half the original dosage every six to eight hours for two to three times (Vet-Kem, 1992). (See also Activated Charcoal, below.)

Oxygen also is helpful. If you can keep the cat alive, eventually its body will eliminate the toxin. On the other hand, a sufficiently large dose will kill the cat before it can be helped, even if you live next door to an emergency hospital.

Prevention of this type of poisoning includes keeping pets away from containers of insecticide. Be sure to safely dispose of empty containers. Carefully wash all sprayers, buckets and other objects which have come into contact with the product. Distribute spray or dip carefully and evenly so that there are no puddles from which the cat can drink. Confine all pets until treated yard areas have dried completely. Do not store insecticides in unlabeled containers. If possible, do not store them at all.

DO NOT mix insecticide unless you have written instructions for that specific product, whether on the label or in a separate folder. One of my clients lost a cat when a friend gave her a bottle of insecticide and said to mix it one part insecticide to 10 parts water (1:10). The label did not give instructions, and the flyer accompanying the bottle had been lost. After the flea dip was applied, the cat went into organophosphate poisoning and died. A later check with the pet store revealed that the recommended dilution was equivalent to a 1:128 solution!

NOTE: Many flea and tick dips which are perfectly safe for your dog may be fatal to your cat. DO NOT use the same product for both unless the directions specifically say it is safe for cats. Cats ingest the material as they groom. What is safe on the outside of the cat may not be safe on the inside!

Organochlorine insecticides include products such as Aldrin®, Dieldrin®, Heptachlor®, Endrin®, Chlordane® and Lindane®. The use of these products is severely limited because they persist in the environment and some are known to cause cancer, but stocks are still sitting around in garages and barns. Toxicity can occur when a pet eats contaminated food, or the compound is carelessly used and the cat gets into it. **Mothballs** contain a related substance which causes similar signs when eaten.

Signs of organochlorine poisoning include twitchiness, restlessness, vomiting, salivation, depression, and incoordination. These signs may be followed by blindness, convulsions, coma, and death. Get the cat to a veterinarian as soon as possible. If the convulsions can be controlled, the cat probably will live.

Toxaphene is an organochlorine insecticide that is often used as a cattle dip. A cat may fall into the vat while cattle are being dipped, or drink some of the material which has dripped off the cattle or run out of a truck where the cattle have been sprayed. Cats are best kept away from cattle dipping or spraying operations. If the cat falls into a vat, it should be washed off immediately with clear water, and then shampooed and rinsed thoroughly. Wear rubber gloves so that YOU are not poisoned by this material. The concentration used on cattle can be toxic to humans. If the cat drinks some of the dip, treat it as described above for organophosphate poisoning, including, if possible, a quick trip to a veterinarian.

Pyrethrins are natural insecticides derived from several species of *Chrysanthemum*. They are used commonly in flea control products. Pyrethrins are fairly safe to use around cats, as mammals metabolize them quite well. Man-made pyrethrin-type compounds are somewhat more toxic. These include products such as allethrin, tetramethrin, and fenvalerate. In some products, the pyrethrins are combined with other insecticides which make them much more toxic. Be sure to read the label so you will know what you are using.

Signs of pyrethrin poisoning include vomiting, diarrhea, salivation, lack of appetite, and difficult breathing. The cat may be hyperactive, staggering and have seizures, or it could be somewhat depressed. First aid is the same as for strychnine (see below). Take the cat to a veterinarian immediately.

Rotenone is derived from the roots of a plant. It is fairly safe when used according to directions. Large quantities can cause toxic reactions in cats. Depression and vomiting are the most common signs. There is no specific antidote for this poisoning. Bathe the cat thoroughly with detergent to remove as much of the product as possible from its coat. Wear rubber gloves. Give activated charcoal. If the cat goes into convulsions, your veterinarian can give drugs to control them.

DEET is a common ingredient in some insect repellents that are used for protection against the deer ticks which carry Lyme disease. It can cause poisoning in cats, and should not be used on cats. If you are concerned about your cat bringing Lyme disease bearing ticks into your home, simply keep it indoors at all times.

Naphthalene is used in some types of **mothballs**. A poisoned cat may show lack of appetite, depression, vomiting, twitching, diarrhea, and dilated pupils. Induce vomiting, give activated charcoal to limit the absorption from the digestive tract, and take the cat to a veterinarian as soon as possible. Their odor is also toxic to cats, so be sure the cat is not shut in a closet with mothballs.

Cats may be poisoned when there is **new construction** in your house or neighborhood. A cat may drink rainwater which is standing in an open, discarded paint or wood stain can. Waterproofing tar from basement walls may rub off on the fur; the cat becomes ill when it tries to lick off the tar and swallows it. Glues, spackling, and solvents are almost all toxic when inhaled or eaten by a cat. A cat may even be accidentally included in a wall because it is sleeping inside as it is being sealed closed. Hand tools and electric tools used around the construction site also can be a hazard to these curious animals. Turn off ALL power tools, even if you think you're going to be right back. Meanwhile, keep your pet away from trenchers, backhoes, and other equipment being operated at the building site. A cat may be lost when it crawls into a vehicle which is delivering building supplies and jumps off many miles from home.

Household chemicals such as **lye** and **bleach** may get on the cat's skin if it is not kept out of the way while you are cleaning. Concentrated solutions of any of these products can be quite caustic to the skin. Flush with plenty of lukewarm water; then, thoroughly wash the cat with soap and water, rinsing well. If the cat drinks one of these products, give olive oil or egg white, but DO NOT try to make the cat vomit. Take it to a clinic immediately.

Acids may be spilled on the cat's skin. Battery acid, swimming pool chemicals, and certain cleaning agents are all strong acids. The cat will be in severe pain when suffering from an acid burn. Flush the area with large quantities of cool water. Apply a paste made of baking soda (sodium bicarbonate) and water. If the cat has ingested the acid, treat as described above for household chemicals.

The **deicer** used on roads, sidewalks, and driveways contains salt and/or calcium chloride, and can be an irritant if your cat gets the material on its feet. If your cat is outside during the winter, it may ingest this substance as it licks its paws. If these products are used where you live, wash the feet with a damp washcloth when you bring the cat into the house.

Ivermectin is a safe antiparasitic drug when used according to label directions. One of the most common products is Heartgard-30® (Merck), which is used to control heartworms in dogs. Toxicity may occur when a product formulated (such as Eqvalan® (MSD AGVET)) for cattle or horses is used in cats. Imagine, for example, the difficulty in accurately dosing a 10 pound cat with a paste wormer made and measured for a 1200 pound horse! Injectable ivermectin, available for large animals, has the same measuring problem. It is easy to accidentally overdose the cat using one of these products.

Signs of ivermectin toxicity include head bobbing, extreme incoordination and dragging of the hind legs, unusual voice changes, lack of appetite, and personality changes (Frischke, 1991). The cat may salivate or vomit. Signs show that the brain is involved, and the cat may have trembling or convulsions or appear to be blind and disoriented. This may progress to weakness, with the cat unable to stand, followed by stupor. As the poisoning progresses, the breathing and heart rates become slow, the cat becomes pale, enters a coma and dies (Lovell, 1990). Take the cat to your veterinarian as soon as possible.

Treatment of ivermectin toxicity may be successful, but may take one to four weeks of intensive, expensive treatment for the cat to fully recover. The message? If you are deworming a cat, use a cat dewormer.

Metaldehyde is the toxic component of baits used for snails and slugs. **Snail baits** often are placed where cats can get them, and are palatable enough that some cats will eat them. A cat that has eaten snail bait may vomit, salivate, and become uncoordinated. Increased heart and respiratory rates, muscular twitching, and convulsions are common. Some cats appear to be blind. About half the cats that eat snail bait die. Give olive oil and/or activated charcoal and take the cat to a veterinarian as soon as possible. The best prevention is to keep the cat away from areas where snail bait is being used. Pelleted snail baits are more easily picked up by the cat, so it is a good safety measure to use a meal formulation instead and place it where cats can't get to it.

Warfarin and **coumarin** are toxic components of some common rodent poisons. The cat may be poisoned by eating the bait, or by eating rodents poisoned by these compounds. These poisons work by inhibiting one of the K vitamins necessary for the blood to clot normally. This results in spontaneous bleeding. The cat may have hemorrhages of various sizes visible in the membranes of its mouth or eyes. Large hematomas can form under the skin if the cat bumps itself or is otherwise injured. The blood may not clot if the cat is bitten or cut. In some cats, a poor appetite, droopiness, or difficulty in breathing might be the only signs.

Anticoagulant toxicity from older formulations of these compounds is most often seen with exposure to small amounts over a period of three to 10 days. One large dose may not be harmful. A cat may eat a whole box of this type of poison ONCE and survive, but a teaspoon every day for a week could easily kill it. Take the cat to your veterinarian. He or she will give vitamin K, and chances are the cat will be fine.

Newer anticoagulant products, such as **brodifacoum** and **diphacinone**, cause similar symptoms. Just one dose may be sufficient to cause symptoms (or death) in cats. Cats can suffer toxicity from eating rodents poisoned with them. Signs may occur two or three days after the rodent is eaten. The most prominent sign is difficult breathing, and the cat will be droopy, with a poor appetite. The cat may show external hemorrhages, as above, or bleed within the chest, abdomen, or from body openings. Prolonged vitamin K therapy (two to four weeks) is necessary if a large amount of one of the newer products has been eaten. Blood transfusions may be needed to save the cat's life.

Vitamin D3 (cholecalciferol) is the active ingredient in some of the newer rodenticides. It is NOT safe when eaten by cats in anything but the smallest amounts. Signs of toxicity include vomiting (which may be bloody) and a severe bloody diarrhea. The cat may have weakness, muscle twitching, nausea, rapid shallow breathing, and abdominal pain. It may be dehydrated, and may drink and urinate more than normal. Organ failure may occur due to calcification of soft tissues in organs such as the heart, lungs, and kidneys. The cat's body temperature may drop as low as 96 degrees F (35.6 C). Coma and death soon follow. Signs may appear one to two days after the cat has eaten the material, and become progressively worse.

Induce vomiting with syrup of ipecac as soon as possible after you know that the cat has eaten a vitamin D3 rodenticide. Take the cat to a clinic. If you wait one or two days until signs appear, it may be too late to save the cat—irreversible damage likely has taken place. In some cases, large amounts of intravenous fluids, as well as other drugs, may be needed to try to keep the cat alive. Treatment may take up to two weeks because the vitamin is held in body fat. As with most poisonings, it's a lot easier to prevent than to cure (Gunther, 1988).

Thallium is another substance which has been used for rodent and predator control. A cat with acute thallium poisoning shows a lack of appetite, vomiting (sometimes with blood), and possibly bloody diarrhea. Chronic poisoning will result in hair loss, along with thickening and ulceration of the skin. Laboratory tests will confirm the presence of this toxin. Early diagnosis and treatment often have good results.

Sodium fluoroacetate (1080) has been used to control both rodents and predators. An extremely potent and long-lasting toxin, its use has been strictly limited in recent years, but stocks still exist and may be misused, either accidentally or deliberately. Cats may be poisoned by eating material containing the compound, or by eating animals that have been killed by it. Within one-and-a-half hours after eating it, the cat becomes restless and irritable.

It may wander aimlessly, meowing, urinating, and defecating. Violent convulsions often occur. The cat may seem to improve, then go back into seizures. Cats poisoned by "1080" usually die within two to 12 hours after signs begin. There is no known treatment and most affected cats die. If you suspect 1080 poisoning, take the cat to a veterinarian as soon as possible. Intensive supportive therapy might make a difference.

Strychnine is used as a rodent (gopher and vole), predator, and skunk poison, as well as being given maliciously on occasion. Cats also can be affected when they eat poisoned rodents or birds.

A cat that is poisoned by strychnine will become nervous and excited, and may salivate. As the poisoning progresses, the cat goes into convulsions, becoming stiff like a sawhorse. Its head will be pulled toward the back as the neck muscles contract. The front legs will be pulled forward and the hind legs stretched backward, like a sawhorse. The cat gasps and chokes as the muscles of the larynx constrict. It may turn blue as its breathing is shut off. The cat will froth slightly at the mouth as it gasps for air, and its lips will be pulled back, exposing the teeth. Spastic convulsions will rack the body, coming in waves. Any stimulation such as a loud noise will start a new wave of convulsions.

There is NO effective home treatment for strychnine poisoning. If untreated, the convulsions become more severe, and the cat dies of asphyxiation—a very unpleasant death. Give activated charcoal, but only if you can do so VERY quickly, before signs appear. Do not attempt to give it if the cat cannot swallow or is already in convulsions (see Organophosphate Poisoning, above). Take the cat to the nearest veterinarian as soon as possible. The cat will be anesthetized to stop the convulsions, and treated to remove the toxic material from the stomach and digestive tract. If the cat survives the first 24 hours, its chances of survival are good. The cat may have to remain under anesthesia for many hours while its body slowly removes the strychnine.

Sticky traps are used to catch both insects and rodents. A cat may stumble into one and become stuck to it. Use butter (margarine does not work as well) or a mechanic's hand-cleaning product to dissolve the adhesive. Then wash the cat in liquid dish detergent, rinsing well. These traps are more messy than toxic, but it is best not to leave the material on the cat.

Antifreeze (ethylene glycol) is very attractive to both cats and dogs because of its sweet taste. A small quantity can be fatal. Antifreeze poisoning occurs commonly in the winter, spring, and fall when people are draining radiators. It can happen if your radiator leaks onto the garage floor or driveway, as the cat may lap up even a small puddle. Ethylene glycol poisoning also can occur when cats drink color film processing chemicals. High blood levels occur within one to three hours after the cat drinks the liquid. A high percentage of cats die if not quickly treated.

Signs of antifreeze poisoning include nausea, vomiting, excessive thirst, excessive urination, abdominal pain, diarrhea, depression, incoordination, and staggering. The cat may have difficulty breathing, a rapid heart rate, a lowered body temperature, muscle twitching, convulsions, blood in the urine, and kidney failure. Eventually, the cat becomes very drowsy, enters a coma, and dies. Take the cat to a clinic as soon as possible. The veterinarian may have to treat the cat intravenously for two to three days and, with luck, may be able to save it. The sooner treatment begins, the better are its chances for survival. Don't wait to see if the cat develops symptoms if you know it has drunk antifreeze. By that time it is almost always too late. Avoid antifreeze poisoning by cleaning up even small spills and carefully storing and disposing of it.

Oxalate poisoning is what kills a cat with antifreeze poisoning. Oxalate crystals in the kidney also can be due to poisoning with other substances, such as ink eradicators, bleach, cleaning agents, photographic solutions, and deicer solutions. Some plants also can cause this poisoning. These include rhubarb (the leaves only, not the stem part which we eat), philodendron, calla lily, caladium, elephant ear, skunk cabbage, Virginia creeper, and garden sorrel. Dumbcane (diffenbachia) also causes the cat to shake its head and salivate. Cats that are fed large amounts of spinach may develop calculi (stones) in the urinary tract.

Dishwashing detergent is useful for removing some tars and toxins from a cat's coat. However, it should not be used on very young kittens or very small, thin-skinned adult cats. Some of these products contain enough ethyl alcohol to be absorbed and cause toxicity. The cat should be rinsed very thoroughly. Other cleansers should never be left unattended in sinks or tubs where the cat may lick them.

Non-stick cookware has a coating which is toxic to mammals, including cats and humans, when it is heated to a high enough temperature to vaporize the coating into the air. Incidentally, this vapor may be fatal to caged pet birds. When animal or vegetable oils or grease are overheated, the products released into the air are similarly toxic. They also may cause severe eye irritation and tearing. Turn off the stove to prevent further heating. Get your pets and/or children out of the house to prevent further inhalation of the material. Then, open windows to ventilate. It may be necessary to call the fire department, some of which will bring large fans to get the toxic smoke out of the house.

Carbon monoxide is a colorless, odorless, non-irritating gas. It is generated by furnaces, stoves, and vehicle exhaust, especially if operated in a confined area with inadequate ventilation. Carbon monoxide poisoning can occur when a cat is carried in the trunk of an automobile. The cat may be depressed, and have an elevated temperature and muscle twitching. The mucous membranes can be either muddy colored or cherry-red. Give artificial respiration if necessary, and administer oxygen if safely available. The cat may have to be hospitalized for a few days of treatment.

Chocolate can be toxic to cats. It contains theobromine, a stimulant similar to caffeine, which can cause an irregular heartbeat. Prominent signs are related to central nervous system stimulation. The cat may be restless, excited, and nervous. It may exhibit panting, vomiting, diarrhea, depression, and frequent urination. The mucous membranes may be bluish. As the poisoning progresses, muscular tremors, seizures, coma, and even sudden death may be seen. Most fatalities occur six to 24 hours after the chocolate is eaten (Hornfeldt, 1987). Signs of chocolate poisoning begin four to five hours after chocolate is eaten. **Caffeine** from soft drinks, coffee, and tea can cause similar signs with an overdose. There is no specific treatment for chocolate poisoning. If you know the cat has eaten chocolate, it is helpful to induce vomiting, even if it is several hours later. Do not induce vomiting if the cat is in convulsions. Give activated charcoal if you have it available. Take the cat to your veterinarian.

Lead poisoning is one of the most common toxicities in pets. It may account for as many as 22% of accidental poisonings in cats (Prescott, 1983), and seems to be more common in summer and fall. Lead poisoning can occur when a cat chews surfaces painted with lead-based paints, or when it licks sanding dust from its coat during house repairs or remodeling. A kitten may get lead poisoning from chewing on a wheel weight or fishing sinker. An adult cat may eat a bird that has been shot with lead pellets.

Lead poisoning is a cumulative process. It comes on slowly and the signs may vary, making it difficult to diagnose. Signs may occur three to 14 days after the cat eats the substance containing lead. The cat may show signs of abdominal pain, and may cry when its belly is handled. It may have vomiting, diarrhea or constipation, and a poor appetite. If the nervous system is affected, the cat will show hysteria, nervousness, and meowing, and may stagger, tremble, and have convulsions. Blindness and deafness can occur.

Lead poisoning is most often seen in cats that are less than one year of age, living in an inner city area where buildings are old, or in a house that recently has been remodeled. Like some insecticides, lead-based paint is mostly off the market, but some still exists. The cat may get dust from old lead-based paint on its coat and ingest it while grooming. If you are sanding or remodeling, keep your cat away from the dust as much as possible. Give the cat frequent baths to help keep the dust off its coat. Removing the source of lead is often enough to allow the cat to recover completely.

Teething and curiosity may lead a kitten to chew items an adult cat would not touch. Glazed ceramic dishes, especially those from Mexico, may not have been fired well enough to bind the lead pigments in the glaze. Lead can slowly leach out into the food or water and be a source of chronic lead exposure. Lead can come from hard water running through lead pipes, solder, lead-foil, lead acetate solutions, linoleum, roofing, and newspaper. Treatment with urinary acidifiers such as potassium iodide or ammonium chloride can cause acute lead poisoning in cats that already have high levels of lead in their bones.

Treatment for lead poisoning involves administration of chelating drugs to help remove the lead from the cat's system. This could take one to two weeks of hospitalization, and can be very expensive. Surgery may be needed if the cat has eaten a solid item such as a drapery weight. If your cat is affected by lead poisoning, and you have young children, consult your physician about the possibility that they were exposed to the same materials. Many large cities have clinics which test children free of charge for lead poisoning.

Arsenic is found in some herbicides and insecticides. The cat may be poisoned by licking its feet after walking in a recently treated area. It also is found in many ant poisons, such as Terro® Ant Killer (Sanoret Chemical). When used properly, a drop or two of the poison is placed on a piece of cardboard. Overzealous users may fill a lid with a large amount, which the cat drinks because of the sweet taste. It doesn't take much to poison a cat because of its small weight—as little as one-tenth of a teaspoon (.5 ml) may be fatal. Arsenic is a component of some rodent poisons, such as Vacor® (Rohm & Haas). It also may be present in wind-borne smoke or dust from some metal smelters.

The most common sign of arsenic poisoning is vomiting, which occurs within minutes. The vomited material may have a garlic-like odor. The cat may be restless, trembling, and weak. It may show severe abdominal pain, along with diarrhea which is sometimes bloody. The membranes can be bluish. In a severe case, irregular heartbeat, staggering, shock, weakness, collapse, coma, and death are likely to occur. Take the cat to a veterinarian as soon as possible. Several days of intensive treatment may be necessary before you know whether the cat will live or die.

Mercury may be found in some marine fish such as tuna. Poisoning may occur in cats that are fed nothing but tuna or similar fish for long periods of time, usually four to six months or more. Kittens that are victims of this metal may be less active and playful than normal. They also may be noisier and more vocal than usual, and may spend more time eating than kittens that are fed beef or other foods. Chronic mercury poisoning also leads to muscle weakness and loss of balance. Treatment, if successful, may take seven to 10 days.

Cocaine may poison a cat, whether given deliberately or ingested accidentally. Signs of cocaine toxicity are those of stimulation of the central nervous system. The cat may salivate profusely, twitch or shake, vomit, have an increased heart rate, and can go into convulsions. The effects of cocaine on the heart can be life-threatening. In addition, fatal respiratory depression is possible with a large enough dose. Take the cat to a veterinarian as soon as possible. And be sure to tell him or her what the cat has eaten. The signs of cocaine intoxication are not specific, and the veterinarian might not otherwise figure it out in time to save the cat. There is no specific treatment for cocaine toxicity. All the veterinarian can do is treat the symptoms that are occurring at the time. If you cannot take the cat to a clinic, and it has not been more than a couple of hours since it ate the cocaine, induce vomiting to remove as much of the material from the stomach as possible. Give oxygen if it is safely available.

Marijuana cigarettes or marijuana-laced foods are rarely fatal to cats, but will cause obvious signs of sickness. These may include depression, drowsiness, lowered body temperature, incoordination, salivation, vomiting, and a slowed heart rate. The pupils of the eyes may be widely dilated. Some cats may become extremely hypersensitive and may die. Even inhalation of marijuana smoke may bother some cats. A mild case may be treated by keeping the cat warm and in a quiet, darkened area until it recovers.

If the heart rate is severely slowed, veterinary treatment may be necessary.

Plant poisonings are sometimes seen in cats. They are more common in winter when both the cat and the plants are kept indoors. Kittens are especially susceptible to poisoning by plants as they chew on anything and everything around them. An older cat, especially if it is the only pet, may become bored when left alone for long periods of time and chew on plants if they are handy. One of the best protections against plant poisoning is to give your cat safe, chewable greens, such as a pot of oats or catnip.

Some decorative Christmas plants are very toxic. Poinsettias and mistletoe may cause irritation and blistering of the membranes of the mouth and stomach. The cat may show lack of appetite, vomiting, and paralysis of the tongue. Mistletoe may cause a slowed pulse. Get the cat to your veterinarian so he or she can monitor the cat's pulse and administer specific antidotes, if necessary. Needles from your Christmas tree may be poisonous to a cat that eats them. Drinking water from the base of the Christmas tree stand also can cause pine tar poisoning. This causes sores on the tongue, a sore throat, irritated stomach, vomiting, diarrhea, and lethargy.

Both flowers and leaves of Easter lily (*Lilium longiflorium*) are poisonous to cats. A single leaf can kill your cat, causing death by kidney failure in two to five days (Buck, 1993). Signs of poisoning include vomiting, depression, and dehydration. Treatment includes inducing vomiting to rid the cat of the vegetation, activated charcoal, and prompt hospitalization. Other offending house plants are: Diffenbachia (dumb cane), ivy, azalea, philodendron, elephant ear, amaryllis, and schefflera.

Diagnosis is often difficult if the cat was not seen eating the plant. If the cat has vomited, look for plant material in the vomitus. Look for chewed edges or missing leaves on your plants. Encourage the cat to vomit.

Most plant poisonings can be successfully treated by your veterinarian. In most cases, symptoms are treated as they occur. The best prevention is to keep house plants out of the cat's reach (how about hanging planters?), or in a room where the cat is not allowed. It also helps to make sure the cat receives plenty of attention, play, and a balanced diet. Some people have reported that spraying house plants with a mixture of vinegar and water makes them unattractive to cats. You also can use bitter apple spray or a mixture of hot pepper sauce and water. Mouse traps or rough bark placed around the base of the plant may keep the cat away. Do this at the first sign that the cat is chewing on your plant. These plants are not poisonous to have in your house—they're only toxic if the cat eats them.

A number of common outdoor plants are also toxic to cats. Among these are apricot, autumn crocus, azalea, bird of paradise, bittersweet, black-eyed susan, black locust, bleeding heart, bluebonnet, boxwood, buttercup, caladium, castor bean, cherry, chokecherry, chrysanthemum, clematis, cornflower, crotalaria, croton, crown of thorns, cyclamen, daffodil, deadly nightshade, death camas, delphinium, eggplant, elderberry, English ivy, euonymus, flax, four o'clock, foxglove, hemlock, holly, horse chestnut, hyacinth, hydrangea, iris, jack-in-the-pulpit, jimson weed (Datura), lantana, larkspur, laurel, locoweed, lupine, marigold, mistletoe, mock orange, monkshood, morning glory, mountain laurel, nightshade, peach, peony, poison oak, pokeweed, poppy, potato, privet, rosary peas, rhododendron, rhubarb (only the leaves), skunk cabbage, snow-on-the-mountain, tobacco, tomato, and wisteria.

Outdoors, yew trees may cause signs of shaking, weakness and collapse, and the cat may have trouble breathing if it eats the leaves. The heartbeat may become fast and irregular, and coma, convulsions, and death can result if the cat is not treated. Try to induce vomiting. Take the cat to your veterinarian so that its stomach can be thoroughly emptied, and drugs for the heart problem can be given if needed.

Oleander and lily of the valley can cause poisoning with symptoms of dizziness, depression, and a rapid, weak heartbeat. If untreated, the cat may stop breathing, and its heart may stop. Induce vomiting and seek veterinary help.

Thistles and cactus can cause a foreign body reaction when they prick the cat or stick to its skin. When the cat swallows the stickers as it removes them, intestinal irritation may occur. If you know the cat has been stuck by these spines, pull them out rather than letting the cat remove them. Give drugs to soothe the bowel and a laxative to help the material pass out of the gut.

Poison ivy does not seem to bother cats. The main problem is that the cat can carry the toxin to YOU on its fur, after picking it up by running through or rolling in the plant. You may be affected if the cat rubs against your bare legs, or you may get it on your hands as you pet the cat. If you know your cat has been in contact with poison ivy, put on rubber gloves and give it a thorough bath with cat shampoo and plenty of water.

Cats are susceptible to most of the same **mushrooms** that poison humans. *Amanita* is perhaps the most toxic genus. If you know (or suspect) your cat has eaten one or more poisonous mushrooms, encourage it to vomit. Take the cat to a veterinarian for further treatment if other signs appear.

Blooms of **blue-green algae** occur on ponds and lakes in the upper Midwest and southern Canada during dry, hot, summers. Pets become poisoned by the endotoxin produced by these algae when they drink water from the pond. Signs of algae poisoning include vomiting, abdominal pain, diarrhea, muscular twitching and staggering, followed by paralysis and convulsions. Death may occur within one to two hours after the cat drinks the water. Encourage vomiting. Give activated charcoal if you have it and if there are no convulsions. Take the cat to a clinic as soon as possible.

Aflatoxin is the name given to a toxin produced by the growth of *Aspergillus flavus* or *Penicillium* molds on feed. They are often found on corn, peanuts, or cottonseed that has molded, whether in the field or in storage. Acute toxicity requires continuous exposure for 20 to 30 days, at a minimum of one part per million in the diet (Morgan, 1985). Signs include weakness, lack of appetite, and depression. The cat may have diarrhea, which may be bloody. The blood may clot poorly, and the cat may show jaundice due to liver damage. Collapse and death may occur within seven to 10 days after signs begin. Symptoms are treated as they occur. See your veterinarian if you think your cat is affected. To avoid aflatoxin toxicity, do not feed any food, even cat food, which has molded. Aflatoxin can be produced in foods which do not look moldy. If your cat seems to have become ill from food, your veterinarian can have the food tested by a laboratory.

Botulism is uncommon in cats, but is occasionally seen. The cat becomes paralyzed, followed by coma and death. If recognized early enough, antitoxin can be given, and the cat might be saved. Cats are somewhat resistant to botulism. These poisonings are best treated by your veterinarian. Prevention includes keeping the cat out of garbage and keeping other people from feeding it spoiled food.

Cats may ingest **pills** or **drugs**, whether by accident or deliberately. The possibilities range from accidental dosages of prescription drugs, whether heart medications or antibiotics, to deliberate dosages of illegal drugs. A partial list would include tranquilizers, amphetamines, narcotics, heroin, etc. Most **human vitamins** have enough iron to be a hazard, and should never be given to cats. An overdose with some of these drugs can easily be fatal because cats are so much smaller than humans.

When the cat and its family move into a new house, it could receive a critical overdose from eating medication found in a corner—perhaps pills which have been left after a party. If the cat gets into medication, take the pill bottle or some of the medication or substance to your veterinarian immediately, along with the cat. Some drugs, such as antibiotics, will cause little or no harm, while a large dose of heart medication may severely upset or kill a cat. Cats and dogs may act together to get in trouble with medication. The cat might get up on the counter and its little feet could push the pill vial off onto the floor. The dog then crunches it open and eats the pills. Don't leave any medication, including common ones such as aspirin, heart medicines, and cough syrups where the cat (or dog or child!) can get them.

Treatment for an unknown drug poisoning is largely symptomatic. Observe the cat carefully, and consult your veterinarian if the signs are anything other than mild and transient. By the way, a cat can eat a month's supply of birth control pills without any harm.

Nonsteroidal anti-inflammatory drugs, such as ibuprofen (found in Motrin®, Advil®, Nuprin®, Aleve®, etc.) can cause poisoning in cats, especially when eaten in large quantities. Naproxen (Naprosyn®) may cause similar signs. With any of these drugs, the cat may be staggering and incoordinated, and depressed or in a stupor. Vomiting can occur, as well as diarrhea (which may be bloody or blackish). Bleeding into the stomach will sometimes occur, and may be life-threatening. If the drug has been deliberately given for several days, the cat may have enough internal bleeding that it also is anemic and pale. Kidney failure can occur. The prognosis for survival is good if the kidney failure can be reversed. In some cases, it may not be completely reversible. If you are sure your cat has consumed one of these products, encourage vomiting. Give activated charcoal and take the cat to your veterinarian for further treatment.

Excessive quantities of **aspirin** can be fatal to cats. This is because they eliminate the drug more slowly than humans. Also, cats are quite small compared to humans. One baby aspirin can be given every other day, and reactions are rare. Check with your veterinarian to see if it is appropriate for your cat. Signs of aspirin toxicity include depression, lack of appetite, vomiting, convulsions, lowered body temperature and death.

Acetaminophen products (Tylenol® and other non-aspirin products) are toxic to cats even in very low dosages. This is because the cat's liver does not have the enzymes necessary to metabolize the toxic by-products produced in their bodies. The toxicity may be seen within four hours after this medication is given. Acetaminophen also is found in many cold medications, and in aspirin-free arthritis pain medicine.

TREATMENT OF POISONINGS IN GENERAL

If you know or suspect that your cat has ingested a toxic substance, what can you do? Begin by calling your own veterinarian or emergency clinic. Ask for recommendations for the particular substance you think (or know) your cat has ingested. This is important because vomiting should be induced with some substances, but is totally wrong for others. Do not bother trying to induce vomiting if you are close to a clinic. Take your cat to the clinic and let the veterinarian take care of it. He or she has injectable drugs which will make the cat vomit almost immediately.

If you cannot get the necessary information there, call the 24-hour National Animal Poison Control Center (NAPCC) (at the University of Illinois College of Veterinary Medicine, Urbana, IL). The number is 1-900-680-0000. There is a $20 minimum charge for this call for five minutes. NAPCC also may be reached at 1-800-548-2423. This number has a $30 minimum charge, to a credit card only, but this fee includes follow-up calls and consultation with your veterinarian if needed. Some manufacturers pay NAPCC to provide information on reactions to their products. If you call about one of these, the call is free.

In general, the cat should be encouraged to vomit if it has ingested a poison. If you know the cat has swallowed a petroleum product such as kerosene or gasoline, or a caustic (acid or alkaline) substance, DO NOT induce vomiting. If the cat has ingested an acidic solution, DO NOT give sodium bicarbonate (baking soda)! The gas-forming reaction can rupture the stomach. With these, give cream, milk, or water to dilute the substance. Also, DO NOT try to induce vomiting if the cat is unconscious or has any nervous system symptoms, such as tremors or convulsions.

The cat will vomit if you give it syrup of ipecac at 1 teaspoon per 5 pounds of body weight, to a maximum of 3 teaspoons (1-2 ml/kg body weight, 15 ml maximum). Do not give more than 1 tablespoon (15 ml) to even the largest cat. The dose may be repeated in 20 minutes if the cat does not vomit with the first dose. Do not give more than two doses. Syrup of ipecac does not work on all cats. It usually can be purchased at a drugstore. If you do not have syrup of ipecac, you can put a couple of teaspoons of salt on the back of its tongue. A third method you can try is to give the cat a half-and-half mixture of 3% hydrogen peroxide and water. Pour it into the lip pouch. Table salt and peroxide do not always work. Syrup of ipecac is better if you have it available. After the cat has vomited, offer milk or cream and take the cat to the clinic as soon as possible.

Activated charcoal is one substance which safely can be given with any poisoning or suspected poisoning. It can be helpful with substances as diverse as organophosphate insecticides, accidental drug overdosages and herbicides. It is safe, and can be kept on hand to use if needed. SuperChar®-Vet (Gulf-Bio-Systems, Inc., 5310 Harvest Hill Road, Dallas, Texas, 75230) is one brand. It comes as a liquid which can be given in an emergency. It should be given to your pet in the bathtub or outdoors, as it can stain. Although this product has sorbitol added, which may have a laxative effect, some charcoal products may cause constipation if not followed by a laxative. Keep this in mind after the initial crisis is past (Buck, 1986). Do not give any oral drug to a comatose or unconscious animal. Burned or charred toast is mentioned in some books as an emergency antidote. It does NOT work. Keeping a bottle of activated charcoal mixture on hand is cheap insurance for both pets and children.

SNAKEBITE

A cat may be bitten when it blunders into or deliberately attacks a poisonous snake. Some cats routinely kill snakes, and their intended victim may be poisonous. The cat may be merely curious and want to see what the snake is. When it reaches out its nose to check it, the cat gets too close and the snake strikes. In northern parts of the country, snakebites are most common in summer (the snakes are hibernating during the colder months), but in the South and Southwest, they can occur any month of the year.

Poisonous snake bites in North America are most often from pit vipers. These snakes include copperheads, the cottonmouth or water moccasin, and some 32 species of rattlesnakes. Pit vipers have a slit-shaped pupil of the eye, much like a cat, in contrast to the round pupil of the non-poisonous snakes. These snakes have two modified salivary glands which produce venom, attached to a sizable pair of fangs, which inject the venom during a bite. Coral snakes also are poisonous, but for the most part they are small and limited to small geographic areas, which reduces pets' exposure to them.

Several factors determine the severity of a poisonous snakebite. The weight, age, and general health of the cat will determine its reaction to the venom. Some species of snakes are more poisonous than others. For example, in the western United States, the bite of the Mojave rattlesnake is generally more severe than that of the Western Diamondback. Bites on the cat's head may be quickly fatal, while those on the legs may give time for treatment. A glancing bite which injects little or no venom may not be a problem, while a head-on bite which strikes deeply into the tissues may be fatal even if you get veterinary help quickly. The smaller the cat, the more likely the bite is to be fatal, other factors being equal.

Snake venom is composed of proteins, including enzymes that dissolve proteins in the victim, destroying capillaries and tissues at the bite site. They also contain neurotoxins, which damage the nerves and may cause paralysis, including the respiratory system. Other components of venom dissolve red blood cells and damage the heart and circulatory system. Coagulation times may be increased, with the blood not clotting normally. In addition, dead tissue at the bite wound offers an ideal place for bacterial growth. Infection and gangrene may occur. If the cat lives through the initial crisis, large areas of tissue may slough, leaving large, ugly ulcers that are slow to heal.

You may see the snake bite the cat, which makes the problem easy to diagnose. Otherwise, you must look for signs that a bite has occurred. Bites occur most frequently on the forelegs, shoulders, head, and neck. If necessary, clip the hair from the area. This may help to tell a snakebite from a wasp or spider bite. One or two fang wounds may be seen, appearing as small punctures. If the snake has struck the cat more than once, several fang marks may be seen. The cat may show extreme pain at the bite, swelling, and discoloration of the area, and may have excessive thirst and other signs of shock. These symptoms are not seen with bites from nonpoisonous snakes. Some people mistake the hole of a draining, swollen abscess for a snakebite. If it stinks, it's probably not a snakebite.

If the venom has gone directly into a blood vessel, the cat may become unconscious immediately, with or without convulsions. The size of the swelling and severity of signs depend on the amount and toxicity of the venom which was injected. The cat probably will have no appetite, and may be listless for several days after a snakebite. A large injection of venom is nearly always followed by a large tissue slough. In some cases, full-blown signs may not develop until several hours after the bite has occurred. If you KNOW the cat has been bitten, it is usually worth having it hospitalized for observation.

It's worthwhile to know the snakes in your area, and to be able to identify those that are venomous. This will keep you from treating a cat that has been bitten by a harmless bull snake, or from not treating a cat bitten by a rattlesnake. The treatment may cause damage, so it is important that it not be given, except as a lifesaving measure. Do not get bitten trying to kill the snake for identification.

FIRST AID FOR SNAKEBITE: Immobilize the cat as much as possible until it can be treated. Unnecessary physical activity will increase absorption of the venom. Do not use excessive heat or cold on the bite area. Do not give tranquilizers, as they may add to the effects of the snake venom, giving a more severe reaction. Do not give painkillers, as they may mask important signs.

THE BEST FIRST AID AND TREATMENT FOR SNAKEBITE IS TO TAKE THE CAT TO A VETERINARIAN AS SOON AS POSSIBLE. He or she has specialized drugs that may make the difference between life and death. The veterinarian may have, or be able to quickly obtain, antivenin. The best first aid for snakebite, whether for your cat or yourself, is your car keys and a cool head!

THE FOLLOWING MEASURES ARE ONLY TO BE USED IF YOU ARE MORE THAN ONE TO TWO HOURS FROM A VETERINARIAN. YOU MAY CAUSE DAMAGE BY USING THEM. IF YOU CANNOT GET TO A VETERINARIAN, THEY ARE WORTH A TRY.

If you cannot get the cat to a veterinarian quickly, begin by isolating the venom. If the bite is on a leg, put a flat tourniquet between the bite and the heart. It should be tight enough to slow the venous and lymphatic flow in the surface tissues. It should NOT be so tight that blood flow to the leg stops. You should be able to easily insert a finger under the tourniquet. When properly applied, it may be left in place up to two hours. DO NOT loosen it at intervals because this could allow the venom to be circulated from the bite area. If you can get to the veterinarian within a reasonable length of time (one to two hours), DO NOT use a tourniquet. In many cases, more damage has been done by a tourniquet than by the snakebite. If used incorrectly, it may result in gangrene and/or loss of the leg!

Articles have been written about using electroshock (as from an automobile battery) for snakebite. Reliable studies have shown that this is NOT helpful, and it may be fatal to an animal as small as a cat by stopping its heart. Don't try it!

If you are not within one to two hours of a veterinarian, it is worthwhile to try to remove as much venom as possible. Apply suction at the fang marks with a snakebite suction cup for at least 30 minutes to remove as much venom as possible. It is not a good idea to suck the venom with your mouth because it may enter your body through any cuts or open areas in the mouth. If you are in ANY doubt about this step, don't. Take the cat to a clinic as soon as possible.

An antivenin is available for the toxins of North American pit vipers. One brand is Antivenin Polyvalent (Fort Dodge Laboratories, Fort Dodge, IA, 50501). If you live in a snakebite area, and have cats (or dogs) which you value for their economic or sentimental value, you may wish to keep some of this on hand. Its main drawback is that it is VERY expensive, and as many as five vials (50 ml) may be needed for a small cat (the smaller the cat, the larger the dose that is needed on a per-pound basis). Ideally, the product works best when injected intravenously. If you cannot do this, intramuscular injection is better than not giving it. Or, if you are close to a veterinarian, take the antivenin to him or her and have it injected. Additional doses may be needed every two hours if symptoms such as pain and swelling remain or recur. The earlier the antivenin is given, the more effective it is.

Your veterinarian may give the cat antihistamines to help delay or suppress allergic reactions which might occur, either from the snakebite or from the antivenin. Antihistamines also help calm the animal and reduce its activity. One drug which is commonly used is Benadryl® (Parke-Davis). An adult cat may be given 8 mg orally every 12 hours, while a kitten should not have more than 4 mg every 12 hours.

The cat also may be given antibiotics to help prevent or reduce infection in the dead tissues. Intravenous fluids may be needed, as well as blood transfusions. The wound should be cleaned as thoroughly as possible, and it may be useful to place a loose bandage over the wound to keep the cat from licking it. The cat should be placed in a cage or small run to limit its activity, and in most cases will be hospitalized for AT LEAST 24 hours.

Bites by coral snakes are uncommon because these snakes are shy and move mostly at night. Because most of them are fairly small, it is not easy for them to get their mouths around a cat's leg. The fangs are in the rear of the mouth, so the snake must bite and hang on in order to inject venom into the wound. The bites tend to be very small punctures. There is generally little or no local reaction at the bite, which makes them hard to find.

Clinical signs may not develop until two to 12 hours after the bite has occurred. However, when signs begin, they rapidly become serious. Treatment may not be successful if it is begun after signs occur—a real catch-22 since you may not know the cat was bitten until signs begin. Death is primarily due to respiratory paralysis. If the breathing apparatus is not completely paralyzed, pneumonia can occur after the cat has recovered from the bite, and it still may die.

If you suspect that your cat has been bitten by a coral snake, it should be treated before any clinical signs occur. The product commonly used is Antivenin® *(Microrus fulvius,* equine origin) (Wyeth). The cat should be taken immediately to a facility which has a respirator, as well as equipment for intensive care, in case its breathing stops. All cats that are bitten by coral snakes should be hospitalized for 48 hours, and carefully monitored. It may take several weeks for the cat to recover completely.

The above mentioned antivenin does not neutralize the venom of the Sonoran coral snake (*Microuroides euryxanthus*) found in southern Arizona and northern Mexico. Treatment is largely supportive. Again, respiratory support may be needed.

Gila monsters (and the related Mexican beaded lizards) are the only lizards in the world which have developed venom. They tend to bite and hang on, probably more from fear of being dropped or flung away than from viciousness. These lizards do not have fangs like the poisonous snakes. They have grooved teeth, from which secretions of their modified salivary glands are directed into the bite wound. In many cases, you may have to pry the Gila monster off the cat. Use a couple of sticks to separate the jaws and watch that it doesn't bite you in the process. Gila monsters can swap ends with lightning rapidity.

If enough venom has seeped into the bite wound, the cat will show severe pain at the bite site within minutes. There may be a severe drop in blood pressure, which may be life-threatening in a small cat. The cat may salivate, have tears running from its eyes, and urinate and defecate frequently. Take the cat to a clinic for treatment. Lowered blood pressure may make it necessary to give intravenous fluids to keep the cat alive. No antivenin is available. Antihistamines do not seem to help. If the cat survives the blood pressure drop, it probably will come through the crisis.

Please don't kill the Gila monster. They are sluggish, basically non-aggressive, and only bite when prodded or annoyed. There aren't many of them left. You are lucky to be able to see one!

INSECT STINGS

These include stings by bees, hornets, wasps, and ants. Multiple stings are common because the insects are found in colonies with large numbers of individuals. The cat may have severe local swelling and pain with the stings. This usually becomes more tolerable within an hour or so after the stings have occurred. If the cat is stung severely around the neck or face, there may be enough swelling that it cannot breathe. This is, of course, a real emergency. Anaphylactic shock may occur. Take the cat to a veterinarian as soon as possible.

If the cat has only one or a few stings, and minimal reaction to them (other than pain and annoyance), you can give Benadryl® (see Snakebite, above, for dosage). Observe the cat carefully for signs of breathing difficulty, severe swelling, or shock. The cat's face may be swollen and comical for a day or two, but one or two stings are usually more annoying than life-threatening, except in an allergic individual.

BURNS

Burns, in general, are most severe in very young or very old cats, and when they involve the head or joints and result in the formation of scar tissue. Burns may occur when hot oil, water, or food spills on the cat in the kitchen, or when it walks into them. Burns occur, for example, when the cat takes a stroll on hot asphalt or on a radiator or stove. Cats seem to be less sensitive to heat than humans and may remain sitting on a hot stove long after their hair begins to singe. Burns can occur from a house fire or by contact with flame. When the cat feels the pain, it probably will run, and may be angry when you catch up with it. Be careful not to get hurt in the process.

A superficial burn only affects the outer layer of the skin. These often are called first degree burns. The skin may be reddened, and may later peel (much as a sunburn does on human skin). These burns may be hard to find if the cat's hair is not burned, or the skin is dark colored. First degree burns may be quite painful, but they need little care and heal rapidly.

Partial thickness (second degree) burns go completely through the outer layer of the skin into the middle layer. The site may be reddened and swollen, and may ooze yellowish plasma. Blistering may occur, especially with burns from flame or scalding liquid. The site is painful, but less so than with a superficial burn (because the nerve endings are damaged and no longer relay pain messages to the brain). These burns heal with little or no scarring IF they do not become infected. Healing usually takes about two to four weeks.

Full thickness (third degree) burns go through the epidermis and dermis. These layers are coagulated and deadened. Portions of the skin may be charred and severely swollen. Dry gangrene can occur, with the entire damaged skin layer peeling off, exposing underlying tissues. Because the nerve endings have all been burned, the area is insensitive. The hair is either gone or pulls out easily. Infection and severe scarring are common. These are severe burns, and should be treated by a veterinarian.

Shock may occur if more than 15% of the skin surface is burned. If more than 50% of the body is involved, consideration should be given to euthanizing the cat promptly, without treatment, for humane reasons. You know how much a small burn from touching an oven or barbecue hurts. Imagine how extremely painful that would be over half the animal's body—and the nerve endings rejuvenate fairly quickly. Euthanasia is the kindest course of action.

FIRST AID: If a burn has just occurred, apply ice compresses or cold water for 20 to 45 minutes. Treatment with cold water is useful within two hours following the burn. You can restrain the cat in a T-shirt or pillowcase with its head sticking out, and run cold water over it. Cold water helps reduce the extent of the burn, and decreases its depth by dissipating heat. It also relieves the pain. Be careful not to chill the cat excessively, thus making the shock worse, or to cause frostbite on the skin by leaving ice on too long.

If you are not present when the burn occurs, you may not know there is a problem for hours or even a day or two later. The cat will act anxious, and show pain when touched. If the skin is light-colored, it may be obviously reddened. Eventually, there will be hair loss. Restrain the cat and very gently clip the hair away from the area.

If the burn is anything other than minor, there is a good chance for infection. Cover the burn with a clean cloth or gauze moistened with a solution of one teaspoon of salt in a quart of lukewarm water. Do NOT use cotton, because the loose fibers become caught in the surface of the wound and are very difficult and painful to remove. Do not put oily ointments, grease, petroleum jelly, or butter on the burn! They don't help, and they make treatment much more difficult. Take the cat to the clinic as soon as possible.

Treatment for severe burns may necessitate intensive care by your veterinarian. It may include administration of fluids to replace those lost through the damaged skin surface, and antibiotics to help prevent infection. Corticosteroids may be given to help reduce inflammation and swelling, especially in the lungs. Lung damage occurs both from inhalation of hot gases and from toxic products and particles in the smoke. Drugs may be given to reduce pain. Infection is the most common cause of death in cats that survive the initial burn.

Chemical burns may be caused accidentally or deliberately by battery acid and many other products stored around the household. If the burn is caused by an acid, it should be neutralized by a mild alkali, such as baking soda dissolved in a glass of water. If the burn is caused by an alkali, it can be flooded with vinegar or lemon juice. Anything more than a small chemical burn should be examined by a veterinarian as soon as possible. If you do not have any of these neutralizing agents handy, or do not know the cause of the burn, rinse the cat in cool water for at least five minutes. Take the cat to a veterinarian as soon as possible.

Burns due to solvents and petroleum products should be handled with care. A cat's skin is very thin, and there is a danger that the products will be absorbed through it. Avoid volatilizing the product if possible, because the fumes may cause pneumonia—in both you and the cat! Wash the cat with dishwashing liquid and be sure to rinse it all off. Dishwashing liquid may be toxic to kittens and should be used with caution. Take the cat to a clinic.

Burns due to flames are most often seen with a house or apartment fire. They also are seen when a cat is deliberately doused with gasoline and set on fire. The odor of gasoline or another petroleum product on the cat is the first clue that such an act of extreme cruelty has occurred.

Burns caused by hot tars or grease are difficult to treat. Carefully remove as much as you can by blotting it off with paper towels or clean rags. Cut the hair away very gently, if necessary, to get the material away from the skin so that you can see how much damage has been done. If you have an ointment containing polyoxyethylene sorbitan, coat the remaining hair and the skin with it. Neosporin® ointment, and some other antibiotic ointments, contain this solvent. If there is just a small spot of tar, you can rub the ointment in, put a bandage over it, and leave it for six to eight hours to soften the tar. If you do not have one of these drugs, rub salad oil, lard, or shortening gently into the hair and skin. Then wash the cat as above. This treatment should be done at home only with small or minor burns. Major ones should be treated at a clinic where the cat can be sedated and supported with intravenous fluids as the damaged tissue is cleansed.

Burns from direct heat occur primarily in association with food and cooking. They may happen when a cat licks a hot barbecue grill, or hungrily gulps dry cat food to which excessively hot water has been added. In this case, the cat's esophagus and stomach may suffer burn injury, in addition to the burns on the mouth and tongue. Scalding injuries can occur from hot grease or food spilled on the cat as it begs near the stove or lies in the middle of the kitchen floor. This is another reason to have a well-trained pet that will stay out from underfoot and not beg!

Friction burns may occur when a cat has a rope or cord dragged rapidly around a leg or over its skin. They also happen when a cat is tied and falls out of a vehicle or trailer and is dragged on the road. Friction burns frequently occur when a cat is hit by a car and skids along the pavement. Similar injuries may occur to the foot pads after vigorous exercise on a hard, rough surface such as asphalt pavement, while trying to cross a road when being chased by a dog. Excessive shearing forces created by sudden stopping and turning may lead to separation and detachment of the entire pad surface. In some cases, it may be necessary to use skin grafts to replace the area damaged by friction burns.

To deal with a severe friction burn, remove as many of the sticks and stones and as much of the dirt as possible. Wrap the injured, abraded area in a sheet or towel dampened with cold water. Take the cat to your veterinarian as soon as possible.

Begin by treating any burn OTHER than tar or grease burns with cold water as described above. Remove hair from the area and clean it very gently. A small burn can be gently washed with chlorhexidine solution. Small burns may be treated by applying an ointment. You can use gentamicin cream, chlorhexidine (Nolvasan®) solution, or silver sulfadiazine cream (Silvadene Creme®). Petroleum-based (greasy) ointments should not be used on a fresh burn. Aloe vera may be helpful on small burns which have just occurred, but should not be used on serious burns.

Small burns usually should not be bandaged. If the cat wants to lick the area, it should be restrained from doing so, either by an Elizabethan collar or a loose dressing or covering. It is very important to keep the burned area clean to avoid infection, so the cat should be kept from rolling in dirt or otherwise soiling the burn area. If you are treating a burn and it shows pus, discoloration, or signs of infection, have it checked by your veterinarian. Some cats may need to be sedated for a few days, or given painkillers to reduce the pain. If a burn is this bad, see your veterinarian.

Sunburn is uncommon in cats. It may occur when a cat is sheared extremely closely and then allowed out in hot, midday sun before seven to 10 days have passed for hair regrowth. Cats with white areas on the end of the nose or on their ears may have severe problems with sunburn. If the cat is both indoors and out, a good solution is to allow the cat out only at night.

ELECTRICAL BURNS

Kittens, especially, may chew electrical wires or phone cords. Christmas is a hazardous time when strings of lights may attract them. This may result in severe burns to the tongue and the membranes of the mouth, in addition to possibly stopping the cat's breathing and/or heart. If the cat is still near the wire when you find it, either knock the wire out of the socket with a wooden stick or with the leg of a wooden chair. Then you can take care of the cat. If it has just occurred, start CPR immediately. In some cases, you can restart a heart that has been stopped by electrical shock and revive the cat. If the cat has a heartbeat, but is not breathing, begin artificial respiration. Take the cat to your veterinarian as soon as possible. The resulting burns in the mouth should be checked by your veterinarian, as there is a good chance for infection.

SMOKE INHALATION

A cat that has inhaled smoke may also have burns on its face, lips, and mouth, as well as singed whiskers and hair. The cat may become unconscious, be hoarse, and have cherry-red membranes in its mouth, either from extreme heat or from inhaling carbon monoxide.

For smoke inhalation, give oxygen if it is safely available. Continue administering it for 30 to 45 minutes. This will help remove much of the carbon monoxide the cat has inhaled. If you think your cat has taken in much smoke, take it to a veterinarian as soon as possible. If you're not sure and are willing to wait and see, observe the cat carefully for 24 hours. Lung edema may occur that long after smoke is inhaled, with the cat making gurgling noises as it breathes, and appearing depressed and weak. Other signs of severe lung damage include aggressiveness or irritability, stumbling or incoordination, drowsiness, collapse, and convulsions.

The lungs can be so damaged that pneumonia follows. If this happens, the cat will show depression, fever, and lack of appetite, and may have trouble breathing. This can occur as much as a week or so after exposure to smoke. In either case, take the cat to a veterinarian as soon as possible.

LIGHTNING STRIKE

Cats are, on rare occasion, struck by lightning. The cat may be walking on a high ridge or may be standing next to a tree or fence which is hit by lightning. The cat that survives may be dazed and staggering or unable to stand. If the cat was wet, it may have burns on its body and on the soles of its feet. First aid consists of letting the cat rest and treating the burns. It may be necessary to clip off some of the hair in order to determine the extent of skin burns. If the feet are burned, bandage them for protection.

FROSTBITE AND HYPOTHERMIA

Hypothermia occurs when the core temperature of the body drops significantly below normal. It may occur accidentally from exposure to cold weather when the animal cannot get to shelter because it is unconscious, injured, caught in a trap, left outside by the owner, or unaccustomed to a new, cold climate. It also can occur when the cat is accidentally or deliberately locked in a freezer or refrigerator. A wet cat exposed to cold (or wind) can easily become hypothermic. It may occur at moderate temperatures if the animal has increased susceptibility to cold because it is elderly or ill. Injured cats can be at risk from hypothermia because of a combination of shock and decreased circulation, forced immobility, and damaged skin surfaces. Smaller animals are susceptible to hypothermia because they have a large surface area in relation to their body volume. Newborn or young kittens (and malnourished or elderly cats) may have smaller reserves of fat, glycogen, and muscle.

As hypothermia progresses, the body core temperature falls and metabolic processes slow. The skin and extremities are very susceptible to frostbite and freezing. Blood vessels in the skin contract in order to shunt blood to the internal organs. The heart rate and cardiac output decrease, and the pulse becomes weak. Urine output from the kidneys falls. Breathing becomes shallow and slow, and the cat may shiver. The cat may become mentally slow, and the pupils may be dilated. Any frozen skin or limb becomes bluish or pale, having little or no feeling. In the end, ventricular fibrillation occurs and the heart stops.

Mild hypothermia occurs when a cat's body temperature is 90-99 degrees F (32-37 C). This may be endured for 24 to 36 hours. Moderate hypothermia occurs at a body temperature of 82-90 degrees F (28-32 C). A cat may survive between four and 24 hours with this body temperature. Severe hypothermia occurs at a body temperature of 82 degrees F (28 C). The maximum survival time at this body temperature is five to six hours. It may be as little as one to two hours if the cat is ill or diseased (Dhupa, 1995).

Treatment begins by returning the core body temperature to normal. Shock must be treated, including giving oxygen. Bring the cat indoors and wrap it in blankets. This is sufficient treatment for a mild case of hypothermia. More severely chilled cats should be placed on hot water bottles (not TOO hot!), in a tub of warm (not HOT) water, or on an electric heating pad. It should be just slightly more than lukewarm. If the hot water bottle or heating pad is too hot, the cat's skin may slough. When a cat with moderate to severe hypothermia is rewarmed, there is a chance of an "after-drop" in the core temperature. First the skin warms up, then the core begins to warm. Take its temperature every 15 minutes for three to four hours to make sure it does not drop again.

Frostbite (cold injury) occurs when body tissue freezes. Frostbite can occur from exposure to cold or windy conditions, or contact with cold liquids, glass, or metal. A cat that licks an ax which has been used to cut meat is the classical example of this problem. Flood the area with lukewarm water to release the cat. Contact with dry ice or liquid nitrogen also can cause frostbite.

Cats are especially prone to freezing their footpads, usually from long-term contact with deep snow or cold surfaces. Frostbitten skin may turn gray, white, or reddish. It may be scaly and small areas may slough. Bring the cat into a warm area. Apply warm, moist towels, changing them often until the area becomes pinkish. Treat with any mild healing ointment. If there is any question about the extent of the damage, take the cat to a clinic for examination. Reduce or remove contact with the cold surface to allow it to fully heal.

Deeper tissues may be frozen if an animal is injured and unable to return home, or is caught in a trap where it cannot move around to keep warm. Damage can be quite severe. Prompt medical treatment may save large areas of tissue, and may make the difference between life and death. If your cat has deeply frozen tissue, DO NOT attempt to thaw it. Keep the frozen areas insulated so they stay frozen, and protect the frozen tissue so it is not injured in transit. Take the cat to a veterinarian as soon as possible. Tissue damage is increased if the frozen tissue is thawed and refrozen.

If you absolutely cannot take the cat to a veterinarian, do the best you can, and realize that the cat may die no matter what you do. This treatment should NOT be attempted if there is any chance you can take the cat to a hospital within six to eight hours. Thaw the frozen tissue rapidly. Use warm, not hot, water—100 to 112 degrees F (37.7-44.4 C). Do this only if you know that you can keep the tissues from refreezing. Otherwise, leave them frozen until they can be permanently thawed. Do not massage or rub the frozen tissues, and do not apply snow or ice to them!

The thawed part will become reddened and swollen. Blisters may occur on the skin. The cat often will attempt to scratch or chew them. It may be necessary to put an Elizabethan collar on the cat. Most veterinarians feel it is better to leave the lesions open than to cover them with dressings, bandages, or damp ointments.

Cats with severe frostbite will need systemic antibiotics to help prevent infection. It may take two to three weeks before it is clear which tissue is healthy and will live, and which is dead and should be removed or amputated. If at all possible, preserve the pads of the feet which have been frostbitten. The cat should have a high-calorie, high-protein diet, in addition to a vitamin supplement. This is especially true if the cat has been suffering from malnutrition, or has been in a trap or shut up in a building and has not had any food for some time.

Frostbite is rare in cats that are healthy, well-fed, and free to move. It is of utmost importance that cats that are kept outdoors in cold climates have enough food to produce sufficient heat to keep their body temperatures normal. Extra fat can be added to the diet if needed to provide enough calories. Be careful to increase the amount of fat in the diet gradually to avoid causing diarrhea. That would remove the benefit of the fat and lower the cat's resistance. Both frostbite and hypothermia are fairly uncommon in long-haired cats because of their protective coats. In general, cats instinctively seek shelter from extreme cold.

ALLERGIC REACTIONS

Allergic reactions may occur with insect bites such as wasp or bee stings. Exposure to other allergens may occasionally produce itching eyes, with tears running down the cat's face. The cat may sneeze and have difficulty breathing. Its face may be lumpy and swollen. In a severe case, the cat can collapse and become unconscious. If this happens, take the cat to your veterinarian as soon as possible. With a mild reaction, you can wait to see what happens—most of them will go away within two to 24 hours—or you can give an antihistamine (such as Benadryl®) for a mild reaction (for dosage see Snakebite, above). Do not use these drugs on kittens or pregnant cats without your veterinarian's approval.

CHOKING

Choking can result when the cat swallows a bone, toy, or piece of food which is too large. This occasionally happens when two cats are trying to eat together. One may wolf its food as fast as possible so the other does not get it. If there are large pieces of meat or bone, a fragment may lodge in the back of the mouth. The cat will make retching motions and paw violently at the side of its face. The problem comes on suddenly, with no previous signs of abnormality. One person can often relieve a cat that is choking. Push the lower jaw open and tilt the head back. USING EXTREME CAUTION, try to remove the object with your fingers. If this does not work, kneel behind the cat, and try a Heimlich Maneuver as you would in a human. Wrap your hands around the body just behind the ribs. Squeeze moderately hard a few times, pressing upward and inward. If the object does not come out, take the cat to a clinic immediately.

Do NOT attempt to relieve "choking" in a cat which has been acting peculiarly. Have the cat examined by a veterinarian. In rare cases, choking or gagging may be a sign of rabies. Don't take a chance with your life and those of family members.

FISH HOOKS AND PORCUPINE QUILLS

Cats are occasionally caught by fish hooks (does that make them "catfish?"). This is especially true if the cat tries to get a cheese ball or fishy-smelling bait off a hook, or is standing in the way of a child's wild cast. Or, it may be gaily chasing that tempting, moving lure on the end of the line. The cat will usually have the hook through its lip or tongue.

Or, the cat may step on a hook and catch it in its paw. If you are close to town, cut the line two to three inches from the hook. Take the cat to a veterinarian and let him or her sedate the cat and clip it out.

If you're not near a clinic, you'll need to take care of it yourself. Roll the cat in a towel to restrain it. If the hook is just barely into the skin, you may be able to pull it out the way it went in (backwards). If it is deeper, you will need to grit your teeth and push the barbed point on through the skin or tongue. If it looks like it will go through one of the large blood vessels on the underside of the tongue, DON'T try to take it out yourself—take the cat to a veterinarian. Those vessels bleed profusely.

After you have pushed the barbed end on through the cheek (or wherever), clip the eye end off with a pair of pliers. Now you can pull the hook through, continuing in the direction it went in. Dab the area with an antiseptic. Watch it for the next week or so to be sure there is no infection at the site. If infection does occur, take the cat to your veterinarian for antibiotic treatment. Be sure doors are closed or the cat is placed in a crate after this treatment, or it may leave the area in its pain.

Rarely, a cat will tangle with a porcupine and end up with one or more quills, usually in the face or paw. If there are only one or two quills, you can restrain the cat and pull them out with a pair of needle-nosed pliers. If there are many quills, take the cat to a veterinarian within 24 hours or so; don't worry about removing them. They look miserable, but as long as the cat is not rubbing against anything, they do not cause any pain. I know—I sat on one once, and it didn't hurt a bit until I slid in and out of my vehicle!

HOUSEHOLD HAZARDS

A cat can be crushed and killed when a sofa bed or recliner is closed. Be sure your cat is not sleeping inside before you shut it. A rocking chair can smash a cat's paw or tail. A cat can pull a hot iron off the ironing board and onto itself, which could cause a fire as well, if the iron falls onto the carpet or floor. Curling irons, electric rollers, and toasters can burn the cat if it touches them or drags them onto itself by getting caught in the cord.

Clothes dryers can be deadly. They are so attractive to cats—warm cozy places filled with lots of soft bedding. Your cat may crawl inside for a nap. Never close the dryer without checking for felines. Cats that are accidentally cycled in a dryer are usually a mess. The cat is thumped and tossed, so it usually has a concussion. Usually, the cat has bitten its tongue as its mouth opened and closed, so the face and coat are a bloody mess. The cat may be suffering from heat prostration. If it has not been in the dryer too long, it may recover. Take the cat to your veterinarian immediately. Don't let your cat get in the habit of sleeping in the dryer, even when it is cold. A cat also may be injured when it gets in a clothes washer.

A curious cat may stroll into an unused refrigerator or freezer, or it may be placed there by a child. While the cat may survive a short stay, a long internment can be fatal. A cat may hop into an open picnic cooler that is sitting on the kitchen or garage floor, and it may close

as it rocks when the cat gets in. A cat can be caught by a garage door as it comes down, and may be severely injured or even killed. Watch your cat until the garage door is completely closed.

Keep your cat away from the fireplace (even if it's not in use), and all heating units. Keep it off the kitchen counters. Besides being unsanitary, the cat could burn its feet if it strolls across a hot burner. A cat may jump onto a barbecue while seafood is being grilled, again burning its feet, or eat barbecue ashes soaked with meat grease. Don't leave a hot oven door open. The cat may be curious about this normally unavailable spot, and may not know it is hot until it jumps onto it. By the time the cat leaves, all four paws may be severely burned. If you want to vent the heat, open the door an inch or two. Keep the door closed while using oven cleaners because they may cause poisoning or chemical burns; the fumes may be harmful, too. If you have a wood stove, never allow the cat on it, even when it is cold. If the cat is accustomed to sitting on it in the summer, it may blithely hop onto the stove in winter while it is hot.

The bathroom contains hazards for cats. An unattended, filled bathtub may drown a small kitten that slips into it and is too small to climb out. The toilet also can drown a cat that falls in. Many of the chemicals used in cleaning the toilet or that are placed inside the toilet tank are toxic to cats. If you have an electric heater in the bathroom, make sure you don't leave bath mats, towels, or toilet paper where they will cause a fire if the cat pulls them down. Also, be sure the heater is not near a bath mat that might catch fire if your cat should spray urine into the heater. It can short out and catch the rug on fire.

Keep all medication tightly shut in the medicine cabinet with all lids on tight. Otherwise, a cat may help itself to the pills out of curiosity.

Plastic bags can be a hazard to the cat that sticks its neck through the handle, runs off, and gets caught on something. A cat that becomes wrapped or trapped in one may suffocate. Office supplies such as computer ribbons, correction fluid, mending tape, and small pieces of paper can be hazardous to cats. As with children, anything that is small enough to be swallowed or chewed can be a hazard.

Aluminum foil and plastic wrap can cause intestinal obstruction if eaten. The cat may fish these items out of the trash if they are soaked with meat juices or blood.

Christmas decorations can be hazardous to your cat. Eating tinsel may cause choking or an intestinal blockage as well as poisoning. Angel hair (spun glass) can irritate the cat's skin and is harmful if eaten. Ornaments with small pieces may come apart and cause choking or intestinal obstruction. Never put a yarn or ribbon around your cat's neck. It's fine to let your cat play in wrapping paper, but don't go away and leave it alone. Keep plastic six-pack can rings away from the cat.

Cats may chew on phone and appliance cords, especially when they are young and teething. One cure is to put some Bitter Apple on a cotton ball and rub it on the cord. The foul taste will keep many cats from chewing. Another solution is to buy a portable phone and put the base station in a cupboard, on top of the refrigerator, or in another location where the cat cannot reach it. Cats also may chew the air hose to an aquarium. This is not a hazard to the cat, but may be fatal to the fish. Try the Bitter Apple on it, too.

Batteries can be hazardous when chewed by cats. If the cat bites through the outer covering, chemicals inside can cause severe burns in the mouth. Store batteries where pets (and children) can't get them. The refrigerator is a good location, and they last longer, too. A button (disk) battery may be fatal if the cat swallows one and it stays in the stomach long enough to dissolve the outer covering.

The cat may use a tablecloth as a climbing post and be injured when it pulls a load of glassware onto its head.

Doors can be a hazard to your cat. A carelessly opened door can allow your indoor cat to escape. Once outdoors, it may panic and flee or hide, becoming lost or injured. Be sure that guests and workmen know the cat should not be let out, or place the cat in a secure place until they are gone. An open door easily can be slammed on a kitten. One of my own kittens followed me out the front door, unknown to me. It closed on the front leg, breaking one of the bones. The cat was successfully treated and recovered well, but if I had been watching, it wouldn't have had to go through the pain. Teach children and adults to watch for cats as they go through doors and screen doors.

Gas stoves may be turned on by an active cat. This could be fatal to you and the cat if it is done at night while you are sleeping. Your gas company may be able to recommend a shutoff valve or safety knobs.

A cat may be trapped accidentally in a shed, basement, closet, cupboard, dresser drawer, or other enclosure for a number of days without any food. A cat that has been seriously undernourished for a couple of weeks may have a low body temperature, and lower heart and breathing rates than normal. Especially if it is summer, dehydration may seriously complicate the problem. If the cat is able to eat and drink, start it on limited amounts of fluids. Give the cat water, or canned beef or chicken broth, a few sips at a time. Do not use bouillon cubes—they're too salty. Then start the cat eating small quantities of a high-quality canned cat food. Give two or three tablespoons every few hours for one or two days until the cat is obviously feeling better. Do NOT let the cat eat all it wants, as the stomach will be overloaded and the cat will vomit everything. If the cat is very weak or ill, it should be taken immediately to a clinic.

FAN BELTS

Getting caught in a fan belt or slashed by the fan blades of a vehicle engine is a truly horrible fate for a cat. At worst, the cat can be killed. At best, it's terribly frightened. In between are all sorts of mangling injuries. The cat may get up on a still-cooling engine to stay warm in cold weather. Or, it may be hiding there or in the wheel well because it is a cozy dark place. One of my friends lost a lovely bluepoint Siamese. The cat was sleeping under the hood on a winter day. The owner got in the car, started the engine, and drove thirty-five miles from her ranch to town. When she made her first stop, the cat ran from where it

had crouched, probably terrified, for the whole trip, and darted away. They never found the cat, which was sad because it was a really special cat.

Make sure your outdoor cat is accounted for before you drive away. Get in the habit of banging on the hood or fender of your car before you get into it. In winter, honk your horn and wait a few seconds before starting your engine. This will awaken your cat if it has gone to sleep on the still-warm engine and give it time to move before you start your car. Be sure your cat is not hiding under your vehicle. Your car may be a normal part of your cat's (or your neighbor's cat's) home territory. To a cat, it's no different from any other hiding place.

SKUNKED

If you live in the country or on a farm or ranch, your cat may be curious enough to check out a skunk. The skunk normally wins and the cat comes home smelling terrible. Begin care by thoroughly flushing the cat's eyes with lukewarm water. Then, apply a mild antibiotic eye ointment or a couple of drops of olive oil. This will help relieve any stinging in the eyes.

You can remove some of the odor from of the cat's coat by giving it a bath in tomato juice. Follow this by a bath in cat shampoo and water. You also can try a rinse of household ammonia diluted 1:10 or 1:20 in water. Be sure not to get this solution in the cat's eyes. These methods may not get rid of all the smell, but they will make it more tolerable. You also can try diluted lemon juice instead of tomato juice. A chemist developed a mixture that you can mix to remove skunk odor: 1 quart of 3% hydrogen peroxide, 1/4 cup baking soda (sodium bicarbonate), and 1 teaspoon dish detergent. Bathe the cat in the mixture, then rinse VERY thoroughly with water (Krebaum, 1993). A product called Skunk-Off® also will help to get rid of the odor—obtain it from your veterinarian, pet shop, or feed store. Believe it or not, the odor WILL wear off in time—if the cat does not contact another skunk!

HIGH-RISE SYNDROME (HRS)

Cats have the ability, when they fall or are dropped, to turn and land on their feet. This is not true if the cat is dropped head- or tail-first, but only when the feet are nearly horizontal. Blind cats cannot right themselves, but deaf cats usually can do so.

With more of our population living in apartments and high-rise housing, greater numbers of cats are affected by high-rise syndrome (HRS), a fall of two or more floors of 12 to 15 feet each. One of the first published reports, from New York City, discussed 132 cats in a five-month period that had jumped or fallen from an upper-story window or patio (Whitney, 1987). The cat may roll out of an unscreened window as it turns over in its sleep. It may be frightened or startled by something inside the room, or it may be tempted by a passing bird or insect. Veterinary hospitals in large cities may treat one or more of these each week.

Amazingly, cats live through falls as many as 24 stories. They have lived through even higher falls if the landing was in some way cushioned, such as a cat that fell onto a canopy from a twenty-eighth story window. Humans and dogs rarely live through falls of three or more floors. As many as 90-95% of cats that survive the first half-hour and receive medical attention will live.

When a cat falls, it instinctively turns in midair so that all four feet are pointing at the ground. The cat orients itself like a diver, pointing its front feet, followed by its nose. The cat remains tense until it reaches the maximum speed (terminal velocity, reached after it has fallen 60 feet). At this point, instinct somehow tells the cat that it needs to relax. This allows the final shock of the fall to be absorbed by the cat's whole body as it lands flat, like a pancake with legs sticking out to the sides.

Three main injuries are seen with HRS. The cat will usually have a bloody nose because its nose has hit the pavement. It also may be because fractured ribs have punctured a lung. The cat usually also has a split soft palate. It may have other fractures, including a broken lower jaw. The skin may be peeled off the lower jaw, and its canine teeth may be broken. These injuries look horrible, but usually heal well if treated immediately. If the cat is unconscious, you may have a couple of minutes to pull the skin back into place. The cat may have a compressed chest; if it is in severe respiratory distress, lay it on its side and gently give CPR. Be prepared for the cat to awaken angry.

The cat will need treatment for shock. Get the cat to a clinic immediately! It may be necessary to drain air and/or blood out of the chest several times in the first 24 hours after injury. The cat may need oxygen to ease its breathing. Most cats with HRS should have a chest X-ray, even if they are not having difficulty breathing, because chest injuries are so common. After its condition has stabilized, fractures and dislocations can be repaired. These are often compounded and can be complicated and expensive to fix. Cats whose hard palates have been split by the crash landing can often be treated conservatively, using antibiotics and a soft diet for three to four weeks. Fractured teeth may need to be removed.

You may not believe that your cat has fallen or jumped from the window when the superintendent brings it home. A bloody nose may lead you to suspect that it has been attacked by a dog, hit by a car, or poisoned. If you live more than two stories above the ground and your cat has a bloody nose, your FIRST thought should be HRS. Because the cat may have air in the chest cavity, it should NOT be anesthetized for the first 24 hours unless absolutely necessary.

To prevent HRS, install tightly secured screens in all windows. If you rarely have a window open other than to repair an air conditioner, the cat should be placed in a carrier while workmen are present. Or, put the cat in a bathroom or closet where it cannot accidentally escape.

Your cat doesn't have to fall out a high-rise window to escape and be injured. Window screens in a home can come loose. Wood framing dries and shrinks or the mesh loosens and the screen may pop off when a cat rolls or leans against it. The cat may leap at or through the screen when a bird flutters its wings nearby. It may attempt an impossible jump from a windowsill to a nearby tree limb.

This can lead to loss of your cat if it gets out and wanders away during the night. It can, of course, lead to more serious injury if you live in a high-rise building. Secure your window screens with sturdy latches, or drive a few nails around the outside of each screen to hold it tightly in place.

BANDAGES AND SPLINTS

A bandage is good first-aid until you can take your cat to the clinic. If you live in a remote area, it may be your only treatment. If at all possible, after you have given first-aid, take the cat to your veterinarian for further care.

Bandages are often essential to help stop bleeding. They also can keep a wound clean and free from dirt and contamination, and keep the cat from chewing and licking at the injury. In some cases, they can support weakened tissues so healing can occur more rapidly and efficiently. A bandage can help control edema and swelling that occurs after the circulation to a leg is damaged by a wound. A splint can immobilize a fractured leg, allowing it to heal.

Keep simple bandaging materials on hand in case your cat is injured. And, who knows, they might come in handy for you or a family member. Gauze sponges are useful; two by two and three by three-inch (5x5 and 7.5x7.5 cm) are convenient sizes. Non-stick pads are handy for use directly on open or bleeding wounds. Telfa Pads® (Curity/Colgate Palmolive) are one example. Plain, porous adhesive tape,

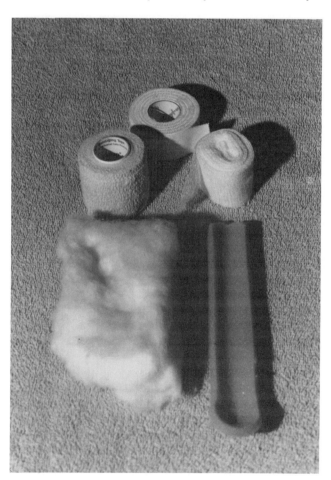

Bandaging materials: spoon splint, roll gauze, adhesive tape, Vetrap®, and cotton.

one-inch (2.5 cm) wide, is useful. Waterproof tape should not usually be used, as it may become damp underneath and become badly infected.

It also is useful to have an elastic bandaging material. Vetrap® (3-M) is a non-sticky elastic bandage often used on horses. It also is handy for cats. Co-Flex® (Andover Coated Products, Inc.) is a similar product. Pull eight or 10 inches off the roll before you lay it onto the leg; then it will not be applied under pressure as you wrap it around the limb. Otherwise, it is easy to wrap it too tightly. Be sure NOT to pull any elastic bandage too tightly. Feel the cat's toes from time to time to make sure they are warm. If the cat is light-colored, they should be pinkish rather than blue. If in doubt, take the bandage off and rewrap it. It's better to replace the bandage more often than to risk losing a foot or leg to gangrene caused by lack of circulation.

Plain roll gauze is sometimes useful; two-inch width is convenient. Roll cotton is used for some types of bandages, and can be purchased at the drugstore. Cotton is available in one-pound (1/2 kg) rolls. Do not place cotton directly on an open wound or a burn.

If your veterinarian has bandaged or splinted the leg, and the bandage comes off, take the cat back immediately. Don't wait until the next day; get it checked promptly. A slipping bandage or loose cast can cause severe damage in only a few hours.

BANDAGING A LEG

A bandage is used to stop bleeding and protect a wound on a leg. If you have to bandage a leg wound, be sure to wrap it all the way down, including the foot. This will keep the cat's foot from swelling below the bandage. Some blood may soak the bandage. Do not worry, as long as it is not actively dripping through. However, if it is dripping, wrap several extra layers of gauze or tape over it, tightening it very slightly.

If you are not going to have a cut sutured, you can wash it with chlorhexidine solution before bandaging. Moisten the hair around the edges of the wound with the solution. Lay a gauze sponge in the cut to keep hair out as you clip it. Clip the hair back from around the edges, about a half-inch on all sides. Then remove the hair-covered sponge and pick out any hairs which have fallen into the wound. Pat the wound out gently with a sponge moistened in the chlorhexidine solution. When the wound is clean, coat it with an antibiotic ointment such as gentamicin or bacitracin-neomycin-polymyxin. Do not do this if you are taking the cat to a clinic for treatment.

Put a non-stick gauze pad over the wound, to keep it clean and to avoid damage to its surface. Wrap the entire leg with roll gauze. Begin two or three inches above the injured area and wrap completely down around the toes, pulling the gauze snug but not tight. When you get to the

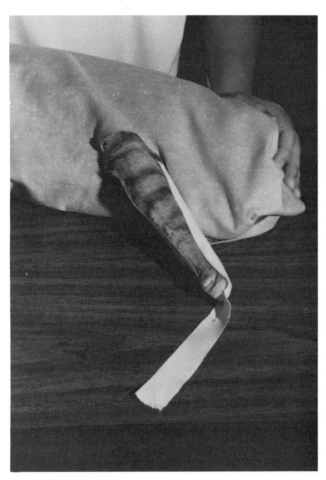

Tape on top and bottom of leg. Top piece is longer than lower one, so that some adhesive is left exposed.

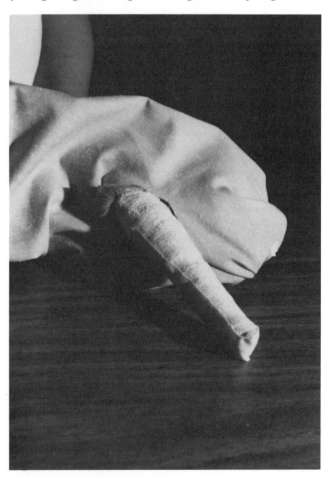

Wrap leg with gauze, at least two layers. Then, stick tape to the gauze on the back of the leg.

bottom (just beyond the toes), give the roll a half twist. The twist will help to get you turned around and headed back up the leg. Then wrap back up the leg to where you started. Using a roll of one-inch adhesive tape or flex bandage, begin wrapping tape about two inches ABOVE where the gauze ends. Starting above the gauze will help keep the bandage from falling off. Don't be afraid to wrap tape onto hair. It helps to keep the bandage in place, and avoids many problems. Wrap tape down over the gauze to the bottom of the foot. Tear the tape off the roll and pat the end down flat. Whether you are wrapping with gauze or tape, be sure to wrap in a spiral pattern rather than in circular rings. Otherwise, the rings may act as tourniquets and cut off circulation in the leg. Overlap each layer between one-third to one-half on the previous one.

Tear a half-dozen strips of tape six to 10 inches long, depending on the cat's size. Place the middle of each strip over the bottom of the toes, and smooth the ends upward on each side of the leg. Do one from front to back, one from side to side, and the others at angles in between. This will give a "bumper" or a "boot," which will protect the toes and help keep the bandage from wearing through.

Finally, begin taping again from the bottom just above the toe area, and wrap 'round and 'round as you did before, spiraling up the leg. Stop where you started the first wraps of tape above the gauze and your bandage is complete.

Most bandages should be changed every three to five days. Change it sooner if it becomes wet or soiled, or if the cat licks or chews enough to dampen it. A small amount of licking and chewing is to be expected. However, if the cat simply won't leave it alone, remove it and check for a problem. When you change the bandage, cut down the side opposite the injury. Use bandage scissors if you have them, or cut VERY carefully with regular scissors, being careful not to cut or poke into the skin. Split the bandage apart midway down the leg, where the tape runs over the gauze and it is easy to start separating it. Then, you can pull each half away from the other until the bandage is free. It may be helpful to cut the hair loose at the top. But cut the hair away from the tape rather than from the leg. Otherwise you will soon have a leg with no hair. You need the hair to protect the skin and to keep the bandage from falling off.

SPLINTING A FOOT

The cat that has broken a toe or a bone in the lower foot can be immobilized by a spoon splint or lightweight wood or plastic molded to the same shape. This type of splint is useful for emergency protection until you get to a veterinarian. Do not use it if you can take the cat to a clinic within six to eight hours.

The best splint for a foot injury is a metasplint or spoon splint, called that because it is shaped like a spoon. It

Put tape overall. Be careful not to get it too tight. Date it so you know when it was applied.

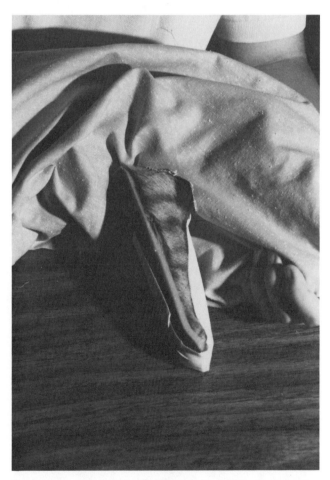

Put tape on foot as for simple leg bandage. Pad the leg with cotton. Place in splint.

allows room for the cat's pads, and avoids the pressure that may occur with a flat piece of wood or plastic. Pad the splint carefully with cotton batting, torn so that it is one continuous, flat sheet. The cotton can extend a half-inch or so beyond the edges of the splint so the sharp edges do not gouge the cat's leg.

Put a small puff of cotton between each pair of toes to keep them apart and to keep moisture from causing sores between them. Don't forget the dewclaw. Put a piece of tape down the bottom side of the cat's leg, sticking it well to the hair. This piece of tape should extend about four inches (10 cm) beyond the cat's toes. Do the same with a piece on top of the cat's leg. The top piece should extend about a foot beyond the cat's toes. Stick the end of the bottom piece to the top piece. Putting the two pieces together will leave a sticky area on the top piece hanging free. This sticky area is of utmost importance in keeping the splint from sliding off the cat's leg. Then dust the cat's hair with boric acid powder or talcum (not cornstarch!) powder as high as you are going to put the bandage. Fluff it well into the hair, especially between the toes.

Wrap the cat's leg with gauze, applied gently. DO NOT pull it too tightly! Two or three layers of gauze are about right. Put one or two thin layers of cotton around the cat's leg. Lay the cat's foot in the splint. Next, pull the tape down and stick the sticky area to the bottom (back) of the splint. Tape over the entire splint, foot and leg, exactly as de-

scribed above for bandaging the foot. Use porous adhesive tape rather than the waterproof kind. Write the date you applied it on the bandage.

For a broken toe, about three weeks in the splint are sufficient. For other broken bones in the foot, four or five weeks may be better. In general, younger animals need to be splinted for less time than do mature ones.

Any splint or bandage must be kept clean and dry. Keep the cat indoors. If you have to put it outside in the morning while there is still dew on the grass, put a plastic bag over the splint. Secure the bag with tape or a rubber band. Let the cat out just long enough to urinate and defecate. Bring it back inside and remove the bag. Also use a bag if it is raining or if there is snow outside. Do not bathe the cat until it is completely healed. If the cat gets wet, the bandage must be changed as soon as possible to prevent infection from developing underneath it.

If the cat licks the bandage, use Bitter Apple spray. This stops some cats but not all of them. Other cats respond well to a very light coating of petroleum jelly, liberally sprinkled with cayenne pepper. Variton Creme® (Schering) keeps many cats from licking bandages. Put a very light coating of it on areas the cat can reach. A product called Ro-Pel® is available (Burlington Bio-Medical, Farmingdale, NY). It is extremely bitter, and is useful to keep a cat from licking.

However, licking may be a sign that the bandage is too tight, or that there is infection underneath. If it has been

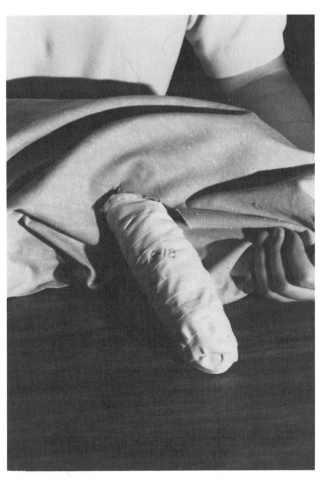

Tape over splint and leg together.

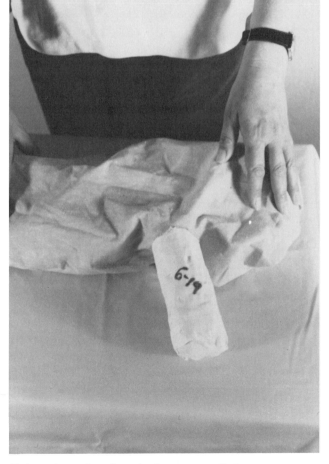

Robert Jones bandage (soft cast or splint).

several days since you have changed the bandage, change it, looking for a problem. If you don't find a problem, and the new bandage is comfortable, then put on the bad-tasting stuff.

SPLINTING THE FRONT LEG

For a front leg, a straight piece of wood, split lengthwise to make a splint, will work well. It should be slightly narrower than the width of the leg, and can be put either on the inside or the outside of the leg. If there is a cut or wound, put the splint on the opposite side. Pad the splint well with cotton. Use clean, soft rags if you have nothing else to use for padding. Be sure to carefully restrain the cat before you begin.

Pull the leg gently to the point where it is nearly straight. Wrap the leg well with cotton batting. If you do not have that, use cloth or blanket material, making it about one-half inch thick. This wrapping should be barely snug, NOT tight, and as smoothly wrapped as possible. Lay the leg on the splint, and wrap snugly over both splint and wrapped leg using gauze if you have it. Wrap a layer or two of adhesive tape over this. If at all possible, use a porous tape, or a product such as Vetrap®. If worse comes to worst, use duct tape or any other tape that is handy. Now that the leg is immobilized, take the cat to the veterinarian. If you can take the cat to a veterinarian within six to eight hours after its injury, don't put it through the pain of splinting the leg. Just keep the cat confined and quiet and get it to the clinic.

SPLINTING THE HIND LEG

To make a splint for the hind leg, use one-fourth-inch plywood. Or, you can use stiff flat plastic or cardboard for an emergency splint. Lay the cat on its side, with the good leg DOWN. Put the plywood on the floor under the good leg and trace around it (it hurts less, and you can move it as needed). Cut about one-half inch (12 mm) inside the lines you have drawn, all the way around. The splint should be smaller than the leg so that the leg will not slide around on it. It should, however, be about one-half inch longer than the leg so that the toes do not touch the ground.

Pad the splint with cotton. Wrap the leg in thin sheets of roll cotton (about half the thickness of the sheet—it usually splits easily), 'round and 'round until you have a padding about a half-inch thick. Put the leg in the best position you can. Put the splint on the outside of the leg, and tape it snugly to the splint with porous adhesive tape, as described above. The leg will shrink with lack of use, and the splint may loosen. It may be necessary to replace it. If the splint has been on for three weeks or so, it is a good idea to unwrap the leg and apply fresh bandage material. As a rule of thumb for any broken bone, immobilize AT LEAST the joint ABOVE and the joint BELOW the break.

ROBERT JONES BANDAGE

The Robert Jones bandage is a thick, bulky bandage made with roll cotton. It can be used to stabilize fractures or dislocations which occur at or below the stifle and elbow joints. It puts enough pressure on the area to prevent soft-tissue swelling, helping to control pain. It also is useful as first aid for fractures, and it may be handier than a solid splint if you do not have wood or plastic material handy. Since it is bulky and porous, it can absorb considerable quantities of moisture if the cat gets into dew or water. It takes about one-half pound (1/4 kg) of roll cotton to make the bandage. Unroll a one-pound roll of cotton. As you reroll, tear it up the middle, leaving right and left halves. The six-inch-wide cotton strips are much easier to handle than the 12-inch roll.

If there is a cut or wound, it should be cleaned with chlorhexidine solution and covered with an antibiotic ointment and a non-absorbent dressing. Put tape on the top and bottom of the leg (see Splinting the Foot, above). Lightly bandage over the wound with gauze and tape. Make sure the bandaging is not too tightly applied.

Begin wrapping with one of the cotton strips at the foot and wrap upward. Leave the cat's two longest toes exposed. If the nails are not colored and you notice that they are turning purple, the bandage is too tight. If the toes are cold, or if the cat licks its toes, the bandage may be too tight or there may be infection underneath. Wrap the cotton up the leg, pulling it evenly snug. Wrap it as far upward as you can, either into the armpit or the groin. Wrap a layer of gauze over this, again working from toes to top. Pull the gauze snug. For this type of bandage, gauze four inches wide (10 cm) works better than narrower sizes. Stop the gauze about one inch (2.5 cm) short of the top of the cotton. This will leave a comfortable cushion of cotton at the top, and it will keep the gauze from sliding over the top of the bandage and cutting into the cat's skin. Then, stick the first two pieces of tape that you applied to the back side of the gauze. This will help keep the bandage from sliding. Put a layer of tape over the entire bandage, again wrapping from bottom to top. You can use either porous adhesive tape or an elastic product such as Vetrap® (3-M) or Elastikon® (Johnson & Johnson).

The bandage is easily removed by carefully slitting the outer tape with a sharp blade. You can then pull the layers of cotton apart, or unroll them. If you are putting on a fresh bandage, leave the first two pieces of tape in place. Just cut it off at the toes, and put new pieces of tape over the top of it to make new stirrups to hold the new bandage in place. This will avoid the irritation of removing the tape and putting new tape on the irritated skin.

Any bandage may rub at the groin or armpit area. It may be necessary to cut a notch in the bandage material to leave room for the cat to move its leg. It also may be useful to dust the cat's skin at the top of the bandage (in the armpit or groin) once or twice a day with baking soda, talcum powder, or medicated (not cornstarch!) powder.

In an emergency, a Robert Jones bandage can be made from layers of blanket, towel, or sleeping bag material. Several layers of material can be laid all over the leg until it reaches about two inches (5 cm) thick. Then, it can be wrapped overall with gauze and tape. Pull the tape fairly snugly, but not so tight that blood circulation is cut off. This type of bandage will give the cat nearly as much protection as would a solid splint.

BANDAGING THE HEAD AND NECK

It may be necessary to bandage the cat's head if it has a hematoma on one or both ears. It is important not to make a head bandage too tight. The lower half of the bandage forms a collar as it encircles the throat, and you should be able to slip two fingers under each side of it. If the bandage is too tight, the cat can have trouble breathing or swallowing. You can slit whichever edge of the collar is tight, cutting one or more slits until you have relieved the discomfort. Then you can lay tape over the cut areas to reinforce them. This procedure will eliminate the necessity of redoing the entire bandage.

If a head bandage slips, it usually will slide to the rear. If this happens, the cat may have trouble breathing. Remove the bandage immediately and try again. The cat may scratch at the bandage with its hind legs, trying to remove it. If this happens, it may be necessary to put an Elizabethan collar on the cat.

BANDAGING THE CHEST AND ABDOMEN

A chest bandage may be necessary if the cat has a penetrating wound, or has damage to the skin in the chest area. The main thing is to avoid wrapping the bandage too tightly. Otherwise, the cat may not be able to breathe adequately. As with a head or neck bandage, you should easily be able to slip two fingers under either edge of it. If you are using elastic tape, be sure to pull it off the roll and lay it on WITHOUT tension. If the cat has trouble breathing, take the bandage off immediately. A chest bandage slips quite easily. To anchor it, the bandage should be stuck to the hair for one to one-and-a-half inches (5-8 cm) at both the front and rear. Again, an Elizabethan collar may be needed to keep the cat from scratching at it.

Bandages on the abdomen should be secured to the hair much the same as those on the chest. The abdomen should not be bandaged too tightly, although it may have a slightly more snug bandage than the chest.

ELIZABETHAN COLLAR

An Elizabethan collar is used to keep a cat from licking at a bandage or splint. Or it may be used to keep a cat from licking at an open wound or skin infection. Ready-made Elizabethan collars are available in several sizes, depending on the size of the cat. The collar must be large enough to go around the cat's neck and meet on the other side, and must extend outward far enough to keep it from reaching around the edge and chewing, licking, or scratching with a hind leg. After the collar is put on the cat's neck and snapped or laced together, it may be tied to the cat's collar or harness with pieces of gauze or scraps of nylon cord. This will keep the cat from rubbing or pawing it off over its head.

If you don't have a ready-made Elizabethan collar, your cat can be a "carton-head." A plastic carton works just as well as an Elizabethan collar. Buy a soft plastic refrigerator carton or a very lightweight, thin, shallow bowl. Get one that is two or three inches deeper than the distance from where the back of the cat's neck meets its shoulders to the end of its nose. Cut a hole in the bottom of the carton. Don't make the hole too large; you want to PUSH it to get it over the widest part of the cat's head. Then it will be loose enough for the cat's neck. Cut a small hole and try it and, if necessary, cut and try until it barely fits on over the cat's head. When you have the hole the right size, punch two holes through the bottom on each side. These will be used for gauze or cord to tie the bowl to the cat's collar. The base of the bowl will be at the cat's collar, and the open end will be toward its nose. The cat is generally able to eat and drink by putting its head down over the dishes. At first, it will stagger around and bump and into everything. Ignore the cat's initial discomfort. It soon will learn to navigate quite well with the bowl. Bowls also work well on some cats that can get around the Elizabethan collar.

You can also cut an Elizabethan collar from a piece of stiff cardboard. Make the outside diameter about three times the width of the cat's head. Cut a small hole in the center for the cat's neck, beginning with one about two inches in diameter. It should be just barely larger than the cat's neck—and that isn't very large! Then make a slit from the center to the outside so that you can try it over the cat's neck. Enlarge the opening to fit, put it on the cat, and tape the slit together to secure it.

Be sure the cat's nails are trimmed so that if it gets a foot past the collar, it can't scratch at the skin, eye, or ear you are trying to protect.

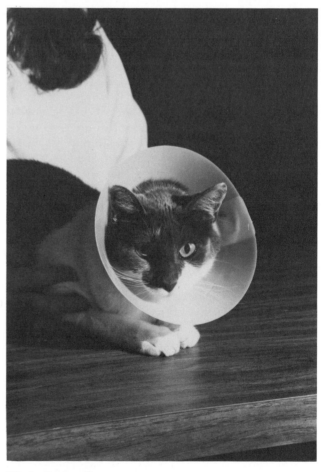

Elizabethan collar.

Chapter 10

GROOMING AND SKIN DISEASES

A FUR COAT

Short hair is genetically dominant in domestic cats, inherited from their African ancestors. Long hair seems to have been selectively bred by humans. A few cats have mutated (then were perpetuated by selective breeding) to relative hairlessness, having only whiskers and a few scattered hairs on their bodies. Their skin feels soft and leathery.

Calico cats are white cats blotched with black and orange. The combination also may be black, cream, and red, or chocolate, lilac, or blue with red and cream. Calicos of all colors are normally female. Male calicos are occasionally seen. No, they're not valuable (there seem to be rumors they're worth a million dollars!); they're just rare. Tortoise-shell cats are a basically black (or blue, brown, or lilac) cat with patches of cream and red; nearly all of them are female, too. Most male cats with the red or orange coloration in these patterns are sterile.

Cats whose coats contain red pigment, such as red tabbies (striped cats), some tortoise-shell cats, and some calicos with orange, often will develop red or brown spots on their skin as they mature. The spots are seen on the lips, eyelids, nose, and ears, and are flat rather than raised like a skin mole. They look like freckles and grow larger as the cat ages. They are normal.

White cats may turn yellowish or dingy as they age. This may be due to staining with urine, blood, tears, saliva, or protein wasting. The use of hydrogen peroxide also may cause the cat's fur to yellow. The yellowing is not removed by shampooing. Have the cat checked by your veterinarian to determine what is causing the color change, as it might be due to a systemic problem.

When the hair is damaged or clipped on a Siamese cat or cat of related breeding, it sometimes grows back a different color, either much lighter or much darker than the surrounding hair. In some cases, the regrowth may be pure white. Some of these cats return to a normal color the next time they shed, while others retain the new color spot for life. If your cat is a show cat and is going to have surgery or has an abscess or skin wound treated, be sure to tell your veterinarian so he or she can clip as little hair as possible.

Some Siamese cats have a hereditary hair loss problem. The kittens are born with a soft downy fur, which they lose several weeks after they are born, ending up almost bald. The Sphynx (Sphinx) breed of cats are bred to be hairless. In either case, the cat is completely lacking in hair follicles, and will be bald for life. There is no treatment that will bring them back.

Some cats appear to have a thinner hair coat between the ear and the eye. It will look the same on both sides. This is because the hair in this area is short and grows directly outward, allowing you to look straight down to the skin. While the cat is shedding, it may nearly bald in this area, and a Siamese may lose most of the color on its face. This is normal for many cats, and is not a problem.

Siamese cats may lose pigment from the foot pads and the leathery end of the nose. This may turn your cat's nose from brown or black to bright pink! The pigment loss seems to occur when the cat matures, around nine to 12 months of age. It may be related to a hereditary white spotting factor in the breed. The cat is not ill, but there is no way to return the original color.

Cats that have been grossly obese (over 20 pounds) and later lose weight may have hanging folds of skin. Those in the anal and genital areas may hold urine and feces. Sores, eczema, and urine scalding may occur, as well as continuing bladder infections. Your veterinarian can take "tucks" to remove this extra skin to make the cat more comfortable and healthier. Be sure the cat stays at a normal weight for the rest of its life.

Because the skin is out and exposed to everyday view, it's usually easy to determine when your cat has a skin problem. Unfortunately, diagnosis of exactly WHAT the problem is may be very difficult. The skin has only a limited number of ways to respond to insult or injury. For this reason, a host of ailments will show the same outward symptoms. The cat may lose hair or itch. It may show crusting or draining sores, tracts (deep, narrow, infected areas below the skin surface) or ulcers, or it may have nodules on or in the skin. Incidentally, itching may also be caused by kidney or liver diseases and mast cell tumors.

Diagnostic tests may be necessary, including skin scrapings, biopsy, culture, and blood tests. In some cases the only solution is to try a number of treatments until one is found that works. Do not hesitate to ask for a referral to a veterinary dermatologist (skin specialist) if your cat's problem is not cured within a reasonable length of time. They are found at veterinary colleges and in larger cities. In a few cases of skin disease, a cause is never found.

Some cats with skin problems will itch severely. Excessive licking and grooming may show that the cat is itching, not that it thinks it is that dirty. If you scold the cat every time it scratches or grooms excessively, you will only train the cat to hide when it wants to scratch. Occasionally, a cat shows severe itching, but careful veterinary examination detects no disease or infection. These animals may benefit from oral antihistamines, such as chlorpheniramine maleate. This also may help some cats that lick excessively or seem to itch for no apparent reason. Chlorpheniramine is quite effective to stop itching after fleas, food allergies, and other treatable problems are ruled out. It has few side effects other than occasional drowsiness, which usually goes away after a few days. The drug can be used for long term treatment (one to two years), if necessary (Miller, 1990). This is in contrast to treating itching with corticosteroids, which often have long-term or fatal side effects.

Occasionally, a cat will scratch or rub a sore at the base of one or both ears. In many cases, this is due to an infection in the ear or ear mites. The cat is just scratching as close to the itch as it can get. So, it is an ear problem, not a skin problem. Similar sores may be seen with fleas.

Most skin ointments do not work well on cats, as the animals just lick them off. At worst, they may be harmful to the cat. Ointments containing gentamicin may be absorbed through a skin cut or abrasion, or licked in sufficient quantity to cause kidney failure. The cat also may cause further damage to the problem area as it scrubs with its tongue. Dips, pills, or injections usually must be used to directly attack the cause of a skin problem. In general, if a skin problem is moist and weeping, treatment will be aimed at drying it. If it is dry and cracking, it is appropriate to soften and soothe it.

GROOMING AND SKIN CARE

Two cats that live comfortably together may groom each other. This is especially true of the neck, where it is difficult for the cat to clean itself. Occasionally, one cat gets into the habit of chewing off the other cat's whiskers while washing. This is not harmful. Cats probably perceive human petting as a form of grooming, and learn to accept and enjoy it.

A short-haired cat requires very little care for its skin and coat. It uses its teeth to comb through the coat, and washes it by licking. A brief brushing with a soft bristled brush or a rubber dog curry comb every day or two will help with grooming and is all the cat should need. This combing will remove dead fur without causing skin irritation. After the brushing, stroke the cat's fur with a piece of velvet, silk, or chamois cloth for extra shine. The cat's whiskers are part of its sensory apparatus and should never be trimmed or cut.

While a few long-haired cats never get mats, most of them cannot groom themselves adequately. There is simply too much hair. Matting is especially a problem on the back of the hind legs, under the belly, on top of the rump and behind the neck and ears—areas the cat cannot reach. Matting is also a problem with cats that are overweight or arthritic, thus physically unable to groom themselves.

Grooming also removes twigs, burrs, and other material caught in the coat of a long-haired cat that lives outdoors. When grass seeds (foxtails, foxtail barley, or cheat grass) mature, their awns can catch deep in the cat's fur, next to its skin; they can work inward, causing irritation and infection. Remove them by working carefully through the coat with your fingers or a wire brush. Don't leave these materials in the coat for very long. They can form the nucleus for a large mat of hair, which probably will have to be cut out. If you live in a rural area where this is a serious problem, you may want to use electric clippers to remove all the hair on the cat's feet—top, bottom, and between the toes. This will allow the awns to fall out rather than poke into the skin. If a grass awn does puncture the skin, it may become infected and form an abscess. Carefully remove the seed with tweezers, and swab the puncture hole with tincture of iodine. Regular cotton swabs may be too large; make a tiny one by wrapping a few fine strands of cotton around a flat toothpick or broom straw.

A long-haired cat should be brushed or combed daily to help prevent matting and remove loose hair. This also helps remove the scurf or dandruff that occurs as particles of skin die and are shed into the hair. Put a towel on your lap and start gently working through the cat's coat. Two tools are helpful for long-haired cats: Use a large metal comb for the body and a smaller metal "flea" comb for the feet. Some people prefer a hairbrush with knobbed tips to avoid scratching the cat's skin. You can use a wire brush to remove the dead hair. Pay special attention to the cat's rump because it usually has a lot of dead hair. A soft toothbrush works well on the cat's head and face. Don't yank the brush through the cat's hair; use your hands to separate the hair and work carefully through it. It also is helpful to begin at the ends of the hair, working inward toward the skin.

If you acquire the cat as a kitten, it is a perfect time to begin grooming. By making it a part of the regular time you spend with your pet, it will learn to enjoy it. The cat may even fall asleep as you comb. Let the cat smell the grooming tools before you begin. Move slowly and gently so you don't scare the cat. If your combing accidentally hurts the cat, it may hiss, bite, or scratch, and probably will try to get away. Stop combing for a moment, but never let the cat jump down from your lap. If you let the cat's ill behavior scare you, soon you will not be able to get near the cat with a comb. Just wait a moment and start combing again.

The skin on the belly, under the legs, and on the backs of the hind legs is very sensitive. Work slowly and gently in those areas. Because of their need for help with grooming, long-haired cats do not make good barn cats unless you are willing to help them with their coats. If the cat's coat is especially hard to comb, your veterinarian or groomer can provide a spray to help untangle it. Corn starch also may help with a tangled coat. Keep it away from the cat's eyes and ears.

It often helps to give the cat a treat after you finish grooming. Some owners even comb the cat while it is eating. Simply kneel on the floor beside the cat and begin combing. This also may teach your cat to tolerate being combed—just comb for a minute or two the first day. Gradually increase the time until you can completely comb the cat while it eats dinner. Don't try to groom the cat when it is hungry. It will be distracted and may associate grooming with an unpleasant wait for food. Other owners wrap the cat in a towel and straddle it. This is a desperation measure which doesn't encourage the cat to enjoy being groomed! You also can put a collar or harness on the cat and attach it with a short piece of light chain to a ring on the wall behind a table, or to a rod extending a couple of feet over the table. You can even use a turntable made for grooming toy show dogs. No matter how many tantrums the cat throws, try not to lose your temper. Deal with the cat calmly, quietly, and firmly. With time, the cat will be trained to accept this operation.

If a long-haired cat is not groomed frequently over a period of several months, it will develop tight wads or mats of hair in its coat. If you are willing to pick away at them, beginning at the outside, you can eventually comb them out without too much hair loss. Or, soak the matted hair all the way to the skin with a dematting product. Allow it to nearly dry. Then, carefully pick and comb out the mat. Or, the mat can be split with a knife (be careful not to cut the cat), then combed out. If you don't want to go to that much trouble, just cut out the entire mat. Electric clippers work well. Ease the clipper head down, under each mat, cutting it gently away from the skin. Or, you can use scissors, carefully sliding them under a mat and cutting perhaps a quarter-inch of its attachment away from the skin with each bite. Do this very slowly and cautiously, as it is easy to cut the cat's skin, especially with an old mat that is closely attached. Be sure not to cut off the cat's whiskers or the long hairs above its eyes.

If the cat has many mats and you can't remove them, there are two choices. You can take the cat to a groomer and let him or her cope with the problem. Or, you can take the cat to your veterinarian. Chances are good the cat will have to be sedated or anesthetized. However, this will allow your veterinarian to do a thorough job of combing out what is possible to comb and clipping out the rest. You will likely end up with a happier cat because it has been sedated. No matter which way you go, you'll probably have a cat that looks like a high-low shag carpet. Just remember that the difference between a good haircut and a bad haircut is three weeks . . .

There is yet another alternative for someone who doesn't want to constantly groom a long-haired cat. It is also a good choice for areas that are hot and/or humid in summer. Have a groomer or veterinarian give the cat a close, all-over clip at the beginning of summer. Or, the cat can be clipped in a "lion shave" which removes fur except on the head, feet, and tail. Either way, the cat doesn't have the misery of wearing a fur coat that it can't unzip and hang in the closet. By winter, it's grown out again—fresh, clean, and comfortable. Don't do this with a cat that you want to show, as a regrown coat may not be perfect for show standards. An occasional cat may be self-conscious for a few days, but if you interact with the cat as you normally do, and don't laugh, it quickly will appreciate the new-found comfort.

Cats that do their own grooming may have hairballs. They occur when the cat swallows hair it has licked from its coat. The hair irritates the stomach until the cat vomits. Hairballs are usually a sign that the cat needs more help with its grooming—brush the cat often and the problem usually will go away (see Digestive System Chapter).

EXCESS SHEDDING

Occasionally, a cat may seem to shed excessively. If you pull on its hair, a large amount comes out, and you may even be able to pull out enough to make a bald spot. This may be due to illness, high fever, or the stress of pregnancy or nursing a litter of kittens. With some indoor cats, constant shedding is due to bright lighting. It may be lessened if you can cut down the number of hours of light to which the cat is exposed to each day.

A shedding cat should be groomed daily. This will keep the extra fur from landing all over your clothing, carpet, and furniture. It will also help to keep hairballs from forming in the cat's stomach as it tries to groom itself.

There is no treatment for cats that shed excessively and are otherwise normal. The cat usually will regain a normal coat in a couple of months. If the shedding is due to illness, skin allergy, parasites, hormone imbalance, fever, or pregnancy, it will stop and the hair will regrow when the cat is again healthy.

BATHING

Most cats don't need baths if they are brushed regularly. Too many baths cause far more problems than too few. If your cat has dry, itchy skin and a scaly coat, try bathing it less often and see if it clears up. Bathe the cat if it is dirty, smells badly, or has parasites in its coat.

A cat may need a bath when it has come in contact with a foreign substance such as grease or road tar. It is especially important to remove petroleum products or paint from a cat's coat. Otherwise, the cat may become ill when it tries to lick the material from its fur. Leaving the material on the coat can cause severe irritation and damage the skin.

If the cat has grease, oil, gum, or tree sap in its coat, pre-treat it by rubbing mineral oil or vegetable oil into the spots before bathing. Or, use a mink oil coat conditioner if you have some handy. Work it in, teasing it gently through the hair with a wire slicker brush or stiff nylon-bristled brush. Then, work in a SMALL amount of watered-down liquid dishwashing detergent. Do this BEFORE you put water on the cat, rubbing the soap into the oil. Be careful when using dishwashing liquid on kittens, as it may be toxic to them. Continue with the bath, lathering well with dishwashing liquid. Be sure to rinse thoroughly so that no soap is left in the cat's coat, or it may become ill when it grooms itself after the bath. Do NOT use paint remover or thinner or other petroleum-based product to remove the grease. They can irritate the skin and poison the cat. After all this washing, the cat may be left with little or no natural oils in its coat, and may benefit from a spritz of an oil-based coat conditioner. Another alternative is to simply clip out the tar or grease spots before the bath, then wash the cat with cat shampoo.

If your cat is very muddy, it may easier to delay bathing. Put the cat in a warm, safe place to dry (such as the bathroom with the heat turned up). After the cat is dry, gently comb out the mud. After brushing, the bath may be unnecessary.

An ideal soap or shampoo should lather well, rinse out easily without leaving a residue in the coat, and remove debris and dirt without removing too much of the natural oils. It should not irritate the skin or eyes. Irritation from shampoo may result from depletion of the natural skin oils, excessive softening of the skin surface, or the mechanical effect of the foam. Some cats may be sensitive to shampoo ingredients. Some shampoos contain soaps that form an insoluble curd in hard water ("bathtub ring") that remains on the cat's coat. This residue will leave the hair dull and tacky-feeling. A final rinse with water to which a little vinegar or lemon juice has been added will help remove the residue or film on the hair. Or, try a different shampoo. It is especially important to rinse the cat well to completely remove any shampoo.

Most shampoos contain detergents, which do not leave a film in hard water, but tend to strip more of the natural oils from the cat's skin and coat. Many detergent-based shampoos have oils, such as lanolin, added to help replace oils lost in shampooing. These oils lubricate the hair, leaving it shinier and easier to comb.

Be sure to use a shampoo made specifically for cats. A product made for dogs may not be safe for cats unless the label says it can be used on both animals. Human shampoos are much too drying for cats, and may contain ingredients irritating to the cat's skin. They may leave the cat itching and scratching, and may start skin problems. Even "baby" shampoo is not good for use on cats. They are much the same as others used by humans except that the pH is balanced to avoid burning the eyes. This still doesn't make them right for the cat's skin, and they cause dandruff in some cats. Cats are far more sensitive to certain chemicals than are dogs. They also lick vigorously at the hair coat, thus ingesting any product put on the hair or skin.

Hair conditioners similar to those sold for people are available for cats. They add shine and body to the hair. They help to reduce static electricity, which can make a long-haired cat's coat snarl and "flyaway." The conditioner may be slightly acidic to help remove any hard water film that remains on the hair. Protein conditioners leave a layer of protein on the hair, giving it more body and shine.

Fatty or oily conditioners put a fine film of oil on the hair, giving body and shine, and making it easy to comb. They contain essential fatty acids and products such as sesame oil. Oily conditioners are sprayed on the coat while it is still damp after the bath, or they may be added to the final rinse water. They will cause the coat to lie flat, and should not be used if you want the coat to fluff. Sesame oil rinse products can be used on cats with dry skin. An after-bath sesame oil spray is available (Sesame Oil Emulsion Spray®, Veterinary Prescription). Examples of moisturizing conditioners available for veterinary use include Hylyt EFA® (DVM) and Humilac® (Allerderm). These products come in handy pump sprayers for use between baths. If your cat's coat is dry, make sure it is getting plenty of fat and fatty acids in its diet (see Feline Gourmet Chapter).

How do you bathe a cat? It all depends on the cat. Some cats can be washed easily in the kitchen sink and rinsed with the spray attachment if they become accustomed to it gradually and gently. Bathing a cat at this height is easier on your back than stooping over a tub. The cat also may be more comfortable at sink height than when you are towering over it in the tub. Washing the cat in the sink can be quick and convenient. Fill the sink halfway with water and put a rubber mat or towel in the bottom to keep the cat from slipping. Have a rag or washcloth handy for washing the cat's face and make sure shampoo, flea products, or conditioners are within easy reach. If your sink does not have a hose or the cat will not tolerate its use, a plastic tumbler is handy for scooping rinse water over the cat. Some cats are bathed easily by putting them BESIDE the pan of shampoo/water mixture and using a sponge or rag to pour the water over the cat. Do the same with the rinse water.

For safety's sake, always keep the cat facing away from you, and keep all objects out of its way. Put the cat in the water at one time. Encourage the cat to lie down in the water by putting a soft pressure on its back. Use one hand to hold the cat, and the other to wet the hair, rub in shampoo, and rinse.

Bathing some cats is a major project in the bathtub, just short of a world war. For the worst ones, it's sometimes easiest to just take off your clothes, get in with the cat, shut the shower doors behind you, and go to work. It is necessary to balance the probability that you will get soaked if you don't undress against the possibility of scratches if you do. In any case, be sure to clip short all of the cat's toenails before starting the bath project. Close all doors and windows in the room where you bathe the cat and where it will dry. This is for two reasons: to prevent escape and to keep drafts from chilling the cat while it is damp.

Be sure you have removed as much dead hair as possible before beginning the bath. Comb and brush the cat thoroughly, and then cut out any mats. If you leave mats, fleas and other parasites may remain underneath. Mats also may keep the area from being dampened, but if water does get underneath, the mats will not dry and may cause an acute moist dermatitis.

Prepare everything before you begin, including towels to dry the cat, a hair dryer if needed, and shampoo and conditioner. When you bathe the cat, prepare to get wet and/or dirty. Put on old clothes and get ready for the mess. If you are using medicated or insecticidal shampoo, you may wish to use rubber or plastic gloves to protect yourself.

It is important to protect the cat's eyes before bathing, especially if the cat is rarely bathed. Put a dab of petroleum jelly, a couple of drops of mineral oil, or a one-fourth inch strip of eye ointment (obtained from your veterinarian) in the eyes just before you begin. Blink each eye open and shut a couple of times to spread the film over the eye. This is especially important if you are using a medicated or insecticidal shampoo. If you bathe the cat frequently and it cooperates while you carefully wipe its face with a washcloth, it is unnecessary to put protective material in the eyes. However, be very careful not to get any shampoo or dip into them. Oily protective materials have the disadvantage that when the cat wipes its eyes after the bath, it may get the material on its fresh, clean coat.

If the cat's ears are dirty, clean them before bathing the cat. Wrap a cloth or piece of paper towel around the end of your finger and gently remove only the material that comes out easily. NEVER use cotton swabs to probe into the cat's ear canals. This only packs dirt down onto the eardrum (and contributes to job security for your veterinarian!).

Before you bathe the cat, place a small piece of cotton in each ear to keep water from getting into them. Don't force the cotton down into the ear canal—just put it in as far as it will go easily with gentle pressure. The goal is not to plug the ears tightly shut, but to keep water from going down into the ear canal during the bath. Remember to remove the cotton after the bath.

Wet the cat's hair completely before adding shampoo. Skin problems are not just "hair" problems. It is important that the shampoo reach the skin, especially if it is a medicated or flea shampoo. This also helps dilute the shampoo so that some areas do not get a concentrated dose while others get less. If you are applying a dip, it is of the utmost importance that it reaches the skin as well as coating the hair. You can use a fillable brush dispenser to squeeze and coat the solution through the animal's coat. Dips should not be rinsed off, but allowed to dry on the hair.

Use warm water for the bath, sudsing the shampoo gently through the cat's hair. Your fingers will work better than a brush for scrubbing the skin. Lather thoroughly, adding more water to make more suds, rather than adding more shampoo. Use the least amount of shampoo which will do the job. This will make rinsing much easier. Rinse VERY thoroughly because soapy residue can irritate the skin. If you are using a medicated shampoo, leave it on the cat for the recommended time in order to get the full benefit. Do NOT cheat on the time! Don't leave the cat while it is "soaking" in the lather. If you do, the cat may rub shampoo into its eyes or try to lick it off.

Wash and rinse the entire cat except the head. Wash the head last, because the cat will want to shake it when you bathe it. Try to keep the shampoo out of the cat's ears and eyes. A sponge or washcloth works better to wash the head than does spraying water over it. Rinse well. If you have a shower with solid doors, this is the ideal time to get out of the way, shut the doors, and allow the cat to shake until it feels comfortable. Then take the cat out and dry it.

Rubbing with towels, dry the cat as much as possible. If it's warm in the house, or there is a sunny window sill, let the cat finish drying by itself. If it's cold, dry the cat with a hair dryer set on the low or warm setting (NOT hot). This is great for cats like Persians with thick, luxurious coats. Keep the cat inside and out of drafts until it is completely dry. REMEMBER TO REMOVE THE COTTON BALLS FROM THE EARS!

Elderly cats and cats fewer than six months of age need special care in bathing. They can become chilled easily, leading to illness. Keep the cat warm and protected for at least three to four hours after the bath. It is worth taking extra time to dry the cat thoroughly.

If you bathe only one or two cats in a household that has several, the dry cats may pick on the wet cats after their bath. Some wet cats seem to lose their confidence until they are dry. Either bathe all the cats on the same day so they will be on equal social footing, or keep wet cats in a separate room until they are completely dry.

Dry shampoos don't work well for cats, and may contain ingredients which are harmful when the cat licks itself. If you decide to try one, use ONLY products specifically labeled for cats.

NAIL TRIMMING

Check your cat's toenails at least once a month. A rough scratching post or piece of wood will help the cat sharpen the nails on its front paws. You may not, however, want your cat to do this since sharp claws can make holes in clothing or pantyhose. The nicely sharpened claws may catch in the carpet or on upholstery, also damaging the cat as it tries to pull loose. Nails which are not trimmed for a long time may grow in a circle, going into the foot pad or side of the leg, causing pain and infection. At the same time, the cat stretches and marks, both by the visual shredding on the post and from scent glands on its feet. If left to its own devices, the cat will chew shredded or ragged nail sheaths with its teeth.

Use nail clippers made for pets. Two basic types are available: One resembles scissors with short ends hooked toward each other like a parrot's beak. The other has a guillotine-type blade—the nail fits into the hole and is neatly cut off. The latter type is my favorite, but use whichever works best for you; they work equally well on the nails. After a long period of use, the trimmers become dull and the blades tend to crush the nail instead of cutting it. This can be very painful for the cat, and it may cause irreversible damage to the nail. When the clippers stop cutting cleanly, buy a new pair. Toenail clippers meant for humans work well for nipping the ends off kittens' claws, but don't work so well on adult cats because they tend to crush the thicker claws.

If you acquire a kitten, it is easy to teach it to allow you to handle its feet and trim its claws. Hold and rub each paw in turn several times a day, while you are holding the cat. Gently push under the pads to squeeze out one claw at a time. Hold the foot firmly, but don't have a tug-of-war with the cat. The goal is to gradually establish that you are dominant over the cat, not to punish or intimidate it. Do this until the cat is comfortable with the procedure. I find it easiest to lay the cat upside down in my lap with its head away from me. If you are trimming an adult cat's claws and someone else is holding the cat for you, it may be easiest to have the cat in an upright position.

Cut off the transparent ends of the claws, beyond where the blood (seen as a reddish or dark center) ends. This area is easy to see on cats with white nails, but much more difficult on cats with dark nails. For dark nails, you will be guided by the angle of the nail—where the curve near the foot changes to the curve near the end (see illustration). In general, you are cutting off less than half the length from the end of the nail to where the skin begins. You also can begin by nipping off a little bit at a time and working gradually toward the cat's foot. Try not to exceed that halfway point.

It is a good idea to ask your veterinarian to demonstrate nail trimming before you attempt it the first time. This can be done when you take the cat in for a vaccination or checkup. After that, it's easy for you to do at home.

Don't forget to trim the dewclaw. This is the vestigial toe (or in some cats, several toes) located on the inside of the leg just above the paw. They may be present on the front legs, hind legs, or both. If your cat has dewclaws, they will need trimming even more than the rest of the nails because they do not receive ANY wear. If not trimmed, they can grow around in a circle and back into the skin at the base, or into the side of the leg, causing infection and pain.

If your cat has long hair, you may have to feel into it to tell whether the cat has dewclaws. If your cat continually snags its dewclaws on furniture or carpet, they can be removed, and will make the cat much more comfortable. If this is done at the same time as neutering, spaying, or other surgery, the cost is minimal. If you have the cat declawed, the dewclaws will be removed at the same time.

If you do trim a nail too deeply, your cat will let you know it. It probably will cry out and attempt to pull its foot away from you. A drop of blood may appear on the end of the nail. Hold the foot firmly, while telling the cat to hold still. Dab the blood away with a tissue or paper towel. When the bleeding has stopped, dab a tiny spot of cyanoacrylate glue (Super Glue®) on the claw. Hold the cat still until it is completely dry. Or, you can touch the bleeding end with a styptic pencil or with ferric subsulfate solution. Both of these are available at the drugstore, and it is a good idea to have some such product on hand before you start the clipping project. Cut the rest of the nails a bit further away from the cat's body.

Two types of nail clippers for cats.

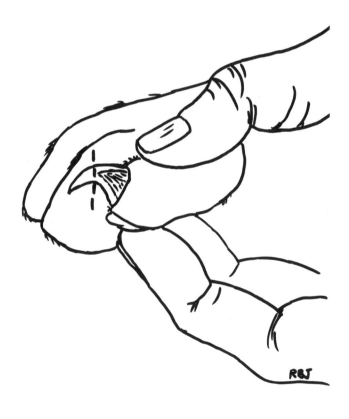

Do not trim nail any shorter than where the angle changes.

Trimmed nails are much less effective weapons, so the cat should not be allowed outdoors, much like a declawed cat.

If the nails are not trimmed, they may become overgrown. This is especially true of the dewclaws. The nail may grow around in a circle and grow back into the skin of the cat's leg. It may bleed or cause an infection which will drain pus, and the cat may limp. Clip the overgrown nail beyond the "quick." Pull the offending pointed end out of the skin (you may need to use a pair of tweezers). The pad or skin may bleed. Swab it with tincture of iodine solution for a couple of days until it is healed.

An outdoor cat may have broken nails. They become split or shredded as the cat races. This is especially true of the dewclaw. The cat may limp or lick at its paw, and may bleed. The ragged claw may be caught in the carpet or on a scratching post. Restrain the cat and carefully trim off the shredded part. If it goes into the "quick," mend it with cyanoacrylate glue (Super Glue®). Be sure to keep the cat still until it is dry. Keep an eye on the area to make sure it does not become infected. If it does, take the cat to your veterinarian.

FEEDING FOR A HEALTHY COAT

An adequate, well-balanced diet will help your cat have a healthy coat. Most high-quality, complete cat foods have all the nutrients necessary for good skin and hair health. Added fat may be needed if you are feeding dry cat food. Some dry foods contain adequate fat, but the fat is not adequately protected by antioxidants and becomes rancid in storage. Extra fat is not usually necessary if you are feeding a canned cat food. In some cases of skin disease, such as seborrhea, added fat may make the skin problem worse. (See below for treatment).

Lack of certain vitamins and minerals can affect the skin. Vitamin A deficiency over a period of time causes major changes in the skin. These include a poor coat with scaly patches on the skin, usually with hair loss. In addition, the cat will have a poor appetite, lack energy, and lose weight. Breeding cats will not reproduce normally. Males are infertile and females may not come into heat or will abort their kittens or have them stillborn. Cats are unable to convert carotene into vitamin A. Too much of this vitamin can cause problems, too. It is stored in the liver and toxicity may result.

Lack of vitamin E causes a disease called pansteatitis, otherwise known as "yellow fat disease." Cats that are short of biotin may show acne and similar dermatitis involving the hair follicles.

A deficiency of iodine can cause hypothyroidism, in which the thyroid gland does not produce adequate quantities of thyroid hormone to keep the cat healthy. One sign of this disease is a short, thin hair coat. Zinc deficiency can cause slow hair growth and a poor, thin hair coat. The skin may be scaly and there may be ulcers along the edge of the lips.

Cats that are fed table scraps and leftovers may not have adequate quantities of fatty acids in their diet. The cat may have a poor, thin hair coat, and dry skin with a lot of dandruff. Some cats will lose noticeable quantities of hair. Vegetarians who feed their own food to their cats may have animals that are severely lacking in the fatty acids needed for a healthy, shiny fur coat. Some cats that receive vegetable oils in their diet, without any animal fat, also will show signs of fatty acid deficiency. Some cheap generic cat foods are lacking in nutrients needed for a good coat. Changing to a good quality food often cures the skin problem (and is cheaper than paying the veterinary bills to diagnose and fix the problem). Occasionally, cats that are fed a good quality cat food made by a reliable manufacturer will have a thin, poor hair coat for no reason. Some of these animals show complete recovery when additional essential fatty acids are added to their diet.

One of the best (and least expensive) sources of fatty acids is pork fat. Bacon grease is one of the easiest, or you can use lard. Mix about a quarter-teaspoonful with the cat's food each day for the first week. Increase it to a half-teaspoonful the second week, three-fourths the third week, and so on until the cat develops either diarrhea or overly soft stools. Then cut back to the amount you gave the previous week. Feed the cat that amount for the next three to four months. If the cat's coat problem is due to lack of fatty acids, it should be greatly improved in that time. If not, consult your veterinarian to determine what is causing the skin problem.

Commercially available fatty acids do not give good results in cats, as opposed to dogs, where they can greatly benefit the animal. However, if your cat has a dry, dull, scaly coat, one of these products may be worth a try—after you have ruled out causes such as improper nutrition or intestinal or external parasites. Try an encoated fatty acid supplement with omega-3 fish oils plus evening primrose oil. For most of these products, it is safe to give a bit more than the label recommends—try up to twice the amount of supplement if the label dosage does not work. Reduce the amount if the cat gets diarrhea.

THE ITCHING CAT

The first step in treating the itching cat is to determine what is causing the problem. Don't begin by giving the cat a bath, as that may aggravate the itching. It may take careful observation to discover that your cat is scratching. You may be gone much of the day and simply not see the cat scratching, chewing, or licking itself. Or, you may have shouted at the cat or otherwise disciplined it when it was scratching. The cat may still be itching, but may hide when it scratches so you can't give the cat a bad time about it! Recognize that excess grooming is not necessarily the result of the cat trying to stay clean. It may be licking because it is itching.

Kittens and young cats that have come from a cattery, pet shop, or shelter may be itching because of a contagious skin disease such as fleas or ringworm. Persian cats are prone to recurring ringworm infections, and may itch because of it. Older cats may itch because of diseases of the immune system, or from skin tumors.

Have you changed anything with the cat recently? New food, new shampoo, or anything else? Any changes in the environment: new carpet cleaner, floor cleaner, insect spray? Is there someone new in the house (human or animal) who could be causing the cat to be nervous? If there is a change, undo it if you can. If not, watch the cat to try to determine what is causing the itching. A cat that has itched for a long period of time without showing any signs of skin disease is usually allergic to something, from fleas to food. Cats that itch very intensively are often infected with mites (see External Parasites Chapter). This is especially true if more than one cat is affected, or if other pets or humans in the same household are itching, too.

Does the itching occur only at a certain time of the year? Most seasonal allergies occur only in warm weather, and are often due to fleas. Or, they may be due to allergies to a plant or pollen, or to a cleaning product or insecticide that you use only during a particular season. Itching occasionally may be seen in the winter due to dry skin because of forced-air heating or dry indoor air.

Cats that have been on the same food for a long time may still be allergic to something in their diet. Unless test feeding has been done, food allergies should not be ruled out as a cause of itching. Be sure to tell your veterinarian if the cat is on any medication, or if it has been given medication for itching in the past. Did it work or not? Also be sure to tell him or her if you have recently traveled to or moved from another part of the country. This may make a difference in the diseases the veterinarian will consider. Has the cat been boarded recently?

Hair loss may occur where an injection (especially corticosteroids) has been given or a skin medication has been used. It may be followed by loss of pigment in the skin, thinning of the skin, and tearing or ulceration. This will heal in time without treatment.

Flea allergy is the only skin allergy that is common in cats. It is perhaps the most common cause of the itching cat (see External Parasites Chapter).

FLEA COLLAR DERMATITIS

Flea collars or flea medallions can sometimes cause a dermatitis around the cat's neck. This is not too common, but when it occurs it can cause severe irritation. You may first notice that the cat is scratching. If you look closely, the area underneath may be reddened and raw-looking. In severe cases, there may be ulcers or pus under the collar, as well as general symptoms that the cat is not feeling well, such as fever and depression.

A mild case can be cured by removing the flea collar. More severe cases may require veterinary treatment, including clipping hair away from the raw sores. The cat can then be treated with soothing antibiotic ointment. It also may be necessary to give either oral or injectable antibiotics to help combat the infection, for one to three months, to heal a severe case of flea collar dermatitis. Occasionally, if the reaction is severe enough or has gone on long enough, the cat will die despite treatment.

Flea collars should not be used on cats that are weak, ill, elderly, pregnant, or nursing, or on cats fewer than about four months of age. Proper fit will help prevent flea collar dermatitis. Make the collar as long as possible so that it will fit loosely, but not so loosely that it will catch on tree limbs or that the cat can get its lower jaw caught under it as it grooms its chest. You should be able to slide a couple of fingers under the collar when it is fitted properly.

Cut off any extra length. Some people believe the collar should be taken out of the package and "aired out" for two or three days before it is placed on the cat. This is probably a good idea and certainly can't hurt.

Do not expose the cat to any other insecticides containing organophosphates for seven days before or after putting on or taking off a flea collar. If you know the cat is going to be scheduled for surgery, remove the collar a week in advance. If your cat is injured and has to have surgery, be sure to tell your veterinarian that it has been wearing a flea collar. Flea collars may be more toxic to cats when the weather is hot or the humidity is low.

If your cat wears a flea collar, check the skin underneath every three to four days to make sure there are no problems. Should your cat have a reaction to a flea collar, use another method of flea prevention.

HAIR LOSS (ALOPECIA)

Hair loss in kittens and very young cats is most commonly due to ringworm or hereditary problems. Young adult and middle-aged cats are prone to allergic skin diseases and psychogenic skin disease (rolling skin disease and lick dermatitis). Elderly cats have problems with hair loss due to tumors, especially lymphoma, as well as hyperthyroidism and Cushing's disease (an excess of adrenal cortical hormone). Diabetes mellitus can cause hair loss, seborrhea (greasy, odorous skin), and pimples on the skin. These symptoms will go away when the cat is treated for diabetes.

Some of the most common causes of hair loss in older cats are ringworm, mange (several kinds), and food and flea allergies. Hair loss also may be due to abscesses under the skin and similar infections. Treatment with some drugs such as oral or injectable corticosteroids (glucocorticoids), or progesterone-type hormones may cause hairlessness. Hairlessness in a localized area may also be due to a vaccination. Be prepared to tell your veterinarian when the problem started, if it is becoming larger or smaller, and any changes or treatment that occurred around the same time. If you have several cats, is only one affected or do several have the same problem?

ALLERGIC SKIN DISEASE (ATOPY)

Allergic skin disease is rare in cats, as opposed to dogs, where it is quite common. Reactions are rarely seen from contact with drugs or chemicals unless the chemicals cause physical damage to the skin. Cats rarely have an allergic reaction resulting in hives. Almost without exception, the most common sign of allergy in cats is itching, whatever the cause.

Atopy refers to reactions in the skin, including itching, which are caused by an allergy to something in the cat's diet, or to a substance which has been inhaled. If humans have an allergic reaction to something they have eaten, they usually break out in hives, or have a stomach ache, gas, or diarrhea. Instead, cats and dogs usually just itch. Atopy is mainly a disease of younger cats. About three-quarters of all cats with atopy first show signs between six months and two years of age.

Allergic reactions occasionally may be seen on the skin of cats infested with internal parasites. The cat may have a poor, rough hair coat and pimples. Its skin may be dry and covered with dandruff, and it may itch. Getting rid of the worms will relieve the skin problem; if the cat is reinfested, the skin disease returns.

Contact dermatitis is occasionally seen, and some cats may be abnormally sensitive to mosquito bites. The cat will have pimples on the ears, nose, and pads of the feet. Hospitalize the cat for seven to 10 days to get it away from its environment. Or, if cost is a problem, isolate the cat at home, keeping it in a room without carpet if possible. Use shredded paper in the litter box rather than cat litter, and make sure no insects can get in through the window screens. In either case, improvement will confirm that there is an allergic problem, but will usually NOT reveal what is causing the reaction. In some cases, it is impossible to determine the cause.

A few cats are allergic to commercial food containing fish. Many foods that are not "fish" flavored still contain fish oil or fish meal as a base. Some fatty-acid coat conditioners also are made from fish oil. Begin by taking the cat off these products. Other cats react to beef, milk products, soy, wheat, horse meat, eggs, corn, chicken, or pork. Or, the animal may be sensitive to preservatives, coloring agents, or other additives in the food. In the cases where food allergies are seen in cats, the most common sign is intense itching, with or without pimples, hives, or ulcers on the skin, especially on the neck and head.

The cat's skin may appear greasy and have an odd odor. There may be hair loss or broken hairs where the cat has licked itself. It may even pull out its fur, leaving broken stubble. The cat may twitch its skin as if annoyed, and scratch at its face, or rub it, possibly causing open sores. Some cats will have eosinophilic granuloma on the lips (see Rodent Ulcer). Atopic cats may have behavioral changes, and may appear withdrawn from contact with their families.

Cats with food allergies almost never show vomiting or diarrhea. When these signs do occur, they may be sudden and severe. Cats have either a skin response to food allergy or digestive-tract symptoms, but usually not both.

A number of diagnostic tests may be needed to rule out other causes of skin disease. These may include a complete blood count (CBC), a stool sample to check for worms and excessive hair, a culture of broken hairs and skin cells to check for fungal infections, and skin scrapings to check for mites. Hair samples will be microscopically examined to determine whether the hairs are being broken by excessive grooming. A skin biopsy also may be needed.

A food trial also may be an important diagnostic test. Neither skin antigen injection tests nor serum testing will accurately diagnose food allergies in cats. Most experts do not consider the radioallergosorbent test (RAST), intradermal testing, or ELISA test accurate for pinpointing food-based skin allergies in cats.

Treatment with corticosteroids usually does not work well for cats with food allergies. If they are given at all, they should be used only for the most severe symptoms. They should be given orally, and preferably only for a short

period of time. Some cats may respond to treatment with antihistamines such as Benadryl®, Chlortrimeton®, Hydroxyzine®, or Clemastine®. Side effects of these drugs include vomiting or drowsiness, and the effects of a particular dosage may vary from one cat to another.

Food allergy can be suspected if your cat develops skin disease soon after a change of diet. However, the majority of cats with food allergies develop them after eating the same food for two or three years. If digestive upsets accompany the itching, this may be an even stronger case for a food allergy.

A special elimination diet is usually used to detect food allergies. A prescription diet such as Nutritional Care™ R251 (Ken Vet, (800)-7KENVET) can be fed. This is a lamb- and rice-based diet which provides a limited number of ingredients. Other specialized diets are available. If you have previously given the cat a lamb and rice diet, use something different for the trial, such as one based on rabbit or duck. Whichever one you use, be sure it does not contain poultry products, whey, yeast, wheat, corn, and other ingredients previously fed. These foods are bland and balanced, and can be fed for a prolonged period of time. Begin by mixing it with some of the cat's regular diet over a period of five to 10 days until the cat is eating only the prescription diet. Do not give any table scraps, treats, or vitamin and mineral supplements, and keep the cat off all unnecessary drugs. Do not give fatty acid supplements containing fish oils, as these may be causing the allergy. Use distilled or de-ionized water as the sole water source.

The cat should be kept on the elimination diet for a minimum of three to four weeks. Many cats take that long to show a favorable reaction. With some cats, as much as eight to 10 weeks may be needed to confirm the allergies. If the special diet cures or greatly improves the cat's problems, it can be kept on this food. Occasionally, a cat may be allergic to lamb, so if the diet doesn't cure it, try one with another meat source before ruling out foodstuffs as the cause of itching. The cat should be kept indoors to avoid exposure to other sources of allergen (or handouts or food stolen from another cat's or dog's dish) during the test period.

If you do not have access to a prescription diet food, feed the cat only boiled brown rice (or potatoes), boiled chicken, duck, or lamb and distilled water. It is helpful to put the meat and rice into the blender, as some cats will not eat whole grains of rice. Home-boiled rabbit is eaten well by many cats. Another diet that can be used is Gerber's lamb baby food and water. Whatever diet you use, it should be something that the cat has not eaten at any time within the last couple of years. Remember to change gradually to the test diet over a period of several days.

Because homemade test diets are deficient in many vitamins and other nutrients, they should not be fed for more than about six weeks. Many young cats on these diets will show calcium deficiency within a month, taurine deficiency in six weeks, and thiamine deficiency within 10 to 14 days (vomiting, lack of appetite). Do NOT supplement with any vitamins while the cat is on the trial diet because the cat may be allergic to an ingredient in them. An outdoor cat should be kept indoors so that it does not supplement its diet with birds and mice. If you need to keep the cat on the "test" diet indefinitely, consult your veterinarian to avoid deficiencies. It is best to change as soon as possible to a commercial diet which is "nutritionally complete."

If you have several cats, you may need to feed an elimination diet to all of them. Otherwise, the itchy cat may steal from its friends' dishes. If the cat has badly damaged its skin, you may have to put an Elizabethan collar on the cat for the first couple of weeks of the trial diet. Antihistamines also may help suppress the itching until the diet is under control.

When the cat acts as though it no longer itches, it can be given its original diet again, for up to two weeks. If it begins scratching again, this proves the existence of a food allergy.

Once it has been determined the cat has an allergy, you can use one of the commercial, balanced hypoallergenic diets (such as R251, Hill's Prescription Diet Feline d/d or Protocol Feline 4c or Cornucopia). Do NOT add anything to it, and do not give ANY treats or table food. It is usually not worth trying to substitute one regular commercial food for another, because ingredients common to both may be causing the problem.

If the cat's skin problem is due to allergies, improvement may be dramatic. Within one to two days, the cat will stop itching and feel better. If you feed the test diet for two weeks and there is no improvement, food allergies may not be causing the problem. Continue feeding the special diet for three to four weeks to be sure.

You can test to find which specific food is causing the skin problem by adding food ingredients back into the diet one at a time, but not more often than one each week. If the cat is going to react, it will usually do so within 24 hours. Finding enough foods to make an adequate diet may take several months. Meanwhile, the cat may become deficient in vitamins and minerals. A vitamin-mineral supplement, preferably with fatty acids included, should be fed daily after the initial month's trial. Cats must have the amino acid taurine in their diet to prevent blindness. Taurine tablets are the best and most reliable source of this essential substance.

Once the offending food ingredient is found, the chance for a complete cure is nearly 100%. Simply quit using any food which includes the offending ingredient. In many cases, even if you don't discover exactly which food item is causing the problem, you can still find a hypoallergenic diet that will stop the skin irritation. The prescription hypoallergenic diets are well balanced and can be fed for the rest of the cat's life, if necessary. These special formulas are not as tasty as regular cat food. You may have to try several to find a balance between what the cat will eat and what its allergies will tolerate. Unlike humans, cats do not usually "outgrow" their allergies.

Adding a fatty acid supplement to the atopic cat's diet may be helpful. Examples are products such as Efa-Vet (Efamol-Vet) or DermCaps (DVM). In some cases, your veterinarian will give a low dose of an antihistamine (such as chlorpheniramine, 2 mg twice daily). This drug should not be given to cats that have heart disease. Some cats will have a secondary bacterial infection on the skin (pyoderma), and may need antibiotics for three to four weeks along with their dietary change.

SUNBURN

Sunburn may occur in thinly-haired, light-colored cats that are outside in the summer. Also called solar dermatitis, it is especially common on the ears of white cats, or those with white ears, especially cats with blue eyes. Long-haired cats seem to be as badly affected as the short-haired models. The first sign is reddening and thickening along the edge of the ear. This may spread over the entire ear, followed by hair loss. Next, the ears may become crusted, scaly, eroded, bleeding, and weeping. This may be very painful for the cat, which adds insult to injury by scratching and clawing at its ears, compounding the problem. If this goes on for a long period of time, the sores may turn cancerous—usually squamous-cell carcinoma. About 10 percent of feline cancers are of this type.

If carcinoma develops, the only cure is for your veterinarian to remove it. Surgery is the most common treatment. In some cases, it may be necessary to remove the entire ear flap to limit spread of the cancer. Squamous cell carcinomas also can occur on the thinly haired area at the base of the ears, the bridge and end of the nose, the lips, and the eyelids. If the location of the tumor is such that surgery can't be done, radiation therapy may be used. The good news is that tumors on the face rarely spread to other parts of the body.

Care of sunburned ears is easy—keep the cat out of the sun. If it is an in/out cat, let it out only at night. Feed the cat in the morning to be sure it comes back in rather than spending the day outside. It is also helpful to coat the ears with a good sunscreen product, but don't use too much as the cat will ingest it while trying to wash it off.

Sunburn also may occur in light-skinned cats that have hair loss for any reason. The animal may have been closely clipped, either when it was groomed, to remove mats, or before surgery. Some females may lose much of their hair when they have a litter. Again, keeping the cat inside during the day can completely prevent sunburn.

BURNS

Burns occasionally happen when cooking grease or hot water are accidentally spilled on the cat. Because of the cat's hair, it may look less severe or even go unnoticed for a while. As with humans, the best treatment is to cool the area as quickly as possible. Turn on the cold water in the kitchen sink. Take the cat with two feet in each hand and hold it under gently running water for several minutes. Or, cool the area with cool compresses or ice packs. Be sure to remove the ice pack for five minutes from time to time so that the animal isn't frostbitten in addition to the burn. Cooling is helpful anytime during the first couple of hours after the burn has occurred.

Minor burns can be treated at home. Gently clip the hair away from the burn. Silver sulfadiazine cream (Silvadene®, Marion Laboratories, available at drugstores) and is one of the best treatments for burns. You can use it with a Telfa® pad under a bandage if the area can be bandaged. Change the bandage twice a day. If the area can't be bandaged, put an Elizabethan collar on the cat so it cannot lick off the medicine and further irritate the area.

If the burn is severe, take the cat to your veterinarian for treatment. The cat may be in shock, and it may be necessary to have the wound cleaned and damaged tissue removed. The heat may damage the pigment cells enough that the hair will regrow white when it is finally healed, or, a large area of scar tissue may be permanently hairless.

FROSTBITE

Frostbite is occasionally seen in cats that live outdoors in cold climates; however, it is uncommon if the cats have an adequate supply of nutritious food. Damage is most commonly seen on the tips of the ears. Occasionally, the tip of the tail may be damaged. The earliest signs include hair loss and scaliness at the tips of the ears. If the freezing is detected soon after it occurs, the ear tips can be thawed with water no warmer than warm bath water. It is important that the ear be kept from refreezing.

If the damage is severe, the tip of the ear may die and fall off, leaving the edge permanently shortened and crinkled. Any soothing ointment can be used on the edge of the ear, including petroleum jelly. In any case of frostbite, when the hair grows back, it may be white, and the ears will be more susceptible to being damaged again by freezing.

SCABBY CAT DISEASE

This is one of the common names for miliary eczema or miliary dermatitis. It is a symptom rather than a disease. In order to treat scabby cat disease, it is necessary to discover what is causing it.

Affected cats have small pimples which break, drain, and form scabs. The disease may start on the back, then spread to the rump, head, and neck. The cat may itch intensely and may scratch continuously. Other cats lick or rub themselves against furniture. Some animals will act annoyed, have a changed personality, growl, and suddenly run or jump as if chased. The cat may twitch the skin frantically.

One of the most common causes is external parasites, including flea allergy. Less commonly, it is due to lice or mange mites. Other causes include bacterial infection, infection with ringworm, or allergic reactions to foods or other substances. Vitamin deficiencies, especially lack of biotin or fatty acids, may be involved. If other humans or animals show signs of skin disease at the same time, fleas or mange should be strongly suspected.

Occasionally, no cause can be found. That doesn't mean there isn't a cause—it just can't be found. Cases without a known cause are sometimes treated with progestogens, which are hormones. In some cats, this treatment will be needed for the rest of the animal's life. There are a number of possible side effects to this treatment, so it should not be used unless other possibilities for cause and treatment have been exhausted.

ACNE

Mature cats may have a skin condition on the chin which is referred to as "acne." This is not related to adolescent acne in humans. The oil-secreting glands on the chin become plugged and turn into "blackheads." This may be due to the fact that a cat usually is unable to wash its chin with its paws when it is taking a "cat bath." Occasionally, signs of acne are seen on the lower lip. Rarely, it also may occur on the upper lip. It is also possible that a cat with acne may produce abnormal waxy or oily material from its hair follicles. Or, the cat may not shed the old hairs properly when new hairs are growing into place.

Acne in cats is seen as pimples or blackheads on the chin. The cat usually doesn't have any itching—the disease is noticed because it is unsightly. Occasionally, the blackheads may become infected. Then, the area will appear reddened and swollen, and the pimples may rupture, draining pus. If the acne has been present for a long time, the cat may have pits or scars similar to those seen in humans with acne.

Some cats with acne may simply have dirty chins as food particles cling to the hairs. For these cats, the cure is simple. Gently wipe the cat's chin with a dampened washcloth after each meal, and then dry it with a soft cloth and powder it. Use cornstarch for a light-colored chin and fullers' earth for a dark-colored chin. For some cats, this may be a necessary part of their everyday grooming. Others may benefit from a change from moist to dry food. It also may be helpful to wash the food dish daily, or to run it through the dishwasher to keep it sanitary.

If there is no infection in the area, it is unnecessary to treat the acne. Just be sure it does not become infected. If it does, take the cat to your veterinarian for examination and treatment. It may be necessary for the cat to be anesthetized in order to clip the hair away from the sores and thoroughly examine and clean the chin. If there are deep tracts, they may need to be drained surgically. A systemic antibiotic, such as Amoxicillin®, is usually given for eight to 14 days. In severe cases, treatment may be needed for six to 10 weeks. In some cats, adding a fatty acid supplement to the animal's diet may help the acne, odd as that may seem. In a few tom cats, neutering may help clear up the condition, especially if the cat also has a case of stud tail.

If the acne tends to become infected, gently wash the chin daily with a mild soap such as benzoyl peroxide shampoo (Oxydex® (DVM), Pyoben® (Allerderm), or chlorhexidine (Hibiclens). Benzoyl peroxide products may be irritating to the skin; if it becomes severely reddened, stop using them. A mild corticosteroid cream, such as one containing 1% hydrocortisone, may help cats that have cysts or form scars on the chin. Salicylic acid solution is helpful to some cats with mild cases of acne (Stri-Dex® Pads, Glenbrook). Warm packs may be held on the chin for five to 10 minutes, three times a day.

Most cats with acne have continuing problems with it. To have a chin free from acne, it may be necessary to cleanse it every two to six days for the rest of the cat's life. In time, some cats recover from minor cases of acne even if left untreated.

BACTERIAL SKIN DISEASE

Pseudomonas bacteria can invade damaged skin, especially if it is covered with a bandage, keeping the area warm and moist. If the area is covered with a slimy green drainage when you change a dressing, have it checked within a day or so. The pus may have a sickly sweet smell. These bacteria may be very resistant to antibiotics and difficult to treat. Wounds should be left open to air rather than bandaged, when possible. Using disinfectants in a wound may delay healing, and sometimes create conditions favorable to the growth of Pseudomonas.

ROLLING SKIN DISEASE

Also called neurodermatitis, feline hyperesthesia syndrome, or neuritis, "rolling skin disease" is common in Siamese or Siamese-mix cats. It is occasionally seen in other purebreds and in domestic cats. Affected cats are usually between one and four years of age, but may be any age. Any cat may occasionally have signs similar to neuritis. In some cats with rolling skin disease, the behavior becomes so overwhelming that the cat cannot go about its normal activities.

Symptoms of rolling skin disease include twitching or rippling the skin of the back, apparent hallucinations, staring with widely dilated pupils of the eyes, licking or biting at the tail, violent swishing of the tail, frantic howling or meowing, and sudden stops to lick as the animal is eating, walking, or running. The cat may run around the house attacking objects, including people. The attacks may somewhat resemble epileptic seizures, as the cat may seem not to know what it is doing, and it may even urinate outside the litter box. The cat may sleep peacefully, but suddenly awaken and attack you. Between episodes, the cat may appear normal or may be slightly upset. Some cats may show personality changes, such as an affectionate cat becoming nasty, or a grouchy cat suddenly becoming loving.

This disease must be differentiated from rabies, which may show similar yowling or voice and personality changes. Cats with rolling skin disease show signs continuously. With rabies, the disease comes on suddenly. If there is ANY question at all about a diagnosis, confine the cat to a carrier or box and have it examined by your veterinarian immediately. Of course, if the cat is strictly an indoor cat, rolling skin disease is the more likely problem.

The cause of rolling skin disease is unknown, but the signs suggest it is a mental illness, possibly due to an unstable personality. It may be due to frustrations or environmental pressures or possibly, brain damage. Or, the cause may be problems with the skin or the nerves in it.

Any medication you put on the skin will soon be licked off by the cat. In some cases where the cat has mutilated its tail, the tail has been amputated; but, the cat may continue to attack the tailhead or the stump. The only drugs that seem to give any long-term relief are those that work on the mind. Phenobarbital is effective (and must be prescribed by your veterinarian). Primidone, which is normally used to treat epilepsy, can be given to cats in small dosages. Within a matter of hours after treatment, the cat may return to its normal disposition. Some cats will need treatment for a long time. After a period of treatment, you can gradually decrease the dosage to the least amount that will keep the animal free of symptoms. Many owners recognize the early warning signs, such as twitching the skin and looking at the tail, that signal that an attack is on the way. They can then administer

medication to stop it. If the cat is damaging its tail, it may be necessary to bandage it until treatment has taken effect, to allow it to heal and prevent the cat from mutilating it.

LICK DERMATITIS

Lick dermatitis is seen in mature cats. Another name for the disease is self-induced psychogenic hair loss or psychogenic alopecia. It is more common in indoor cats than in ones that live outdoors. The cat will pick a spot on its coat and chew and lick at it until the hairs are short and stubby, or until it is bald. Some animals worry at the spot until it also is reddened and ulcerated or oozing pus. The spots are usually on the feet, flanks, or belly, where the cat easily can reach to lick. Other cats will end up with a hairless strip down the back and sides of the rump. One distinction is that the cat has created the lesion itself. Some cats are closet cases, only scratching or pulling their hair while hiding from their owners. The hair pulling may be quite symmetrical from one side to the other, leading to suspicions of endocrine disease, in which areas are sparsely haired or completely bald rather than having stubble or broken hairs.

Some cases of lick dermatitis are seen in cats that were weaned too early or hand-raised as orphans. If the cat was given attention when it showed the behavior, it may have been reinforced, making it a learned behavior that continued. Begin by ignoring the actions, after you have thoroughly examined the cat for obvious signs of skin problems. Only give attention when the cat is not licking.

It is important to eliminate disease as a possible cause of these bald areas. Your veterinarian probably will want to check the cat for ringworm. In ringworm, hairs in the stubble area are easily pulled out, while with lick dermatitis they are not. An obese cat may lick at the area around the tailhead because it cannot reach back to wash its perineum. Gently washing the area once or twice a day may stop the frantic attempts to clean itself. Be sure the cat doesn't have fleas, lice, or other external parasites. Cats with feline leukemia may show excessive grooming.

You can try putting an Elizabethan collar on the cat for two to three weeks; this may keep the cat from chewing or licking. If the areas show improvement during this period, you have a diagnosis.

Now the bad news. Most cases of lick dermatitis seem to be psychological problems, originating in the cat's mind, especially after a change in its lifestyle. This may include moving to a new home, boarding in a kennel, new animals in the neighborhood coming into the cat's yard, or having new pets or persons in the household (such as a new baby). Lick dermatitis is frequently seen in purebred cats, especially Siamese, Abyssinian, and Burmese, which tend to be sensitive and high-strung. They may lick because they are bored, nervous, or lonely for attention from people. Ignore the cat so as to not reward it for this behavior.

Cases which are caused by changes in the cat's environment sometimes may be reversed by undoing whatever has changed. However, since it's difficult to return a new baby, the only thing that can be done is to treat the symptoms. Treating the lesions themselves usually does little or no good. Rarely, products such as Variton ointment, smeared directly on the lesion, are helpful.

If caught early in the behavior, some cats may be stopped by a loud noise, squirt of water, shake can, or other diversion, preferably not directly associated with people around them. Some cats stop the behavior when given a compatible cat for a companion.

As with rolling skin disease, for most cats the only treatment that seems to work is drugs that lessen the animal's anxiety. Diazepam (Valium®, at 1-4 mg once or twice daily) is commonly used. Phenobarbital works on some cats that are not affected by Valium, but it can make the cat sleepy. Elavil® (an anti-depressant drug) and Acepromazine® (a tranquilizer) may work with others. These are all prescription drugs that must be obtained from your veterinarian. They can give considerable relief to the animal, but you may need to treat the cat for the rest of its life. Side effects may include drowsiness, staggering and/or constipation. Since the cat is otherwise healthy, and drugs used for treatment can cause undesirable side effects, you may choose to live with the problem. With some cats, once the original stimulus is removed, the medication can gradually be withdrawn.

Megestrol acetate (a hormone) is sometimes used to treat lick dermatitis. This drug can be quite effective, but it can have severe side effects. Make sure the risks are worth the benefits (see Nursing Chapter for more information).

Some cats will suck on their own skin. This is probably a variation on lick dermatitis. Sometimes a product such as Bitter Apple can be applied to deter the animal from this sucking. Occasionally, older kittens that are kept with their mother may nurse her for a year or more. Sometimes, this can be stopped by putting Bitter Apple on her mammary glands. Whatever you put on the mother to make the "kitten" stop nursing must be something that is safe for the mother cat when she cleans herself.

Occasionally, a cat will chew at its tail until it is completely mutilated and must be amputated. The cat may then chase the "phantom" tail. These cases are sometimes seen when the owner rewards the cat by picking it up or paying attention to it when it exhibits the bizarre behavior. They sometimes disappear when ignored. It's worth a try.

STUD TAIL

Stud tail, also called tail gland hyperplasia, is a disease seen almost exclusively in mature purebred male cats that are sexually active. It is especially common in the Siamese, Persian, and Rex breeds. Rarely, it may be seen in males that have been neutered and in females, both spayed and unspayed. Oil-secreting glands on the top of the tail are overactive, resulting in blackheads. The oily secretions from the glands form a waxy, scaly yellow-to-black coating on the skin and hair on top of the tail, and the hair may be matted. This does not seem to cause the animal any discomfort, pain, or itching. It just looks bad, especially on a white-haired cat. Rex cats also may have this greasiness in the skin folds around their claws.

Castration of the male cat will cure the problem in many individuals. You may need to wash the cat's tail once or twice a week with a shampoo such as benzoyl peroxide (Pyoben®, Ailerderm, Inc.), or one containing sulfur compounds. Other cats respond to daily washing of the affected area with any cat shampoo. Carefully pat the area dry with a soft cloth. Then, dust it with cornstarch for a light-colored cat or fullers' earth for a dark-colored cat. Do not use an ointment or salve on the area. Most cats lick these materials off their skin immediately, and moisture from the saliva keeps the area from drying and may allow further infection. Progestogen compounds may help control the skin disease, but may adversely affect a breeding male. Some cats do not overcome stud tail, no matter how they are treated.

Confinement in small quarters such as catteries may discourage the cat from grooming properly. Getting it outdoors where it has space, fresh air, and sunshine may encourage the cat to clean itself normally. Treatment of stud tail is mainly for cosmetic reasons, and is not absolutely necessary if you don't mind looking at the cat as it is.

RODENT ULCERS

Rodent ulcer also is known as feline eosinophilic granuloma complex (EGC), eosinophilic plaque, or collagenolytic granuloma. This is a skin disease that occurs in the mouth, on the lips and chin, and sometimes on the feet or down the rear legs. A small ulcer may start on the lip and spread until the entire chin is ulcerated.

The cause of this disease is unknown. It has been suggested that the cat's canine teeth damage its lips or that damage is caused by the rough tongue as it licks and grooms itself. Others may be due to a sharp canine tooth which irritates the skin on the lip, causing an erosion that later becomes an ulcer. Chronic food or inhalant allergy and chronic low-grade bacterial infection also have been proposed as causes. Other veterinarians think it may be an autoimmune disease in which the cat becomes allergic to certain components of its own skin. Some cases appear to be due to mosquito or gnat bites. Others seem to be inherited. Flea allergy also may be a cause. Be sure the cat is flea-free, and that it stays that way by treating your other animals, your house, and your yard. Consider this to be a case of flea allergy until proven otherwise.

Cases are seen in cats from six months to about nine years of age, with most being around one year. Twice as many females have the disease as males. Sometimes, more than one kitten from a litter will be infected. Except for this skin problem, affected cats usually feel and act healthy.

Rodent ulcers may recur from time to time, healing and then returning, or occurring elsewhere on the body. Open sores on the edge of the lips are one of the most common symptoms. They are rounded, reddish or reddish-brown, raw-looking, and may have a shiny surface. The hair is gone from the area. The majority of rodent ulcers are seen on the upper lip, and may occur on both sides or just one side of the mouth. Other lesions may extend into the mouth, occurring on and around the tongue. Sores are occasionally seen on the pads of the feet, making the animal quite miserable.

Other rodent ulcers are similar in appearance but may be raised, fiery-red hairless areas. They may occur on the mouth or anywhere else on the skin, especially the abdomen and inside the thighs. The cat appears to itch miserably, and may scratch, chew, or lick at the area until it is raw or bleeding.

Another form of rodent ulcer, called linear granuloma or collagenolytic granuloma, shows up as firm, rounded white, yellow, or yellowish-pink, hairless, raised sores. These are often seen on the back of the hind legs, and may form a line of firm lumps. In some cats, they will be seen as nodules in the mouth or in the armpits or chest wall. They may cause a thickening or swelling of the lower lip or chin, giving the cat a "pouting" look. In kittens, they may not cause a problem. Other cats may itch and scratch until their skin is raw.

A form called indolent ulcer is most commonly found on the upper lip. Sores are rounded, shiny and golden yellow, red, or brown, with a firm white or pink border. The center is sunken and ulcerated. While these lesions are ugly, they do not seem to cause pain. Sensitivity to food bowls has been proposed as a possible cause. Abrasion from the tongue or teeth also has been suggested.

It is important to distinguish rodent ulcer from squamous cell carcinoma, which may look similar and may be fatal if neglected. For this reason, it is a good idea to have this type of lesion checked by your veterinarian. A biopsy may be needed to confirm it. Ulcers on the tongue and around the mouth also may occur from uremic poisoning, and this may be the first sign that the cat is going into kidney failure or has diabetes.

Many treatments for rodent ulcer have been tried. Bad-tasting ointments have been used, but the cat licks them off. Bandages and Elizabethan collars will keep the cat from licking while they are on; the moment they are removed, the cat begins licking again.

Corticosteroid drugs, given in high dosage for a period of 30 days, seem to work well for some rodent ulcers. Prednisolone at the dosage of 1/2-1 mg per pound can be given twice daily, or a corticosteroid injection may be used. It is very important to withdraw the drug gradually at the end of the treatment period to let the cat's adrenal glands resume production of hormones. Progesterone (a reproductive hormone) has been used with some success. The ulcers may recur when the medication is stopped, and some animals may need to be on one of these drugs indefinitely. Work with your veterinarian to use the lowest dosage that will control the sores, as either one of these drugs can have serious side effects when given for long periods of time.

Some rodent ulcers have been treated by injecting small quantities of corticosteroids directly into the sore, once a week for a month. This treatment often is used with single sores when medication given orally or by intramuscular injection does not work.

Rodent ulcers that do not respond to medical treatment are often treated with electrocautery, cryosurgery (freezing), or laser surgery. They may be treated by routine surgical methods if the location is such that there is enough skin to suture together afterward. Any of these methods may result in permanent deformity of the mouth. Radiation and laser therapy have been used on rodent ulcers that could not be healed by any other method. They are sometimes successful.

Rodent ulcers almost never heal by themselves. They should be treated early and aggressively in order to achieve a complete cure and prevent recurrence. If the sores are not treated completely, they tend to return; they are much more resistant to treatment the second time. If your veterinarian advises giving pills for a month, don't quit when the sores begin improving. Treat the cat until all medication is gone. If rodent ulcers repeatedly return, the cat should be checked for flea allergy, as well as for allergies to foods and inhalant allergens. Putting the cat on a hypoallergenic diet may provide some relief. A 2% solution of erythromycin (used for the treatment of human acne) may be put on the lesion, using a cotton swab. The bitter taste of this drug may cause the cat to salivate for several minutes after it is applied (Freiman, 1991). Some ulcers in the mouth area may be impossible to cure.

DANDRUFF

Dandruff is not common in cats, but may be seen occasionally. It is usually accompanied by dry skin and a dry hair coat. Some cats also may have itching. It may be caused by hot, dry air indoors in winter because of central heating. If this is the case, it may be cured by humidifying the air and/or turning down the thermostat. Some cats may have dandruff because of a fat deficiency in their diet. Other cats may have dandruff because of parasites on their skin, especially lice or mange mites. Ringworm may cause dandruff. A cat that is poorly nourished also may have dandruff. Using a human shampoo to bathe the cat can cause dandruff in some cats. The dandruff itself cannot be treated, because it is just a symptom. Don't try to use a dandruff shampoo made for humans, as that may worsen the problem. Try to eliminate any of the obvious causes. If that doesn't work, have the cat examined by your veterinarian. Severe cases of dandruff may result from a mange mite called Cheyletiella (see External Parasites Chapter).

ABSCESSES AND OTHER SWELLINGS

Abscesses are one of the most common skin problems in cats. They usually occur because the cat has been bitten or scratched by another cat. The resulting puncture wounds then become infected. Abscesses are most common in male cats that have not been neutered. They fight with other males, either over a female in heat or to defend their territory. Abscesses are most common on the base of the tail, the tail, and the back. They also may occur on the feet or face, or elsewhere on the body.

The bite or claw marks that cause the abscess usually go unnoticed because of the cat's fur. Obvious signs may occur suddenly. If the bite is on a foot or leg, the cat may limp or hold it up. The area may show pain and swelling, or the animal may show no pain. If the abscess has broken and drained, the first sign may be pus or moisture on the cat's skin. It may wash and groom the area so much that the fur is constantly wet. If pus is draining out, it may be yellow, white, greenish, or brownish-red. It often has a foul odor. The cat may have a fever and be unwilling to eat, as well as being depressed and inactive.

When you check a swelling you think might be an abscess, the cat should be held by someone who is competent to restrain it or wrapped in a towel or blanket. Otherwise, the cat may try to bite or claw you because of its pain. Carefully feel around the swelling. Early in its development, an abscess may be quite firm. Later, the skin at the top of the swelling, called a "point," will become thin. It may be reddish-purple. The area may feel warm to the touch when compared with the surrounding skin.

Abscesses rarely heal by themselves. In an area where the skin is loose, such as over the back, untreated abscesses may break and drain, heal closed, refill with pus, and repeat the cycle. This may continue until the animal's entire back is covered with thickened, scarred skin. This skin may never grow normal hair again, causing the cat to have a thin, ragged coat, as well as spending many months in misery. Bacteria from the abscess may spread to the bone in the area, causing an infection of the bone (called osteomyelitis), or to a nearby joint, causing an arthritis. It may cause a pus-forming infection in the chest, abdomen, or sinuses. Rarely, coccidioidomycosis, a fungal disease, can cause swollen lymph nodes and draining skin lesions which may look like abscesses.

If you know your cat has been bitten by another, it should be treated promptly with antibiotics, whether by injection or orally. If given within about 24 hours of the bite, this often will prevent an abscess from developing.

Full veterinary care for an abscess may include surgery to clean out the pocket of infection. This usually must be done with the cat fully anesthetized. The infected area may be cleansed or surgically removed, and then sutured partially or completely closed, sometimes with a drain tube placed in the site. Antibiotics will, of course, be given. Ask the cost before you have treatment done—complete therapy is sometimes quite expensive.

Some owners prefer to treat abscesses themselves, and this can substantially reduce the cost of care. You must, of course, be sure the problem is an abscess and not a fracture, blood clot, or tumor. If the suspected abscess is on a leg or foot, with the cat carefully restrained you should be able to hold one end of the bone under the swollen skin in each hand and check if the bone is complete. Compare it to the same bone in the normal leg. If you have ANY doubt, have the cat examined by your veterinarian. Swellings on the side of the face may occasionally be due to a tumor or inflammation of the salivary gland.

If you feel a softened area or thinned skin, the "point" of the abscess, you can confirm it by using a hypodermic needle. An 18-gauge, 1 inch needle is fine. Again, the cat should be firmly restrained by wrapping it in a towel. Clip the fur from the swollen area and for a half-inch around the base of it. Cleanse the clipped spot thoroughly with chlorhexidine solution, or wipe it several times with cotton balls moistened with rubbing alcohol. Push the needle into the highest spot of the swelling, perpendicular to the skin. Go JUST through the skin so that the end of the needle is in the cavity of the swelling—about a quarter- to half-inch. Wait a moment and see what comes out. If it is pure blood or clear, golden, straw-colored serum, the swelling is a blood clot. Leave it alone and it will disappear with time. If it is an abscess, pus will usually flow out of the needle. Occasionally, the pus is thickened into clots that do not come through the needle; you will see it caught in the end of the needle when you remove it.

If the swelling is a tumor, it will feel "meaty" and firm rather than having a "point." If after clipping the swollen area, it is discolored—angry red or purplish-blue—there may be a large area of infection. If either of these are seen, take the cat to your veterinarian. An abscess which is not yet ready to be opened also can feel meaty instead of fluid-filled.

If the swelling is an abscess and you have removed pus from it, it needs to be drained. Using a sharp surgical blade or knife tip, make an X-shaped incision JUST through the skin at the point of the abscess. Push the blade through, nicking cleanly through the skin about one-eighth inch long. By this time, pus should be oozing out of the opening. If it is not, you must reevaluate the other possibilities: tumor, abscess not ready to drain, or a blood clot. If pus is coming out, the area must be opened for adequate drainage. Make an X-shaped incision, about one-quarter inch long, through the skin at the point of the abscess. DO NOT try to be kind to the cat by making a tiny incision. You will not be able to clean it out adequately, and it will close over on the outside before it is healed on the inside. You will be right back where you started, with a cat with an abscess. Open the area so that you can EASILY get a cotton swab into the hole.

Swab out the hole with strong (7%) tincture of iodine. Move the swab completely around the hollow. Dab off pus and excess iodine with paper towels. Try to keep it out of the cat's fur, as it may become ill from trying to clean it out by licking it. When you are finished, press dry paper towels against the skin, pushing out as much iodine and pus as you can, and cleaning as much of the material as possible from the skin.

The bacteria in some cat abscesses may cause infection or illness in humans, especially if you have a cut or scratch on your hand. Wear disposable gloves while treating a cat with an abscess. Clean up areas touched by the pus with household bleach or another appropriate disinfectant. Dispose of pus-contaminated papers by burning or secure them in a plastic bag before putting them in the trash. Soak any cloth towels that have pus on them in water to which household bleach has been added; then wash them with hot water and detergent. Or, throw them away.

Clean out the abscess twice a day, using the iodine. The object is to keep the cavity open and draining. It should become gradually smaller, and each day you should be able to swab a little less deeply into the hole. If the hole in the skin suddenly closes over or forms a scab, pick it off and keep swabbing. If you let it close over before it is healed from the inside, you will be back where you started.

Some veterinarians treat cat abscesses by flushing them with hydrogen peroxide. This makes fancy bubbles, but I believe it does little to cleanse or heal the wound. This is a matter of opinion and personal preference. Putting antibiotic ointment on the outside of the skin also is nearly useless in healing abscesses.

Instead of an abscess, a bite on the cat's leg may produce a more generalized and widespread infection called cellulitis. This is similar to a large abscess that spreads widely under the skin and does not want to come to a head. It may be very serious by the time the cat finally appears ill, and intensive medical treatment may be needed. The infection can enter the bloodstream, causing a septicemia ("blood poisoning"). This may cause damage to the cat's kidneys, heart, and other internal organs. It may not make the cat ill at the time, but may shorten its lifespan by a significant amount. In rare cases, the infection may be so serious that it kills the cat. A cat that is bitten on a foot or the tail may have a chronic infection in the bone which may be difficult or impossible to treat. Occasionally, it may be necessary to amputate the cat's tail.

If you are treating an abscess or cellulitis yourself, you MUST be able to give antibiotics to the cat. The cat may receive an injection of procaine penicillin or a similar antibiotic. Then, tablets such as ampicillin or amoxicillin tablets are commonly used. Amoxicillin tablets are usually given at a dosage of 5-10 mg per pound of body weight (11 mg/kg), once or twice a day. Ampicillin is used at the same dosage, two or three times daily.

Mycoplasma-like organisms may cause chronic abscesses under the skin of some cats. These abscesses usually contain reddish-brown, relatively odorless pus. They also may be difficult to heal when handled with the usual medical or surgical treatment. These particular abscesses heal quite rapidly when the cat is treated with tetracycline, given orally.

Plague may cause abscesses, especially on the legs and in the lymph nodes around the jaw. The cat will have a high fever. If you live in an area of the southwestern United States where plague is a problem, it is especially important to treat any abscesses promptly and carefully, because if it is plague, it can be spread to humans by contact with pus, or by sneezing as the cat becomes ill. It is important to keep the cat isolated and to wear rubber gloves when handling the abscess. The best prevention in these areas is to confine your cat to the house, and your dog to the yard, and to avoid either of them having contact with strange animals that do not live in your household. Continuous and vigorous flea control is a must. Think of these measures in terms of cheap protection for yourself and your family against what can be a fatal disease.

In North America, feline leprosy (also called mycobacterial granuloma) is restricted to the northwestern U.S. and adjacent areas of Canada. It is also seen in New Zealand, parts of Australia, and Great Britain. It seems to be caused by Mycobacterium lepraemurium, which causes rat leprosy. It is more commonly seen in younger cats during the winter months. The disease shows up as one or more nodules on the head and/or legs. They may or may not ulcerate and drain. The disease is treated by surgically removing the nodules. If your cat has abscesses which are firm and meaty, or which drain and do not heal after treatment with antibiotics and swabbing, have it examined by your veterinarian.

Abscesses which do not heal well, or heal and recur, may suggest that the cat has a damaged immune system. This may be due to infection with feline leukemia virus, FIP, FAIDS, Hemobartonella, or another disease organism.

The cat should be tested for these diseases. Many cats with these viral diseases have continuing abscesses because their weakened immune system is unable to deal with bacteria that they otherwise could overcome.

Nodules in the skin may be caused by foreign bodies such as hair or grass awns which have penetrated the skin. As the body attempts to get rid of the foreign material, a draining tract or an abscess may form. In many cases, the offending material may go unnoticed when the area is cleaned or drained. Tracts which continue to drain also may be due to a bone, metal or wood fragment, fungus infection, or other cause. These problems usually are treated as abscesses. When they do not heal, they should be checked by your veterinarian to determine exactly what is causing the problem.

Abscesses are rather easily prevented. Begin by neutering your male cat. While this is most effective if done before the cat is sexually mature, many cats still have fewer abscesses (because they do less chasing around and fighting) if neutered after they are mature. Keeping the cat, whether male or female, at home and separated from strange cats will go a long way toward preventing abscesses.

TUBERCULOSIS

Tuberculosis occasionally may be seen as a skin disease in cats, usually in barn cats in areas where it is common in cattle. The cat may have one or more bumps, abscesses, or plaques on its head, neck, or legs. Nonhealing ulcers may be seen on the nose, lips, or eyelids. Or, a draining abscess may occur under the eye or on the neck. Swelling may produce a deformity or bump on the bridge of the nose or on the forehead, resembling a parrot's beak. The pus has a foul odor and is usually thick and greenish or yellow. Tuberculosis is a disease that humans can catch from an infected cat. For this reason, if a cat has tuberculosis, it should NEVER be treated, but should be euthanized, for the safety of all the other people and animals around it.

RINGWORM

Ringworm (dermatophytosis) is the name given to the skin disease caused by a fungus. Microsporum canis causes about 98% of ringworm in cats. Ringworm may be found in cats anywhere, anytime. It is perhaps more common in purebred cats, probably because they are raised in catteries with large numbers of cats. Cats may be coming and going from these colonies, for breeding or to and from shows. This increases the chance for exposure to the microscopic spores which cause the disease. Inbred cats may have a lowered resistance to the disease organisms. Ringworm also may be seen in cats from pet shops or animal shelters, where numbers of animals from different sources are gathered and sanitation may be poor. The animals may be handled by a number of different people, some of whom can easily be infected with the disease. Ringworm is more common in areas with high humidity and warm temperatures.

Ringworm also is more common in long haired cats than in cats with shorter coats. Some veterinarians believe ringworm is more common in Himalayan and Persian cats, as well as in Siamese. Some Persians are prone to deep-seated, persistent infections which heal slowly and poorly. It is much more difficult to see hairless spots on a long haired cat, as well as to be sure that an infected animal is thoroughly treated. Some long-haired cats will have a hair coat that looks thin and tattered all over, rather than having distinct bald spots. Ringworm is more common late in summer through early winter. Some experts believe that poor nutrition contributes to ringworm. While this has not been proven in cats, it is certainly true in horses—they have more ringworm late in winter when their hay may be severely lacking in vitamin A. Cats that have deficient immune systems or other diseases are more susceptible to ringworm.

Ringworm may be seen in tiny kittens, two to three weeks of age. They are probably infected shortly after birth. Signs of ringworm begin two weeks to a month after the cat is infected. Older cats acquire the disease from cats, dogs, and humans, especially children, who are infected with ringworm. Cats become somewhat resistant as they grow older. Tom cats may get ringworm during their fights with other males. At first, the spots may look like claw marks or scratches with scabs, but instead of healing, the areas become larger, with hair loss.

Typical signs of ringworm start with bare, scaly spots on the face. Some lesions will have a thin, whitish-gray crust, while others have moist scabs. They may be tiny at first, but enlarge until they form somewhat circular areas. There is a sharp edge where the hairless skin joins the skin which still has its normal fur. The eyelashes and whiskers may fall out, and their loss may be the first sign of ringworm. A cat with only one bare spot will still have infected areas elsewhere on its coat. Occasionally, older cats show a type of ringworm on the chin with hair loss and reddening of the skin. In another kind of ringworm, the cat's skin is covered with little brown-colored crusts, with the hair growing through in ragged patches or clumps. The cat does not have bare spots, but its coat is poor. As the cat washes, it spreads the infection to other parts of the body, usually from face to feet and then over the rest of the body. Occasionally, ringworm may cause changes in the skin or hair color, with or without hair loss. Cats with ringworm may or may not show signs of itching.

The cat's claws should always be checked. Nails that are infected with ringworm will be whitish, instead of their normal shining, grayish color. The surface of the claw will be ragged, chalky, or crumbled-looking. The fungus may infect only one or two nails, or they may all be involved. Occasionally, tumors which have spread to the toes may be mistaken for a fungus infection.

Approximately 60% of ringworm infections are brightly fluorescent when examined under an ultraviolet ("black") light called a Woods lamp. The infected hairs (or broken-off hairs) may glow whitish, yellowish, greenish, or a dull gray color, especially at the end nearest the skin. This must be distinguished from a light purplish color given off by dandruff, scabs, claws, and some medications. If the ringworm involves a claw, the entire nail may glow brightly. Compare it to the other, presumably normal nails. Cats that show positive under a Woods lamp do not need further testing before treatment.

The other 40% of ringworm cases do NOT fluoresce under a Wood's lamp. For these, it is necessary to take a few hairs from the lesion and put them in a special culture medium to see if the fungus will grow. It may take a week or more to get results from this laboratory test because fungi grow very slowly. The hairs also may be examined under a microscope, where the fungi may be seen. Because ringworm can have such varied signs, it should not be ruled out in cases of feline skin disease or hair loss without thorough examination, and laboratory culture if necessary.

If the cat is not treated, ringworm may eventually clear up by itself, assuming that the animal's immune system is normal. This may happen within one to three months, or it may take up to three years. Almost any treatment will "cure" a mild case, while nothing will work on the worst of infections. Many cats that recover without treatment remain carriers for the rest of their lives, although they do not show any signs of the disease. Other cats from catteries will go through life with a thin hair coat and permanent "dandruff," spreading ringworm along the way. When examined with a Wood's lamp, these carriers will show fluorescent spots all over their bodies. For the sake of your other pets, your family members and yourself, ringworm should be treated.

Ringworm is easily spread, both from one cat to another, and from cats to dogs, humans, horses, or other animals with which they come in contact. Any of these animals (including us!) may get it from one of the others, and spread it to still another. A child may bring ringworm home from school and give it to the cat, that gives it to the dog, that gives it to the neighbor's child. The first sign may be a rounded, reddened, possibly itching area on your arm, leg, face, neck, or scalp. Consult your physician if signs appear. Adult humans are fairly resistant to ringworm. The spot or spots usually heal with a few treatments with a topical medication such as tolnaftate (Tinactin®). Children have less resistance to ringworm, and the disease may cause considerable annoyance, especially if it gets onto the child's scalp.

If you have small children who cannot (or will not) avoid handling the cat, it may be advisable to have your veterinarian hospitalize the cat for a week or two until the treatment begins to take effect. This will give you a chance to get the disease under control if it has already affected the children, and to clean up areas which have been contaminated by the fungus. Your physician may recommend that you euthanize the cat. This is certainly not necessary, as the disease is completely treatable in almost all cases. All it takes is time, medication, and sanitation!

If the cat has more than a few small lesions, its hair should be completely clipped off when treating a case of ringworm. This makes healing more rapid and effective, as well as removing much of the infected material, to help prevent spread of the disease. It also makes it easier for medication to reach the skin. It is especially important with long-haired cats and those that have a severe case of ringworm.

Shaving can be done when treatment with griseofulvin is begun, or several days later, when the drug has had a chance to begin to work. The clipping is usually done under complete anesthesia. Your veterinarian will wear disposable protective gear such as a gown, mask, and gloves. The procedure will take about half an hour, and must be done in an area where the hair will not blow around or be lost. The cat is placed on newspaper or cloth which also can be thrown away or burned so that the infective hairs cannot cause ringworm in other animals or humans. The cat can be clipped using a #10 blade or scissors. The clippers are steam sterilized after being used on a cat with ringworm, to prevent spreading it to other animals. Or, they are soaked in alcohol. Obviously, the cat may look rather ragged after clipping, and the lesions may look noticeably worse for one to two weeks until the hair begins to grow back.

The skin may be treated with 2% lime-sulfur dip (such as Lym-Dyp® (DVM)) applied twice a week for four weeks. Tamed iodine (povidone iodine), three tablespoons per gallon of water (40 cc/liter) can be used. Or, you can use a solution of household bleach (such as Clorox), 1 part bleach diluted in 20 parts water. Chlorhexidine (Nolvasan® Fort Dodge Laboratories) does not seem to be particularly effective against ringworm when used on the skin (DeBoer, 1995). Be careful not to get any of these products into the cat's eyes. Sponge the solution through the cat's coat, or dip it into a pan or sinkful of the mixture. Do not rinse, but let it dry on the hair and skin. Restrain the cat so that it cannot lick off the medication as it is drying. An Elizabethan collar can be put on until the cat is dry.

Ointments such as tolnaftate (Tinactin®) which work very well on humans, are nearly useless on cats. They simply don't work. Clotrimazole (Veltrim®, Haver-Lockhart) works well on cats if they don't lick it off. It can be used if there are only one or two spots. Apply it twice daily to the bare spot and about half an inch (1.2 cm) into the surrounding hair. Continue to treat the cat with topical medications for a week to 10 days after the last clinical signs are seen and hair growth begins in the bare spot. Treating the cat systemically, however, generally gives a better permanent cure, and helps avoid ending up with a cat that becomes a carrier animal or in which the disease recurs.

Animals that do not improve with topical treatment should be treated with systemic medication. Your veterinarian probably will use a drug called griseofulvin. This drug is given orally and is absorbed from the cat's digestive tract. From there, it goes into the skin and nails, where it makes the new hair and nail growth resistant to attack by the fungus. This works especially well for cats that usually lick off any medication put on their skin. The drug is given at a dosage of 25-50 mg per pound body weight daily (divided into two doses) until the claws or skin are negative for fungi.

Giving the griseofulvin with a fatty meal (such as tuna in oil) helps increase its absorption from the gut. Side effects include lack of appetite, itching, nausea, vomiting, and diarrhea. If any of these occur, check with your veterinarian immediately. This is not a serious problem—it just may be necessary to decrease the dosage of the drug for that cat, or to divide the daily amount into three or four doses. Rarely, griseofulvin can cause anemia and/or bone marrow depression, as well as jaundice, staggering, and depression. Severe side effects may develop when griseofulvin is used in cats

that are positive for feline leukemia. It should not be used on them. Reactions are rare, but the drug is probably best used for cats that do not respond to routine treatments.

Griseofulvin should not be given to cats in the first half of pregnancy as it may cause deformities in the kittens or cause them to be stillborn. Other pets that are exposed to an animal with ringworm, but do not have signs of it, may be given a two-week preventive course of griseofulvin. They also may be dipped or rinsed when the infected pet is treated. Animals that are not visibly infected should be treated before handling or rinsing the cat with ringworm. A few cats may have ringworm that is resistant to griseofulvin.

Itraconazole or ketoconazole are oral drugs which are sometimes used to treat cats that are resistant to griseofulvin. They also should be given with food. These medications have numerous side effects, including lack of appetite, weight loss, depression, diarrhea, vomiting, and jaundice. They also should not be used in pregnant cats.

Treatment usually takes at least three to four weeks, and sometimes up to eight weeks. It is important that no daily treatments are missed. The cat's coat may appear normal within two or three weeks after treatment begins. Because the fungus spores which are already on the hair or nails are still alive and able to cause infection, it is essential to continue treatment until the claws or fur are completely grown out. For this reason, the animal should be treated for two weeks to a month after the bare spots are gone. Some infected nails may not be healed after a year of treatment.

When the cat is being treated with griseofulvin, it is not absolutely necessary to also use medication on the skin. However, if you do, it will help to shorten the time that the cat needs to be treated, by as much as half. It also will help reduce the chance the cat will infect another animal or human, or reinfect itself. Some cases recur because of reinfection from another cat, dog, or human. All animals in the house should be treated at the same time if the ringworm does not clear up quickly. Treatment always is more likely to be successful if the skin is directly treated at the same time.

Failure of ringworm to respond to griseofulvin may be because the dosage is too low or the cat has not been treated long enough.

If the claws are infected, it may be necessary to treat the cat with griseofulvin for up to six months. In addition, you may need to soak the cat's nails for 10 to 15 minutes in chlorhexidine solution (Nolvasan®, Fort Dodge) or in 2% lime-sulfur dip on a daily basis. These dips are continued until two weeks after the cat tests negative for the fungi. Lime-sulfur dip will discolor jewelry and stain paints and some woods. It has an odor of rotten eggs, which lessens as it dries. It may turn a light-colored cat's coat temporarily to a bright, mottled yellow, or it may make the cat's coat and skin dry enough that its use must be stopped. Other than these few disadvantages, lime-sulfur is a good, safe, inexpensive treatment. If these treatments do not cure the ringworm, declawing may be the only permanent cure.

A vaccine is available for treating ringworm due to Microsporum canis (Fel-O-Vax MC-K™, Fort Dodge). It is said to reduce clinical signs in as little as two weeks by stimulating the immune system to fight the disease. The vaccination also may help prevent this ringworm. A few cats will form a small lump at the injection site, which goes away within a week and does not cause any long-term problems. This vaccine is used in addition to, not instead of, routine treatment. Cats that are vaccinated before they are infected may still become infected, but have smaller, less inflamed lesions.

Cats that have just recovered from ringworm sometimes can relapse badly if treated with corticosteroids. This is especially a problem with long-acting drugs such as methylprednisolone. Healing may be delayed in cats with compromised immune systems. Cats with severe ringworm that does not respond to treatment should be checked for other diseases.

Sanitation in your home is important because ringworm is fairly contagious to children, although usually self-limiting in adult humans. It can be spread by contact with one of the hairless lesions, or by a few infected hairs, which can remain infective for a year or longer. If possible, the infected pet should be isolated in a cage or in an easily-cleaned room, such as a bathroom, until medication begins to take effect.

Vacuuming all floors and upholstered furniture will help remove contaminated hairs and fungus spores. Do it daily until the infection is controlled. You can vacuum the cat, too, if it will tolerate it. Discard the vacuum bag after each use. Wipe all hard floors and surfaces with diluted bleach solution. Hard surfaces, such as tile or counters and litter boxes, can be washed with a disinfectant solution such as household bleach. The clothing you are wearing when handling the cat, as well as its bedding, can be soaked in a solution of household bleach (one part bleach to 10 parts water), or you can "cook" it in boiling water for 20 minutes. Use the same treatment for brushes and toys. Even with the best of cleaning, it is difficult to eliminate the spores from the house with one cat in the household, and even worse with more than one. If you have the cat(s) concentrated in one room, the heating and ventilation ducts and ceiling also should be vacuumed, preferably before cleaning the floors. Chlorhexidine is not effective against ringworm on the skin.

Anyone who handles the cat should wash his or her hands with soap and water. They may first be rinsed in alcohol. Better yet, wear plastic or rubber gloves while handling an infected or suspect cat until it is known to be cured. Do not touch any part of your body, or another animal or person before washing. The disease is easily spread by objects, so bedding and toys used by the animal should be washed with a disinfectant solution such as household bleach (see above). Treating the infected individuals in a household usually will control the disease. Good sanitation goes a long way toward getting rid of ringworm in a cattery. Vacuum all vehicles used to transport cats. Disinfect all hard surfaces, cages, and crates. Disinfect or remove all toys and grooming tools. Colony owners may be quick to blame visiting cats for the disease, but it is more likely to exist continuously within resident animals. Keeping litters separated, reducing stress, and lowering the number of cats will help control ringworm as well as other diseases. New cats should be isolated and cultured for ringworm before they are introduced into the group. While waiting for results, they can be shampooed or dipped with lime-sulfur dip every five days. Vaccinating against ringworm is probably not necessary in a household, but may be the only way to stop it in a cattery.

CLAW PROBLEMS

Problems which affect only one claw or only the claws on one foot are often due to injury, tumors, or infection, especially from bite wounds. Problems which affect both feet suggest an underlying systemic disease such as feline immunodeficiency virus infection, feline leukemia, or other abnormality of the immune system which lowers disease resistance.

Bacterial infections of the claws and the skin folds around them are fairly common in cats. The area around the base of the claw, or the skin between the claws, may be reddened and painful. It may be draining pus. This generalized infection should be distinguished from an abscess, where there is a definite pocket of pus (see Abscesses, above). Bacterial cultures and/or a skin biopsy may be performed to diagnose the exact problem, determine which bacteria are involved, and pick a specific antibiotic for your cat's problem.

If it is not possible to culture the claws, trimethoprim-sulfa may be tried; it is often successful in treating these cases. Using electric clippers or curved scissors, hair should be clipped away, as completely as possible, from the affected skin and the base of the problem claw. Soak the cat's foot in lukewarm water to help remove any pus or crusty material and reduce the pain. Or, gently hold a cloth soaked in lukewarm water over the area. Carefully remove any loose material or exudate, and pat the foot dry with a soft cloth or tissues. Then, use chlorhexidine (Nolvasan®) solution for soaking the affected area. Keep the disinfectant in contact with the sore foot for three to five minutes. Again, pat it dry, removing as much of the disinfectant as possible so that the cat will not swallow it when it licks its foot.

Brittle, shredded nails occasionally are seen in cats. The most common cause is a long-term, low-grade infection, although sometimes no infection is present. They may occur in a cat that is very old, as part of the aging process. Nothing can be done to cure them, but you can make the cat more comfortable by trimming its nails frequently so the ragged edges do not catch on carpet and fabrics. Using a nail clipper often shatters the affected nail, so it is best to shorten it with a nail file, if possible.

If the nail shatters down to the quick, it will be very painful to the cat and may become infected. File off as much of the torn nail as you can. Then, mend it with cyanoacrylate glue (Superglue®), coating both the nail and the quick with one or more thin layers, allowing it to dry completely between coats. Press the claw out and hold it out until the glue has dried. You MUST keep the cat restrained through this process so the foot does not become stuck to anything. The glue will gradually wear off as the claw grows out. Meanwhile, it will protect the area against infection, moisture, and litter box mess. Or, you can bandage the foot and keep it covered for a couple of days. Most cats tolerate the glue better than they handle being bandaged, and the glue does a much better job.

Occasionally, a young cat may have fragile, crumbly claws. If there are no nutritional problems, it is probably genetic, and there is no cure for it. Another common disease which can infect the claws is ringworm (see above). When a cat has a chronic claw problem which, for any reason, cannot be cured after a reasonable attempt, declawing will give a permanent cure.

OTHER FUNGAL DISEASES

Sporotrichosis is a fungal disease that occasionally affects the subcutaneous tissues of the cat (as well as many other animals). It may begin with one sore or nodule and end up as ulcers and/or crusty, non-healing sores on one or more of the cat's feet. From there, it may spread to the head, back, and upper part of the tail as the cat grooms itself. Antibiotic treatment fails to cure the lesions, and the cat may become very thin as the disease progresses.

The organism which causes sporotrichosis is often found in the Missouri and Mississippi River Valleys, as well as in coastal regions. It occurs naturally on plants, hay, and in the soil. It is spread by rough or thorny vegetation. For this reason, it is often called "rose gardener's disease." It also may be spread by animal bites or insects. The cat may contract it from contact with another cat or from scratches from thorns or a penetrating foreign body. This disease is contagious to humans and other animals. Once diagnosed, it is important to keep the cat confined until it is under control, and to wear gloves and protective clothing while treating or handling it. Touch the cat and the secretions as little as possible (also see Werner, 1993). Ketoconazole and itraconazole are drugs used to treat this disease, but some strains may be resistant. Prognosis is guarded because drugs used for treatment are very toxic. Smaller, non-invasive masses can be removed surgically. This may eliminate the disease if it is diagnosed early.

Valley fever (coccidioidomycosis) is a fungal disease found in the soil of desert regions of the southwestern United States, especially the low deserts of Arizona and the San Joaquin Valley of California. The spores are spread from disturbed soil by wind during dry seasons. It is a significant problem in dogs, causing pneumonia and involvement of the bones. More than half the cases in cats involve the skin, including draining sores, abscesses, swollen lymph nodes, and lumpy granulomas under the skin. The cat also may have a poor appetite, weight loss, and fever. A few cats will have bone lesions. Cats seem to be fairly resistant, and cases are rare, usually occurring in middle age. Ketoconazole is the most commonly used medication, and it may be necessary to treat the cat for as long as two to three years. If stopped too soon, many cats that seemed to be cured will relapse (Greene, 1994). It is possible that the drug only suppresses the organisms rather than killing them. In some cases, treatment may not be successful (Greene, 1995).

SO YOU'RE ALLERGIC TO CATS

Many humans are allergic to cats, including myself. What can you do if this is the case and you still love and want to live with cats?

Some people have fewer problems with Siamese cats. It may be possible to convince a breeder to let you try a Siamese cat in your home to see if you can live with it. The trial should be at least a week (unless you have problems sooner). If you can tolerate the look and feel of one of the hairless breeds of cat, such as a Sphinx cat, this may be a solution.

Keeping the cat well groomed may help. It's best to have someone other than the allergic person do the grooming. Brush the cat daily, or even better, teach the cat to allow you to vacuum it. Keeping the floors mopped and vacuumed also will help keep the dander under control. If you live in a house without carpet, with only hard floor surfaces that can be wet mopped daily, this may make life easier.

It's best to keep the cat strictly out of the bedroom. Keep the door closed at all times so that the dander doesn't blow in there. Good filters in your forced-air heating or air conditioning system also may trap dander and keep it from blowing from other parts of the house into the bedroom. Electrostatic precipitators help in some houses. It may be worth trying one, at least in your bedroom, so you have pure air to breathe at night.

Some people benefit from having injections to desensitize them to the cat antigens. This is a long-term therapy where shots are given one or more times a week. It eventually may enable some people to tolerate cats. Consult an allergy specialist if you are interested.

For many years it has been considered that allergies are due to shed hair and skin debris (dander). Recent research suggests that the allergy may instead be due to the cat's saliva and the secretions from the sebaceous glands at the roots of the coat hairs. As the cat licks its hair, saliva dries, falls off in flakes, and becomes part of the environment, stimulating allergies. Because the secretion flakes are very small, they can stay airborne for a long time and float throughout the house. Frequent bathing can dry the animal's skin and coat, producing greater amounts of dandruff, flakes, and scales. Heated houses with their low humidity dry out the cat's coat, adding to the problem. Urine also contains antigens which stimulate allergic reactions. It may help to have a non-allergic person change and clean the litter box.

A company named Allerpet™ has developed a product which helps to cleanse the cat's skin and fur. It is wiped over the cat's coat once a week with a sponge or washcloth. The product is said to remove the flakes which cause allergies, making it easier for humans to tolerate cats. (Allerpet, Inc., P.O. Box 1076, Lenox Hill Station, New York, NY 10021). A brochure on pet allergies is available from Allerpet. Tranquilizers have been put into cats' food to help reduce their effects on humans. This doesn't help humans and only results in a sleepy cat.

Having outdoor cats that you can "visit" is an alternative that works for some people. Many people can tolerate contact if they don't live with the cat 24 hours a day. This is a much better alternative if you live in the country than if you live in a city, where the cat can get into a great deal of trouble (as well as being a nuisance to others).

Chapter 11

EXTERNAL PARASITES

- *Fleas*
  - *Sex and the Single Flea*
  - *Flea Allergy*
  - *Flee, Flea*
  - *Fleas and Your Cat*
  - *Flea Control Products*
  - *Fleas and Your Dog*
- *Lice*
- *Ticks*
- *Mange*
  - *Cheyletiellosis*
  - *Notoedric Mange*
- *Red Poultry Mites*
- *Maggots*
- *Cuterebra Infestation*

FLEAS

Fleas are hard-shelled, six-legged wingless insects. The adults, which you may see on your cat, are reddish, brown, or black. While they are only about one thirty-second of an inch long (less than 1 mm), they may leap as much as eight inches high and 12 inches distant (20cm/30cm). These prodigious feats are due to their extremely strong legs.

Fleas reproduce quickly. One mating pair, which may live as long as a year, can create 250,000 progeny in that year. Fleas do not do well in very cold areas such as the northern United States and parts of Canada, nor do they thrive in hot, dry climates, or in areas with cold winters such as Colorado and Wyoming. Fleas do not survive or reproduce well in altitudes of more than 5,000 feet. However, all other locations seem to be perfect, from the flea's viewpoint. Fleas don't go away by themselves. If you ignore the one or two fleas you found on your pet, soon you will have plenty of them!

Fleas are perhaps THE most predominant external parasites that infest cats. *Ctenocephalides felis*, the most common flea species in the United States, infests both cats and dogs. If animals aren't handy, these fleas are not above nipping the nearest human! They will die in one-and-a-half to two months without a blood meal from a dog or cat; human blood does not have the needed components for reproduction, so a cat flea may bite a human but cannot live on one. *C. canis*, the dog flea, is sometimes found on cats in the United States. The human flea, *Pulex irritans*, is often found on cats or dogs, especially in Mississippi and Georgia.

Fleas which otherwise infest poultry also are seen on dogs and cats in the southeastern United States. The "stick-tight" flea that infests poultry or birds (*Echidnophaga gallinacea*) is a large flea that sometimes infests cats that prey on birds. These fleas stick tightly to the cat's skin. Remove them by hand or use any of the insecticides mentioned below.

Different species of fleas infest wild animals, but do not seem to affect domestic cats and dogs. Fleas can serve as intermediate hosts for parasites, such as tapeworms, and for infectious diseases, such as plague. They can carry the tapeworm *Dipylidium caninum* to a small child (or the cat itself) that accidentally swallows a live or dead flea while grooming. In a household with a number of cats, fleas can carry the blood parasite *Hemobartonella* from one cat to another.

Small kittens may lose enough blood to fleas to become anemic. Healthy cats may support a constant small population of fleas without too much damage. This is not to say that it does them any good or that they should not be controlled! If the cat is ill and doesn't groom itself, flea numbers may greatly increase, further contributing to ill health. Fleas also may cause serious allergy problems (see Skin Disease Chapter).

SEX AND THE SINGLE FLEA

Understanding the life cycle of the flea helps in understanding how to get rid of them, both on the cat and on the premises. Adults of *C. felis* must have a meal of cat or dog blood in order to reproduce. Then it can mate and lay eggs. Given a choice, the adult flea will spend its entire life on the dog or cat, unless it falls off or is removed by scratching.

Cats that have fleas will scratch all over their bodies and lick and groom incessantly. A cat that scratches only at its cheeks until there is a raw spot below or in front of one or both ears may have ear mites or an ear infection instead of or in addition to fleas. It is NOT normal for a cat to spend much of its day scratching or grooming.

The female flea lays small whitish eggs, mostly on the cat or dog's hair. Eggs fall off into the pet's bedding, the carpet, the lawn, and everywhere else the pet goes. A female flea may lay 20 to 30 eggs per day and several hundred during her lifetime, especially if she has frequent blood meals. The eggs incubate two to 14 days before hatching.

Flea eggs hatch into tiny whitish maggot-like larvae. The larvae feed on organic material such as dandruff from the pet, dried blood, or feces from adult fleas. The larvae burrow down into lawn, carpet, or cracks in tile or flooring. They grow and molt twice, in a time span of one week to six months. This may occur in as little as two to three weeks inside your house, where there is no sunlight, drying or freezing. Now the flea larva is in the third stage in which it spins a white cocoon. In a few days, a pupa is formed inside the cocoon.

Favorable conditions for speedy completion of the life cycle include a high relative humidity (70-85%), and a temperature of 65 to 85 degrees F (18.3-29.4 C). These are nearly year-round conditions in much of the southern and southeastern United States! Vibrations from a person or pet moving around near the pupa stimulate it to emerge as a young adult.

Under ideal conditions, the flea's entire life cycle from egg to young adult may be completed in two to three weeks. It may take as long as a year if conditions are less favorable. The instant the flea emerges from its cocoon, it begins looking for dinner . . . your cat, your dog, you. . . . From egg to death of the adult, the flea's entire lifetime may be around six to 12 months. If its surroundings are suitably humid, the flea may live four to 12 months without a meal. Fleas spend as much as 90% of their life cycle somewhere other than on host animals. It is surmised that adult fleas prefer to stay on the host animal if at all possible. However, at any given time, only about one flea in a hundred will be an adult. The rest of the population will be in the egg, larval, or pupal stages. These immature stages MUST be eliminated in order to control of the that you can see!

Fleas especially like areas around the cat's head or tail because they are more moist, but they may be found anywhere on the animal. When they bite the cat, they make a tiny hole in the skin with their mouthparts and eat the blood seeping from the skin. At the same time, some of the flea's saliva gets into the wound. This is the antigen that can stimulate the cat to have a case of flea allergy (flea bite allergy, actually). If the fleas are carrying plague or typhus, this is where they "inject" it into the cat. The bite also causes itching, resulting in the cat scratching or chewing at the area. After the cat has been bitten a number of times, it becomes allergic to the bite, and has a rapid allergic reaction at a bite site. At the same time, the damaged skin may be invaded by bacteria or fungi which normally inhabit the skin surface, adding insult to injury.

Fleas are often difficult to spot, even on a short-haired white cat. It may take some time and effort to find them. Put your cat on a light-colored surface such as a white bed sheet. Fluff the cat's hair back and forth with a brush. Use a fine-toothed flea comb to check next to the skin, especially on the head and neck, under the belly, and on the cat's rump. Watch for reddish or brown specks that look like coarsely ground pepper. These are flea droppings ("flea dirt"), and confirm that fleas have recently been on your pet, even if none are now present. If you aren't sure about the specks, put a few of them on a piece of white paper and add a small amount of water. If they turn reddish after a minute or two, it confirms they are blood-filled flea droppings. You also may see small whitish specks. They are flea eggs.

FLEA ALLERGY

Flea allergy (flea bite dermatitis) is the only skin allergy common in cats. The cat becomes allergic to the flea's saliva, which flows into the wounded skin each time one of the pests steals a blood meal. Because it takes some time for this reaction to develop, flea allergy is rarely seen in cats under six to seven months of age, and becomes more common in cats three years of age or older. When an older cat is exposed to fleas for the first time, it is likely to have a severe reaction.

If you live in the southern or coastal states where fleas live year-round, the cat may have a year-round reaction. In the northern states, the allergy may be more of a problem in summer and fall. Cats that have seasonal itching are prime suspects for flea allergy.

Flea allergy can cause intense itching. At first, small red pimples are seen at the sites of flea bites. Later, the cat may have "whiteheads," especially on the belly, groin, and over the hips. In some cases, the cat's entire body may be involved. If the cat bites, chews, and scratches because of the itching, the skin may become infected, with reddening and pus. A cat that scratches mainly at the hind part of its thighs and tailhead should be considered to have fleas until proven otherwise!

Because of the allergic reaction, each flea bite may cause itching for several days. Also, fleas can bite the cat and then drop off, remaining in your carpet. Thus, the fact that you only see a few fleas on the pet does not mean that they aren't the cause of its misery. If members of the household have flea bites, your cat may have a flea allergy problem, even if you don't find fleas on it.

A cat with flea allergy may wash, groom, and scratch itself until its hair is sparse or entirely gone, especially over the back and top of the tail. The skin may be dry, itchy, inflamed, or reddened, and it may be a different color where it is most damaged. There may be seborrhea, an excessive production of skin oils, that may result in greasiness and a foul odor, or dry skin and dandruff. The cat may have pimples or pustules with reddish-brown crusts, especially on the neck and back. Or, it may have raised, moist, ulcerated plaques, mainly on the inside of the thighs and on the belly. In the worst cases, the skin down the legs to the hocks, and on the thighs, flanks, and abdomen may be involved. It may become thickened, dark-colored, and scabby or crusty. Cats that have large amounts of fleas may be anemic from blood loss.

A cat that grooms or chews to excess may have serious hair loss. Some of them may bathe so much that the coat is thin and ragged. Others will attack one specific area, leaving it completely bald. Bare spots are usually seen on the top of the back, the upper part of the tail, and the inside or rear of the thighs. The cat may chew only when alone, so you may think the hair is falling out or not growing properly. You can put an Elizabethan collar on the cat for two to three weeks; when the hair begins to grow back, it will confirm the role of excessive grooming as part of the cat's skin problem. Meanwhile, check for fleas. However, a lack of fleas on the cat does not rule out a few flea bites as the cause of the problem, especially in a cat that grooms excessively.

If the cat has any fleas, and is scratching or grooming excessively, the problem should be considered a flea allergy unless ALL fleas are totally eliminated and the problem is still present. Flea allergy is THE most common cause of severe itching skin disease in cats.

Intradermal skin testing can be useful in diagnosing flea allergic skin disease. It is not effective for desensitizing the cat. Currently, there is no flea extract that seems to be more than 50% effective in reducing a cat's sensitivity to flea bites.

The only effective treatment for flea dermatitis is to control the fleas. Total control is the only measure that will give total relief. A single flea bite can cause a reaction, with the usual itching and misery, in the allergic cat. All cats and dogs on the premises must be treated at the same time, and the house or yard should be sprayed (see below).

If you can't keep the cat (and any other pets you have) indoors and get the fleas under control, it may be impossible for the animal to gain any relief. Or, it may be possible to keep the cats inside, while aggressively treating your yard, as well as controlling fleas on your dogs.

Frequent injections of corticosteroids or the same drug in pills, given by your veterinarian, may provide some relief from symptoms. Unfortunately, life-threatening side effects are almost inevitable with long-term use of this type of medication. Antihistamines such as chlorpheniramine may give long-term relief to some itching cats, with fewer side effects. They are not, however, as effective as corticosteroids. Side effects may include excessive thirst, drowsiness, and excitability. These drugs may provide the animal some relief while flea control measures take effect. They are NOT a substitute for flea control.

A flea collar will NOT control flea allergy dermatitis. The flea collar will work only when the flea is already on the animal; thus, the flea has a chance to bite before the collar kills it, and the cat has an allergic reaction despite the collar. Injecting flea antigen to desensitize the cat has been tried, but is very expensive and usually does not work. If you have tried treating the flea allergy while being diligent about eliminating fleas, and the cat does not gain significant relief, return to your veterinarian. A cat that is allergic to fleas also may be allergic to other substances. It is also a good idea to patch-test your allergic cat with any dip or insecticide you are planning to use, to make sure there is no allergy to it.

Occasionally, cats may be allergic to insects other than fleas, such as *Culicoides* flies or mosquitos. They may have either miliary dermatitis or crusting and/or an ulcerative skin condition on the ears and nose and around the footpads. They may or may not be itching (Fadok, 1995). The best treatment for these cats is to keep them indoors when the insects are feeding, usually at dusk and dawn. If you can't do this, the cat should be treated frequently with pyrethrin gels or foams.

FLEE, FLEA

Read and strictly follow the manufacturer's instructions for any products used to control fleas. If you don't, you may be creating a hazardous situation for your family and pets and be breaking the law!

It is a good idea to consult your veterinarian about current flea control techniques. He or she can recommend a combination of products for your cat (and dog), house, and yard, which are compatible and effective. Other factors may influence the choice of products, such as whether you have small children or exotic pets. Each program must be tailored individually for the size of the indoor and outdoor areas which are involved, as well as the time of year. It will depend on whether you live in an area with freezing temperatures part of the year, or whether the climate is moderate year-round. Also, some insecticides work well in one part of the country, but are nearly useless in others because the pests have developed resistance to them.

Because of the mobile, on-the-pet, off-the-pet nature of fleas, it does little good to treat your house but not the yard, or to bathe the cat and leave the car in which it rides untouched. It's much more effective simply to declare war on the little pests, and dedicate one day every two weeks for a month or so to eradicating them. Then, utilize a maintenance program one day every two to three months. Remember, off-and-on measures don't work.

Reinfestation is the biggest reason for failure in flea control. Fleas reenter the house, carried by the cat, the dog, and people. Some people wonder why they should fight fleas in summer when the cat just goes outside and picks up more of them. Why not wait until the weather cools and take care of it then? Because it won't work. While you wait for cold weather to arrive, fleas become firmly entrenched in your house and yard, reproducing like crazy, and guaranteeing you a long, hard battle to eliminate them. Fleas can remain frozen for a year or more and thaw out, good as new. Each flea you don't get this year means dozens for next year. Meanwhile, your pet has suffered several months of needless misery, especially if it is allergic to flea bites. Most household flea problems start with a few fleas infesting the pet, and multiply from there. The key strategy is to act before the few become many.

Prevention should begin before the flea season starts in your region of the country. Don't wait until you have a visible, miserable infestation. Pets should be dipped or treated as soon as the first fleas are noticed, and the premises and house sprayed no more than two-and-a-half weeks after treating the cat (or dog).

Sanitation is an important part of flea control, both indoors and out. It should be done before any insecticidal products are used. Indoor vacuuming helps remove flea eggs and larvae from carpeting. Vacuum carpets and corners, under the sofa and chair cushions, inside closets, and between mattresses and box springs. When finished, spray insecticide into the vacuum cleaner bag and discard it.

CAUTION: It is not safe to put moth balls in a closed vacuum cleaner bag while using it; the fumes which are generated may be toxic and explosive. Do not put a piece of insect strip or flea collar in the vacuum cleaner bag, as the vacuum's air flow may spread unsafe levels of the product throughout the house.

Steam cleaning carpet is quite effective in removing and killing the eggs and developing stages of fleas. Ask the cleaning company to use an insecticide in the cleaning solution. Or, you can buy the appropriate product when renting a steam cleaning machine. Mop the floor using normal household cleaners. Take special care to clean dirt and debris out of cracks and corners. This will keep flea eggs and the organic material on which larvae feed from accumulating. Caulk holes and cracks in the walls and mopboards to eliminate a large number of fleas. They're in there, but won't be able to get out.

The cat's bed should be washed thoroughly and dried at as hot a temperature as possible to kill fleas that have fallen off the animal. Do the same with throw rugs, sofa throws, and pillows the cat uses. If your cat lies on your bed, wash all that bedding, too. If you use disposable bedding for the cat, throw it away once a week during the initial phase of the flea war. Discard it in a sealed plastic bag, preferably after spraying with an insecticide. Clean hard surfaces where the cat sleeps, such as a television, window sill, end table, or hard floor.

Outdoor cleanup is equally important before you treat the premises with insecticide. Mow the lawn, and rake all dead leaves, weeds and thatch from the lawn and yard. Houses on pilings and house trailers on blocks require special treatment and cleaning in the crawl space to eliminate trash which harbors fleas. Remove rotting lumber, and treat your woodpile along with the rest of the yard. Haul away debris so the fleas go with it. Bermuda grass and similar lawns have surface runners which make good living places for fleas. It is more difficult to control fleas in these lawns than in bluegrass and ryegrass turf. Places where the cat (or dog) sleeps outdoors need special treatment, both in cleaning and in treatment with insecticides. If your dog has dug holes in the yard or under its house, they should be treated for fleas.

For more information on cleaning up for pest control, and a wealth of general advice on pet cleanup, read, *Pet Cleanup Made Easy* by Don Aslett (Writer's Digest Books, 1507 Dana Avenue, Cincinnati, Ohio, 45207). I highly recommend this book to any pet owner!

Controlling fleas indoors may involve a spray to kill adult fleas (called an adulticide), and an insect growth-regulator hormone, such as fenoxycarb or methoprene, which kills flea larvae. These will reduce the number of applications needed to keep the pests under control. Methoprene keeps the fourth-stage flea larva from forming a pupa. It is effective for 75 to 90 days, and can be used safely in your home on that schedule to control fleas.

Using sprays such as Diazinon® or Permethrin® inside the house and in the yard can greatly reduce the flea population. Chlorpyrifos, while effective, can be cumulatively toxic to cats. Make sure the liquid has completely dried before allowing a cat onto a treated area. If a powder has been used, be sure the cat does not get it on its feet and lick it off. It is best to keep cats out of the treated area for 24 hours. Chlorpyrifos should not be directly applied to cats (Buck, 1991).

A product called sodium polyborate can be used to help control fleas indoors. It is a desiccant (drying agent) rather than an insecticide, and must be applied by a professional exterminator licensed by Rx For Fleas, Inc. It may last a year or more in a carpeted home and up to six months on tile or hardwood floors. This may be the best choice if you have small children, fish, birds or other exotic pets in your home. Pyrethrins may be added for immediate kill of adult fleas. Occasionally, there may be some dust, and shampooing the carpet will void the product warranty. The initial cost is expensive, but the one-time fee may be less than the total of repeated exterminator visits throughout the year. Similar products are available for homeowner use. These may or may not be effective, and some of them may damage no-stain carpets. They should not be used in households where the cat (or the owner) has a respiratory problem. Dust from some these products can cause attacks of asthma in humans and respiratory difficulties in animals.

Never use an outdoor chemical inside your house, and don't use chemicals on your cat that aren't specifically labeled for cats. If the cat is running loose outside your yard, it won't do much good to treat your own yard because the cat will carry fleas home from elsewhere.

Warmth and high humidity favor the growth and survival of fleas. Households with a number of cats, as well as catteries, should be kept as cool and dry as possible. Don't use a swamp cooler for cooling. Cats comfortably tolerate temperatures as low as 55 degrees F (13 C). Outside buildings, plant vegetation that needs little or no irrigation, to keep the humidity low.

Meanwhile, you have to treat, AND KEEP ON TREATING, until you have killed all the fleas which hatch from eggs on your pet and premises. Then, your job is to keep the cat from becoming reinfected. This is why one intensive campaign, with careful cleaning, will make a good start toward safe, effective elimination of fleas. Many flea control programs begin with treating pets, house, and premises on day one, day 14 , and again on day 30. After this careful beginning, you can treat every two to three months.

Which product should you use? Literally hundreds are available, from shampoos to foggers to mists to dusts—and everything in between. There is no such thing as a perfect flea control product. As with any pesticide, these chemicals must strike a delicate balance between toxicity to the pest and toxicity to people, their children, and their pets. And, pesticide resistance in fleas is an ongoing challenge, just as it is with other insects.

Below is a sample program for a household with young children, and with sensitive pets such as birds or cats. This program can be used when cats or dogs are treated with organophosphate insecticides such as fenthion or cythioate, PROVIDED you choose a house and yard insecticide different from organophosphate or carbamate. Many organophosphates are toxic to cats, especially in dips and powders. Ronnel® and Malathion® are safe for use on cats, but only at concentrations lower than those used on dogs. Be sure to follow the dilution carefully.

Day 1. Thoroughly clean house. Spray all surfaces, crevices, and the bottom couple of feet of the drapes and walls with an insecticidal spray. Do NOT use one which contains carbamates or organophosphates. Before spraying, remove birds, fish, and other pets from the area, as well as their food and water dishes. Be sure to cover or remove all human food, too.

Air the house well before you (and the pets) return. Several hours after spraying is completed, wash food and water containers and fill them with fresh contents. Wash any people dishes and utensils that were exposed to the insecticide.

The entire house must be sprayed at one time. Otherwise, fleas just move from one room to another. When spraying the dog house and garage, use products made for indoor use. If you have sprayed the house with a microencapsulated (slow release) product, avoid vacuuming as long as possible to allow the microcapsules to work.

Clean the yard. In the evening, cover it with a spray or dust (dusts or granular products can be applied with a fertilizer spreader). Be careful to work the material into corners and crevices, around plants, into bushes, and under low trees. Also, treat the children's sandbox. The next day, water the insecticide in thoroughly. Allow the area to dry completely before you return your pet (or children!) to it. Be sure to spray the dog house inside and out—roof, ceiling, floor, and walls—and the crawl space and the area under the porch if the dog or cat goes there. Products containing an organophosphate can be used, providing the label says they are safe for cats, and that you keep the cat from walking in the yard for the recommended length of time.

Treat your cat at the same time with a product appropriate for cats. Do not give the cat (or dog) fenthion or cythioate on the same day you treat the premises or house.

Day 14. Same as day one, including the cleaning.

Day 30 or 31. Repeat the entire process again.

From then on, clean and treat the house every two to three months just like day one. Every two weeks, retreat the yard and premises, cleaning as necessary. Do this as long as the nighttime temperature is above 50 degrees F (10 C).

Treat your cat by dipping or shampooing it. Again, be sure not to use an organophosphate or carbamate insecticide on the cat at the same time you are using these products to treat the house or yard. Otherwise, your cat may receive an overdose. If you are using a pyrethrin-type product in the yard, this can be used on the cat (or dog) at the same time without problems. Pyrethrins are very safe products. Microencapsulated products last for varying periods of time, and are made for use on both the premises and on animals. Consult product directions for reapplication intervals.

Carbamates and organophosphates belong to a class of chemicals called cholinesterase inhibitors. If you are looking for a product without these, it may say, "does not contain cholinesterase inhibitor." Both can be quite toxic to cats if overdosed. Be extremely careful to measure them precisely and apply them as directed by the label. Signs of toxicity include salivation, vomiting, diarrhea, sweating, gasping, and death. A cat that has been poisoned should be washed thoroughly to remove as much insecticide as possible from the fur. Wear rubber gloves to avoid absorbing the insecticide yourself.

If the cat has NOT been treated with a carbamate or organophosphate insecticide, products such as Malathion® are good for yard use. Foggers containing methoprene use insect growth hormones to kill the larvae, and can be used in conjunction with any other insecticide.

You can call an exterminator to treat the house and premises, while, at the same time, you take the cats and dogs to the veterinarian or groomer for a dipping or treatment. Be sure you know which product each one is using. However, cleaning before the exterminator arrives is essential. Exterminators sometimes treat only the perimeter of the room, which does not get rid of the fleas. It is necessary to treat the carpet, furniture, under the furniture, one or two feet up every wall, and the lower part of the draperies to reach all the areas where fleas commonly hide. Treat all rooms in your house, whether your pet frequents them or not. You probably have carried some fleas around on your body, moving from room to room, and you do not want to leave any safe haven for the pests. Discuss the job you want done with the exterminator to be sure there is a complete understanding of how thorough you want the treatment to be. Ask what insecticide will be used so you can tell your veterinarian or groomer. Make sure the product used is safe for use around cats.

FLEAS AND YOUR CAT

Fleas LOVE cats! The free-roaming cat is one of the biggest factors in keeping itself, your dog, and your home well supplied with fleas. It does little good to confine your dog, treat it for fleas, treat the premises, and let your little four-legged feline flea taxi run loose. The cat goes freely from one yard to another, where the tiny pests hop on for a ride home. Your best efforts at flea control will come to nothing if your cat roams through your neighbors' untreated yards, reinfesting your house and yard.

The single easiest thing you can do to help reduce your flea population is to keep your cat indoors! It is not harmful to do so. Cats that live in single-cat households and those that are kept indoors are at very low risk from fleas.

Cats that live in your carefully treated house and remain in your insecticide-treated yard also can be free of fleas. However, feral cats cruising through your yard at night may reinfest it with fleas even with the best control program.

FLEA CONTROL PRODUCTS

This section is merely an overview of flea control formulations which are available. New products are being developed every day, and old ones are being removed from the market.

Be sure that whatever flea product you use is specifically labeled for use on cats, or is recommended by your veterinarian for use on them. Don't take the word of a pet shop employee that it's suitable for cats. Many products meant for dogs are toxic to cats, and using one of these may be fatal. Chlorpyrifos and Blockade® (Hartz Mountain) have been found to be toxic to cats. DO NOT use these products on your cat (Whitley and Melman, 1987). Remember, anything you apply inside or outside your house will eventually end up inside the cat when it grooms itself.

A flea comb with very fine teeth (30 or more per inch) can be purchased at the drugstore or pet shop. This comb is one of the simplest and safest flea treatments, especially for tiny kittens and puppies. Comb against the direction of hair growth. Use it along with cleaning and spraying the house or premises to minimize the flea load until young animals are old enough to tolerate being treated with insecticides.

Flea control products come in a wide variety of forms: shampoos, dips, dusts, powders, sprays (both water- and alcohol-based), mousses (foams), foggers, mists, and any other form that a manufacturer thinks might entice you to buy the product. You should have no problem finding product(s) for your particular situation.

Shampoos are primarily used to clean the cat's skin and haircoat. They may contain pyrethrin-type products to kill fleas present at the time the cat is bathed, but generally do not have any residual effect for flea control. For that reason, shampoo won't kill fleas that jump on the cat after it is bathed.

Shampooing may be followed by a dip or spray that has a residual killing action. If you plan treatment after bathing the cat, be sure to dry it with a towel so that the dip or spray isn't diluted by water in the cat's coat. Some flea shampoos do contain an insecticide with residual action, such as carbamate insecticides. If you are using one of these products, do not dip or spray the cat, or treat the premises at the same time with a carbamate or organophosphate-type product.

Dips are meant to have some residual activity against fleas. For that reason, they are not rinsed out of the cat's coat. The cat should not be towel dried after the dip is applied. Allow it to dry naturally or use a blow dryer. Confine the cat while the fur dries so the cat does not rub the dip out of its hair. Watch that the cat does not lick its coat while the insecticide is wet, as an excessive amount of it may be ingested, resulting in a toxicity. Before dipping, protect the cat's eyes with a dab of eye ointment or drop of salad oil in each one. Most dips should not be used on kittens fewer than four months of age unless recommended by your veterinarian.

Dipping may be done in a vat of prepared insecticide. Many veterinary clinics and animal shelters in the south keep a vat mixed up and ready at all times. Or the "dip" compound may be sponged onto the cat. In any case, apply it gently and carefully to the cat's face, using a sponge or saturated cloth. In addition to the residual effect, dips immediately kill fleas when the cat is well saturated (so the product makes contact with the fleas). Dips soak into a thick or matted hair coat more effectively than sprays. Wear rubber gloves while applying the dip.

Be sure to mix the dip according to directions. With insecticides of any kind, it's not true that if "a little bit is good, a lot is better." A "lot" may be fatal. Most dips cannot be stored for more than about a day after they are mixed; then, they lose effectiveness. Mix each batch just before you are ready to use it. Be careful when discarding leftover dip so that you do not put it where an animal might drink it, or contaminate a water supply. Some dip insecticides will kill fish, so be careful that it doesn't run into a stream.

Because some cats may be extremely sensitive to chemicals used in flea-control products, test any new product which will be applied directly to your cat's skin. Apply it to no more than one-third of the cat. Check the cat several times in the next 12 to 24 hours, watching for redness, swelling, itching, or irritation. If there is no reaction, you can use the product on the entire cat, according to label instructions.

Dusts or powders were once the most common method of flea control on pets, but have been largely replaced by sprays. Some dusts are useful for treating carpet and other flooring, furniture and vacuum cleaner bags before they are discarded. A flea powder containing 5% carbaryl can be mixed half-and-half with talcum powder. This gives a 2 1/2% product which is safe to use on kittens (and puppies). Carbaryl is fairly safe for cats, but may stain the cat's fur and any carpet or furniture it contacts. Powders may not work well on cats with dense undercoats such as Persians, or on cats with very sparse coats. They may dry the cat's fur.

Sprays or mists give a quicker kill of adult fleas living on the cat than do dusts or powders. They also are easier to apply to the underside of the cat. Pump-type sprayers may be tolerated well by even shy cats. The alcohol base of some sprays may irritate cuts or sores on the cat's skin, and may make the cat drool profusely. If this occurs, change to a water-based spray, which is also less drying to the cat's coat. These products are usually pre-mixed and ready to use straight from the sprayer. Sprays which contain pyrethrins do not build up, so they are good for frequent use.

Even if the label says it is safe, it may be risky to use flea spray on a kitten, especially one fewer than six weeks of age. Instead, dilute a water-based natural pyrethrin spray with water, dip a flea comb in the mixture, and comb fleas off the kitten. Bathe the queen and rinse her thoroughly so the kittens do not lick or suck the insecticide from her coat.

As you are spraying, lift the cat's coat with a comb. This allows better penetration of the spray. The cat should be well dampened but not soaked. If your cat doesn't tolerate spraying or dipping, use a Brush-Ette®: The spray, which is poured into the handle, flows out through hollow bristles into the cat's coat. Many cats that will not tolerate sprays will permit brushing with this brush. Use a spray from time to time on your grooming tools to kill fleas that might linger there.

Aerosol flea sprays also are available. Some can be used on either cats or dogs, if the pet will tolerate the noise and blowing air. They usually cost about twice as much as pump spray products. If you are concerned about the environment, find an aerosol that doesn't use a fluorocarbon as the propellant.

Sprays that are meant for animals can be used on the cat's bedding, or on your furniture or carpet. However, they are usually much more expensive than sprays meant for that purpose. And, they often contain coat conditioners, repellents, and other ingredients that are wasted on your carpet. Flea repellents, as such, are not helpful in a flea control program. The goal is to get rid of the pests, not redistribute them from one animal to another or to your house, where they can continue to multiply and pester your pets.

When applying spray to a cat, be sure it does not get into the eyes, nose or mouth. Puff a bit of spray onto a cotton ball and wipe it around the cat's face. Use a routine each time you spray so you don't miss any spots. Be sure to spray between the toes and footpads where fleas can hide. As much as possible, try to keep the cat from licking itself after the spraying.

Many sprays are formulated for use in the kennel or yard. The concentrated form is often called an emulsifiable concentrate. These products are usually applied with a garden-type sprayer after diluting them with water to the proper mix. Most of them contain either carbamate or organophosphate insecticides, which give a reasonably good residual insecticidal action; otherwise, it would be necessary to spray every day. They often have a strong and rather unpleasant odor. Do NOT use a yard or kennel spray on your cat. It may contain compounds as carriers which are harmful to the cat, or the product itself may be harmful. A few products are available which can be used either as dips or premise sprays. If you use one, read the label carefully to avoid giving your cat an overdose. The concentrations may change for different uses.

Ready-to-use sprays diluted in water are generally less expensive than those diluted in alcohol. They are slow to dry on both pets and fabrics, but do not catch fire. Water-based sprays do not soak into a greasy coat.

Alcohol-based sprays are much more expensive. One advantage is that they dry quickly. Also, the alcohol easily penetrates the flea's shell, giving a rapid kill. They also work well on cats with greasy coats. However, they catch fire easily, so the freshly treated cat, furniture, carpet, and other items must be kept away from fire and flame. In addition to the fire hazard, there are several disadvantages to alcohol-based products: The alcohol may dry out the cat's coat; it may be irritating to inflamed or injured skin; and it may damage some plastics and wood finishes. It is very important that sprays with an alcohol base be applied in an area with good ventilation.

Sprayers used for diluting and applying insecticides should be washed well with soap and water after use. Otherwise, seals and hoses may be damaged by long-term exposure to the organic solvents.

Foams or mousses are now available for flea control. These may be the best flea products yet invented for use on cats. Spray the foam onto your hand and then rub it into the coat (use rubber gloves!). Some of them contain microencapsulated pyrethrins, giving long-term release of the insecticide. One problem with foams is that they may create a peculiar spiked hairdo on a long-haired cat. Examples of foam products are Sectrol Two-Way Flea Foam® (Animal Care Products/3M) and Sectillin™ Flea and Tick Mousse® (Bio-Ceutic), which can be used on both cats and dogs.

Foggers or bombs are used indoors. They are popular because they are easy to use, but may not be the most effective choice. While the label on the can may say it will treat several thousand square feet, in reality most of the fog falls within 15 or 20 feet of the container. The material does not go into the corners of rooms or through doors very well. For these reasons, it is usually more effective to use one smaller fogger for each room. Foggers also do not penetrate behind draperies and under furniture, including tables and chairs. If you have a serious pest problem, it is best to spray under furniture, behind drapes, and behind items in closets before fogging. Sprays are more effective than foggers, and can be used in areas such as under furniture cushions, in closets, and under furniture, which most need treatment.

The insecticides contained in foggers are effective against fleas, as well as ticks and mites. They have the added advantage of getting rid of flies and moths. Most foggers contain an organophosphate insecticide with residual action, which, on the carpet, often is effective against the larval stages of fleas. Until you are sure you have the flea problem under control, it is a good idea to spray and fog every room twice a month. Usually, if combined with good sanitation, this can be done for three treatments, followed by a two to three month schedule for fogging and spraying.

Flea collars are plastic strips impregnated with an organophosphate insecticide which is released slowly. Flea collars only kill the small percentage of fleas which are near the cat's head; most fleas are on the back, hind legs, and tail. They are convenient, but are a negligible part of the flea control picture. They don't do much by themselves, and they can cause more problems than they cure.

If you buy a flea collar, make sure it is fresh and change it at the recommended intervals. Be sure there is at least an inch of space between the cat's neck and the collar to allow the cat to pull free if it gets caught. A breakaway collar which releases if the cat gets caught is an excellent safety feature. Never use a flea collar on a kitten fewer than four-months-old, or on a cat that is sick or does not have fleas. Flea collars are no help to cats with flea allergies, as the flea is already on the cat and biting before the collar can kill it. Check the cat frequently to make sure there are no sores, reddened spots or bald spots under the collar. The drug from a flea collar can accumulate and cause toxicity in the cat. If the flea collar becomes wet, it can release much more insecticide than it is supposed to. Remove it immediately if the cat is out in the rain or dew-dampened grass or if you are giving the cat a bath. If you suspect your cat will need surgery, remove the flea collar immediately. But BE SURE to tell your veterinarian that you have done so, as this information must be considered when administering anesthetic to the cat.

Flea Egg-Control Collars (Ovitrol®, Vet-Kem) are available. They break the flea life cycle by stopping the development of flea eggs and larvae, and are said to sterilize adult female fleas. Flea-growth inhibitors are not insecticides as such and are very safe for use on cats. When used along with treatment of the home and yard, long-term flea control can be successful. Vet-Kem's Flea Infestation Prevention Pack™ is guaranteed to control fleas for eight months.

Electronic (ultrasonic) flea collars have been sold for use on cats. The high-frequency sound waves are supposed to reduce flea numbers or keep fleas off the cat. One study showed that an average of 98% of the fleas were still on the cats after one week of treatment (Dryden, 1989). In addition, they may annoy a cat that has normal hearing. Don't use them.

Systemic treatments are available for fleas on dogs. They are not approved for cats, and are generally not safe for feline friends except when used by a veterinarian in special circumstances.

Insect growth regulators are among the latest entries into the flea-control arsenal. Fleas on cats can be controlled by products such as Ovitrol Plus (Vet-Kem®, Zoecon Corp., Dallas, TX). This type of product contains a hormone, methoprene (Precor® Insect Growth Regulator), and natural pyrethrins. It can be used on the cat's fur, and will kill flea eggs which have been deposited there. This will help prevent outdoor cats from reinfesting your house with fleas. The hormone keeps flea pupae from changing into adults, and they eventually die without reproducing. Pyrethrins give a three- to five-day residual action against adult fleas, and methoprene kills fleas for a longer period of time. Using this type of product once a month on all cats and dogs in the household will go a long way toward flea control. Retreat as often as necessary to kill adult fleas. If fleas are especially serious, it may be necessary to dip, mousse, or shampoo the cat before treating with this type of product. In problem areas, you also can treat the cat every five to seven days on a year-round basis, using a long-acting pyrethrin product. Methoprene is good to use in areas where babies will be crawling. It also is available as a fogger.

A non-toxic, once a month liquid flea control product, lufenron (Program®, Ciba-Geigy), is available for cats more than six weeks of age. It is mixed with moist cat food and fed as a treat. This product is not an insecticide. Think of it as "birth control for fleas." The flea sucks blood from a treated cat, and lufenron is deposited in the eggs. Most of them do not hatch and the few larvae that do soon die. The same product is available for dogs. When used on all pets in the household, lufenron should give long-term flea control. If you are just starting to attack a flea infestation, use standard insecticides and insect-growth regulator products to help kill adult fleas that are already in the environment until the lufenron can take effect.

A biological control product is available for use on soil or sand outdoors. A nematode (a type of very small worm) has been found to be parasitic on flea larvae and cocoons. Flea eggs are not susceptible, but the larvae are attacked by the nematodes when they hatch. The nematodes are mixed with water and sprayed with any convenient sprayer. These natural flea predators are non-toxic to children and pets. Their effect on your yard is said to last up to four weeks in damp weather, after which they need to be reapplied. The lawn must be watered at least weekly to keep the nematodes alive. Temperatures higher than 95 degrees F (35 C) or lower than 45 degrees F (7 C) are fatal to the nematodes. When the predators have killed all the available flea larvae, they die and biodegrade. Brand names include Interrupt™, (VPL, P.O.Box 34820, Phoenix, Arizona 85067), Bio Flea Halt™ (Biosys) and Bio Safe™ (Ortho).

Flea traps can be used because fleas, like other insects, are attracted to light. You can make a flea trap by setting a lamp (safely secured so it will not tip) over a pan of water. Put a few drops of dishwashing detergent into the water to break the surface tension so the fleas will sink and drown. Or you can buy a trap which has a light and uses a sticky surface to catch the fleas. One example is the Pulvex Flea Trap (Zema Corporation, P.O. Box 12803, Research Triangle Park, NC 27709, or at your pet shop or feed store). Traps can be used in one room until you no longer catch fleas, and then taken to another room. Be sure to rotate the trap through each room about every 15 to 20 days to catch the new crop of pests as they hatch and mature.

Citrus extract (d-limonene) is derived from the peel of citrus fruits and used in sprays and other formulas for external use. Some of these products have caused toxic reactions in cats. If you wish to use them, Hill's VIP Products is one reliable brand which is available. They seem to be fairly effective at killing fleas, but do not offer the residual insecticidal action of pyrethrin products."

Natural" flea-control products vary from somewhat helpful to totally useless for anything except separating you from your money. Giving the cat sulfur or garlic does not help control the flea problem. In addition, anemia may be seen in cats that are fed garlic pearls. Doses of thiamine (one of the B vitamins) have been proven to be ineffective against fleas in dogs (Halliwell, 1982). It does not seem to be any more effective in cats. Brewer's yeast has been suggested, but a study at the School of Veterinary Medicine at the University of California at Davis found that the effect is only temporary, and of no lasting value.

Ultrasonic boxes for use in the house are not helpful, and may eventually cause damage to your ears. Fleas do not have ears, so the ultrasound doesn't bother them. They are attracted by the cat's body heat, the vibrations as the cat moves, the change in light level caused by the cat's presence, and the increase of carbon dioxide in the area from the cat's breath. The same conditions stimulate pupae to hatch into adults.

Diatomaceous earth, boric acid, and silica gel are sometimes recommended for flea control. They act to kill fleas by drying out their body fluids. Boric acid is found in 20 Mule Team Borax laundry detergent. Diatomaceous earth is used in swimming pool filters and can be purchased from pool suppliers. These products have a very abrasive structure, and can rapidly cut through and damage carpet fibers and furniture upholstery. They do seem to be fairly effective, however, at killing fleas. Sodium polyborate is used as a household treatment under the name Rx for Fleas, Inc. (1-800-666-3532).

A number of companies make integrated lines of flea control products for your cat, dog, home, and yard. Examples are the Vet-Kem® Flea Control Guarantee Program (Vet-Kem® Div. of Zoecon, Dallas, TX 75234), and Pitman-Moore's Defend™ Flea and Tick Control Products. Available from your veterinarian, they are made to work together, safely and effectively, and usually work better than a random bunch of bottles from the drug or grocery store.

There are NO short cuts to flea control. It must be done thoroughly and completely. There is NO point at which flea control is "finished." Parasites come back, whether your animals bring them, or whether you accidentally carry them home from the park.

FLEAS AND YOUR DOG

What is a section on flea control in dogs doing in a cat book? Fleas LOVE cats, but they also like dogs, and it does little good to control them on one type of animal in your household without treating the other. Some products that are not normally used on cats do a great job of flea control on dogs. They can be helpful in getting your pest problem under control.

Systemic flea control products are used in dogs to control fleas, ticks, lice, and other sucking and biting pests. They kill the pest when it feeds on the dog's blood or body fluids. One of these products, Proban® (Haver) is given orally as a liquid or tablet. It contains an organophosphate insecticide which spreads throughout the dog's body and works quite effectively to kill adult fleas on the dog. It is not currently approved for cats, and should not be used on them.

If your cat sleeps with or grooms your dog, be sure your veterinarian does not use Defend® EXspot® on the dog. This powerful insecticide (permethrin) is placed on the dog's back. The cat may ingest enough to make it ill. This insecticide should not be used on cats, but can be effective on dogs whose feline housemates are less intimate.

If you have a large acreage and the dog ranges widely, it is difficult to treat the entire property with insecticide. It may be more realistic to treat an area about 50 feet outward from the doors the dog uses. Keep a can of flea spray close to the door, and use it to spray the dog's legs as it goes out and in. This will cut down the number of fleas the dog brings indoors. Dogs seem to be more susceptible to flea allergy than cats, but fleas may be more attracted to cats. This means that in some homes the cat carries the pests home and the dog itches. Flea allergies can be a serious problem for cats (see Skin Care Chapter).

LICE

Lice are wingless insects that live their lives on their favorite host animal. They are flattened from top to bottom, and are often brownish or dirty gray in color. They are rarely found on cats unless the animal is ill, anemic, or elderly. Lice also occur when cats are overcrowded, stressed, malnourished, or kept in dirty conditions. Lice and their tiny eggs (called "nits") may look like fine dandruff clinging to the cat's hair. Some cases of lice cause severe itching and hair loss, while others show almost no symptoms. Cats that scratch may have thickened skin with surface scrapes and hair loss. Lice may be especially numerous in mats near the ears and elsewhere on the body. Cats with large numbers of lice may be weakened and anemic, and some become grouchy and hostile.

Felicola subrostratus is the most common biting louse which infests cats. The common dog louse, Trichodectes canis, is occasionally seen on elderly cats in poor health or on kittens. If your dog has lice, be sure to check your cats. Cat lice do not live on humans, but may crawl on persons in close contact with the cat.

You may be able to diagnose a case of lice by holding a sheet of clean white paper under the cat. Scratch and rub vigorously down to the cat's skin. If lice are present, the tiny (about one-sixteenth inch (1 mm)) cigar-shaped insects will fall onto the paper. Lice move by crawling rather than hopping. They go from one cat to the next by direct contact or through infested carpet or bedding.

Lice are treated with the same medications as for fleas, above, and the surroundings also should be cleaned and treated. Clip off hair mats before treating the cat. Retreat the cat once or twice a week, for at least three to four weeks. This will kill new lice hatched since the last treatment. Factors contributing to the infestation should be corrected.

TICKS

Ticks are arachnids (eight-legged) rather than insects (six-legged). Tick larvae have only six legs. All ticks have four stages in their life cycles: egg, larva (seed ticks), nymph, and adult. All stages of both sexes are parasites and feed on blood and lymphatic fluids. The adult male has a hard shell which does not expand after feeding; however, adult females, nymphs, and larvae swell to several times their original size after a meal. Ticks may hibernate through the winter, becoming especially active in the spring when searching for a meal.

Ticks are larger than fleas, ranging from about one-sixteenth inch in length (1 mm) to a blood-filled female tick which may be a half-inch (1.3 cm) long. They are usually brown or grayish, hard-shelled, and flattened. A blood-filled female may look like a glossy bead hooked to the skin at one end. In the woods and wilds, ticks are carried by wild rodents and deer. Ticks can climb onto a cat that is walking through a grassy or wooded area, or they can hitch a ride home on your dog, drop off, and climb onto your cat. Ticks are usually not a problem if both your cats and dogs are kept indoors. They are a minor problem in suburban cats. Ticks can be a significant pest to free-roaming rural pets, although cats seem to have fewer ticks than dogs. Perhaps cats pick off some of them while grooming. You may feel the tick as a lump on the cat before you see it.

The tick burrows into the skin and begins sucking blood. If the cat has enough ticks infesting it, a life-threatening anemia may occur. Ticks also carry several diseases, including Lyme disease, Rocky Mountain spotted fever, and tularemia. Indeed, they are more likely to cause disease by carrying it from one animal to another or to you than by the damage they cause the cat.

Pets are occasionally affected by Lyme disease, which is relatively easy to treat if detected early. Left untreated, it can lead to arthritis, meningitis, and damage to the heart and kidneys. If you live in an area where Lyme disease occurs, your cat is far more likely to act as a taxi, bringing ticks inside that later crawl onto you, giving you the disease, than the cat is to contract it. Or, the tick may crawl onto your carpet, and later climb onto your dog, giving it Lyme disease. You may detect the tiny stage of the tick, the nymph, which is considered to be most infective, by rolling a masking tape lint roller over the cat's coat, especially the head and body. Or, you can use a flea comb on the cat. If you live in Lyme disease country, diligent, continuing tick control on your pets and in your yard is a necessity to keep you and your family from getting the disease. Easier yet, make the pet(s) strictly indoor animals and make life safer for everyone.

If a tick attaches to your cat, use a pair of blunt tweezers to remove it. Either wear rubber gloves or cover your fingers with a paper towel to keep from getting any material from the tick on your skin. This will help prevent you from acquiring any disease from the tick. Do not use your fingers to remove the tick. Many ticks are too small to effectively hold, and squeezing them too hard may cause a pumping action, pushing infected material into the pet. Grasp the tick as closely as possible to the skin. Pull upward with a firm, gentle, steady pressure. Do not jerk or twist the tick, as you may break it apart, leaving the mouthparts in the cat's skin. If mouthparts do end up left in the skin, they will fester out, much like a splinter.

Do not let the tick, or any fluid from it, touch your bare skin, as disease-causing agents could enter through your mucous membranes, or through any cut or scratch. Do not puncture, squeeze, or crush the tick if you can avoid it. Dispose of the tick by immersing it in a disinfectant such as alcohol or household bleach. Disinfect the site where you removed the tick. Then, thoroughly wash your hands and the tweezers with a disinfectant such as 1:32 bleach in water. Hydrogen peroxide is NOT an adequate disinfectant. Applying home remedies such as petroleum jelly, kerosene, gasoline, nail polish remover, or a burning match in an attempt to remove the tick are not effective.

MANGE

Mange is the name given to skin disease caused by one of several microscopically tiny mites (arachnids). Severe mange is often seen in dogs, but is very rare in cats. Demodectic ("red") mange can cause dogs to be nearly hairless, and may affect several dogs in one litter or group. It is common in the southeastern United States. In the rare cases when demodectic mange infests a cat, the animal is usually suffering from another illness which has left it weakened and susceptible. Examples are feline leukemia, FIV, diabetes mellitus, and feline distemper. Demodectic mange in cats tends to be a more mild disease than in dogs. It may show up just on the head (ears, chin, bridge of the nose, and around the eyes). Very rarely, it covers the body, with hair loss or reddened, crusty areas. Some cases may be symmetrical from one side of the cat to the other, suggesting endocrine disease or neurodermatitis. Chronic demodectic mange cases may include darkening of the skin. There is little or no itching with one type of demodectic mite, while another causes extreme itching. Mild cases usually resolve themselves without treatment.

It is assumed that demodectic mange is usually transmitted from the queen to her kittens shortly after birth. Many, perhaps most, normal cats have a number of Demodex organisms in their skin with no signs of disease. Demodectic mange does not seem to be contagious between adult cats or to humans or other animals. (Treatment: Veterinary Medicine Magazine, Dec. 1994, p. 1117).

Sarcoptic mange is also very rare in cats, usually seen in animals with suppressed immune systems. It is common in dogs, and pet pot-bellied pigs, and can infest humans, causing severe itching.

Cat fur mites (Lynxacarus radovsky) occasionally infest cats in Florida, Puerto Rico, and Hawaii. These mange mites do not burrow into the skin like the others, but live on the surface. This infestation is recognized by a "salt and pepper" scurfiness or scaliness on the skin and among the hairs. The cat may also have scabs and sores on the skin surface. The disease is spread from one cat to another, but may not involve all cats in a household. Humans are not affected by cat fur mites.

Grain mites (harvest mites, chiggers, Trombicula autumnalis) may infest outdoor cats. The mites live in fields and forests in decaying vegetation. Small rodents may carry them to cats (that may occasionally carry them to humans). The cat's ears, face, feet and belly may be crusted, and it may itch severely. The skin may be scaly and hair loss may occur. This disease is usually seen in the summer and fall. The mites' red-orange larvae cause the itching, but may be gone by the time the animal is closely examined.

Your veterinarian will diagnose mange by taking a scraping from the cat's skin. In some cats this may cause a little bleeding. It is necessary to help diagnose the disease and is not harmful to the cat.

Lime-sulfur (1.6%) dip once a week for three to nine weeks will usually cure these types of mange. The premises should be treated as for fleas, above.

The drug ivermectin, an injectable wormer which is used in dogs, cattle, and horses, is not approved for use in cats. However, when given in carefully regulated amounts by your veterinarian, it can be safely and effectively used to treat cases of mites and mange (especially sarcoptic mange) which do not respond to other treatment. If nothing else works, it's worth a try, and may cure your pet's misery. In excessive dosages, ivermectin products can be toxic to cats, and should never be used on kittens. Do NOT use cattle, horse, or dog wormer on your cat. There is a great possibility you might kill it. Ivermectin usually works well on sarcoptic and notoedric mange, but generally does not affect demodectic mange.

Corticosteroids should never be given to cats infested with any kind of mange mites. They will lower the body's defenses against the mites and may allow them to spread.

CHEYLETIELLOSIS

Cheyletiella species are large mange mites which spend their entire life cycle on their host animal. They infest the skin surface of rabbits, dogs, and occasionally, cats, feeding on skin debris. When this infection is seen in catteries, it is often called "walking dandruff." Signs are most common in kittens. The cat's haircoat may be filled with white scales and flakes of skin. The cat's back is often the most severely affected, but grooming may remove much of the debris, making it more difficult to find mites. The top of the cat's head also may be badly affected. The cat shows little or no itching. Cats that do not have symptoms may be carriers, spreading the highly contagious disease to people or other cats around them, and should be treated accordingly.

It is sometimes possible to see the white mites walking on the skin by using a high-powered magnifying glass. You also can use a piece of clear tape; stick it to the dandruff on the cat's coat, remove it, and examine it. Or, you may be able to see the mites if you comb through the cat's hair with a flea comb and examine it with a magnifying glass. Occasionally the mites can be seen crawling in and out of the cat's nostrils. Mites may be difficult to find because of the cat's careful grooming.

This type of mange can be treated with some medications which are effective against fleas, such as a single treatment with 0.2% Malathion® in water dip or a carbaryl shampoo. Lime-sulfur dip also works well and is ideal for kittens, pregnant or nursing queens, or cats that are ill. Bathe the cat gently to remove scales and crusts before medicating it. Treat the cat with lime-sulfur AT LEAST three times, one week apart. Treatment may be needed for four to eight weeks until mites are no longer found. Not all flea products are effective against this mange when used alone. Whatever product is used, repeated treatments are the key to the cure. Treat all pets on your premises. Flea-control products which contain pyrethrins are useful as well as safe. Your veterinarian may treat this mange with two or three injections of ivermectin (see Mange, above).

These mites don't live more than a couple of weeks when removed from the pet. Spray the premises with a product such as Malathion® as its residual action will help kill the mites. It may be necessary to treat every two weeks for a total of six to eight weeks to eradicate them. Use the same control methods as you would for a flea infestation.

Cheyletiella mites can accidentally infest humans who come into contact with the pet. Since they do not reproduce on humans, the irritation goes away within three weeks after the cat is treated and no longer providing mites.

NOTOEDRIC MANGE

This type of mange is rare overall, but is common in a few areas such as northern islands in the Florida Keys. It also is called feline scabies, but can infest rabbits, dogs, and foxes. The most prominent sign is intense itching. The cat scratches and licks vigorously, leading to complete hair loss and raw, bleeding skin. First signs may appear on the tips of the ears, then on the rest of the face and neck. Sores may be seen on the feet, probably because of the cat's washing, and on the tail and perineum because of the way it curls up to sleep. In young cats, the entire body may be covered. Small pimples and grayish or yellow crusts may be seen on the skin. Badly affected cats may have thickened and darkened skin. Secondary bacterial infections may occur, and severe cases may be fatal.

Your veterinarian will diagnose notoedric mange by microscopic examination of skin scrapings. Treatment is the same as for cheyletiellosis, above. All animals in the household must be treated. Under the right humidity and warmth, mites can survive for a few weeks in the environment. This mite can infest humans and cause severe itching.

RED POULTRY MITES

The red poultry mite, Dermanyssus gallinae, is often seen on farms where chickens are raised. During the day, it lives in roosts and nests, coming out at night to feed on the chickens. It may occasionally infest dogs, humans, pet birds, or farm cats, especially those that live in or around poultry housing. These small whitish-gray or blackish mites may be seen crawling on the cat's hair, using a magnifying glass. They are red only if they have had a meal of blood. Crusty, bumpy sores and pimples resembling those from cheyletiellosis (see above) are seen around the cat's lips and elsewhere on its face. There is severe itching, especially on the back and feet. The cat can be treated with lime-sulfur dip or any product approved for use on cats that will kill fleas. For the good of the poultry, people, and other pets, the chicken house and yard should be carefully cleaned, and the poultry should be treated to eliminate the infestation.

MAGGOTS

Common blow flies normally lay their eggs in dead carcasses and rotting meat. If the cat is ill or injured, or its hair is matted with blood, urine or feces, these flies may lay their eggs on the soiled hair. This happens when the cat is outdoors part or all of the time, and is seen in warm weather. It is more common with longhaired cats that are unable to groom themselves, and on whom cuts or bite wounds may go unnoticed. The masses of white or yellow eggs hatch within 12 hours, and the larvae ("maggots") begin to eat the soiled material. As they move about on the cat's skin, they produce enzymes which dissolve protein, causing severe irritation and damage. As this activity causes holes in the skin, the maggots may move in and out of the holes, eating the damaged tissue. The skin may end up with numerous small holes, or a few large, ragged-edged sores. The odor is unbelievably foul, like rotting meat, and this may be the first sign you notice.

If the numbers of maggots are large, the tissue damage may be severe and large amounts of toxins may be released. Some cats die from the resulting toxicity and infection.

Take the cat to your veterinarian for treatment, if possible. If not, GENTLY clip all hair away from the sores and one to two inches outward, to make sure you have found all the openings and tunnels created by the maggots. Clean the area with chlorhexidine, gently flushing out all holes and cavities. All maggots MUST be removed. You can do this with tweezers or forceps, being careful not to tear or break them apart. Treat the inside of the wounds with an antibiotic solution or ointment (without a steroid), or swab them out with 7% iodine. Spray the rest of the cat's haircoat with an insecticide used for killing fleas. If the cat is toxic because of the worms' secretions, veterinary care may be necessary to save its life.

CUTEREBRA INFESTATION

Larvae of the rodent or rabbit bot-fly may infest cats. This larva is also called a warble, bot or grub. It is most common in farm kittens or young outdoor cats with thin, delicate skin. They are especially seen in late summer or early fall. More than a couple of the larvae may be fatal to the kitten by putting severe stress on the cat's immune system or by causing secondary infections. The adult flies usually are not noticed. Female Cuterebra lay eggs in or near nests of rodents or rabbits. These hatch into infective larvae in response to body heat given off by an animal. A kitten may pick them up by playing near a burrow. The tiny larvae, one-sixteenth inch (1 mm) long, usually enter the kitten through the skin of the mouth or nose, but also may go in through cuts in the skin. They then will migrate to various locations under the surface of the skin.

The larvae may grow to as much as an inch long and one-third inch in diameter (25 mm x 8 mm). They may be grayish, brownish, or black. The sores or swellings containing the larva are commonly seen on the skin of the chest and neck. You first will notice a thick-walled abscess under the cat's skin. The grub may have made a breathing hole through the skin—circular in shape, with smooth edges. It does not look like a cut or injury. Pus may ooze out through the hole, and you may see the larva squirming under the skin.

Do NOT squeeze the sore because rupture of the worms may result in anaphylactic shock, which may be fatal. The breathing hole has to be surgically enlarged to permit removal of the grub (or grubs). Take your cat to your veterinarian. If this is impossible, have someone hold the cat securely, or roll the cat in a towel. Clip the hair from around the lump. Using a very sharp knife or razor blade, make a tiny slit, starting at the edge of the hole and working away from it like the spoke of a wheel coming from the hub. A slit one-eighth to one-quarter inch long (3-6 mm) should be sufficient. The larva can then be VERY carefully squeezed or lifted out. Don't rupture the worm or the sac around it! The abscess can be swabbed out with 7% iodine solution to remove any pus which is present. Continue treating as you would any abscess until the hole has healed from the inside (see Abscesses in Skin Disease Chapter).

Chapter 12

INTERNAL PARASITES

- *Ascarids and Roundworms*
- *Hookworms*
- *Whipworms*
- *Tapeworms*
- *Treatment for Intestinal Worms*
- *Pinworms*
- *Toxoplasmosis*
- *Coccidiosis*
- *Giardiasis*
- *Lungworms*
- *Liver and Pancreatic Flukes*

Signs of worms may include a bloated abdomen, loss of appetite, failure to gain weight, diarrhea or vomiting, a rough coat, bloody stools, and worms in the feces or vomit. Tapeworm segments may look like grains of rice on the hairs of the hind end or in the feces. Cats can also have worms without any visible signs.

To determine if your cat has worms, a veterinarian will need a fresh stool sample. You can easily pick one out of the litter box and take it in a clean plastic carton or bag, or piece of plastic wrap. Don't use your bare hand, even if the piece is dry! One small piece (or a couple of teaspoons if the cat has diarrhea) is sufficient. Just turn the bag inside-out over your hand, pick up the sample, turn the bag back over the sample and close it. Take the closed bag to a veterinarian. If you have several cats, assume they are all infested, unless some are "new" to your household.

ASCARIDS AND ROUNDWORMS

Toxocara cati is the most common ascarid (a type of roundworm) that affects felines throughout the world, both domestic and wild. *Toxocara canis* and *Toxascaris leonina* are other ascarid species seen in cats. The worm eggs can live for several months in cat feces in your yard, especially in warm damp climates. As many as a quarter to half of city or farm cats in a given area may be infected. The best mouser may be continually plagued with ascarids.

Cats become infected by eating infective larvae or by eating rodents, especially mice, that carry these worms. After the cat ingests the worm larvae (or eggs with larvae), the larvae burrow through the wall of the cat's stomach. One to two days later, they enter the mesenteric veins, then the liver, and via the bloodstream, the lungs. They puncture the airways, are coughed up and swallowed by the cat, again

entering the stomach wall. After further maturation they enter the cavity of the small intestine and lay eggs which pass in the cat's feces. All of this can happen in as few as 10 days, or it may take up to three weeks if the cat has eaten an infested rodent. Ascarid larvae may form cysts in the cat's muscles. When an infested queen becomes pregnant, larvae are released from the cysts; they may be passed in her milk, causing worm infestation in her nursing kittens.

Incidentally, young puppies may test negative on fecal exams even though they are infected with *Toxocara*. In areas where these worms are common, puppies should be routinely treated, preferably at three to four weeks of age and again in a few weeks (Schantz, 1994, p. 1024). This will keep the puppy from passing worms to your cat, your children or yourself.

Kittens and young cats often show signs of ascarid infection, including slow growth, dry ragged hair coat and a sagging potbelly. Enough adult worms may be present to block the intestine, occasionally causing death, or they may penetrate the intestine, causing peritonitis. Older cats usually develop some degree of immunity to ascarids. They may carry worms and shed eggs, but rarely show clinical disease.

Queens that have larvae encysted in their muscles may infest each succeeding litter. Regular worming does not eliminate the problem because the medication cannot get through the cysts; wormers kill only the adult worms in the intestinal tract. A routine worming program for kittens and adult cats can help avoid infesting new queens with ascarids. Good sanitation will help prevent ascarid infection in adult cats. Keep litter boxes clean.

Your veterinarian has many effective drugs which, when given orally, will kill both immature and mature ascarids. Piperazine adipate is given at 100 mg/lb (200 mg/kg). Pyrantel pamoate at 2.5 mg/lb (5 mg/kg) also works well. Be SURE not to overdose with piperazine. It is safe at the recommended dosage.

Children can be infested with ascarid larvae by accidentally eating soil contaminated by feces from an infected cat or dog. Kids who deliberately eat dirt are especially at risk. Worm larvae migrate through the child's body, causing a condition called visceral larva migrans. Signs include coughing, asthmatic wheezing, weight loss, fever, and an enlarged liver. In rare cases, they may travel to the eyes, causing blindness, or into the brain, causing nervous system disturbances. These conditions are rare, but may be seen where play areas are badly contaminated by feces from infected animals. For this reason, it is important to keep children's play areas free of animal waste. Sandboxes should be covered when not in use, and children should not be allowed to dig in flower beds used as toilets by neighborhood cats. Cats (and dogs) should be routinely dewormed to keep them from passing eggs in their stools.

A few cats may be infected with large intestinal roundworms (*Strongyloides* species). They are most common in the southeastern United States, especially from Florida to Texas. The most frequent symptom is mild to severe diarrhea, lasting from a week or two to several months. Cats may be weakened, and if untreated, may die. These worms are not contagious to humans.

HOOKWORMS

Hookworms (*Ancylostoma* and *Uncinaria* species) are tiny intestinal parasites, less than a half-inch long. They suck blood from the intestinal wall, and when they detach to move to another site (five to six times a day), leave a wound that bleeds for some time, causing further blood loss. They can easily take enough blood from a cat to cause anemia, although infestations in cats are usually less severe than those in dogs. In a kitten, the blood loss can be fatal. Hookworms are especially common in hot, wet areas of the central and southern United States. They are more common in cats between one to five years of age.

The cat becomes infected by eating hookworm larvae. They mature in the cat's intestines and produce eggs which are passed in the feces, infecting other kittens or adult cats. Hookworm larvae may enter young kittens by penetrating the skin; they travel via the bloodstream to the lungs, are coughed up, swallowed, and mature in the small intestine. In older cats, they migrate to the lungs, are trapped in the muscles, and remain encysted there. Hookworms may live one and a half to two years.

Hookworm infections are difficult to detect. Cats with hookworms may have intermittent vomiting or diarrhea; black, tarry stools; and little or no energy. The cat may be thin, growing more slowly than normal, and have a poor, rough haircoat. Some cats may have pale gums from anemia, but this is less common than in infested puppies.

Hookworms may cause skin disease during their migration. This is usually seen on the feet, especially between the toes, and may cause tender, painful feet. Skin areas which come into contact with the ground may be reddened and sore. The skin lesions do not respond to antibiotics, and do not heal until the cat is treated for the worms.

The only way to diagnose hookworms is to take a fresh stool sample to a veterinarian. As with many roundworms, drugs such as fenbendazole are effective; a second treatment is usually given three to four weeks after the first. The cat should show definite improvement within two to three weeks after the first treatment. Cats that are severely anemic may need intensive care, including a blood transfusion, to stabilize them before deworming.

Hookworms which infest cats can also infest dogs, causing severe disease. When the larvae puncture human skin, they can cause a disease called cutaneous larva migrans. This usually occurs when people walk barefoot in moist areas or swim in contaminated waters. The thickened, reddened skin lesions can itch severely.

To prevent hookworm infestation, a cattery should be kept dry and clean of feces. Although hookworms are almost impossible to control on shady, moist soil, an infested yard can be treated with 10 pounds of borax per 100 square feet soil (Sosna, 1992). The cat(s) and dogs should have routine fecal exams and be dewormed if necessary.

WHIPWORMS

Whipworms (*Trichuris* and *Capillaria* species) have a direct life cycle. Cats are "infected" when they consume food or water contaminated by whipworm eggs which contain larvae. The eggs are very resistant to sunlight or drying, and can remain viable for a year or more. Recent evidence suggests that cats are not actually infected, but are merely passing eggs through the digestive tract which were taken in while eating prey. Symptoms are rarely seen. When noticed, they are similar to those of lungworms. Cats that show symptoms can be treated with drugs such as mebendazole. These worms are almost never contagious to humans.

TAPEWORMS

Tapeworms (cestodes) are likely to be seen by the owner of an outdoor cat (and some indoor cats). Segments look like white, grayish, or yellowish, flattened grains of rice. They may be seen on the skin and hair around the anus, under the tail, or on the feces. When the segments are dried, they may look like small brown or gray dried crusts, much like uncooked grains of rice. Although tapeworm segments or eggs are not usually found on routine fecal examination, a veterinarian will usually take your word that you have seen segments.

The life cycle of the most common tapeworm of both cats and dogs, *Dipylidium caninum*, is typical. Tapeworm segments are passed in the cat's feces. They rupture, spreading egg packets throughout the cat's environment. Flea larvae eat the tapeworm eggs, mature, and return to the cat for a blood meal. When the cat feels a flea crawling on its coat, it chews at it with its teeth, and may swallow the flea. The tapeworm larvae are released in the cat's digestive tract, develop into adults, and the adult tapeworm head segments attach to the wall of the intestine. There they mature and pass new egg-filled segments, repeating the cycle. Adult tapeworms may reach one to two feet in length. Segments which break off and pass down the digestive tract are what you see. They may still be alive and moving across the cat's skin or through its hair. This is one of the few parasites that is more common in city cats than in rural felines. Their incidence is closely related to the number of fleas in the environment.

Taenia taeniaformis is a similar tapeworm whose intermediate host is usually a rodent or rabbit (rather than a flea). *Echinococcus multilocularis* is a tapeworm common in foxes and coyotes (and in the rodents they eat) in the North Central states and in tundra areas of North America, extending as far south as Ohio, Indiana and Illinois (Schantz, 1994, p. 1026). Both cats and dogs are susceptible to these worms, which can cause serious disease in the lungs or liver (called hydatid disease) when carried to humans. The incubation period in humans is long (up to 10 years) and about half the cases are fatal.

If this disease is common in your area, prevent your pet from eating rodents, and use careful sanitation to avoid hand-to-mouth transfer of eggs. Hand washing is particularly important. Praziquantel is a drug which will remove both adult and juvenile tapeworms. All your cats and dogs should be treated every three months.

Diphyllobothrium latum is a very large tapeworm, as much as 36 feet (12 meters) long. It is common in the Great Lakes area of North America, but areas of incidence are small and isolated. It is more common in humans than in cats. Freshwater fish are the intermediate hosts. Cats (and humans) become infested by eating fish or fish viscera. Fish should be thoroughly cooked before they are fed to felines (or eaten by humans!).

Mesocestoides species are normally found in birds. Infective intermediate stages occur in insects. When cats eat these bugs, the tapeworms become established outside the digestive tract. They develop in the peritoneal cavity, causing chronic weight loss, emaciation, and death.

The tapeworms commonly seen in cats generally cause little harm. However, massive quantities of tapeworms can drain enough nutrients from the cat to leave it malnourished and thin, with a poor, ragged coat. This is uncommon. Diarrhea may also be seen.

It's repulsive to see the segments crawling around your cat's hindquarters, or on your clothing after your cat has departed. Tapeworm eggs also may be passed into the environment, where they are picked up by intermediate hosts, such as insects. When eaten by a child, they can cause intestinal disease. Your cat should be treated if it has tapeworms and is around small children.

Several drugs are available to remove tapeworms from cats. Droncit® (BayLabs, Shawnee, KS 66201) is available to veterinarians in tablet, paste, and injectable forms. Epsiprantel (Cestex®, Beecham Labs) will remove *D. caninum* and *T. taeniaeformis* from cats with one dose. Fenbendazole (Panacur®) can be given for three successive days at 20 mg/lb (50 mg/kg). Some cats will eat the medication mixed with their food. Dead tapeworms are usually not seen in the feces because they are digested before being passed, so absence of worms doesn't mean the medication was ineffective.

Cats that eat insects or mice may become reinfested, and will need treatment from time to time. This does NOT mean the treatment didn't work. It means the cat was reinfested, probably for the same reason. If the tapeworms are *D. caninum* (carried by fleas), you MUST control the fleas to keep the worms from recurring. Plan on treating the cat as often as needed. Tapeworms may recur in as little as three to four weeks. Many outdoor cats need treatment three to six times a year. Prevention, of course, begins with keeping your cat indoors and controlling fleas, roaches, and other insects, and rodents which may carry tapeworms. Also, tapeworm eggs can be carried by flies that have fed on infected feces.

TREATMENT FOR INTESTINAL WORMS

In general, treatment begins by having a fecal sample checked to determine the specific worms. Wormers are poisons, designed to be more toxic to the worms than to the cat. Because of that toxicity, they should not be used routinely or lightly. The most specific and effective wormers are available only to and through veterinarians. Because wormers may be harmful to your cat if they are given with other medications or pesticides, be sure to tell your veterinarian if you are using a flea collar, flea powder, or medication on your feline, or if your home and yard have been recently treated.

Many types of wormers are on the market, including injections, pills, chewable tablets, and pastes. Some are safe enough that your veterinarian will sell them to you and let you administer them yourself. Other drugs are so toxic that they can only be administered safely in a clinic. Be sure to weigh your cat before going to the clinic so the veterinarian can determine the proper dosage. It is very important to administer all the prescribed medication. A few weeks later, take another stool sample to the clinic to be sure the worms are gone. Although this is not necessary if the cat had tapeworms, the cat may be reinfected if its lifestyle has not changed.

Remember, if your cat has an emergency in the middle of the night, the veterinarian who knows you is more likely to get out of bed and care for your cat. Give the veterinarian a profit on the worming and he or she will be more willing to meet your emergency needs. There's nothing wrong with being a good and valued customer.

Don't bother with over-the-counter worming medications. Most of them treat only one or a few types of the worms that may infest your cat, as well as being limited in their effectiveness. If you are wrong, you have subjected your cat to a possibly toxic drug without doing it any good. Some of the over-the-counter wormers are extremely poisonous. One of the most common ingredients of these products, toluene, was abandoned by veterinarians over 20 years ago because it was too toxic, as well as being ineffective.

If your kitten is ailing, some people will say "it just needs worming." Worm medication is not safe enough to be used indiscriminately. And, if the cat is ill, worm medication may weaken or injure it to the point of death.

A positive fecal sample does not necessarily mean that worms are the cause of the cat's diarrhea or illness; there may be another disease. Also, a negative fecal sample does not always mean the cat is wormless, as female worms may not have been producing eggs at the time of the sample.

All parasites which inhabit the digestive tract shed some stage of their life cycle, whether egg, larva or segment, in the feces. An incubation period is needed before the feces stage becomes infective to another animal, whether of the same species or an intermediate host. This period may range from two to six days to several months or more, depending on environmental conditions. This time in the parasite's life is an easy and effective point at which to break the cycle of infection.

There is no better preventive measure than cleaning up the animal's feces and promptly disposing of them. If done daily, this can greatly reduce the cat's risk of reinfection and can limit the spread of parasites to other animals (or humans).

When you acquire a new cat or kitten, have a fecal sample checked for worms. If they are present, you can have the cat treated immediately so it does not spread worms to other pets or contaminate your yard. Then, if you keep the cat indoors, you can greatly reduce the chances that it will become reinfected. In areas where worms are a constant problem, be sure to take along a stool sample at checkup time, or when the cat is ill.

Children can catch some kinds of hookworms and roundworms by playing in a sandbox or yard that has been contaminated by a cat or dog. Humans can become infested with tapeworms if they accidentally eat a flea, the host which carries them. Keep your child's sandbox covered when it is not in use for play. Teach your child to wash his hands before eating, especially after playing with a pet or outdoors in the yard. Don't let pets sleep with children if they have external or internal parasites of any kind.

PINWORMS

Pinworms are NOT a parasite of cats and dogs; thus, children don't get pinworms from them. Pinworms are passed only between humans, usually because small children are careless about sanitation and don't wash their hands after using the toilet or before eating. A misinformed physician may want you to get rid of the cat or dog because the child has pinworms. Don't do it if pinworms are the only problem. Your pet isn't to blame.

TOXOPLASMOSIS

Toxoplasmosis (caused by *Toxoplasma gondii*) is a disease found throughout the world. *Toxoplasma* is a protozoan parasite, a single-celled animal (much like an amoeba) which must live part of its life cycle within the body of another animal. In addition, it forms cysts and spores which can live outside the host, waiting for another suitable victim to come along. In the cyst, it can live in warm moist soil for more than a year. This organism is important, more because it can spread to humans than because of how it affects cats. In some areas, nearly 60% of stray cats carry *Toxoplasma* organisms. Strays are more commonly infected than domestic cats, probably because of their hunting and scavenging feeding habits.

Toxoplasma has an extremely intricate life cycle. In its intestinal stage, it is passed in the cat's feces to infect children who play in a sandbox or pregnant women who change dirty cat box litter. In this stage, it can also be eaten by cattle, sheep, hogs, and goats as they graze in contaminated grass. This causes a disease in the animal's muscles, resulting in contaminated meat. It is also found in venison and meat from other wild animals, including pronghorn, moose, and especially bears. *Toxoplasma* can also be passed via unprocessed cows' or goats' milk. Humans eating undercooked meat, especially beef or pork, can become infected. After the infection has entered the intestine, it goes to other body tissues, to be passed by a pregnant animal to her offspring (whether human or sheep) via the uterus. This can be an important cause of stillborn lambs in some areas, which can in turn infect carnivores and scavengers that eat the carcass. Or, it may be taken in by rodents, reptiles or birds and passed back to a cat that eats them.

Cats are much less contagious to other cats than to other animals. Among cats, the queen can infect her kittens while they are in the uterus, and they can pass oocysts in their feces shortly after birth. Oocysts are an immature, infective, environmentally resistant stage of *Toxoplasma*. If the disease is present in her intestine, kittens can pick up the disease if they use a common litter box. If the queen hunts, she can bring it home in infected prey, including mice and birds, to infect her kittens when they are weaned and begin eating meat. There is no evidence that an immune queen can pass immunity to her kittens while they are in the uterus.

Toxoplasmosis in cats may appear as a sudden, acute disease that kills young kittens. In an infected litter, kittens that are a week or two old may all die. Older kittens become progressively more resistant, and those that reach three to four pounds in weight will usually live to adulthood.

The acute form of toxoplasmosis primarily affects cats that are two weeks to two or three years of age. The most prominent sign of acute toxoplasmosis is difficulty in breathing, due to a rapidly worsening pneumonia. The cat may grunt as it attempts to catch its breath, but usually does not cough, and is droopy as it usually quits eating and loses weight. A fever of about 104 degrees F (40 C) may rise and fall, but never drop to normal despite antibiotic treatment. This form rarely lasts more than two to three days, although a few infected cats may live up to three weeks. The cats usually die, no matter what treatment is used. The more rapidly the disease comes on, the less likely it is to be successfully treated.

Chronic toxoplasmosis affects many different systems, especially the eyes and brain, causing many different signs. The iris (colored part of the eye) may be reddish and fuzzy-looking, and may have cream-colored pus floating in front of it. The pupils may differ in size from one eye to the other. The cat's eyes may roll uncontrollably from side to side. It may blink more than normally or may be blind. The cat may grind its teeth, be sleepy or restless, or show a personality change to viciousness or excessive affection (rabies should also be suspected). Other symptoms include loss of appetite, weight loss, diarrhea, vomiting, muscle pain, icterus, staggering, convulsions, and swollen lymph nodes. Anemia is common in chronic cases, and symptoms may mimic many other diseases. Chronic toxoplasmosis can occur after low-dose exposure. It is also seen in cats that are immunosuppressed, as from feline leukemia, feline immunodeficiency virus infection (FIV), or animals that have been treated with corticosteroids or other immunosuppressive drugs.

Your veterinarian will diagnose "toxo" by a combination of laboratory tests and, possibly, chest X-rays. Blood tests and/or fecal exams are usually needed to confirm the diagnosis. After infection, cats that recover will have blood antibodies against the disease. Because this makes it difficult to tell whether the infection is current or past, a positive blood test for toxoplasmosis is not a reason to condemn the cat.

When kittens fewer than three to four months of age eat the infective stage of the toxoplasmosis organism, they usually die. Older kittens usually get a mild form of the disease. Their bodies then develop resistance as the immune system reacts against the parasites. This keeps them safe from illness unless they are stressed by other disease. Cats seem to be immune to reinfection for at least six to 12 months after initial infection. However, this may leave the cat in a carrier state where the organisms do not harm it, but are passed in its feces, where they can infest other animals or humans. Older cats may show signs of toxoplasmosis that was probably acquired while they were young. Lowered resistance allows the disease to become evident.

Infection with the feline leukemia virus or FIV commonly plays a role in allowing a cat to become ill with toxoplasmosis. More than half the cats with toxoplasmosis may be positive for these diseases.

It is important to treat cats with toxoplasmosis as soon as possible, in an attempt to kill the parasites before they kill the cat. Sulfa drugs are commonly used, especially sulfadiazine-trimethoprim (Tribrissen, Burroughs Wellcome), and treatment should be given for about three weeks. Triple sulfa is also used. Folic acid should be given as well—one-third of a package of baker's yeast each day by mouth or in the cat's food. If the cat has excessive gas in the intestine, reduce the amount of yeast. Clindamycin may also be used to treat the disease. It is effective but vomiting may occur as a side effect (Wolf, 1991). In some cases, it can be controlled by stopping treatment for 24 hours, then restarting at a lower dose which is gradually increased.

Toxoplasmosis is a significant disease because it can be transmitted to humans. Cats shed the infective stage (oocyst) in their feces. They don't shed them for long (as little as two weeks and only once during the cat's life), but while they do, great numbers are passed. The disease passes to humans as children eat or put their hands in their mouths after playing in soil that has been contaminated by infected cats. Perhaps more common is to contract the disease by eating raw or undercooked meat from hogs, cattle, goats, or sheep that have ingested plants or feedstuffs contaminated by cats.

Most human cases are very mild, and similar to influenza. Fetuses and infants can be infected, sometimes with damage to the eyes or brain. People whose immune systems are compromised, such as AIDS patients and people on corticosteroids or immunosuppressant drugs, can also be infected. In AIDS patients, toxoplasmosis causes a serious infectious encephalitis. Pregnant women are at risk because of the danger of transmitting the disease to the fetus. Cats can cause severe disease outbreaks in goat dairies by defecating in soil and feed bunks. Infected does then pass the disease to their kids (or to humans) via the milk. Keep cats from picking up the organisms by keeping them from hunting or eating raw meat.

You can help avoid infection by toxoplasmosis by eating only thoroughly cooked meat in which no red or pink color remains. Cooking meat to 151 degrees F (66 C) will kill organisms in the meat, as will freezing meat at −4 degrees F (−20 C) for a few days. Wash hands, cutting boards, and utensils with soap and water after handling raw meat. Thoroughly wash all vegetables which will be eaten raw to remove any possible organisms. After working in garden soil or touching raw meat, wash your hands before touching your face, smoking, or eating. It is helpful to wear gloves while gardening or changing a litter box. Children's sand boxes should be covered. If the sand becomes contaminated by cat feces, replace it. Keep trash

cans covered to keep animals from scrounging scraps. Promptly remove dead animals or meat trimmings so cats or pigs cannot get them. Aborted fetuses and membranes from goats and sheep should be handled carefully. Wear gloves and bury or incinerate them. Keep grain containers covered so cats cannot contaminate feedstuffs. Feed only commercial cat food or thoroughly cooked meat to your cat. Cats that live outdoors should be well fed. They won't hunt as much, reducing their risk of eating infected prey.

Cleaning litter boxes every 24 hours will keep the *Toxoplasma* organisms from reaching their infective stage. Cat feces should be burned, flushed down the toilet or put in the trash. Do not bury them in the garden because they might contaminate vegetables or infect children playing in the dirt. No disinfectant works well against toxoplasmosis organisms. Rinse the litter box daily with boiling water. If possible, a woman who is pregnant (or a person who is immunosuppressed) should not change the cat's litter box. If there is no choice, wear disposable gloves. It is especially important that the litter box be changed daily in a household where someone is pregnant or has immune system problems. If your cat has toxoplasmosis, extra care should be taken in cleaning the litter box for two to three weeks while it is being treated.

Cats can be tested with serological tests. In terms of contact with humans, cats that are seropositive are probably less of a risk in the household than negative animals. This is because they have previously been infected and already stopped shedding oocysts. Unless they are immunosuppressed, their infection is unlikely to be reactivated.

The average household cat is less dangerous to the owner than once thought. Veterinarians who have been in practice for 10 years or more, during which they have handled known positive cases, usually still test negative for toxoplasmosis. In New Zealand, 70% of adult humans are seropositive without clinical signs of illness (Lynch, 1993).

COCCIDIOSIS

Coccidia are single-celled microscopic protozoan parasites belonging to a number of different species which live in the cat's intestine. They are transmitted when a host animal such as a cockroach, mouse, sheep, or other animal eats feces from an infected cat. The coccidia develop partially in this host, and when the next cat eats the host animal, it becomes infected. Like toxoplasmosis, this disease is most severe in young kittens, which may be infected while nursing.

Coccidiosis is usually noticed because of diarrhea, which may be bloody or filled with mucus. Severe cases may be depressed, feverish, dehydrated, and anemic because of the blood loss. The cat may be ill for several days. A kitten may have feline distemper or another complicating illness, and the coccidia in the feces are incidental. It is important to get an accurate diagnosis, ruling out other causes of diarrhea before coccidiosis is diagnosed. Like toxoplasmosis, coccidiosis is often treated with triple sulfa or sulfadiazine-trimethoprim (Tribrissen®, Burroughs Wellcome). This medication does not kill the coccidia, but "cripples" them enough to allow the body's defenses to heal the cat. The cat does not develop an immunity to the organism, and the disease may quickly recur if it is stressed or has a damaged immune system. Overcrowding and dirty conditions raise the infection rate.

Good sanitation is important if infection with coccidiosis is a problem. Moist conditions are favorable for the coccidia, so cleanliness and dryness are critical, as is control of insects such as cockroaches. This disease is not a public health problem with humans, but good sanitation should be maintained to keep it from being spread to other cats or from cats to other hosts and back again.

A type of coccidia called *Sarcocystis* can cause serious illness in calves. If your farm cats are infested, they should all be treated to help eliminate the disease. As with toxoplasmosis, be sure that feed is kept clean and that cats are not allowed to defecate in feeders or stored grain.

GIARDIASIS

Giardia are protozoal intestinal parasites found in many animals throughout the world in tropical and temperate climates. They are spread when the cat eats foodstuffs contaminated by feces from infected animals. Severe infections can result in maldigestion, malabsorption, and chronic diarrhea.

Younger cats are most easily infected, especially under the crowded conditions and stress of multi-cat households and catteries. They develop a diarrhea which may be watery, greasy, or contain mucus. The cat may pass gas and have a swollen abdomen and rough haircoat. *Giardia* infections in otherwise healthy adult cats are probably common, although self-limiting and without symptoms. Cats that are immunosuppressed may be very ill.

Some *Giardia* infections can be difficult to diagnose by lab tests. Favorable response to treatment with metronidazole (Flagyl®) or similar medications will confirm the diagnosis. Some drugs used to treat this disease are mutagenic and should not be used in cats that are pregnant. Infected cats seem to be more hazardous to other cats than to humans; however, infants are more susceptible than adults. If you have one infected cat, all felines (and probably the dogs) in your "herd" should be treated. Maintain good sanitation to avoid the risk of infection to people in the household.

LUNGWORMS

Lungworms are occasionally seen in cats. The most common feline lungworm is *Aelurostrongylus abstrusus*. It infests cats worldwide. Infective third-stage larvae are carried by snails or slugs, which are eaten by the cat. Or, the cat may eat a bird, frog, or rodent which has eaten an infected slug or snail. The larvae are carried in the bloodstream and filtered out in the lung tissue. There they develop into adults, living in the smaller air passages. As the worms become adults, they produce eggs which are coughed up, swallowed, and passed in the cat's feces.

The majority of cats with lungworms do not have any signs of illness. Cats with large quantities of lungworms, or those with suppressed immune systems, may show wheezing and a mild cough which does not cease. Some cats may have fatigue and difficulty in breathing with exertion, as well as sneezing.

If the infection goes on long enough, the pulmonary artery may become enlarged and, on radiographic examination, may look similar to feline heartworm disease. Diagnosis is made when the veterinarian finds worm eggs in a sample of the cat's feces. Worm eggs may also be found in material coughed up by the cat or washed from the cat's trachea. Treatment is difficult and may not be fully successful.

A lung fluke, *Paragonimus kellicotti,* occasionally seen in cats (and dogs), has a complex life cycle. Eggs from this worm are picked up by snails, develop into the next stage, and are then ingested by freshwater crayfish, crabs, or similar crustaceans. When the cat eats the infected crayfish, young flukes develop in its small intestine. They pass through the intestinal wall, the diaphragm, and the chest cavity, ending up in the lungs, where they form nodules. The disease is more often seen in outdoor cats.

A cat with lung flukes may show little or no sign of illness. However, a badly infested cat may wheeze and gasp with exercise or excitement, and may have a soft cough, salivate, or cough up blood. Diagnosis for flukes is the same as for lungworms. Treatment can be successful. Keep the cat from eating the host crustaceans to avoid this infection.

Capillaria aerophila is another lungworm which infests cats. Many infections with this worm go unnoticed. When signs are seen, there is usually a persistent dry cough (see Whipworms, above).

Nasal worms (gapeworms) are found in many cats in the Caribbean, especially Puerto Rico. Cats may have no symptoms or they may have severe sneezing, open-mouthed breathing, coughing, and nasal congestion. Reddish-brown worms, sneezed from the nose, are diagnostic. The disease, which can be treated with fenbendazole or mebendazole, is not contagious to humans.

LIVER AND PANCREATIC FLUKES

Liver flukes are small flattened parasites (one-third inch long) with a complex life cycle. Eggs are shed from the gall bladder and bile ducts into the feces. Larvae hatch from the eggs and enter snails, which are eaten by lizards, toads, and crustaceans. The cat becomes infested by eating these animals. Liver flukes are found in hot humid areas such as Hawaii and the southeastern United States, especially Florida. In the Caribbean, severe cases are called "lizard poisoning."

Cats infested with liver flukes show general signs of illness, including lack of appetite, weight loss, and occasional vomiting. The cat may have a swollen abdomen and jaundice. Treatment with drugs such as praziquantel (20 mg/kg body weight) is usually successful. Prevent this disease by keeping your cat indoors.

Pancreatic flukes live within the pancreatic ducts of cats, foxes, and raccoons. In the United States, they occur in the Missouri, Mississippi, Tennessee, and Ohio River Valleys and nearby areas. The life cycle is thought to be similar to that of liver flukes, and feral or stray cats seem most affected. Weight loss and vomiting are the most common signs. Again, prevent the disease by keeping the cat indoors.

Chapter 13

EYE PROBLEMS

- *Eye Emergencies*
- *Corneal Injuries and Ulcers*
- *Glaucoma*
- *Eyelid Problems*
- *Prolapse of the Eyeball*
- *Conjunctival Problems*
- *Tear Staining*
- *Cataracts*
- *Blindness*

Cats cannot see in total darkness, but they can see, probably with some fuzziness, in very dim light. This is because the mirror-like back part of the eyeball lining (the retina), is reflective. Light rays pass through the retina, then bounce back from this mirrored area, increasing the cat's ability to distinguish objects in dim light. This reflection is what you see when you catch a cat's eyes in the beam of your headlights.

Siamese cats may be cross-eyed. Some seem to see normally, while others have poor vision from associated developmental abnormalities (Johnson, 1991). Crossed eyes are an adaptation that allows the cat to see as well as possible; for that reason, they should not be corrected. They should not be bred as the trait is inherited.

EYE EMERGENCIES

This brief list describes emergencies involving the eye and gives instructions for coping with them. In all cases, after you have given first aid, take the cat to a veterinarian as soon as possible.

As a general rule, if it isn't fairly easy to examine an injured eye, DON'T try to do so. If you fight the cat or put too much pressure on the eye, you may rupture it. This is especially a risk if the cornea or sclera (the white part) is cut or weakened.

In most cases, if you need to bandage an injured eye to protect it, you should bandage both eyes. Otherwise, the normal eye will try to move and will cause unwanted movement of the injured eye. Gently wrap the cat's entire head with gauze or a clean cloth, going around the eyes and under the jaw, then behind the ears to keep the bandage from sliding off the head. Be sure not to bandage so snugly that you choke the cat. Moisten the area over the injured eye with saline or contact lens solution, if available; if not, use cool, clean water.

The cat may aggravate an eye injury by trying to wash its face or by rubbing it with a paw. If necessary, you can "hobble" the cat by taping its front legs together. Tape around one leg (not too tightly!), leaving about three inches of tape; then go around the other leg. Next, tape along the center tape again, and back around the first leg.

Injuries which penetrate the globe of the eye, or cuts on the eyeball. Bandage the eye, but be sure there is no pressure on the cornea. If a small object such as a splinter is penetrating the cornea, DO NOT REMOVE IT. You may cause irreparable damage by trying to take it out. Hobble the cat so it cannot paw the eye, and have someone hold the cat while you drive to the clinic. Let the veterinarian remove the object.

Acute corneal ulcer or abrasion. This may be due to an injury or fight. If you look at the cornea from the side, you may see a scalloped or dished-out spot, or a long, deep scratch. The cat may wash its face or rub its eye with a paw. The eye may be reddened and tear-filled, and the eyelids may be in spasm, clamped tightly shut so you can't see the eyeball. The cat may be in obvious pain. There is no need to bandage the eye if you can quickly take the cat to a clinic. If it will be several hours, bandage the eye as above.

Prolapse of the eyeball. This occurs when one or both eyes have popped partially or totally out of the eye sockets. The eye may be in front of the lid, which cannot close over it. It looks horrendous, but is surprisingly painless for the cat if the skull is not fractured. Keep calm. Wrap the cat in a blanket or towel, being careful not to touch the eye. Go to the nearest clinic. If you can't get to the veterinarian within 10 to 15 minutes, bandage the eye as above. Do not attempt to replace the eyeball. If you apply pressure, it may cause further damage.

Descemetocele. This is a condition where a small piece of membrane from within the eye protrudes through a hole in the cornea (the clear covering of the eye). It will be seen as a small bulge on the cornea which obviously comes from within the globe itself. Treat as for prolapse, above.

Acute Glaucoma. This is a sudden increase in fluid pressure within the eyeball. If untreated, it can lead to permanent retinal damage and blindness. With prompt treatment, chances for a cure are good. The cat may hold its eye closed and seem sensitive to light. Excessive tear production may occur. The eyeball may appear larger than normal, and the blood vessels in the sclera (white area) may be swollen and red. The cornea may be clouded or reddish. The pupil may remain dilated (wide open) even if you shine a bright light in the cat's eye. The cat may have trouble seeing. Glaucoma is extremely painful for some cats. Others show little or no pain, which may mislead you into thinking it is not serious. Don't be fooled—it IS serious. Sight may be lost if it is left untreated for as few as three days.

Uveitis. The cat's eye may be red or "cloudy," and the color of the iris (the colored part of the eye) may change. The cat may hold the eye closed and may not want you to examine it because of pain. Tears may run down the cat's face and it may try to avoid bright light. The blood vessels of the sclera may be very enlarged and reddened ("injected"). If you can open the eye, the pupil (opening) may be constricted. Uveitis can occur with several diseases, including feline leukemia, FIP, FIV, toxoplasmosis, and high blood pressure due to kidney failure. If uveitis is not treated promptly, it can lead to glaucoma, cataracts, and/or retinal detachment. Any of these may lead to permanent blindness.

Eyelid lacerations. Cuts or tears can bleed profusely. If not sutured, they can cause permanent scarring, deformity of the eyelid opening, and damage to the cornea from facial hair rubbing on it. Apply a bandage or clean cloth to put gentle, direct pressure on the bleeding area. Cold compresses are also helpful to control bleeding.

Chemicals splashed into the eye. Flush the eye GENTLY for five to 10 minutes, using plenty of clean water. Use a garden hose or pop the cat into a sink or bathtub. If necessary, get in with the cat to hold the eye open and facing the water.

Orbital abscess. This infection may be a single large sack of pus present in the bony orbit behind or beside the eyeball, putting pressure on it so that the cat appears "bug-eyed." It may also be a diffuse infection called cellulitis, or be due to an object or bite wound which has penetrated the area from the skin, mouth, or conjunctival sac. Infection may spread from an infected upper molar tooth or sinus. Signs, including fever, usually appear suddenly. The eye may bulge outward or turn at an odd angle, and the sclera may be reddened. The cat may object if you try to open its mouth. Take the cat to a veterinarian within 24 hours.

Sudden vision loss. This may occur from problems within the eye such as a detached or degenerated retina. Vision loss can occur from inflammation of the optic nerve or from hemorrhage within both eyes when the cat is hit by a car or otherwise injured. It also can occur with some poisonings and brain tumors. Take the cat to a clinic as soon as possible.

CORNEAL INJURIES and ULCERS

The cornea is the clear window-like part of the eye through which the animal sees. As you look at the cat, it is the most obvious part of the eye. This delicate tissue is easily injured by a claw as cats fight or play. Chemicals, infections, or mechanical injury also can cause corneal damage.

The first sign of a corneal injury may be the cat holding its eye partially or completely closed. There may be running tears that make the surrounding hair wet. The conjunctiva—the pinkish membranes of the eye—may be reddened and puffy. If you open the cat's eye and look across the cornea from the side, you may see a scraped or punctured area—a spot where its shining perfection has been marred. A magnifying glass may help you see the scraped surface.

Minor corneal injuries are very painful but will heal by themselves. Use an antibiotic eye ointment (without a corticosteroid) three or four times a day. You may need to put an Elizabethan collar on the cat to keep it from washing its face and irritating the eye with a foot.

Occasionally, a thorn, piece of a claw, or splinter may be embedded in a corneal laceration. If you see ANYTHING embedded in the cornea or sticking through a hole in it, DO NOT remove it. Pulling on it may cause the contents of the eyeball to come out, permanently damaging the eye. This is an EMERGENCY—go directly to the nearest veterinary clinic, where the object can be removed under anesthesia. Transport the cat wrapped snugly in a towel so that it cannot claw at the object.

Larger cuts on the cornea should be sutured by a veterinarian, who will use very tiny stitches to repair the eyeball. In many cases, the cat's sight can be saved by prompt repair. If you can take the cat to a veterinarian, DO NOT put any ointment in the eye, as this may keep it from healing at the suture line. This is because many eye ointments have an oily base which is good for the surface, but not for cut or torn edges.

Ulcers occur when the corneal surface is scratched or scraped, leaving a shallow, scooped-out area. Like corneal abrasions, this may happen when the cat's eye is clawed. They can be caused by smoke, chemicals, burns, soap or cleaning agents, or viruses, especially feline herpesvirus. They also can happen if inward-turned hairs rub the eye each time the cat blinks.

As with cuts on the cornea, you may be able to see an ulcer by looking sideways across the cat's eyeball. Your veterinarian can tell how deep and large it is by staining it with a dye called fluorescein. It turns the damaged area a bright orange-green.

Treatment for shallow ulcers is the same as for corneal abrasions: an antibiotic eye ointment used three to five times a day. Keep this up two or three days after the lesion looks healed.

A corneal abrasion or ulcer should heal completely in three or four days. If not, return the cat to the clinic for a checkup. Also take the cat to the clinic if the lesion worsens, even within the first day or so. Rarely, antibiotic-resistant strains of bacteria such as *Pseudomonas* may infect the injured eye. Improperly treated, they quickly invade the eye, resulting in its loss. If the infection worsens rapidly, have it checked immediately.

In some cases, it is necessary to anesthetize the cat and put in a few stitches to hold the eye shut until it is healed. This is an easy solution because it's difficult to bandage a cat's eye other than temporarily. The eyelids make a safe, clean natural bandage which also supports the surface of the eyeball. You may need to put ointment in the corner while the eye is stitched shut.

Deeper corneal ulcers can be very serious. A cut or scratch which penetrates the cornea easily can become infected, preventing it from healing. The cat may blink its eye continuously or be unable to open it because the eyelids are in spasm. Take the cat to a clinic immediately. It may be necessary to suture the eye shut to keep the contents from coming out, and several weeks of treatment may be needed before you will know if the eye can be saved.

GLAUCOMA

Glaucoma in cats, as in humans, occurs when fluid pressure within the eyeball is increased. Normally, a gentle circulation occurs within the globe of the eye. Fluid is produced and the same amount is drained away—pressure remains constant. Glaucoma occurs when there is too little drainage or too much fluid production. It produces blindness as increased pressure presses on the retina and optic nerve. If pressure persists long enough, the animal becomes permanently blind.

Feline glaucoma is usually secondary to disease within the eyeball. It may occur after the eye is injured, especially if the lens is loosened from its normal position and flops out of place or floats loose within the eyeball. Occasionally, a tumor or growth within the globe, especially from lymphosarcoma, may cause glaucoma. Some researchers feel that Persian and Siamese cats have a hereditary form of glaucoma, often occurring in both eyes (Gionfriddo, 1995, p.266).

Many cats with glaucoma have a cloudy cornea. You may notice a red color within the eyeball, due to red blood cells floating inside. Or, you may see whitish or yellowish exudate, which is usually pus. The eyeball may appear larger than normal. The pupil may stay dilated. It may not change in size if you shine a bright light into the eye. Some cats will be in severe pain while others show none. The iris (the colored part of the eye) may be a different color than normal. The conjunctiva may be reddened and the eye may weep tears. The cat may be blind.

The hallmark of glaucoma is increased pressure within the eyeball, measured with an instrument called a tonometer. Unfortunately, glaucoma usually comes on gradually in cats and can cause blindness before the eyeball is swollen enough to be obvious.

Glaucoma must be distinguished from an eyeball pushed forward by an abscess or tumor behind it. An abscess may be due to an infected root of an upper molar tooth or a foreign body which has penetrated the mouth or throat. Unfortunately, most tumors of the globe are malignant. In either case, the eyelids may not close over the eyeball, and the cornea is in danger of drying and permanent damage.

Glaucoma which has just occurred is a true emergency. If your cat's eye is swollen, bulging, or larger than the other eye, take the cat to your veterinarian as soon as possible—hours count. The veterinarian will prescribe drugs to reduce pressure in the eyeball. Then, a cause can be found, and if possible, be corrected.

In some cases, the pressure within the eyeball can't be reduced. The eye may be blind and extremely painful. Surgery may increase drainage within the eye. If the lens is out of place, it can be removed. If pain persists and surgery does not help, it may be necessary to remove the eyeball to give permanent relief. The cat is already blind. Your cat will still be a useful, happy pet after it heals and will easily adapt to life with one eye with your help and understanding.

EYELID PROBLEMS

The eyelid may grow to the cornea after an infection, especially with feline herpesvirus (FHV-1, rhinotracheitis virus). This may result in blindness if not promptly treated. FHV-1 may cause infection in adult cats, lasting five to 10 days. This may occur in only one eye. Initially, it is treated with idoxuridine (Stoxil or Herplex) ophthalmic drops, often in combination with other eye drops. Some cats may shed virus highly contagious to other cats. After recovery or after exposure at birth, virus may remain dormant for years, coming to life in your isolated adult, indoor cat. Vaccination against FHV-1 does not give complete protection against this eye infection, but it does help (Fischer, 1995).

Cats that have red or cream-colored hair coats may develop small brownish patches as they age. These occur along the edges of the eyelids, lips, ears, and pads of the feet, becoming larger and darker as the cat ages. They are

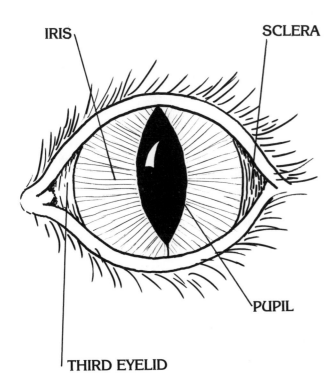

Structures of the eye.

normal and do not cause problems. Squamous cell carcinomas are slow-growing tumors seen in cats with white skin around the eye area (see Tumors Chapter).

Cats may be born without part of the eyelid, giving a slit-shaped eye opening which closes poorly. Other cats, especially some wrinkle-faced Persians, may have an eyelid or fold of skin on the face rolled inward. The cornea is irritated as the hairs turn under and rub on the eyeball. This can lead to ulcers or blindness. Signs include watery, runny eyes. Tears may spill down the cat's face, leaving it wet and stained. The cat may blink continuously or hold its eye partially closed. A piece of eyelid or fold can be removed surgically to make the lid lie more normally. Or, a skin graft may ease the irritation. If just a few eyelashes are involved, they may be removed with electrolysis.

The eyelids may be cut or torn, either by another cat in a fight or by getting caught on a bush or nail. They should be sutured by a veterinarian so the lid edge remains as normal as possible.

The third eyelid is the little membrane in the inner corner of the eye. It helps protect the cornea and spread tears across the eyeball. Normally, it is tucked away, and rarely noticed. In some cases, it may come partway over the eyeball. This can occur if the cornea or conjunctiva are irritated or injured. It also may happen with a tumor or abscess behind the eye, or if the cat is thin or dehydrated.

Both third eyelids may come partway over the eye in some cats, mostly under two years of age. The cause is unknown. Some cases may be due to virus diseases or internal parasites. Some veterinarians believe it is common in cats that eat large numbers of moths ("millers"). It also may occur in cats that are petted and handled excessively, or while the cat is grooming, eating, or defecating. The cat should be examined to rule out treatable causes. If the cat is healthy, there is no reason for concern, and no treatment is needed. It usually returns to normal in a few weeks or months. The third eyelids also will come partway across the eyeballs if the cat is tranquilized or sedated. This is normal and will disappear when the cat sobers up.

PROLAPSE OF THE EYEBALL

Cats are often injured when hit in the head by vehicles, kicked, or bitten by a dog. There may be bleeding behind the eyeball. The bone surrounding it may be fractured. The blow rips muscles that hold the eye in the socket, pulling them loose and allowing the eye to pop out of the socket. It may be squeezed out between the eyelids. This is especially a problem with Persians, whose sockets are shallow compared to the size and volume of the eyeball. Wrap the cat in a blanket or towel and take it to a veterinarian immediately. Under anesthesia, the veterinarian will replace the globe and suture the eyelids together. Sutures are left in place for seven to 10 days.

In some cases, the vision may be saved if the eye can be replaced before the nerves to it are damaged. In others, even prompt replacement will not help. The cat will be permanently blind but the eye will look fine cosmetically. Still others will have enough damage that the cat is in continuing pain and the shrunken, shriveled eye will later need to be removed. In most cases, it's worth replacing the eye to see how it heals before removing it. Removal also prevents sarcomas which later may develop in the useless eye.

CONJUNCTIVAL PROBLEMS

Conjunctivitis (sometimes called "pinkeye" or "red eye") is an inflammation or infection of the thin membrane which lines the eyelids. The conjunctiva starts at the edge of the cornea and continues around to the edge of the eyelid. Conjunctivitis can begin with irritation from wind or foreign objects. It can be one of the first signs of upper respiratory infection, especially if the cat has been recently kenneled or shown, or been to a clinic or shelter. Infections are perhaps the most common cause of feline conjunctivitis. Glaucoma sometimes causes redness of the conjunctiva. Because this pressure can cause blindness, the cat should be thoroughly checked if conjunctivitis does not clear up within a few days of simple treatment.

When kittens are born, their eyelids are firmly closed. They open between three and 15 days of age. If they do not open by 16 days of age, or open partially, conjunctivitis may be present. Instead of opening, the eyes become infected. Pus forms and may ooze from the corners of the lids. Gently moisten the joined area with a tissue or soft cloth dampened with warm water to soften the scabs and wipe away pus. With your fingernail, pick off any crusts that remain. Pull the lids gently apart. Put antibiotic eye ointment into the opening. Continue using it for a couple of days after the eyes open. If they do not open, wait a day and try again. Eyelids that do not open normally may be surgically opened by your veterinarian, usually after about 16 to 20 days of age. If pus drains from the lids after antibiotic treatment or if they do not open normally, take the kitten to the clinic immediately. Permanent damage can be done to a cornea that is soaked with pus under the closed lids, and the kitten may be blind. These kittens often have bulging eyelids with no drainage.

While most conjunctivitis is caused by bacteria or viruses, some is caused by a related organism called mycoplasma. Infection may be passed from a queen to her kittens at or shortly after birth, or contracted later from carrier animals. Mycoplasma is common in catteries but rare in single-cat households. Signs are first seen around two or three months of age. The cat's eyes may be reddened and swollen. They may be sensitive to light and squinting. Cats usually do not sneeze unless also infected with herpesvirus. This conjunctivitis is best treated with tetracycline eye ointment. Improvement is often seen after only one or two days of treatment. Be sure to treat at least three to five days after signs are gone (fourteen days is even better). Mycoplasma conjunctivitis might be passed to humans, so keep children from handling the kittens until their eyes are healed. Wash your hands with soap after handling the cats.

Conjunctivitis in older cats has similar signs, no matter what the cause. The eyes are reddened and the membrane becomes thickened and puffy. Some conjunctivitis looks like bits of cottage cheese on the membranes. The cat may blink its eye excessively, or hold it slightly closed. Tears may run out, making a wet spot on the face. The cat may groom continuously at that side of its face, washing and further irritating it. Pus or crusty deposits may be seen at the inner corner of the eye.

Simple conjunctivitis can be treated with an antibiotic eye ointment used three or four times a day for two or three days. If the infection does not clear up in this time, the cat should be examined by a veterinarian. Conjunctivitis which does not clear up with antibiotic treatment or returns at frequent intervals, may be due to resistant bacteria. Culture and sensitivity testing may be necessary to allow treatment with an antibiotic specific to the bacteria. Or, it may be caused by a virus, some of which can be treated with special ointments.

Conjunctival adhesions occur when a fold of the conjunctiva grows to the eyeball. Kittens are occasionally born with them. It may happen in an older cat, especially with a small injury to the eyeball that goes unnoticed. Your veterinarian usually can correct it with a simple surgical procedure.

Conjunctival hemorrhage is seen as a large, blood-red spot on the white part of the eyeball. It is more definite and prominent than the "red-eyed" look of conjunctivitis, and nearly always due to trauma. The cat may have been hit by a vehicle, kicked by a human or large animal, or bitten around the face by a large dog. It can happen if the animal is handled roughly or nearly strangled.

Conjunctival hemorrhage by itself does not cause any damage to the eye and does not require treatment. It is, however, a sign that something has happened to the cat's head. Watch for signs of concussion, such as dopiness, staggering, or a tilted head, and for signs of overall injury such as difficulty in breathing or lack of appetite. If other problems appear, have the cat examined by your veterinarian.

TEAR STAINING

Normal tear ducts take excess tears from the eyes and drain them inside the nasal passages. Some purebred cats have trouble with tear staining because the shape of their eyelids is abnormal. One example is the Persian cat, with its unusually shortened face. The tear ducts are distorted and do not drain properly, but let the tears flow down over the facial hair. Bacteria grow on the damp hair, causing reddish, yellow, or brown discoloration. The resulting stain is ugly but usually harmless.

In some cases, surgery may be successful in relieving the overflow. In other cats, part of the duct system is missing. Or, the animal may have damaged tear ducts from adhesions, as after herpesvirus infection. No treatment works for missing or damaged tear ducts.

If you don't wish to have surgery done, or if it will not help, frequent cleaning of the face may keep the staining and bacterial growth under control. Wipe it several times a day with a damp cloth. Mild eye drops will cleanse the eyes. Cream bleaches, available at pet shops or groomers, may lighten the stain. Putting the cat on a course of treatment with tetracycline may help, but usually must be repeated several times a year. These actions reduce the growth of the bacteria which color the tears, but only give temporary improvement.

CATARACTS

Cataracts look like grayish or white lines, stars or cloudiness deep within the cat's eye. They occur in the lens from a number of causes, including injury, especially if the cornea is damaged. Cataracts may occur from infection or inflammation within the globe, and are occasionally seen in cats with diabetes mellitus. Any cat that suddenly develops cataracts should have its blood sugar level checked. Surgery is usually not successful with diabetic cataracts. Cataracts sometimes occur when corticosteroids are given for a long time. They may go away if the animal is taken off the drugs.

Young cats may have cataracts which develop as the cat grows. They often occur in both eyes, but one may be worse than the other. If the underlying retina and the rest of the eye is normal, the animal's vision may be helped by cataract surgery. Some developmental cataracts will clear up by themselves, by six months to three years of age.

Senile sclerosis is a normal change within the eye, commonly confused with cataracts, which occurs with aging. It is seen in older cats, usually more than seven years of age. It is bluish or grayish and quite uniform in appearance, much like frosted glass. Distinct lines are not seen. This does not affect the cat's vision, and nothing need be done.

BLINDNESS

Blindness may occur in cats because of injury or damage to one or both eyes. It may happen because of a taurine deficiency in the cat's diet (see Feline Gourmet Chapter), or because of a detached retina from injury, anemia, or diabetes mellitus. Blindness may be secondary to high blood pressure (usually due to hyperthyroidism or chronic kidney disease) or glaucoma. Or, it may occur gradually as the cat ages. Fungal diseases may cause blindness. Histoplasmosis, blastomycosis, and toxoplasmosis all can damage the retina. An eye that has been prolapsed from the cat's head may be so badly damaged that it must later be removed.

Owners frequently do not notice that the cat has gone blind until they rearrange the furniture or move to a new house. As long as the cat is in its old home, it knows where things are. This is particularly true when the cat gradually becomes blind.

The first sign of blindness may be when the cat bumps into an object. I did not notice that one of my cats had become blind until he walked into a mop bucket. Had the cat run into it while playing, I would have thought him careless. But, he bumped into it at normal walking speed. Then I observed him closely, silently opening a lower cabinet door as he approached; he bumped into it. Further examination showed that retinal disease had caused the blindness.

When the cat has gradually become blind, you may notice changes in the normal social order among your felines. The blind cat had been very dominant over my other cat, a female. He would eat first at the food dish, and when they passed, she would get out of his way. Suddenly, there were fisticuffs at the food dish as she thumped him on the head with her paw. When he walked near her, she would hiss and scuffle with him.

Cats normally signal dominance with eye contact. The dominant cat, by staring at the submissive one says, in effect, "I am going to eat first, then you can eat," or "Here I come, I am going to walk here, and you need to move out of the way." The blind cat could no longer direct his gaze to stare down the other one. So, he gave a mixed signal by not staring but still approaching (James, 1982).

An adjustment period occurred between the two animals. The dominant cat learned to lift his chin slightly as he walked, which did two things: It directed his unseeing gaze upward so the female did not take accidental staring as a threat. It also allowed him to "lead" with his whiskers as he walked, using them to feel objects before his nose impacted. In the end, the two cats changed order, so the formerly submissive cat became dominant, and vice versa.

No care other than ordinary consideration is needed for a cat that has become blind. I tried to minimize the number of boxes or odd objects left on the floor. When I picked up the cat and held him, he was occasionally disoriented when placed back on the floor. After he was blind for some time, this disappeared. I think he navigated mostly by sound: The refrigerator is over here, TV over there, etc. I had to be careful that I didn't leave an outside door open, as he considered it a great adventure and would stride across the yard and into the street, head held high, marching bravely forth to meet the world. He lived another seven years in darkness, a truly special pet.

Chapter 14

EAR PROBLEMS

- *Ear Flap Problems*
  - *Tumors on the Ears*
  - *Hematoma of the Ear*
- *Ear Mites*
- *Ear Infections*
  - *Middle and Inner Ear Infections*
- *Vestibular Disease*
- *Deafness*

How do you know if your cat has ear problems? It may constantly scratch its ear (or ears), and there may be a reddened, sore, scratched, partially hairless spot below the ear. This is where the cat has scraped the hair off and scratched its skin while trying to scratch inside the ear. Treating the affected skin will do no good until the ear is treated. The ear may be swollen. There may be flaky or greasy material inside the ear, and it may have an unpleasant odor. The cat may shake its head, rub its ear on the furniture, or shake or tilt its head to the side.

EAR FLAP PROBLEMS

Injuries to the ear flap are common in cats that live outdoors because as they play or fight they encounter the teeth or claws of another cat. Tom cats on the prowl have the most problems. A fresh cut will bleed a lot. Wet a cloth in cold water, wring it out, and use it to put pressure on the cat's ear for 10 minutes or so to stop the bleeding. If the cat shakes its head or paws at the ear and restarts the bleeding, bandage the entire head. This will put pressure on the ear flap to stop the bleeding. Larger cuts should be treated to prevent infection. If appearance is a concern, as with a show cat, you should have the cut sutured promptly. Otherwise, an antibiotic ointment applied two or three times a day will help speed healing.

Bites which occur lower on the ear may cause infection and abscesses. If you notice the bite before an abscess begins, three to six days of antibiotic treatment may prevent infection. If an abscess occurs, it may be necessary to drain and clean it.

Rarely, injury may fracture the ear cartilage where it attaches to the skull. In addition to other damage to the head, the entire ear may droop downward, and the cat will be unable to raise it at a sound. The cat may hold its head downward or sideways, and the eye on that side may be sunken into the head. This is an emergency and immediate treatment is needed. It is impossible to reattach the ear cartilage if it is completely severed, and eventually it may be necessary to amputate the ear.

Cats that live in cold northern climates may have rounded ends on their ears, without the crusty scabs of skin cancer. This may be due to frostbite at some time in the animal's life. Ears that recently have been frostbitten may be pale at first, followed by reddening. They may then become scaly and dried. The scrotum and tail also can be affected.

TUMORS ON THE EARS

White ears commonly are sunburned, especially if the animal lives outdoors. The climate doesn't need to be particularly sunny. An Oregon cat is as likely to have sunburned ears as an Arizona cat. After the ears are irritated and sunburned for a number of years, the cat may develop a form of skin cancer called squamous cell carcinoma. There is some evidence of a hereditary predisposition to the disease. Rarely, it may be seen in cats under a year old; usually they are middle-aged to elderly.

The first sign of skin cancer on the ears may be yellowish, weeping, crusty spots along the outer edge. At this point, the disease may be stopped in many cats by keeping the animal indoors. Use a soothing ointment or petroleum jelly on the edge to keep it softened. If the cat continues to go outdoors during the day, the lesions will progress. They will crust, break, drain, and fall off again and again until the entire ear flap is eaten away; then it starts into the base of the ear. As with other cancers if left untreated, it can spread to lymph nodes in the area and eventually to other organs such as the lungs, although spread from the ears seems less common in cats than in other animals.

Surgery can be done to remove the cancerous edge from the ear. A generous portion must be cut away to be sure all damaged tissue has been removed. If the cat is allowed outdoors in daylight, the cancer will probably reappear.

Tumors are occasionally seen in a cat's ear canal, where they may go unnoticed for a long time. They can interfere with air circulation in and out of the ear canal, giving the cat continuing problems with bacterial or fungal ear infections. Ceruminous gland tumors are fairly common; most are malignant. These tumors usually occur deep in the ear canal near the eardrum. They may not be found until the cat is sedated and thoroughly examined.

Tumors within the ear canal can be quite difficult to remove surgically, although this is generally the best treatment. In some cases, it may be necessary for the surgeon to slit open the ear canal to reach the offending mass. Tumors that are attached by a small stalk are relatively easy to remove. It is a good idea to have the tumor mass checked, to determine whether it is malignant or benign, before deciding whether further treatment is needed.

HEMATOMA OF THE EAR

Hematomas (blood clots) of the ear are fairly common in cats. Hematomas occur when one cat bites or claws another, rupturing a blood vessel under the skin of the ear. Or, the cat may be hit by a vehicle or bitten on the head by a dog. This also can happen when the cat shakes or claws at its ear, rupturing a blood vessel. Shaking or clawing can be due to an ear infection or a foreign object or parasites in the ear.

A hematoma usually occurs on the inside of the ear. Blood fills a pocket, separating the skin from the cartilage. The area will be swollen and extremely tender. The cat may continue to paw or shake its head. It occurs suddenly, and usually feels the same temperature as the surrounding tissues. This is in contrast to an abscess, which develops over a day or more and may feel hot. With an abscess, the cat may have a temperature, be droopy, and fail to eat, but these signs usually aren't seen with a hematoma.

Surgery is the best treatment for these "blood blisters." Take the cat to your veterinarian to have the blood clot removed and sutured. In some cases, a small plastic drain tube may be placed into the blood-filled pocket. The veterinarian also will deal with the cause of the problem (if it's not due to injury) by treating the infection or mites or removing the foreign body.

If the blood clot is not treated, chances are good it will shrink, causing the ear to wrinkle into a "cauliflower ear." Some people find this unattractive, although it is usually not a functional problem except in a show cat. Even with treatment, some ears will wrinkle to a certain extent. Also, the blood clot is a good growth medium for bacteria. If left untreated, the hematoma may become infected, abscess, break open and drain.

Don't try to puncture the swelling yourself to empty it. When the pressure is reduced, the bleeding will continue. And, you might cause an infection in the cavity. If you cannot take the cat in for surgery, make a small roll of gauze or paper towel which will fit vertically inside the cat's ear. Tape around the gauze and the outside of the ear, as if you were taping around a finger. Be very careful not to wrap the bandage too tightly. Then, tape under the cat's chin to support the bandage and help keep it in place. Don't wrap it so tightly that the cat can't eat or drink. You will probably have to put an Elizabethan collar on the cat and/or hobble its legs to keep the cat from pawing the bandage. If it is more convenient, flatten the cat's ear to the head, wrong-side upward, and tape it to the skull, again bandaging under the jaw. If parasites or infection are present, you will need to treat them, too.

EAR MITES

Ear mites, caused by the mite *Otodectes cynotis*, are perhaps the most common cause of irritation and infection in cats' ears. Fifty to 80% of ear infections in cats are caused by ear mites. Ear mites are very contagious to other cats, and also to dogs. They also occur in ferrets, foxes, raccoons, and other carnivores. Rarely, they can infest humans (Wills, p. 313). Ear mites are especially a problem in catteries. A kitten may begin life with ear mites that it acquires from its mother within the first few days after birth, and may have a severe infestation by the time it is several weeks old. If you have one cat with ear mites, you can assume any other cats or dogs in your household also are involved.

Mites are spread by close contact between cats and probably by contact with contaminated furniture, bedding, carpet, etc. Stress and, especially conditions that promote respiratory infections seem to favor ear mites. A few cats may carry mites without any symptoms, acting as carriers to spread them to others.

Adult ear mites live mainly in the ear canal and feed on surface debris and tissue fluids, including blood, and on inflammatory material stimulated by the mites themselves. The life cycle of mites is completed in as little as two or three weeks. They can live for about two months.

Some cats do not show any signs of ear mite infestation, probably because of natural resistance to the parasites. More commonly, however, the cat will be shaking its head and acting restless. One or both ears may be pulled downward or held at an odd angle. The cat may scratch

PINNA

EAR CANAL

EARDRUM

VERTICAL PART

HORIZONTAL PART

Structures of the ear.

its ear until it bleeds. In some cats, the pain and itching may be severe. Occasionally, the cat will scratch a one to two-inch diameter spot below or in front of the ear, worrying at it with a hind claw until the hair is completely gone and the area is reddened and raw. There may be matching spots on each side of the face, and distinct scratches may be seen. The cat may be grumpy and growl if you try to touch it. You may first suspect ringworm or some other skin disease. In reality, the problem is not the face—it's the itching ear. The mites may migrate outward from the ears, causing reddened, itching, hairless spots on the rump, tail, and neck.

Large quantities of thick, waxy material may be visible inside the ear. This is usually brownish or black and may have a foul odor. It may resemble coffee grounds. In rare cases, the cat may have a loss of balance. This occurs when the ear mites penetrate the eardrum, infecting the middle ear. Rarely, the cat may vomit or go into convulsions. Ear mites that are neglected for a long time may lead to more serious infection by yeasts or bacteria. This can progress to perforation of the eardrum, infection deep within the ear, and even brain involvement.

Do not assume that your cat has ear mites just because the ears are infected. You must see the mites as tiny white or grayish slow-moving specks to confirm that this is indeed the problem. It may be helpful to look closely with a magnifying glass and a flashlight.

If you've confirmed that the cat has ear mites, proceed to treatment. Massage the medication gently into the ear, working up and down the cat's ear and the side of its face. Put the cat where it won't cause any damage if it shakes oily medication on the walls or furniture. An ear drop such as one containing dexamethasone, neomycin, and thiabendazole (Tresaderm®, Merck) is usually very effective in eliminating ear mites. Drugs such as Mitox™ (SmithKline Beecham) or Mitaban also work well. Multiple treatments of rotenone also are effective. In resistant cases, your veterinarian may give ivermectin by injection under the skin. The dosages are critically small, so don't try this yourself. Side effects of ivermectin, although rare, may include shaking and blindness. They should be considered before you automatically treat with this powerful medication. Using ivermectin directly in the ears has no reported side effects, but may take longer for a cure.

Whichever you use, the massage will help work the solution down to the eardrum. The cat's shaking will help remove debris. Treat the cat twice a day for two or three days at first. Then, treat the cat daily for 10 to 14 days. This helps break the mites' life cycle and get rid of them. Wait a week, then repeat the treatment for another week.

Meanwhile, treat all your other cats and dogs on the same schedule. Wash bedding, using hot water and bleach or disinfectant. Dust both cats and dogs with a flea powder (be sure to use one that is made for cats). Or, you can use one of the mousse-style preparations to treat the cats and take the dogs to be dipped as you would for a flea problem. This helps kill mites that have migrated elsewhere on the animals. Mites often accumulate at the base of the cat's tail where they migrate when the cat sleeps with its tail wrapped around its ears. Treating all the animals at one time helps eliminate the problem once and for all. Otherwise, you will treat ear mites in one cat, next week in another, next month in the dog and back around again, indefinitely. Just treating the ears with mite-killing medication is rarely effective in eliminating them. Treat the premises as you would for a flea infestation. Flea collars have no effect on ear mites.

Incidentally, kittens born to some queens have more trouble with ear mites than those born to others. Cats that have immune system problems or are infected with feline leukemia have greater trouble with ear mites. These findings suggest that a degree of immunity against the parasites is found in some cats.

Notoedric mange is occasionally seen as an ear problem. It causes intense itching, and the skin of the ears will be crusty and scaly. The cat may scratch its ears enough to draw blood, and the face and paws also may be affected (see External Parasites Chapter).

EAR INFECTIONS

Overall, cats have far fewer ear infections than do dogs. This is probably because their upstanding ears allow better ventilation, and allow them to shake out most objects that fall or are blown into the ear canal. Also, most cats have less hair in their ears, again allowing for better ventilation and less dirt collection. Ear infections may accompany parasitic diseases such as ear mites (see above). Skin diseases, hormonal imbalances, and allergies may bring on ear infections. Or, they may occur alone, caused by bacteria, yeasts, or fungi. Infection in only one ear is usually caused by a polyp in the middle ear, a bite wound, or a tumor within the ear canal.

Signs of ear infection include waxy or oily material inside the ears, easily visible among the wrinkles and folds. In a severe infection, yellowish or greenish pus may be seen. The ears are often quite reddened and may have a foul odor. The cat may be headshy, moving away when you try to touch it or pet its head. In severe cases, the cat may have trouble chewing. As with ear mites, there may be severe itching and irritation. The animal may scratch at its ear badly enough to cause a hematoma. It may shake its head violently or rub it on the carpet. With a severe ear infection, the cat may carry its head tilted, and may stagger while walking. If the infection goes on long enough, the cat may have trouble hearing, or become deaf.

Ideally, treatment for an ear infection would include veterinary care with sedation and thorough cleaning of the ear canal (all the way to the eardrum) to make sure there are no foreign bodies in the ear. The drainage would be cultured to discover what organisms are present so they can be specifically treated. To clean ears, many veterinarians use a Water-Pik® set on the very lowest setting and held well away from the ear. A rubber-bulb ear syringe also can be used for ear cleaning, or, a 12- or 20-cc syringe with a short length of soft rubber tubing on the end. The cleaning solution is squeezed VERY gently into the cat's ears, and suctioned out. This is repeated until the flushing solution is clear. If the solution comes out the cat's nostrils or the cat chokes on it, a ruptured eardrum is indicated. If you are cleaning the cat's ears and this happens, take the cat to your veterinarian. Many infections can be treated by cleaning alone.

The ears may be cleaned with lukewarm water. A cleanser that contains acetic acid (vinegar) and boric acid and is pH balanced to avoid burning also can be used. DermaPet® is an example of such a cleaning solution. Do not use any ear solution which contains alcohol. And, solutions such as chlorhexidine disinfectants (Nolvasan®, Fort Dodge) or products containing salicylic acid should not be used in the ears. They may be toxic to nerve cells in the inner ear, resulting in deafness. Whatever solution is used, it should be lukewarm—not cold nor hot!

Cotton swabs should NEVER be used to clean the ears. They may cause damage, and may pack dirt and wax down into the ear canal. At worst, they can cause rupture of an infection-weakened eardrum. Cotton balls can be used to cleanse the outer part of the cat's ear, and to wipe away cleaning solutions after rinsing the cat's ears.

A topical antibiotic is then used. Ear drops are much more efficient than ointments, which take longer to dissolve the waxy material and are less effective in moving it out of the ear canal. Tresaderm drops are often used. Domeboro Otic (Dome) can help to acidify the ear canal and is useful in healing infection. If you have nothing else available, make a mixture of equal parts of vinegar (preferably white vinegar) and a light salad oil. The vinegar will help to acidify the cat's ears, making them unfavorable for the growth of bacteria and fungi. The oil will help to liquefy the wax and move it out of the cat's ears, as well as drowning any ear mites that are present. Don't let the cat shake this "dressing" on your clothing or carpet.

If the cat has a severe ear infection with a large amount of pus and considerable pain, don't even try to treat it yourself. The ear canal may be damaged, or the ear drum may already be punctured. Attempts to treat or clean it yourself may cause serious problems. Take the animal to your veterinarian.

In half to three-fourths of cats with long-term ear infections, the eardrum may be ruptured, or it may have been ruptured in the past. This necessitates care in the type of products used to clean the ears. Contact with some ear products may kill cells in the middle or inner ear, causing deafness or loss of equilibrium. The cat may lack alertness, and be difficult to waken. It may not react to specific sounds, and the voice may change.

Excessive moisture in the ears keeps the skin soggy and allows organisms which normally grow in the ears to multiply in excessive numbers. This may predispose the cat to an ear infection. NEVER use powdered ear medications. They stick in the ear and may contribute to the problem rather than helping to cure it. A cat with a reddened ear flap (pinna) may have an allergy which will contribute to or even cause the ear infection.

MIDDLE AND INNER EAR INFECTIONS

Both of these are common in cats. They usually occur when an ear infection spreads through the eardrum and inward. Or, they may come up the eustachian tube as a complication of an upper respiratory infection or sinusitis.

The first sign of a middle or inner ear problem may be a change in equilibrium or balance. The cat may tilt its head sideways or downward on the affected side. It may be incoordinated, and stagger, stumble, fall, or roll over with little control. The eyes may roll rhythmically from one side to the other, again without control by the cat. The neck and head may be flexed downward. Rarely, one side of the face may be paralyzed. If the condition persists for a period of time, the cat may walk with its legs spread, crouch down, or even crawl because it is too unstable to walk upright.

Polyps occasionally occur in the ear canal or in the middle ear, especially in young cats. Their cause is unknown, although some may be due to inflammation. The cat may show the same signs as with an ear infection, including ear scratching, head shaking, head tilting, and a pus-filled or waxy discharge. The third eyelid may be pushed partway across the eye. Large polyps in the middle ear may cause rupture of the eardrum. X-rays may be needed to determine the extent of involvement. Surgery is usually the treatment of choice. Afterward, even if the surgery is successful, the cat may have a head tilt and staggering for as many as two weeks.

None of these middle and inner ear problems are ones that you can treat at home. They may not be curable even with veterinary care, depending on the cause and how long it has affected the cat. Take the cat to a clinic as soon as possible.

VESTIBULAR DISEASE

Vestibular disorders are fairly common in cats. The vestibular apparatus is used to help all animals keep their balance and equilibrium. It is a part of the inner ear. The cat begins by holding its head tilted to one side. It will show an involuntary rolling of the eyeballs from one side to the other. The cat may have a sudden loss of balance, toppling over onto one side, and may be unable to walk in a straight line, turning only in circles. This condition, called idiopathic vestibular neuropathy or feline peripheral vestibular syndrome, can occur suddenly in an adult cat, for no apparent reason. It is not life-threatening, but can look very scary when it affects your cat. There usually is no discharge from the ears or nose. Laboratory tests are completely normal. These cats are usually much improved in two or three days. Most affected cats recover completely in two or three weeks without any treatment. A few cats will have attacks in the future, but the majority of them never have signs again. Some animals will have a permanent head tilt. Take the cat to a clinic as soon as possible, because you can't easily differentiate this from a middle or inner ear infection.

DEAFNESS

Kittens are born deaf as well as blind, although they can respond to loud noises even before their ear canals open (around five days of age). Hearing is fully developed by the time the kitten is a month old. Deafness is seen as a hereditary problem in white cats. Cats with a completely white coat that have two blue eyes are almost always deaf from birth or shortly afterward. Cats that have one blue eye and one yellow eye are less often deaf, and white cats with yellow eyes usually can hear. White cats of Burmese or Siamese parentage may not be deaf. If the cat has a black or gray smudge on the head, or spots on the body, it is less often deaf, even if the spots fade as the cat ages. (For more on deafness in white cats, see Delack, 1984). Deafness is uncommon in cats of colors other than white, although I owned a tortoise-shell female that was deaf.

Some antibiotics can cause deafness when given in high dosages or for long periods of time. These include kanamycin, streptomycin, gentamicin, and neomycin. Disinfectants may cause deafness if they are put into an ear with a punctured eardrum. These include iodine compounds, alcohol, chlorhexidine, and others.

Many deaf cats are deaf in only one ear. They can hear sound but cannot tell its location. This is perhaps the most common deafness in cats, and you may not even notice it. Test your cat's hearing by asking someone, with back turned to the cat, to make a loud noise with keys, or whistle or shout. Do this facing away or around a corner from the cat. Otherwise, it may respond to movement rather than to sound.

Older cats do not become deaf as often as dogs do, although in some cats, hearing becomes less acute after about 13 to 15 years of age. You may not notice if your cat gradually becomes deaf. The cat easily may become accustomed to not hearing, and may compensate well enough that you may not notice the loss. Some older cats that are deaf lose their fear of previously frightening objects such as the vacuum cleaner. An older cat that goes deaf may instinctively stay closer to home, not straying far from its yard. It may be less difficult than you think to convert the cat to a strictly indoor cat. The only problem is the cat might try to escape, or sit by the door, meowing. A deaf cat that is brought into the house may seem more destructive than normal because it cannot hear things falling over.

Tiny kittens that are deaf may not survive, as they cannot hear their mother calling. They may die of cold or starvation. Deaf kittens may not awaken for feeding unless they are physically nudged by their mother or littermates. They may be more aggressive when playing because they cannot hear the protests of their littermates when they are too rough. They may cry loudly when apart from the other kittens because they depend on their littermates for security and behavioral cues. It may be difficult to awaken the kitten by talking, but it may be startled by touching, and may even bite when awakened.

Outdoor cats that are totally deaf are at great risk, as they cannot hear a car or dog coming; euthanasia is often the kindest course. If kept indoors, the majority of deaf cats live normal lives as perfectly suitable pets. A few cats are anxious or timid, jumpy, and paranoid, and will require a great deal of care. The deaf cat will feel vibrations on the floor to know when someone is coming, and will learn to recognize different persons visually. Be careful when you awaken the cat, as it may respond by clawing first and asking questions later. Many owners find that a deaf cat is more mellow and less excitable than a cat that can hear. Some of these cats also are less afraid of strangers.

You may need to compensate for the cat's deafness in a few small ways. Instead of calling its name, get the cat's attention by turning a room light on and off, stamping your foot on the floor, or wiggling your fingers in front of its face to get its attention. When you have the cat's attention, shake your finger or make some similar gesture to say "No!". You also can discipline the cat with a water squirt bottle, or by throwing ping pong balls at the cat. If there are several cats in the household, the deaf cat will take many of its cues from the others. Living with a deaf cat is usually not much of a problem. Cats that are deaf from hereditary causes should not be bred so as not to perpetuate and spread the defect.

Chapter 15

HEART AND LUNG PROBLEMS

- *Heart and Blood Vessel Problems*
  - *Signs of Heart and Vascular Disease*
  - *Heartworms*
  - *Aortic Blood Clots*
- *Blood Problems*
  - *Blood Clotting Problems*
  - *Anemia*
  - *Blood Parasites*
  - *Blood Transfusions*
- *Respiratory Problems*
  - *Lung Disease*
  - *Mycotic Pneumonias*
  - *Inhalant Allergies (Atopy)*
  - *Diaphragmatic Hernia*

HEART AND BLOOD VESSEL PROBLEMS

The normal heart rate in a resting, relaxed adult cat is usually between 120 and 240 beats per minute. It is a good idea to take your cat's pulse several times over several days to determine its normal pulse. A cat with a heart rate consistently above or below those values should be checked by a veterinarian as it may indicate a cardiac arrhythmia (irregular rhythm). A normal cat should have a steady, rhythmic heartbeat without skipped beats.

Abnormalities of the heart and associated structures are usually termed "heart disease." These may include inflammation of the heart muscle (myositis), extra beats, abnormally fast or slow heartbeat, skipped beats, leaking (insufficient) valves, or narrowed (stenotic) valves. Heart disease also may include blockage of the coronary (heart) arteries or heartworm disease.

Hypertrophic cardiomyopathy is one of the most common and severe forms of heart disease. In this condition, the heart muscle becomes overgrown and damaged. A taurine deficiency in the cat's food can cause dilated cardiomyopathy, in which the heart muscle becomes enlarged, flabby and inefficient. If it continues, the cat will die. Most cats more than 10 years of age have a condition called valvular endocardiosis, but it seldom leads to symptoms or heart failure.

SIGNS OF HEART AND VASCULAR DISEASE

Cats with heart failure often breathe more rapidly than normal and appear to have difficulty breathing. Cats with heart disease rarely cough. This is in contrast to dogs with congestive heart failure where the most common sign is a continuous moist cough. The cat may have fluid in the chest cavity, which also shows up as difficulty in breathing. The abdomen may fill with fluid, appearing swollen and rounded. The cat may be weak or droopy and less active than normal, as well as showing fatigue or fainting or collapse after exertion. Some cats show only non-specific signs such as poor appetite, weight loss or loss of muscle mass, or lethargy. On some cats, you may be able to feel a rumbling or vibration, as opposed to the regular heartbeat. To check this, put your fingers on each side of the cat's lower chest or cup your hand around the bottom of the chest, just behind the front legs. Make sure the cat is not purring!

Kittens with heart defects may be stunted and gain weight poorly. They may show weakness and fainting as they try to play or follow their mother. These kittens do not improve by themselves and are too small to be good candidates for surgery. After a diagnosis of a heart defect is made, euthanasia is the kindest treatment.

If you notice any of these signs, have the cat examined by your veterinarian. These obviously aren't conditions which can be treated at home. Heart and circulatory problems in older cats can be diagnosed by a number of methods, including use of the stethoscope. An electrocardiogram (EKG or ECG) measures the electrical energy generated by special nerve tissue within the heart which makes the heart muscle contract and expand. Irregularities in the electrical impulses can be found, and they may tell which area is affected and what is happening there. Other tests may include phonocardiograms, echocardiograms (ultrasound examination of the heart), cardiac catheterization, blood tests, dye injection, and X-rays.

Abnormal calcium or potassium levels in the blood may cause unusual heart rhythms (called cardiac arrhythmias). A lack of oxygen in the blood, or medications such as digoxin, also may cause them. Arrhythmias can be treated by treating underlying disorders such as low blood potassium or taurine levels, or with special medications to stabilize the heartbeat. Hyperthyroidism which has led to heart damage also can be treated. This condition is more common than previously thought.

Unfortunately, the majority of cases of heart failure do not have treatable causes. The cat generally needs a heart transplant and there is no reasonable way to do this. Treatment for heart disease usually means managing the symptoms to make the cat's remaining time as comfortable as possible.

Medication such as digitalis derivatives may be used to stabilize the heartbeat. If the veterinarian "digitalizes" your cat, the animal may need to be hospitalized for several days until a dosage is established. You may need to consult your veterinarian from time to time to adjust the cat's medication after it returns home to normal activity and routine. New medications are continually being developed which are increasingly effective in treating heart disease. Diuretics are used in some cases to reduce fluid retention in the animal's body and relieve the load on its heart. In some cases, a pacemaker may be implanted to regulate the animal's heartbeat.

Cats that are anemic may have an increased heart rate. If the area around the nose is white-haired and the skin is normally pink, it will appear to be pale or even "white as a sheet" in the anemic cat. If the cat is Siamese or dark-colored, open the mouth to see its "color," which should be pink. If the cat appears anemic, it is important to consult your veterinarian to determine the cause. In most cases, anemia is not a disease in itself. It is merely an obvious and blatant symptom of something else.

Cats that are hyperthyroid have an excess of thyroid hormones circulating in their blood. One of the consequences of this is an increased heart rate. Other signs include weight loss despite a normal or increased appetite, soft stools, and occasional vomiting. The cat may be hyperactive. Hyperthyroidism may occur with an overgrowth of the thyroid gland, called adenomatous goiter. Currently, the most successful treatment is to remove the thyroid glands if the cat is healthy enough to tolerate surgery. If not, drug or radiation therapy may be used to reduce the amount of active thyroid tissue.

Heart disease may be caused by abnormalities in the lungs which result in an increase in blood pressure in them. This pressure causes the heart to work harder, trying to push its normal quota of blood into the lungs. If this situation goes on long enough, it will result in failure of the right side of the heart. Asthma attacks, pneumonia, and blood clots in the lung also may cause this type of heart disease. If it is caught in time and the underlying cause is corrected, the heart disease may be reversible. If not, it may lead to eventual stretching and weakening of the heart muscle and, ultimately, heart failure.

Dilated cardiomyopathy (DCM) is a disease in which the heart muscle becomes weak and flabby, like a limp balloon, instead of being a springy and tough pump. Low concentrations of the amino acid taurine in the diet may be the cause. When a taurine supplement is added to the diet of a deficient cat, the heart may gradually become stronger. Taurine may be lacking in homemade vegetarian or all-meat diets (see The Feline Gourmet Chapter). It is most common in young to middle-aged cats.

When the cat has heart disease, the body tries to compensate for the reduced blood flow. The heart begins to beat faster and work harder. The muscles of the heart may thicken (or in some conditions, the heart chambers become enlarged) as it attempts to pump more blood. The kidneys may retain sodium and water, trying to increase blood volume and pressure. Temporarily, the animal may

compensate with increased blood flow, and no signs of heart disease are seen.

As the condition progresses, the heart may be unable to compensate. The cardiac output is not sufficient to supply oxygen to the tissues and meet the body's other needs. Then, blood backs up behind the failing heart, creating pressure which causes congestion and fluid accumulation. This condition is called congestive heart failure. If the heart failure involves the left side of the heart, fluid builds up in the lungs. The cat will cough, breathe with difficulty, and be weak. Some cats will be depressed, dehydrated, and have a low body temperature. If the failure occurs on the right side of the heart, the cat will have congestion and fluid in the chest and abdomen. Both sides of the heart are affected in some cats. Heart failure may make other internal organs, such as the kidneys, liver, and gastrointestinal tract less efficient.

Treatment may include emergency stabilization at the veterinary clinic if the cat is seriously ill. Fluids, anti-clotting medication, taurine, diuretics, and drugs to stabilize heart function may be given.

Nutrition is important in helping to manage heart disease. Providing a food with controlled levels of certain nutrients helps to reduce the workload on the heart while maintaining the nutritional needs of the animal. As with humans with heart disease, a low level of sodium helps keep the animal from retaining fluid. However, palatability may be a problem with some low-sodium cat foods. It also is important that the diet be palatable enough that the animal will continue (or resume) eating. The food should have moderate levels of high quality protein. Extra B-complex vitamins and potassium help replace valuable nutrients lost because of diuretic administration. Conversely, a cat with a heart problem usually needs fewer calories than a healthy cat of the same weight. It is critical that the cat have an adequate amount of taurine in its diet. Your veterinarian can help you design the correct diet.

If at all possible, the cat should be medically stabilized before trying to change its diet. Some medications used to treat heart failure cause an upset stomach. Your cat may associate this upset with its new diet and thus, fail to eat it. Gradually change the cat to the new diet over a period of three days to two weeks. It may be helpful to mix a little new food with the old food, and gradually change the proportions of the two foods until only the new one is being fed. Or, you can add small quantities of low-sodium foods (see below) to the new food until the cat is eating well. It may be helpful to sprinkle a salt-free seasoning such as garlic powder (NOT garlic SALT!) on the food to help tempt the appetite. Warm the food to increase its flavor. Feed small quantities of the new food four to six times a day so that it is fresh and tasty each time. Feed only the diet recommended by your veterinarian. NO extra treats!

Cats with heart disease should not be given foods with high sodium levels: milk, cheese, ice cream, bread, cereal, carrots, peanut butter, potato chips, heart, kidney, liver, whole eggs, salted fats (butter and margarine), salted snacks such as pretzels, and prepared meats such as bologna, ham, salami, and hot dogs. Permissible table foods include unsalted beef, chicken, domestic rabbit, lamb, horse meat, fresh water fish, oatmeal, rice, corn, and egg yolks. Do not give pet treats, as most are VERY high in salt.

It is important that the heart patient have fresh, clean water available at all times. If you have a household water softener, the water may be too high in sodium for your cat. The water should have less than 150 parts per million of sodium. If it contains more than that, give your cat distilled water, especially during the first couple of weeks of treatment. You may have to flavor it with a little unsalted beef broth or something similar. If you do not have softened water, determine the sodium content of your tap water by calling your city's water department. Or, have the water tested if you are on a well.

Provide a quiet, calm, comfortable environment for your heart patient. Avoid extreme changes in temperature. If you take the cat to the clinic or boarding kennel in cold weather, make sure the traveling crate is well bedded with towels or rags. Warm your car before putting the cat in it, and be sure to cover the crate with a towel or blanket as you take the cat to the car. Be sure the cat avoids stress, excitement, or extreme exertion. Do not allow the cat to become overweight. If it is already overweight, work with your veterinarian to help the cat lose weight.

HEARTWORMS

Heartworms can lead to congestive heart failure. Cats are quite susceptible to heartworms and a high percentage of cats that are bitten by mosquitoes will become infected. However, even in areas where large numbers of dogs have heartworms, few cats are infected. This is probably because most mosquitoes seem to prefer dogs. In an area where heartworms are a problem in dogs, the incidence in cats will be less than 10% of that in unprotected dogs. Heartworms have been considered rare in cats, but are being found more often, perhaps because tests are better and veterinarians are looking for them!

Heartworms are a serious problem in dogs in some of the wetter parts of the United States. In the past, heartworms were confined to the southeastern United States. Now they are found in every state. However, in climates that are dry or cold, infected areas may be as small as a few square miles, usually in lowlands or valleys. Animals outside this area are safe. The pockets of infection may be due to large numbers of infected dogs.

Heartworms are spread by mosquitoes which have taken in infected blood. They pass infectious larvae in their saliva from an infected dog to another dog, a cat, or a human (after a couple of developmental stages). For that reason, heartworms are usually found in cats that live outdoors, especially toms, probably because they roam, and are exposed to the mosquitoes.

Because the worms are not naturally cat parasites, the infestations are usually light —only one to 10 adult worms may be present inside the heart, although each worm may be as long as five to 10 inches (12.5 to 25 mm). It can take up to eight months for the larvae to migrate and become adult worms in the cat's heart. Many cats probably have

self-limiting infections, in which the worms never get far beyond the site where they entered the skin. As few as two worms may be fatal. This may be due to the relatively large size of the worms and small size of the cat and its heart and blood vessels.

Part of the damage from heartworms is caused when they roughen the lining of blood vessels in the lungs. The inside diameter of the blood vessel becomes smaller, making the heart work harder as it tries to push blood into the lungs.

Cats with heartworms may have few symptoms (or none). However, heartworms can cause blood clots, which in turn cause varying symptoms depending on where in the body they become lodged. The cat may suddenly have asthma and wheezing, coughing, or trouble breathing. A frothy nasal discharge is sometimes seen, and the cat may be weak and listless. In some cats, gagging or vomiting is the only symptom. The abdomen may fill with fluid and become enlarged. The cat may be lethargic, with a lack of appetite and weight loss. Feline heartworms will occasionally stray into the brain and cause central nervous system illness, including depression, head tilting, turning in circles, and convulsions. The cat may die suddenly without any symptoms or sometimes after a bout of peculiar howling.

Because heartworm disease is so uncommon in cats, it is also difficult to recognize. Negative results on tests for heartworm antigen or for microfilaria in the blood do not rule out heartworm infection in cats. Current tests do not always detect heartworm infections, even in dogs. The Knott's test, widely used in dogs, does not work in most cats. Radiographs showing changes in the arteries in the hindmost lobe of the lung are often used for diagnosis. Ultrasound (echocardiograph) tests also are used.

Adult heartworms sometimes can be successfully treated in cats, especially with intensive hospital care, although it can be difficult. The drugs used to kill the worms are toxic to cats. Adverse reactions are frequent, and cats sometimes die suddenly during the treatment. Cats are prone to clots from the worms which are killed by the treatment, possibly because of the small size of their blood vessels. Because of this, the mortality rate from treatment is much higher in cats than in dogs. Surgical removal is sometimes used. Treatment is most successful if the disease is diagnosed before the blood vessels are permanently damaged and before the cat is too weak or ill to be treated.

The cat should be caged or similarly restricted from activity for four to six weeks after treatment. As many (or more) cats may be saved by simply allowing the disease to run its course as are saved by currently available treatments. The life span of the adult worms seems to be short in cats (two to three years compared to six or seven years in dogs), and the cat may outlive the heartworms without drug treatment.

Heartworm infestations in cats are usually self-limiting, again because the cat is not the normal or natural host. Almost no cats have sufficient numbers of microfilaria (heartworm larvae) in their blood for mosquitoes to pass them on to other animals. If they do have microfilaria, they only are present for a short period of time, usually fewer than two months. Because of these factors, heartworms do not easily spread from infected cats to other animals. It is unnecessary to treat the cat with a drug to kill the microfilaria, called a microfilaricide (Otto, 1980).

Cats in problem heartworm areas, especially those living outdoors, can be put on once-monthly heartworm preventives (Heartgard 30® Plus) if recommended by your veterinarian. These medications are not needed by cats that are kept indoors. Because the disease is rare in cats, most authorities do not recommend routinely giving preventive medication. If heartworms are present in your area, additional prevention includes keeping the cat indoors during mosquito season, especially at night, and controlling mosquitoes inside the house. There is no danger of infection from a cat or dog to a human.

AORTIC BLOOD CLOTS

Blood clots sometimes occur in the hind part of the aorta. They may form because of disease changes within the heart, especially hypertrophic cardiomyopathy. Or, they may be due to infection in the lining of the heart or the muscle itself. Clots break off from the damaged tissue and flow with the blood down the aorta as it divides to the hind legs. When it reaches the point where the aorta divides, it lodges and stops. It is joined by a growing mass of clotted blood as circulation to the area slows down and finally stops. As the clot grows larger, the blood supply to the hind legs will continue to diminish.

A cat with an aortic clot may appear lame, and may be incoordinated and staggering. It may seem to be weak in the hind end and may drag one or both hind legs. The Achilles tendons may be stretched until the cat's feet lie flat to the floor like a rabbit's hind feet. If this goes on for some time, the hair may be worn off the bottoms of the hind feet. At worst, the hind legs may be completely paralyzed.

It is more common for the blood clot to occur suddenly. The cat may be an indoor animal that has not been outside and has had no chance to have an accident. It may be limply paralyzed in the hindquarters, and occasionally a fore leg may be affected. The hind legs and the pads of the feet may feel cold to the touch. If you feel inside the hind legs for a femoral pulse, there will be none. The cat's temperature may be below normal. It may have trouble breathing and the membranes may be bluish in color. The cat may cry out and writhe in pain. This is an emergency. Take the cat to a veterinary clinic as soon as possible.

If the cat lives through the initial crisis, the muscles of its hind legs will become hard, swollen, and painful. The clot may shrink enough that blood will flow past it, reestablishing circulation. Or, smaller blood vessels in the area may become enlarged and take over functions formerly carried out by the now-clogged vessels. The cat will start dragging itself along, slowly regaining use of the hind legs. Some cats will return to a normal gait after a period of time. Others regain only partial use of the legs, walking

permanently "down on the hocks" much like a rabbit. Calluses will form on the hocks, and the cat will walk like this for the rest of its life.

Surgery is rarely done for these blood clots. Cats in this condition are poor candidates to survive emergency surgery. The clots are almost certain to recur if the original cause is not corrected.

BLOOD PROBLEMS

BLOOD CLOTTING PROBLEMS

Hemophilia is a disease caused by hereditary lack of one of the blood factors necessary for clotting. If the cat is injured, or if surgery is done on the animal before the problem is diagnosed, bleeding may be severe. Or, you may notice bumps under the animal's skin due to bleeding where the cat has bruised itself.

Hemophilia is fairly rare in cats. When diagnosed, it can be treated by transfusions of blood or plasma. Since the problem is hereditary, any related animals that are being used for breeding should be tested and removed from the breeding program.

Cats occasionally may have blood that does not clot normally because of something they have eaten. Warfarin and coumarin, found in rat and rodent poisons (such as D-Con®), can cause poor blood clotting. Symptoms are similar to those of hemophilia, above. The cat may bleed into the abdomen or bruise easily. Or, a minor wound may bleed for several hours to a day or more. The newer anticoagulants are almost 100% fatal if enough is eaten to cause clotting defects, but they are nearly 100% treatable if caught in time. These products may stay in the body three to 12 weeks, so treatment is essential.

Severe liver disease also may cause poor blood clotting. If there is enough liver damage to result in clotting problems, the cat probably will be icteric, showing a yellow color in the membranes of its eyes and mouth, and also may show other signs of illness. Feline leukemia virus also can cause clotting problems.

ANEMIA

Anemia is a symptom rather than a disease. Membranes in the eyes, mouth, and tongue are abnormally pale or completely white. The skin on the tip of the nose, pads of the feet, and ears is white instead of the normal pinkish color. Anemia is due to a lower than normal number of red cells in the circulating blood. It also may be due to a lower than normal amount of hemoglobin in the red blood cells. Hemoglobin is the oxygen-carrying pigment that gives the blood its normal red color. The cat may become quite anemic before you notice the problem. It may have a poor appetite and little energy. Anemia may be seen with illness, injury or stress. In one study, nearly three-fourths of cats with anemia were carriers of the feline leukemia virus. Cats with feline immunodeficiency virus are also usually anemic.

Anemia can be caused by simple blood loss, such as when the cat is injured and bleeding has occurred. However, shock is usually more of a problem with this sort of injury than is anemia. Internal parasites, especially hookworms, can cause continuing blood loss as the worms suck blood from the intestinal lining. Intestinal tumors or ulcers also may damage the lining, resulting in chronic blood loss. Heavy infestations of fleas may suck enough blood from small kittens to make them anemic.

Anemia can occur when more blood cells are destroyed than are being manufactured in the bone marrow. This is seen with autoimmune hemolytic anemias. The body somehow decides that the red blood cells do not belong to it, and rapidly destroys them. This destruction may be seen with parasites such as *Hemobartonella* that live in the blood cells. It occurs in most cases of feline leukemia. Destruction of red blood cells also can be caused by several drugs and toxins. Medication containing methylene blue can cause anemia in cats.

Griseofulvin, chloramphenicol, trimethoprim-sulfa, and acepromazine are medications which can occasionally cause anemia due to bone marrow suppression. Poisoning with acetaminophen (Tylenol®) and similar products can cause anemia. As little as half a tablet may be toxic. If the cat is accidentally or deliberately given this medication, take it to a veterinarian as soon as possible. Onions, if given to a cat in large enough quantity, may cause anemia and even death. Zinc (present in most coins) can cause anemia in cats. An angry cat that chews on a galvanized fitting on a cage or cat carrier may take in enough to cause severe blood cell destruction within the blood vessels.

Anemia may result from certain vitamin deficiencies, which may occur when a cat is fed a homemade diet. Lack of folate can cause anemia. Folate is present in adequate quantities in commercial foods, however, cats that are ill or eating inadequate quantities of food may run short because it is not well stored in the body.

Immediate treatment for severe anemia usually includes a blood transfusion to help replenish the missing red blood cells. Intravenous fluids may be given to help restore the cat's blood volume and counteract dehydration. Bone marrow transplants may even be used. The next course of action is to determine the cause of the anemia and treat it specifically, whether it is a bacterial or viral disease, an autoimmune problem, cancer, dietary, or something else. Bone marrow examination may help determine the cause of anemia.

BLOOD PARASITES

Feline hemobartonellosis is an infection caused by a rickettsial organism, *Hemobartonella felis*, which lives within the cat's red blood cells. The disease is also called feline infectious anemia. It is worse in older cats than kittens, and is more common in cats that are outdoors or feral. It is especially seen in the spring, when cats are mating and fights and bites occur. Hemobartonellosis spreads when one cat bites another or licks blood from the other cat's fur. It can be passed from the queen to her litter, although exactly how this occurs, whether through the uterine wall, during the birth process, or in the milk, is not known. The disease also may be accidentally spread via blood transfusions. Hemobartonellosis is almost always secondary to stress or another disease, especially feline leukemia, feline immunodeficiency virus, and unhealing abscesses, all of which weaken the cat's defense mechanisms.

Symptoms first may be seen about a month after the cat is infected and may last for a few days to several weeks. They can be general, such as weakness, depression, lack of appetite, weight loss, fever, and pale or slightly yellowish mucous membranes. The cat may have a rapid heartbeat, and vomiting is often seen. It may take two to four months for the cat's red blood count to return to normal.

Hemobartonellosis is diagnosed by laboratory examination of a blood sample. Several samples may be needed to detect the organisms. Animals with complicating diseases are more seriously ill than those with hemobartonellosis alone, and more of them die.

About a third of cats infected with hemobartonellosis will die if they are not treated. Treatment with oxytetracycline for three weeks usually clears up the infection. If the cat is severely anemic, a blood transfusion from a healthy donor may be needed. Because treatment does not completely eradicate the parasite, the cat remains a carrier for the rest of its life. The carrier state also may follow natural recovery. However, having the disease does not give a lasting immunity. If the cat becomes immunosuppressed for any reason, it may recur. Corticosteroid treatment may allow the parasites to prosper and attack the blood cells, quickly bringing back symptoms. Reducing risk factors will give the best chance for a long and healthy life. Flea control will help to prevent stress and occurrence. The cat should be kept indoors to reduce the possibility of contact with other cats, as well as stress that might reduce its resistance (Espada, 1991). Avoid overcrowding if you have more than one cat. This will reduce stress and fighting, helping to prevent other cats in the household from contracting the disease.

Cytauxzoon felis is a protozoan parasite which affects feline blood cells. It spreads to cats from wild animal carriers via ticks. It is seen in heavily wooded rural areas in Missouri, southeastern states, Texas, and Oklahoma. Most cases occur in summer when ticks are common. Early signs include depression, lack of appetite, dehydration, and fever. After three or four days, the temperature drops to normal or below normal before the cat dies. The cat also may show anemia, jaundice, and swollen lymph nodes. Cats affected with this disease almost always die within one to two weeks after symptoms begin. No treatment has been found which changes the fatal course of the disease. Cytauxzoonosis does not seem transmissible to humans or other animals, including cats.

BLOOD TRANSFUSIONS

An anemic cat may need a blood transfusion. This may be because of a severe infestation of internal parasites, ticks, or fleas. It may be needed when the cat has surgery and loses blood during the operation or has acute blood loss for any reason. Or, it may be necessary because the cat has feline leukemia, cancer, kidney or liver disease, or vitamin K deficiency, or is a hemophiliac. A blood transfusion may save your pet's life in any of these situations.

Blood is taken from healthy donor cats that are kept in isolation, or at least separated from other cats (lone house pets). This helps to ensure they are not infected with any disease. The donor cat is also tested for diseases such as leukemia, again to be sure that its blood is normal and healthy. As when humans give blood, the procedure is safe for the donor cat. Some experienced donor cats do not even require anesthesia. One of my cats would sit calmly, purring, as he made his contribution to help save another cat's life. Six weeks is the norm between donations, although a cat could give blood every three weeks if necessary. In general, a donor cat should weigh at least 10 pounds and preferably more. It should be at least a year old, but no more than 10 years old. The cat also should be mild-tempered so that giving blood is not stressful.

Cats have one of three feline blood groups or "types." Donors that are used frequently often are typed to determine which one they have. Blood is usually crossmatched to be sure donor and recipient are compatible so that damaging reactions can be avoided.

RESPIRATORY PROBLEMS

Respiratory difficulty is an emergency in the cat. Cats that are having trouble breathing may be upset and aggressive. If roughly handled, they may die from stress. If oxygen is available, put a clear plastic bag over the cat's head, leaving it open around the neck, and gently flow oxygen into it. This may help calm the cat and relieve its distress enough for you to take it to your veterinarian or emergency clinic. If you don't have oxygen, handle the cat as little as possible and as gently and quietly as you can.

Cats may have polyps in the nose or throat. Symptoms vary with their location and size. Polyps may become large enough to cause difficulty in breathing, noisy breathing, sneezing, nasal discharge, and coughing. If large enough, the cat may have difficulty swallowing. Your veterinarian must anesthetize the cat to examine it. Surgery is the best treatment.

A cat with feline infectious peritonitis (FIP) also may have inflammation of the pleura, the lining of the chest cavity. The thorax may fill with fluid, causing labored breathing.

Pyothorax is a condition where the cat's chest fills with pus. It may be caused by a bite wound, a wound which penetrates the chest cavity, or from any other source of bacterial infection. Bacteria may spread from infected gums or ears. The cat may have a fever. Symptoms may not occur until the disease is quite advanced. By that time, it is life threatening.

Chylothorax occurs when the major lymphatic channel in the chest, called the cisterna chyli, is ruptured or torn. The chest fills with milky, fat-filled lymph. About a quarter of these cats will cough. Chylothorax may be due to trauma or cardiomyopathy. Some cases are due to heartworms, while no cause is found for others. Weekly drainage of the fluid and a low-fat diet may make the cat more comfortable, but rarely allows the vessel to heal. Surgery sometimes cures chylothorax, depending on the cause (Donner, 1991).

Cats with FIP, pyothorax, or chylothorax have similar symptoms. The cat may sit in one spot for quite some time before moving to another. It may sit uncomfortably upright rather than lying down, or may lie with its chest higher than the abdomen. Breathing may be labored and shallow, and the heartbeat may be faster than normal. Symptoms may come on over a long period of time, as many as one to six months. These conditions are all difficult to treat. Treatment must be immediate and intensive, yet without stressing the cat. The veterinarian may lightly sedate the cat and drain the chest cavity to help it breathe more easily. The cat may need antibiotics, corticosteroids, oxygen, and intravenous fluids, all of which usually require hospitalization. If there are no complicating infections, such as feline leukemia, the cat may recover. Otherwise, it may die.

Asthma is occasionally seen in cats. Allergic bronchitis and bronchial asthma occur when the small passageways in the lungs become overly responsive to inhaled substances. Airways become constricted and may be plugged with mucus. Eventually, the bronchial walls become thickened.

The cat may wheeze, cough, and gasp, usually with the neck stretched forward, especially when breathing out. There may be shallow, rapid breathing, or a sudden, hacking, gagging dry cough. Some asthmatic cats wheeze and cough much of the time while others do so only occasionally. In severe attacks, the cat may have fluid in the lungs, which makes breathing difficult. Some cats have extreme respiratory distress, which may include openmouthed breathing and blue-colored mucous membranes. The cat appears normal between episodes.

A cat with asthma should be handled with care. If stressed, it may die. If you have oxygen, place the cat in a box or bag (not airtight) and start a gentle flow into it. This may be enough to stabilize the cat and save its life. If you know the cat has asthma, this may be better than rushing it to the clinic. The cat will usually quit gasping within 15 to 30 minutes, and should then be taken to the veterinarian for treatment. A severely asthmatic cat may be placed on corticosteroids to keep the condition under control. The least possible quantity should be used. In many cases, the cause is never known and the condition can only be controlled.

Cats occasionally have allergic rhinitis. This cat looks like a human with hay fever. It has a clear, watery discharge from the nose and sneezes a lot. It may even have red, watery eyes. This is usually due to something in the environment.

Common causes of both asthma and rhinitis include scented home products such as deodorants and sprays, powdered carpet deodorizers, perfume, aftershave, and talcum powder. Household dust and pollen also may cause problems. Remove offending products from the household. Asthmatic cats frequently belong to smokers. Quit smoking for the good of your cat (if not for yourself!). It is even worse for cats than humans because most of them never get out of the house to breathe fresh air. In many cases, when the humans (including guests) in the household stop smoking, the cat's asthma disappears.

Some cats will have chronic rhinitis/sinusitis. This infection of the nasal passages and sinuses often occurs after one of the feline upper respiratory tract diseases (see Vaccinations Chapter). The virus permanently damages the fine bones within the nose. This is followed by bacterial infection. The cat will sneeze (often in unstoppable fits), wheeze, and breathe noisily and with difficulty. There is nasal discharge, often thick and gray or yellowish, from one or both nostrils. Cats with these symptoms should be checked for feline leukemia and FIP. Treatment may help temporarily, but is not usually successful for the long term. The cat may need antibiotic treatment from time to time for the rest of its life. A few cats may show improvement after intranasal vaccination with modified live virus vaccines for upper respiratory diseases (calicivirus and herpesvirus). Surgically draining the sinuses has been done, but does not lead to a permanent cure. Overall, the chances for a complete cure with any (or all) available treatments are poor. However, it can usually be controlled so the cat can live a comfortable life.

LUNG DISEASE

Pneumonia is uncommon in cats. When it does occur, it is usually secondary to another infection such as feline pneumonitis. Pneumonia also may be seen in cats suffering from immunosuppression (usually due to feline leukemia virus). It is sometimes seen after the cat is injured, such as being hit by a car. Feline calicivirus occasionally can cause a viral pneumonia.

Mineral oil given to a cat as a laxative or for hairballs may be inhaled into the cat's lungs and cause a pneumonia which is usually fatal. This happens because the cat can't taste the oil, and can't feel it in its mouth. So, the cat inhales the oil instead of swallowing it. NEVER give mineral oil for hairballs.

Tumors are occasionally seen in the lungs, usually in cats 10 years of age or older. Unfortunately, by the time the tumor visibly affects the cat's breathing, the disease is usually too advanced to be successfully treated.

Cats are occasionally infected with lungworms that live within the smaller passages in the lungs. Lungworms are often found while diagnosing other more serious illnesses. It is difficult to differentiate this disease from chronic allergic bronchitis.

Gapeworms (nasal worms) occur in as many as half of the cats in Puerto Rico and throughout the Caribbean, but are not found in the continental United States. These parasites live in the nasal passages.

Toxoplasmosis is another parasitic infection which may infest the lungs, and many other systems of the body (see Parasites Chapter for discussion of these infections).

MYCOTIC PNEUMONIAS

Mycotic pneumonias in small animals are caused by several species of fungi found in soil or decaying plant materials. A few of these species are *Candida*, *Aspergillus*,

and *Penicillium*. These diseases also are called systemic mycoses because they can spread throughout the pet's body. The cat usually becomes infected by inhaling spores or fragments of the fungi. These same organisms also infect humans, but seem to be more common in dogs than humans, probably because their noses are closer to the ground. These diseases are occasionally seen in cats.

Because the cat's nose is usually the route of infection, the respiratory system is often the first to be involved. Symptoms of infection are similar in all mycotic diseases. They include lack of appetite, lack of energy, emaciation, and fever. The cat may have trouble breathing but usually does not cough. Fortunately, most mycoses occur in rather well-defined geographic areas, which helps in diagnosis. Some of these diseases show symptoms other than pneumonia, but pneumonia is common to all of them. They are more likely to occur in cats with other illnesses or damaged immune systems (for example, those with FeLV, FIV, or panleukopenia). Treatment rarely works and most infected cats die.

Cryptococcosis is perhaps the most common fungus disease which can affect cats. It usually infects the nasal cavity and sinuses. The cat may sneeze and have a nasal discharge, which may be pus-like, grayish, or tinged with blood. Skin ulcers may occur on the face, and the disease may spread from there throughout the body, including the bones and kidneys. It may spread into the brain, leading to various symptoms, including blindness, circling, staggering, paralysis, and convulsions. The cat may have a poor appetite and weight loss, but there is usually no fever. Cats with symptoms affecting the nasal cavity and skin may recover. Those with nervous system involvement usually do not recover. The prognosis is poor, but a few cats may recover if treated with ketoconazole or similar drugs.

Cryptococcosis is found worldwide in soils, particularly those contaminated by the feces of birds, especially pigeons. The cat is infected when it inhales dust contaminated by bird droppings. About a quarter of cats that are infected with cryptococcosis are chronic carriers of feline leukemia. The immune suppression caused by FeLV or FIV may be a factor in the development of the disease.

Feline histoplasmosis can affect cats of all ages, but is more common in cats fewer than four-years-old. Cats in general are quite resistant to histoplasmosis. Most of them develop non-specific clinical signs as the disease spreads throughout the body. These include fever (which may come and go), depression, lack of appetite, weight loss, and pale mucous membranes. About half of the affected cats will show signs of pneumonia, including rapid, labored breathing. Some cats may have infection in the bones, with swollen limbs and lameness. The disease is diagnosed by laboratory tests. If discovered early, it can sometimes be treated, although treatment seems less successful than in dogs. Histoplasmosis is mostly found in the Mississippi and Ohio River valleys and the Appalachian Mountain Range.

Blastomycosis is another fungus which can affect cats. It is also more common in younger cats. The most common signs are those of respiratory system involvement, including difficult, rapid breathing. A few cats will cough softly. Symptoms of nervous system involvement may include staggering, blindness, and convulsions. The cat may have vomiting, diarrhea, kidney damage, lack of appetite, weight loss, and fever. Again, diagnosis is by lab tests. By the time symptoms are seen, the cat is usually in the final stages of the disease. For that reason, it is very difficult to treat and the outlook for infected animals is poor, particularly if the nervous system is involved. Most blastomycosis occurs around the Mississippi River and the Great Lakes.

Coccidioidomycosis (valley fever) rarely causes respiratory symptoms in cats, perhaps because a cat that is ill tends to be less active and is less likely to cough or have difficulty breathing. It is more often seen as a skin disease (see Skin Disease Chapter) or with occasional bone involvement (lameness). Cats seem to be highly resistant to this organism. Valley fever is found in the southwestern United States, especially in desert areas of Arizona and California.

Treatment of mycotic pneumonias and other systemic mycoses can be complicated by misdiagnosis. These diseases often appear to be something else. When a cat does not respond to routine treatment with antibiotics, further tests should be run to either confirm or rule out the presence of a mycotic disease. X-rays may show masses in the lungs, thoracic or abdominal lymph nodes, or lesions in the bones.

Antifungal drugs can be used to treat all of these diseases. The drugs have many toxic side effects and must be administered and monitored by a veterinarian. The course of treatment may run two to three months or more. Laboratory tests are needed to monitor the kidneys, as some of these drugs are toxic to them. In many cases, it's a race to kill the fungus before the medication kills the cat, depending on how badly it is infected before treatment is begun. Surgery may be required to clean out lesions in the bone, or remove some of the lymph nodes. None of these diseases is easy to treat. Treatment is long, involved, expensive, and only successful perhaps half the time, depending on the infectious agent, the cat's overall condition and ability to resist, and other factors. There is no prevention for mycotic diseases, except good luck. Keeping the cat in good health helps maintain resistance to fungal diseases, and keeping the cat indoors may help reduce the chance for exposure to the fungal organisms. Cats with fungal respiratory diseases are not considered to be contagious to humans. However, cats with blastomycosis involving the skin should be handled with care to avoid infection.

INHALANT ALLERGIES (ATOPY)

Allergies to the same pollen, dust, and molds that cause humans to sneeze and sniffle also may affect your cat. Inhalant allergy (which veterinarians call "atopy") results when the cat becomes sensitized to these substances. Symptoms may occur as young as six months of age, up to around two years of age. It is thought that many cats inherit the tendency toward atopy.

Pollens and mold spores descend in cool air, causing many cats to react more at night than during the day. They also may have more difficulty in damp or rainy weather. Access to a damp basement, house plants, or musty fabrics may put the cat in contact with mold spores. In the South, these molds may be a year-round problem. As with humans, house dust can cause problems. The cat may be allergic to human or animal dander. Thus, your cat may be allergic to your dog —or to you!

A cat with atopy may develop a reaction in the bronchial tubes in the lungs, resulting in asthma. It may wheeze or sneeze, and often worsens with exercise. In some cases, the cat also may show signs of allergic dermatitis, such as hair loss on the face and neck, rubbing the face with the feet or on carpet or furniture, and a thin scruffy coat (see Skin Diseases Chapter). Inhalant allergies cause far more skin problems in animals than do hay fever-like symptoms —just the opposite of humans.

Skin testing does not accurately diagnose food or flea allergy, but it is fairly accurate for the inhalant allergens. Your veterinarian will sedate the cat and clip the hair from a patch on its belly. Specific test antigens will then be injected in a grid pattern. After a period of time, the veterinarian will note which injections swell or become reddened, showing a positive reaction. While blood tests (such as RAST and ELISA) are available to test for allergies, many veterinarians believe they are not yet reliable.

After your veterinarian finds the cause of the cat's allergy, desensitization may be recommended. This involves injecting a tiny quantity of the offending substance into the cat once or twice weekly. The dosage is gradually increased, allowing the cat's immune system to become "accustomed" to the offending substance. When the diagnosis has been correctly made, improvement is slow but steady. A course of treatment for a year or so may be needed, followed by maintenance dosages from time to time for the rest of the cat's life. Your veterinarian also may recommend a fatty acid supplement. Added to the cat's diet, it will help prevent dry skin, which may have contributed to the itching.

Fun note: Cats commonly purr when they are content and happy. It seems you can even see them smiling at times. However, veterinarians often see injured cats that are purring, so there are other occasions when they make this sound. It is unknown exactly how it is made. The cat's vocal cords are used for the rest of its range of sounds, from meowing to screaming and yowling on the back fence at night. Some speculate that purring comes from the pair of "false vocal cords" or vestibular folds. It may be caused when contractions of the laryngeal muscles interrupt the air flow over these folds when the animal is content and relaxed. Or, it may be due to contraction of the laryngeal muscles partially closing the glottis, causing pressure to build. Air movement through this opening may cause the purring. Others speculate that the purring sound comes from a blood vessel when the blood flow speeds up. No one really knows!

DIAPHRAGMATIC HERNIA

A diaphragmatic hernia is a tear in the diaphragm, the muscular partition between the chest cavity and abdomen. The cat suddenly has trouble breathing, especially if it has just been hit by a vehicle or fallen from a height. In some cases, signs may not show up until months later when organs from the abdomen move forward into the chest cavity, causing breathing difficulties. A cat with a long-standing diaphragmatic hernia may sit upright more than usual, or lie with its front end much higher than its hind end.

An X-ray usually confirms the diagnosis. Surgery is then done to repair the tear. Anesthesia is more risky because of the damaged respiratory system, and a few of these cats die in surgery. This may be due, as much as anything, to complications from the original injury. However, surgery is the only option if the cat is to have a chance at a normal life.

Chapter 16

<u>URINARY TRACT AND LIVER PROBLEMS</u>

- *Feline Urologic Syndrome (FUS)*
- *Cystitis*
- *Urinary Incontinence*
- *Feline Inappropriate Elimination (FIE)*
- *Acute Kidney Failure*
- *Chronic Kidney Failure*
- *Miscellaneous Kidney Problems*
- *Liver Problems*

FELINE UROLOGIC SYNDROME (FUS)

Feline urologic syndrome (FUS) is a common cause of illness in cats. The term FUS refers to a group of symptoms. One veterinarian suggested it should stand for "feline urinary signs," which are seen with inflammation in the lower urinary tract—namely, the lining of the bladder, the urethra, or both. FUS includes problems with urination, urethral obstruction and blood in the urine. FUS is not, by itself, a specific disease. The latest buzzwords seem to be Feline Lower Urinary Tract Disease (FLUTD) or Lower Urinary Tract Disease (LUTD), terms which encompass all causes of lower urinary tract symptoms. FUS will be used here because it's handy and simple. A common cause (or result) of FUS is the formation of urinary stones (urinary calculi). This disease process is called feline urolithiasis.

Cats are probably susceptible to urinary problems because of their background. Ancestors of house cats came from the deserts of North Africa. In the hot, dry climate, cats' bodies adapted to concentrate the urine, excreting much less water with mineral wastes than other animals. Even today, cats may wait up to two or three days between urinations. Mucus, bacteria, and minerals may combine to cause FUS. Viruses, fungi, tumors, damaged nerves, and congenital defects in the urinary tract may also cause or contribute to FUS.

About one cat per 100 in the overall population will have some type of urinary tract disease in any given year. Male and female cats are affected about equally. Male cats are more likely to experience complete blockage because of the small diameter of the urethra. Small stones can easily plug this tiny tube. Females usually have an infection in the urinary bladder (cystitis) rather than a complete blockage. Neutered males seem slightly more susceptible than intact males. Persians are more prone to develop FUS than other breeds, while Siamese may have less. Younger cats, between one and six years old, may be have more FUS, but it can be seen in cats of any age.

Indoor cats may be more likely to have FUS than outdoor cats, perhaps because they are less active, reducing water intake and frequency of urination. The extra time the urine spends in the bladder may allow crystals to form. Outdoor cats are more likely to have FUS in the winter if they do not have fresh water available at least twice a day, especially if they are eating dry food. A cat that cannot get to the litter box because of an aggressive cat in the house may suffer from FUS. This also can occur when the litter box is so dirty that the cat will not use it regularly. And that's the cat's definition of dirty, not yours!

Formation of crystals or calculi in the urine requires three conditions: a sufficiently high concentration of crystal-forming minerals, a urine pH (acidity) that favors the occurrence of crystallization, and enough time in the urinary tract for crystallization to occur. Stone formation cannot occur unless all three are present. Conversely, any decrease in these factors helps prevent FUS. A urinary tract infection which adds bacteria or sloughed cells to the urine can contribute to the formation of urinary calculi.

Stress may help trigger FUS. The breeding season is very stressful to many tom cats, who may howl at the window, run around all night, and fight. The tom is probably not eating and drinking normally. Also, hormones associated with the breeding season may help start FUS. Overweight cats that do not urinate often enough also seem more susceptible to FUS.

Abrupt dietary changes may trigger FUS. For example, the owner of a cat that is usually fed one or two meals a day of canned cat food goes away for a couple of days, leaving a bowl of dry food. The cat, unused to the different mineral content, will take a few days to adjust to drinking enough water to compensate for what it usually gets in the wet cat food. Before he can adjust, the cat's urethra plugs and the owner finds the cat dead. Sudden changes from a cat food that is high in meat, producing acidic urine, to one that is high in vegetable matter and producing alkaline urine also may cause blockage.

Symptoms of FUS include frequent or difficult urination, blood in the urine, licking the external genitalia, and pain in the lower abdomen. Occasionally, a male cat will let out a mournful howl as he tries to urinate. The temperature is usually normal. If the cat has been plugged for some time, it may be depressed, because of the increased blood urea nitrogen level. The cat is not processing enough urine to flush toxic wastes from its body.

If your cat is thin and your hands are sensitive, you may feel a large, firm, round object in the abdomen, just ahead of the pelvis. This overly swollen bladder occurs in cats that are "plugged." Feel it gently, so as to not cause it to rupture.

Cats with urinary tract infections or blockage may urinate in odd places, because the cat finds urination painful. It may associate the pain with the litter box and search for another place, hoping urination will not hurt. The cat may sit on a cool, smooth surface such as a sink, bathtub, or tile floor. If your normally housebroken cat urinates in one of these places, look for an infection before becoming angry.

The cat first strains to urinate, leading you to think it is constipated. It may not squat normally, but may strain, hunched over, with its haunches slightly raised. The cat may be unable to urinate, or only dribble small amounts, perhaps tinged with blood. Later, as the bladder becomes overfilled, the cat shows abdominal pain. The cat may be lethargic and reluctant to move, as well as ceasing to eat, becoming depressed and vomiting.

If not treated promptly, this backup of pressure may damage the kidneys and lead to kidney failure. Uremic poisoning and electrolyte imbalances can cause coma and death. If not treated, the bladder may rupture, and the cat will die. All of this can take less than 48 hours if the urethra is completely blocked. THIS IS AN EMERGENCY. If your male cat shows these signs, get him to the clinic within the next two or three hours. Tomorrow morning may be too late. If your veterinarian can't see you at that hour, either find another one or take your cat to an emergency clinic, NOW!

The veterinarian will do one of several things. The swollen bladder may be tapped with a large needle through the abdominal wall to immediately relieve pressure. Because the cat is in pain and does not welcome handling, a sedative or short-acting anesthetic is given before a catheter is passed to allow urine to flow from the bladder. The catheter may be left in place for 12 to 24 hours or more. This prevents the cat from becoming plugged again, and allows reopening if necessary. A bacterial culture and sensitivity test may be done. Opening up a plugged male cat takes a great deal of skill and patience.

A cat that is depressed may need electrolyte fluids to help flush the toxic blood urea nitrogen out through the kidneys. Fluids may be given either intravenously or under the skin. Antibiotics may be given, usually for two to three weeks. It is very important to give ALL the medication. Antispasmodic drugs may make the cat more comfortable. Other medications may be used to encourage the cat to drink more water, stimulate bladder function, and increase the volume of urine produced. Intensive care may be needed to save a cat that has become "plugged."

The bladder may rupture because it has been critically overfilled due to the blockage. This is a very serious problem. The veterinarian may X-ray the cat to determine if the bladder has ruptured. If the damaged area is small enough to heal by itself, peritoneal dialysis may be used.

A catheter is placed in the cat's abdomen and special fluids are flushed into and out of it. These remove the urine and accumulated toxins. Dialysis for several days may save the cat's life and allow the body to heal. If the tear is large, abdominal surgery will be necessary to repair the defect. The cat has perhaps a 50/50 chance of survival.

In the past, the majority of feline urinary tract stones were due to a mineral called struvite. Cat foods are now formulated to reduce this occurrence. Special cat foods also are available to remove struvite stones from cats that tend to form them. Meanwhile, the number of stones formed from other minerals has increased. Stones or sand grains may be sent for laboratory analysis to better determine how to manage your cat's particular problem. Occasionally, stones may form in the kidney. Some kidney stones occur without symptoms, while others cause abdominal pain and blood or pus in the urine.

A male cat that has had more than two episodes of FUS, or that has an especially serious case, may have a damaged urethra. A narrowed area of scar tissue may catch any small bit of crystalline material or mucus, becoming plugged again and again. Surgery, called a perineal urethrostomy, may be necessary. The end of the cat's penis is removed and a new urethral opening is created just below his anus. With careful reconstruction and good luck, the cat can function normally, urinating much like a female. Some of these cats will continue to have numerous bacterial urinary tract infections. This may be due to persisting causes of infection that led to the surgery.

Because the cause of FUS is unknown, it is difficult to treat. Many cases would heal without any treatment IF the cat does not have bladder stones and IF it is not plugged. Most owners don't want to stand by and wait and watch the cat in misery and risk fatal complications, so the cat is treated to make it more comfortable and help prevent recurrence.

Great advances have been made in producing special cat foods which prevent future occurrences of FUS. One of these foods should be fed after the first episode of FUS. It may be necessary to use it for the rest of the cat's life. This is a cheap price to pay to keep FUS from recurring. Your veterinarian will recommend a food based on the type of crystals or stones found in the cat's urine. Because cystitis (a bladder infection) may be the first sign of another episode of FUS, a cat that has recurring cystitis should be put on a maintenance diet for the health of the urinary tract.

Initially, excess magnesium in cat food was thought to be the major factor in the formation of stones in the urinary tract. However, recent research has shown that excess magnesium and phosphate in the diet are critical only when the food produces an alkaline urine. When the urine is acidified, which is normal with most good quality cat foods, this is not a problem. Quality foods are formulated so they do not have excess magnesium. Feeding a special, low magnesium diet to a cat that has never had FUS is unnecessary unless recommended by your veterinarian.

The ash content of a cat food is directly correlated with the magnesium content with dry and soft-moist foods. The ash content of canned foods, however, has little correlation with its magnesium content.

Most veterinarians believe that a quality dry food which is high in calories and fat, and is highly digestible, is no more likely than a canned food to cause FUS. The food should, of course, be nutritionally complete. Some foods which meet these requirements include both dry and canned Science Diet Feline Maintenance® and Prescription Diet Feline c/d®, canned Prescription Diet s/d® (Hill's Pet Products) and Friskies Buffet Beef and Liver® (this flavor only, Lewis, 1987). Waltham™ Veterinarium™ Feline Control pHormula™ is another diet that meets these criteria. The dry specialty foods are only four to eight cents more expensive per day than the best selling dry cat foods. This is some of the cheapest insurance you can buy against one of the worst problems that can afflict your cat.

Meat-based cat foods acidify the urine easily and efficiently. If you feed a grain-based cat food, make sure it is specially formulated to produce acidic urine. Liver or foods which contain liver should not be fed to cats with a urinary tract problem. Feed only the diet which your veterinarian recommends. Do not add vitamins, minerals, table scraps, or treats. Cats in their natural habitat have a diet high in quality protein, with plenty of fat and very little vegetable material other than that in the gut of their prey. No one yet knows how to formulate a food to perfectly replace the cat's natural diet—a cat food equivalent to ground wild mice, with a few chopped birds thrown in for variety.

In the normal cat, the urine is slightly acidic except during a short period after it has eaten; the normal pH (acidity) is between 6.0 and 6.4. After FUS, the pH should be kept at 6.6 or less. Some veterinarians prefer it to be less than 6.4 when the cat is fed free-choice. When you are checking the cat's urine for acidity, it should be done three to five hours after the cat has eaten. Otherwise, the reading is meaningless. Also, the pH of the urine may change after it is passed. For this reason, pH should be checked as soon as possible after the urine is voided. If the cat has not eaten for 18 hours or more, the pH will usually be 6.0, regardless of the diet. The pH is easily checked using pH paper from the drugstore; it changes color to indicate urine acidity. Dietary management is directed toward maintaining this acid condition. Feeding food free-choice helps to keep the urine evenly acidic throughout the day. Even with the best diet, it may be impossible to eliminate all cases of FUS.

Drugs called urinary acidifiers are sometimes given to maintain an acid urine. Acidifiers are used only for cats whose urine stays alkaline when a diet formulated to produce acidic urine does not do so after the cat has been on it two to four weeks. However, it is both more effective and less expensive to keep the pH of the urine low with cat food than by using acidifiers. Acidifiers must be given in the proper dosage, and the cat must eat all the medication and all of the food, if they are mixed. This doesn't work if the cat picks at its food or doesn't eat it all. Acidifiers work better when given with a meal. If you stop medication and the cat's urine becomes alkaline again, it is likely that the stones and/or blockage will recur. Ascorbic acid (vitamin C) and sodium acid phosphate have no effect on feline urine acidity. Methionine is effective, if the cat gets the full dosage. It takes about 1500 milligrams per cat per day to maintain an acid urine. With today's high-quality commercial cat foods, urinary acidifiers are rarely needed as diet is less often implicated in FUS.

It is possible to make the cat's urine overly acid, or to keep it too acid for too long. This may occur if the cat is given medication to acidify the urine and fed an acidifying diet at the same time. The cat may suffer acidosis, osteoporosis (loss of bone mass), and weakness due to potassium loss. Certain minerals can form crystals in acidic urine, so it is possible to cause one problem while curing another. The long-term effects of urinary acidification are not fully known. Some cats are placed on drugs to acidify their urine, and may need to be on these drugs for the rest of their lives. This does NOT mean that these drugs are completely without side effects. Your veterinarian should carefully monitor their use. Anything that decreases the cat's water intake or urine output can lead to the occurrence (or return) of urinary problems. If you have to board your cat, make sure the kennel is aware of the cat's problems, and the possibility that FUS may recur.

Maintaining a larger urine volume helps dilute minerals in the urine and flush out crystals or sandy grains that form in the bladder. Be sure the cat has water available at all times. Some cats will only drink fresh or running water, while others prefer water that has been standing for several days. If the water is dirty or has an unpleasant flavor, the cat may not drink it. If your water is softened or has a bad flavor, you may need to give the cat distilled or demineralized water. Try different kinds of containers. Some cats prefer stainless steel bowls rather than glass dishes. Put water dishes in several convenient places in the house because cats have favorite drinking areas. Broth or bouillon may be given. If you normally give the cat milk, dilute it half-and-half with water until the cat is recovered.

Special cat litters are available which change color according to urinary acidity. This makes it easy to tell if the urinary tract infection has returned. Similar litter may be used with some diabetic cats to monitor their urinary glucose levels.

CYSTITIS

An infection of the urinary bladder, called cystitis, is more common in female cats. The cat may not be eating well, and may urinate outside the litter box. Frequent small urinations may be tinged with blood. Some of these infections may be caused by viruses, or perhaps started by them. Bacteria are rarely seen with disease in the lower urinary tract (see FUS, above). Cats produce highly concentrated acidic urine containing large amounts of urea, which may help protect against bacterial infection.

Some cases of urinary tract infection resolve spontaneously with or without antibiotics in five to seven days

(Ross, 1990). Meanwhile, it may be quite annoying to you that the cat is urinating in several places. If the cat continues to pass blood in the urine, if it fails to get better in five to seven days, or if it has more than one episode of FUS within a three month period, take the cat to your veterinarian.

URINARY INCONTINENCE

Incontinence is the involuntary loss of urine, and is commonly seen in elderly animals. Rarely, incontinence is seen in cats from birth, usually due to anatomic deformities. Manx cats may suddenly have urine dribbling for no apparent reason. Cats that are infected with feline leukemia virus may show urinary incontinence. The reason for this is unknown.

Urinary incontinence may be due to a number of problems. These include changes in bladder and urethral tone, urinary tract infection or obstruction, tumors in the bladder or elsewhere in the urinary tract, neurological dysfunctions, degenerative conditions, or behavioral problems. It also may be due to conditions which cause excessive urine production and the necessity to get rid of it. The most common of these are diabetes mellitus and kidney failure. Drugs such as diuretics may increase urine production enough that the cat has excessive urgency and can't make it to the litter box in time. Corticosteroids may be given to a cat during the summer for allergies, and it may be incontinent during the summer, but fine in the winter. Male cats that have had a perineal urethrostomy (a male cat that has been surgically repaired so that he urinates like a female) because of FUS may have trouble holding urine.

Senility may make the cat forget its training, or it may have trouble remembering the location of the litter box. The cat may be weak or in pain, partially blind, or have poor balance, which makes it difficult to get to the litter box. As the cat ages, it may lose muscle mass, including that of muscles that control urination, leading to incontinence. Urinary tract infections or obstructions may cause severe urgency so the cat cannot make it to the litter box in time.

Urinary incontinence often occurs as leakage or dribbling. The cat may be able to control urination while awake, but leave a wet spot where it has been relaxed or sleeping. If the cat urinates in its bedding, it is probably having a problem with incontinence. If the urine is away from the bed, the cat probably is not incontinent, but is trying to make it to the litter box. Some incontinent cats may trail drops of urine across the floor as they walk.

In most cases, finding the reason for incontinence is a job for your veterinarian. Provide as much information as possible. When, where, and how much does the cat urinate? How much water is the cat drinking? Has the cat had kidney disease or FUS? Your history will be important to the diagnosis. The veterinarian probably will do a urinalysis to see if there is any infection in the urinary tract, and other tests as needed. Once a diagnosis is made, treatment may include retraining, medication, or management. A low-salt diet may be helpful to some cats.

FELINE INAPPROPRIATE ELIMINATION (FIE)

Feline inappropriate elimination (FIE) is the latest name for what used to be called "peeing on the floor." FIE may be due to a physical problem or a behavioral problem. It is one of the most common causes for owners' dissatisfaction with pets. Your veterinarian will begin to diagnose the problem by taking a complete history—where and when does the cat eliminate in the wrong place? This will help to distinguish among: 1) cats with a urinary tract infection (FUS) or other physical disease, 2) cats that are urine marking (spraying), and 3) cats that are urinating normally but outside the litter box. A cat that is usually housebroken and suddenly starts urinating in your presence may have FUS. Defecation outside the litter box will be discussed later in this section.

Inability to control urinary function may be seen with fractures in the pelvis or tail. This may heal with time, but you will need to empty the cat's bladder by gently squeezing out the urine until healing occurs. Spinal disease may cause incontinence, and it may occur with feline leukemia. Cats with diabetes may urinate in the wrong location because they are passing a large quantity of urine and cannot make it to the litter box. Diabetes can be diagnosed from laboratory tests. Some cats will spray because of impacted anal sacs.

At the very minimum, the cat should have a complete urinalysis. If a urinary tract infection is found, further tests, such as a urine culture, may be needed in order to treat the infection with the appropriate antibiotics. X-rays will rule out bladder stones.

A cat that has had a painful bladder infection (cystitis or FUS), constipation, painful diarrhea, or colitis may associate pain with its litter box. It may learn to go elsewhere to avoid the pain, then continue to do so after it is well. If the cat has a urinary tract infection, it may have a continual urge to urinate. Even if the cat wants to do so, it may be unable to make it to its litter box in time. Then, after the cat has urinated in the wrong places for a period of time, the smell of the urine will encourage the cat to urinate there after it is healthy.

Inappropriate elimination, whether urination or defecation outside the litter box, or spraying, is often the first indication that you have too many cats for the size of your house or apartment. Cats normally live as solitary animals other than at mating time or when they fight at the border of adjacent territories. It has been estimated that a free-roaming cat needs a territory of one-tenth of a square mile. This is equal to several city blocks. Thus, a house or apartment with more than two or three cats could feel oppressively crowded to its feline inhabitants.

If the spraying or use of toilet locations outside the litter box began after you added a new cat to a multi-cat household, you may have reached a socially excessive number of cats for the one cat that is especially insecure. You may have to remove the newest cat in the household, or find the shy cat a home where it will be the lone cat. If urination seems to be directed at a particular person's clothing or bed, it may be helpful to have that person feed the cat a tablespoon or so of tasty canned cat food several times a day. Meanwhile, other persons in the household can reduce their contact with the cat until the problem is solved.

Households with 10 or more cats are guaranteed to have a number of urine marking (spraying) cats. Urination in places other than the litter box is sometimes seen in multi-cat households when one or two dominant cats keep a subordinate cat from getting to or using the litter box. This situation often can be remedied by having litter boxes in more than one location, or by reducing the number of cats in the household.

Also, cats are creatures of habit. Confusion and change in the relationships of the humans and animals around them can be very disturbing. Inappropriate elimination can occur when a new pet or person enters the house, or when one leaves. In some cases, the cat never returns to normal after such changes, even if they are reversed. If you are going to keep a cat in an atmosphere of change, it's best for it to begin when it is a kitten.

FIE can occur when there is some physical change in the home, such as new furniture or carpet. It also can happen when you bring in used or antique furniture, rugs, outdoor furniture, a lawn mower, or fabrics upon which another cat has urinated. Other cats outside the house or disturbances such as construction also could upset the cat. Some cats are insecure and are easily disturbed by changes in their environment. They express their feelings in one of the few ways they have available. It may be helpful to spend some "alone" time with the insecure, problem cat. Confine your other cats in a separate room. Let the insecure cat out into the rest of the house for at least three to four hours at one time. Give the cat its own litter box and food and water dishes at this time, along with plenty of attention. Later, confine the cat and allow the rest of the cats to have the run of the house. This may reduce the territorial stress enough that the cat will stop urinating outside the litter box.

The cat may be emotionally upset because there has been some disturbance in its environment and may urinate outside the litter box to mark its territory. The litter box may be in an area that is too noisy or is in a main traffic area where the cat has no privacy. Children may upset the cat with their busy activities. The cat may find a rumbling washer or dryer an unpleasant fixture in its bathroom. If you have had the cat examined to eliminate physical reasons for the behavior change, look for psychological changes.

Both male and female cats (especially intact toms) may start spraying, which is also called urine marking. Spraying is a means of communication. It is used when the cat is territorial (although cats don't mark and defend strict territories as do dogs and some other animals), aggressive, or highly aroused. It also is used in sexual situations such as when female cats are in heat and the neighborhood males are marking as a part of their courtship. Spraying is normal behavior for intact males, who begin the behaviors at puberty. Tom cats that do not spray may not be successful breeders as they may be subordinate to other cats in the area. Female cats also may mark when they are in heat. Any cat, including neutered males and females, may begin spraying during breeding season when intact cats are leaving scent everywhere.

The typical spraying cat is an intact male that backs up to a vertical surface such as a wall or door, or upright objects such as furniture or stereo speakers. He steps in place with his hind legs, holding his tail stiffly over his back, jerking it back and forth, and sprays urine on the vertical surface. Others will be males or females who either spray or squat. In any case, the quantity passed is less than that of a cat that is normally emptying a full bladder. A cat that is marking usually also continues to use the litter box. Urine marking may be stimulated by sexual situations, such as the cat smelling a place where another cat has urinated or one the cat has previously marked.

Cats may mark with urination or defecation in an area where the owner's scent is strongest, often a bed or chair. The cat may somehow feel it useful to associate its smell with yours, and may do this when you are on vacation and ask a neighbor to look in. Cats of oriental breeds, such as Persians, may be more prone to spraying as a protest. This may occur when the cat is frustrated or feels it has been denied your attention. The cat also may feel more secure when it surrounds itself with its own odor. Cats that spray may be more active at night than those that do not spray, and they may appear more aggressive toward their owners.

One of my cats urinated on my pillow and bedspread after being moved to a new house. Shutting him out of the bedroom and paying more attention to him outside it stopped the problem before it became a habit. Cats are more prone to urinating on mattresses which are lying on the floor, or on waterbeds. This may be a type of marking behavior.

A cat that is marking from protest should mostly be ignored. Make sure that YOU initiate contact, whether it involves feeding or affection, much as you would with an overly-demanding dog. Give extra attention to a cat that is spraying from insecurity. This cat may become worse before improving.

Another hazard may be associated with spraying. When a cat, male or female, sprays into an electrical outlet, the wiring may short out and cause a fire! Covering the outlets with plastic caps may help, but urine can still run behind them. Fires have been started when a stud cat sprayed into a wall heater or other electrical appliance.

Most people don't want to keep an intact male cat unless they are in the cat breeding business. Even then, the tom cat is usually confined to a cage or run so his spraying is in an area which is easily cleaned. If you allow a mature tom to run freely in your house, there is a good chance he will spray on the walls, drapes, and furniture. Once in place, the strong urine odor is almost impossible to remove. Even outdoors, toms aren't much fun. They usually mark on walls, bushes, and trees around your yard until it reeks. Neutering will prevent most of these cats from marking.

Neutering males reduces spraying in about 90% of the cats. It also removes much of the unpleasant odor of tom cat urine. If the cat is not neutered, this is the first step. A male cat of unknown history that appears to be neutered may still have one or both testicles up in his abdomen (cryptorchidism). This animal will have a strong urine odor and annoying marking behavior. Female cats may urine mark while they are in heat; spaying may eliminate the problem. If the female sprays on a year-round basis, spaying probably won't cure her problem.

If the cat is already neutered, try to reduce situations that trigger marking. Keep outside cats away from your windows and doors, where they can spray and leave scent. Repellents may keep cats away from the yard, walls, and windows. Closing the drapes so your cat cannot see others may be helpful. Having too many cats in your house can initiate spraying, or keep them spraying in competition with each other. This is done as each cat attempts to mark out a piece of territory to call its own. Moving the most aggressive cat to a place where there are no other cats will sometimes solve the problem. As a last resort, the olfactory nerves may be severed. This works more than 50% of the time.

Discipline is only effective if you can do it WHILE the cat is in the act of elimination, and if it is done EVERY time you catch the cat doing it. Punishing the cat by shouting only will make it avoid you and sneak around to eliminate. Try to use a noise that is not associated with you, such as clanging a pot, slapping a countertop with your hand, or throwing a pillow or shoe near (not on) the cat. Or, try a spray bottle or squirt gun. This may startle the cat into stopping the urination, and give you a chance to carry the cat to the litter box and encourage it to finish the job there. Stay with the cat until it has finished and praise lavishly.

Punishing the cat more than a few seconds after it has messed or taking it to the soiled spot later does not work. The cat does not remember what it did that is resulting in discipline. If you punish the cat and then take it to the litter box, this will make things much worse. The cat will associate you and the litter box with unpleasant circumstances. Some cats react to punishment by becoming even more nervous and are more likely to mess outside the box. The cat may learn to soil only when you are gone, or it will learn to fear your arrival. The fact that the cat "looks guilty," runs away, or hides does not mean that it is making connection between the mess on the floor and your return. It only means that the cat expects a furor when you come home. For these cats, moving them VERY quietly to the litter box or out the door may be more effective than punishment of any kind. Also, the cat that "looks guilty" may not be the culprit!

Keeping the cat out of a room where it has been soiling is usually only a temporary solution. When you allow the cat back into the room, it probably will go back to eliminating in the same location. It is more effective to continue to allow the cat into the room while changing its preference for that place.

It may be helpful to keep the cat confined to a small space for five to seven days. An airline crate or cage is a good place to start the retraining. It should be just large enough for the cat to lie down flat on a bed in one end, with a litter box in the other end. This gives the cat a choice of using either the litter box or its bed as a toilet. The cat should stay in the crate 24 hours a day for at least two weeks. For the first day or two, the cat may cry, howl, or claw the walls, and you may prefer to put the crate in the garage or basement so you can sleep. Keep track, if possible, of the time when the cat eliminates. You might find, for example, that the cat uses the box only in the evening. When the cat is out of the crate again, take it to the litter box at that time and encourage the cat to use it.

After the confinement period, when the cat is using the litter box regularly, take it out when you can directly watch it, keeping the cat in your sight at all times. If the cat begins to squat, scratch, or sniff around the floor as if it is going to urinate, punish it as above. Then take the cat to the litter box, and praise the cat for using it. Begin with one room and gradually allow the cat out into the rest of the house.

Putting the cat's food and water dishes in the area where it sprays may help stop urinating or spraying. Whether full or empty, place the dish on the soiled spot until the cat's next meal. If the cat has soiled in several different areas, split the meal into as many dishes as needed to cover the soiled areas. One owner reported using 15 dishes before curing the problem. After the cat has gone at least five days without soiling outside the box, slowly begin to remove the extra dishes, one at a time. If the cat soils the area again, again feed in all the spots until the behavior stops. This program may take as many as six weeks, but if you persist it will usually work when the problem is mental rather than medical in origin.

THE BEST THING YOU CAN DO TO CONTROL ODOR AND KEEP YOUR CAT USING THE LITTER BOX IS TO CLEAN IT DAILY. Picking out the solids will make the litter box more pleasant for you and the cat. Clumping litters allow solidified urine to be easily picked out. Change the litter completely every two to four days at most. Don't just stir litter. This spreads the odor throughout and denies the cat a clean toilet area. There is a happy medium between having a little odor in the pan to keep the cat using the area, especially early in its training, and having a box clean enough that it will continue to use it. Once the cat is using the box again, gradually extend the time between box cleanings. Ask yourself how often accidents have occurred. A cat that goes outside the litter box once may not be a problem, while a six-year-old cat that has never consistently used the litter box probably never can be completely trained.

When a cat urinates outside the litter box, or in a different part of the house, this is usually because that area is more attractive than the litter box. It may have a more suitable texture. It may have odors from another cat's elimination. It may be cleaner than the litter box, more secluded, or further away from an eating or sleeping area. Changing abruptly to a different kind of litter can cause as many as 50% of cats to stop using the box. Test a new litter by offering it in a separate box near the one already being used.

If the cat is urinating on a horizontal surface, there will be a large amount of urine and the cat usually will scratch in an attempt to cover it. In this case, the cat has come to prefer a toilet location other than the litter box. It is not done for sexual or territorial reasons. Treatment of this cat involves making the chosen location less attractive and the litter box more attractive. As with spraying, if you catch the cat in the act of urination, punish it by spraying with water or throwing a pebble-filled can close to it. Drug treatment will not be helpful to these cats. It is sometimes helpful to cover the floor where the cat is urinating with material that will make it unpleasant, such as aluminum foil or plastic.

Be sure to keep the litter box clean. If you have several cats, it may be helpful to have as many litter boxes as you have cats, plus one. Try large litter boxes filled deep with litter. Other cats may prefer a box with just a cup or two of litter. This makes it easy and economical to change the box frequently. Some cats are offended by scented litters (the same ones that are supposed to smell "good" to humans), and will not use them. They may also object to litter box deodorizers. In most cases, it is better to control odors by keeping the litter box clean than by trying to cover it up with a scent like chlorophyll, mint, or citrus. If elimination problems began at the time you changed to a scented litter, simply change back to your previous litter. Some cats do not like litters that give out odors when dampened.

Check the cat's foot pads to be sure they are not irritated or thickened by the litter. Some substances may be uncomfortable to the cat's feet. Indoor cats have more tender pads than those that run around outside. If you have a plastic litter box, you should replace it occasionally. This is because continuous contact with urine will change its odor.

Your cat just may not like the kind of litter you are using (litter aversion). You will usually know this within a day or two after you try a new kind of litter. The cat may fail to scratch or cover feces. Then, it may stand outside the box and scratch at the side of it, the floor, or a nearby wall. It may stand on the edge of the litter box to avoid getting its paws in the litter, and the cat may shake it from its paws. The cat may jump in, quickly dig a hole, eliminate (with or without covering) and jump out, as if trying to finish as quickly as possible. Litter aversion may be seen from the time the cat is a kitten. A cat that does not like its litter or something about the litter box and that does not scratch in the litter may scratch vigorously when it urinates elsewhere in the house.

Some cats with litter aversion prefer a fine-grained, sand-like "clumping" litter. Others prefer sand if you have access to it, or you can use sand meant for children's sandboxes. The next choice may be regular clay litter. Some cats do not like plastic litter box liners. If you do use them, be sure to get the correct size for your litter box.

Try different types of litter in two to six different boxes at the same time. Try plain clay litter in one box and a trial kind in the second box. Let the cat have each pair of litter types for three or four days; then change one kind, keeping the plain litter in the other box. A suitable clay litter needs a mixture of small granules to absorb liquid waste and larger granules that allow the cat to scratch and cover easily. Large-grained litter also may be less dusty. Some long-haired cats prefer a coarse-grained litter that does not cling to their hair. Also, the right mixture of granule sizes keeps litter from tracking across the floor on the cat's feet, which can be very important to humans! Some cats will use one litter for defecation and urinate in a different location with another type of litter. Many cats like clay litters or clumping litters, and will not use scented litters.

Others cats prefer sawdust or perlite. Some cats like corncob litters (such as FIELDfresh®), alfalfa litters, or litters made from grass (such as Cat Country Organic). These litters are made from natural ingredients, are lightweight to handle, more absorbent than clay, and dust-free. They are biodegradable and can be flushed or composted in your garden (just don't grow root vegetables in that spot). These litters are not harmful if the cat accidentally swallows some while grooming itself. Some cats will resume using the litter box if you offer wood chips or cedar shavings, sand, or shredded paper. A few cats may use unshredded newspaper for a toilet, to the point of using the paper wherever they find it around the house.

If the cat wants to urinate on carpet, it may be helpful to offer carpet scraps, old throw rugs, or rags in the litter box. If the litter box is on a smooth, hard surface, try setting it on a carpet scrap, or putting scraps nearby. You might even build a four- or six-inch wide "deck," level with the edge of the cat box, and cover it with carpet. This should be a last resort, as it would be better to train the cat away from carpet altogether. Other cats may urinate on soiled clothing left on the floor or in the bottom of your closet. Keeping dirty clothes picked up and placed in a hamper or closed container may cure these animals. Some cats will urinate in an open suitcase as you are packing. Perhaps they sense the change in routine associated with travel. Either keep the suitcase closed or shut the cat out of the room.

Try different locations for the litter box, preferably away from the current feeding area. Keep it as secluded as possible so the cat feels isolated from humans and other pets. Many cats will not use a hooded litter box which holds the unpleasant odors inside.

Cats that use potted plants for toilets may use potting soil if you offer it as litter in the cat box. If they are cats that are both indoors and out, they may return to being housebroken if allowed outdoors more often. It's hard to explain to one of these cats that it's permissible to use soil when it is outside, but not when it is indoors. You may eventually be able to use a mixture of potting soil or peat moss and clay litter in the litter box. Putting large wood chips or rocks over the surface of the pot may keep the cat from digging in it and using it for a toilet, and save the plant from being fertilized to death. It may help to put tacks or small nails around the edge of the planter if it is made of wood, or drive small sticks into the soil inside the planter. Then wind pieces of string or yarn between the nails. This may deter the cat from digging in the soil and using it for a toilet. Having only hanging plants may be an alternative.

Carefully evaluate the cat's situation to try to determine why it is soiling in places other than the litter box. It is often easier to change the environment than to train the cat. Some cats just are not picky about where they eliminate, and can be very difficult to correct. Changing the location of the litter box, the location of the box, or cleaning it more frequently may correct the problem. If these changes do not correct the problem, consult your veterinarian, who may be able to offer suggestions or refer you to a feline behaviorist.

Occasionally, a cat may urinate or defecate in the bathtub. It may simply prefer a cool, smooth surface for this function. A cat that is normally litter box trained and suddenly urinates in a bathtub or sink may have a urinary tract infection. Have the cat checked before trying behavioral corrections.

Some behaviorists believe the cat may be trying to mimic the owner's actions in the bathroom. Moving the litter box into the bathroom, while leaving water in the sink and tub, may be helpful. Keep the box there until the cat resumes using it. In some cases, the cat may be using the sink or toilet because it is cleaned promptly! Humans clean it as soon as they find the mess, while being far less likely to clean the cat box as regularly. Try cleaning the cat box more often.

Thoroughly clean and wash the litter box. Fill it only about two-thirds full of litter. Then prop up one end so it has a slight slope bare of litter. This will give the cat a smooth surface and litter to paw after it has defecated. A cat that soils on a tile, linoleum, or bare wood floor may use an empty litter box propped up this way so that urine will run away from its feet. You also can try covering the bottom of the tub with newspaper, aluminum foil, or plastic garbage bags to keep the cat from using it. Or, you can leave a couple of inches of water standing in it until the cat is retrained to the litter box.

If the cat is defecating outside the litter box, it is important to determine if it is ill. If the cat has diarrhea it may be unable to make it to the litter box. Try to determine the reason for the mistake and correct it. It may be necessary to treat the cat or to change foods if some ingredient is causing the diarrhea. If you are feeding the cat free-choice, change to feeding twice a day. Watch the cat carefully from about 20 minutes to an hour after feeding, so you can guide the cat to the litter box. It may help to play with the cat and give it attention for five minutes twice each day. Cats that are orphans, poorly socialized, or are runts of the litter may have digestive upsets that show up as potty problems; extra attention may be helpful. Conversely, a few cats have this behavioral problem if they are petted too much. Until the problem is corrected, stroke the cat for only a couple of minutes at a time. After that, encourage the cat to play with a toy.

Cats that are in pain, whether from urination or defecation, may go outside the litter box, hoping to avoid the pain. Constipation may cause pain, which the cat associates with the litter box. A cat laxative may cure this behavior. Cats will sometimes defecate in an unfinished or crumbling basement where soil is exposed. Repairing the area, then painting the concrete so that it is smooth, may work.

Some cats have a strong, unpleasant fecal odor. Often, this is caused by their diet. For these animals, avoid cat foods made from dairy products or seafood. Do not feed soft-moist foods. A high-fiber diet reduces fecal odor for some animals. Others have problems with foods that contain soybeans or large amounts of cereal grains. Try changing the brand or type of food you are feeding the cat. Anal gland odors are present in some cats, and may cause a strong unpleasant odor from time to time. A natural yucca derivative is available ("N.O.C.™, Nutritional Odor Control," *Veterinary Forum*, Oct. 1990). It can be placed on top of the food for a cat with nasty fecal odor, and may reduce the odor emitted by its feces. If dietary change or use of one of these products does not fix the odor problem, take the cat to your veterinarian.

Thoroughly cleaning the carpet may help remove the odor so that you do not smell it. Place the cat in another room while cleaning the soiled area. However, this may not keep the cat from using that place. Something about the area was attractive to the cat before it started using it, and this attraction may keep the cat using it even after it is cleaned. On the contrary, cleaning the spot may make it even more attractive—ever notice how a cat will rush to use a freshly cleaned litter box?

The carpet and floors must be thoroughly cleaned to eliminate odors. Remember that the urine has soaked deep into the carpet, through the padding, and perhaps into the flooring. Use enough of the cleaner, in a wide enough area, to cover all areas possibly soaked with urine or feces. In most cases, this will take an amount equal to or greater than the amount of urine. Allow the odor neutralizer to dry naturally without blotting. If you have a continuing problem with feline odors, you might consider pulling up the carpet, allowing the floor to dry completely, and treating the floor with a wood (or concrete) sealer. All in all, it's a lot easier to cater to your cat's desire for a clean litter box than to clean the carpet every week.

It can be difficult to remove cat urine odor from carpet or other fabric. White vinegar (mixed half-and-half with water) and detergents (such as Ivory Liquid) will effectively remove odor from carpet on a temporary basis, but it is not permanent. Do not use products which contain ammonia; it is naturally present in urine and its odor may encourage the cat to keep using the spot. Woolite® Rug Cleanser (spray foam product) removes the odor, but leaves the rug smelling like the cleaner. Rubbing alcohol may help to cover the odor. Test it in a small spot, as it may cause fading on some carpets.

Several products are made specifically for removing cat odor from carpets. A product such as F.O.N.® (Summit Hill Labs., Navesink, NJ) or Outright Pet Odor Eliminator® (The Bramton Co., Dallas, TX) will help eliminate odor, even with tom cat urine. These sprays may make some cats happier with their litter boxes. Some products do not work well if vinegar mixtures have been used previously. Some cats will avoid an area that has been sprayed lightly with perfume or Scope® (Proctor & Gamble) mouthwash. Club soda may be helpful if you don't have any of the other products handy (Beaver, 1989).

It may help to use odor neutralizers or repellents such as mothballs, commercial pet repellents, or solid citrus air fresheners. Bars of soap or lemon peels also may help to keep the cat away from the toilet area. Hanging strips of aluminum foil or putting cat toys there may be helpful.

Some cats will tolerate one teaspoon of apple cider vinegar put into one feeding each day. This may change the urine odor enough to keep the cat from wanting to mark the same spot again.

Diazepam (Valium®) can sometimes help decrease the cat's anxiety about the presence of others so that it returns to using the litter box. Two months of treatment work in many cats. Other cats may need six to 18 months of treatment, after which they can be taken off medication and do not begin spraying again. The cat may stagger, and the dosage may need to be adjusted for each individual. A drug called buspirone also may show favorable response in as little as a week. This drug does not cause the staggering, sedation, or dependency which can occur with diazepam. It has been successfully used to treat urine marking and spraying, and works with inappropriate urination when combined with behavioral modification. Megestrol acetate (Ovaban®) can be used to decrease the cat's aggressive tendencies, and is useful when anti-anxiety treatments fail. These drugs are not approved for use in cats and must be used only under the direct advice of your veterinarian. They are not always effective in eliminating spraying, but if you have tried everything else, they may be worth a try. Gradually wean the cat off the medication every two or three months to see if it can get by without it.

If nothing else works, the hormone progestin may stop some cats, especially males, from spraying. If the spraying is caused by anxiety, such as from new pets or visitors in the house, tranquilizers or anti-anxiety drugs may be helpful. Alprazolam (Xanax®) has been recommended to stop spraying in cats, at a dosage of one-half tablet twice daily (Mandelker, 1990).

Basically, there are no drugs that are completely effective for curing elimination problems in cats. If drugs are given, they should be gradually withdrawn every month or two to determine if the cat has stopped the marking behavior.

If your cat goes in and out through a cat door, it may invite friends in for dinner (or they may come in uninvited) and they may spray. The invaders may make your cat feel it has no secure place, and that there is no difference between indoors and out. Then your cat feels the need to spray to remark your house as its own. The solution is to close the cat door and make your cat a strictly indoor cat, giving it a secure hideaway. A cat that is overly nervous may come indoors to excrete rather than doing so while outdoors.

A cat that is accustomed to going outdoors may stay inside and mess there because of "bully" cats that harass it at its outside toilet place. Bad weather may cause the cat to stay indoors beyond the endurance of its bowels or bladder. These cats can be cured by providing a litter box inside the house. Incidentally, cats can dig only in loose soil. If the soil is hard, their retractable claws cannot break the surface. Cats that live in desert areas may get out of the habit of burying their wastes if they live outdoors and there are no loose soil areas nearby.

When you have tried all the cures for inappropriate elimination, including hormone therapy, and nothing works, you can make the cat into an indoor-outdoor animal if you live in an area where traffic is not too heavy. Put the cat outside, but feed it around the same time every day so it will remain in the neighborhood. When the cat has learned to eliminate outdoors, you can begin to allow it inside the house when you can supervise its actions.

Cats may be unwanted visitors to your outdoor flower beds or planters. They see your entire yard as one gigantic litter box. Freshly planted flower and vegetable beds are especially attractive since they are clean and the soil is nicely loosened. Because cats like bare soil, it may be helpful to cover the bare spots. If you are having particular trouble, it may be worthwhile to sod instead of seed a new lawn area. It sometimes helps to cover the soil with a mulch such as shredded bark, lawn clippings, leaves, or pine needles. This may be quite helpful in large open areas that cats find irresistible. Chicken wire is useful for flower beds and the areas around trees to keep cats from digging there and to encourage them to go elsewhere. You can use the wire in large areas, anchored with rocks, or cut smaller pieces and leave them lying on the ground. As the plants come up, raise the wire until they are three inches or so tall; then remove it.

For one or two garden spots that are frequented by cats, sprinkle red or cayenne pepper on the ground, or spray a pepper mixture on the plants. Make it by grinding up a half dozen hot peppers and three or four cloves of garlic. Put this in a container, add a few drops of dishwashing detergent (the liquid kind), add water, and mix it well. Spray this around the perimeter of your garden and/or lawn. Cats will find the smell unpleasant and go elsewhere. Both these treatments need to be renewed after each rainstorm. Used coffee grounds, crushed eggshells, mothballs or ashes from your wood-burning fireplace may keep cats away. If the cats come over a fence on the way into the garden, it may help to apply Tanglefoot (from a garden supply store) around the top of the fence. Cats dislike the sticky feeling and may quit climbing the fence.

ACUTE KIDNEY FAILURE

Acute kidney failure comes on suddenly, and can occur because the blood supply to the kidney is inadequate or interrupted. All of the body's blood supply is filtered through the kidneys, and their large volume of very tiny blood vessels are easily damaged by lack of blood flow. Acute kidney failure also can occur because of a toxic insult to the kidneys. Unfortunately, some of the most useful antibiotics and painkillers (including aspirin and acetaminophen (Tylenol, etc.)) can cause kidney damage in cats. This is also true of drugs such as amphotericin B (used to treat systemic fungal diseases) and many drugs used for cancer chemotherapy. Antifreeze is also a major cause of kidney failure in cats. Anesthesia for long surgical procedures may cause kidney failure in elderly cats.

Cats with acute kidney failure are severely depressed, weak, lethargic, and dehydrated. They quit eating and may have bad breath, vomiting, diarrhea, and sores on the tongue. These cats are extremely ill. Prompt, aggressive treatment may get the cat through this acute episode, but the cat will have to be hospitalized, at least at the start of treatment. It will be given large amounts of fluids to flush the offending toxins out of the kidneys, and to reestablish blood flow through them. Peritoneal dialysis may save the cat's life, allowing the kidneys to regain function. In this procedure, special fluids are put into the abdomen and then drained out to remove toxins. A liquid diet such as Formula V™ RenalCare™ Feline Liquid Diet (Pet-Ag, Inc., Elgin, IL 60120, (800)323-0877) may be fed for several weeks until the cat is stabilized.

In many cases, the cat that survives the acute episode will recover. After a period of several weeks, it will stabilize and may live a reasonably healthy life, even though it may need a special "kidney diet" (see Chronic Kidney Failure, below).

CHRONIC KIDNEY FAILURE

Chronic kidney failure (chronic renal failure, CRF) is one of the most common conditions to afflict cats that are middle-aged and older. As many as one-third of elderly cats seen in veterinary clinics will show some degree of chronic renal failure. This condition comes on slowly and is invariably fatal. In humans, kidney transplants and dialysis keep patients alive. In cats, these measures are not practical. Although the cat will eventually die, the majority of them can live a reasonably good quality life, surviving for months or even years. Early diagnosis allows management to ease the kidneys' load, making the animal's life both longer and better. Many times, it is impossible to tell what originally started or caused the kidney failure. This is not absolutely necessary to its treatment. Abyssinian cats are prone to a disease called renal amyloidosis, which causes a chronic kidney failure requiring similar management.

Poor body condition and dehydration are the most common symptoms of chronic kidney failure. The cat may be drinking more than usual and urinating more than normal. It may urinate more often than usual at night. The symptoms come on gradually over a long period of time. The cat may have a poor appetite, weight loss, depression, weakness, and vomiting. Its coat may be dull and rough. The tongue and gums may show red, rough ulcers, and it may have a peculiar bad breath from the uremia. The mucous membranes may be pale.

Any cat more than seven- to 10-years-old should be routinely checked for kidney disease because it is so common. At the very least, a urinalysis should be done. Kidney function tests such as a blood urea nitrogen (BUN) and/or a serum creatinine test should be done, ideally, twice a year. A kidney biopsy, X-rays, or ultrasound also may be needed. They can give additional information as to the exact nature of the kidney problem, but if you cannot afford them, begin treatment based on the results of the lab tests.

Treatment of chronic kidney failure is aimed at slowing its progress. A cat with chronic kidney failure will need a diet with lowered protein levels (less than 28%), reduced phosphorus, and restricted dietary sodium (salt). The diet should have as few preservatives as possible because many of them are high in sodium. Excess salt in the diet may raise the amount of calcium in the urine and make stones recur. If given over a period of time, it may result in high blood pressure, which can cause blindness in cats.

Examples of kidney diets are Prescription Diet® Feline k/d® and CNM. The reduced quantity (but high-quality) of protein in these foods reduces the load on the kidneys. Twenty-22% protein is quite adequate for cats with chronic kidney failure, but it usually should not drop below this level. The cat feels and looks better and often becomes more active. It may be more alert mentally, and its coat may return to being soft instead of dry and scruffy. Palatability is important, and strong fish, cheese, or meat odors often tempt the cat to eat. To start the cat eating the new diet, or if the cat loses weight, add a little unsalted butter, chicken or turkey fat, or beef tallow. You also can add a small amount of potassium chloride (the "un-salt" type of product)—about the same amount as you would salt your own food. The cat must, of course, have fresh, clean water available at all times. If an infection is present, antibiotics may be needed.

Low potassium levels are a common problem in cats with chronic kidney failure. It is necessary to balance a lowered potassium level in the diet to ease the load on the kidneys while remaining aware of the possibility of dropping the level so low that the cat has severe muscular weakness or even collapse. Your veterinarian will balance the cat's dietary potassium with supplementation if needed. Be sure to let the veterinarian know if your cat shows signs of drooping head or neck or difficulty in walking. Fluid therapy also may cause potassium deficiency. These cats may have difficulty maintaining normal calcium levels, and may lose bone calcium, developing a disease sometimes called "renal rickets." At worst, the bones may become soft and rubbery, and the cat's jaw may bend when touched.

About a third of cats with chronic renal failure will have anemia. The cat may have a poor appetite, weakness, and lethargy. The more severe the anemia is, the more intense the symptoms are. This anemia is treated with male hormones and blood transfusions. Replacement of hormones that are missing from the kidneys with a synthetic substitute (recombinant human erythropoietin) may be lifesaving for some cats. An improved blood count will result in better appetite, weight gain, more normal activity, and a return to a normal mental state. There is a risk that the cat will form antibodies against the drug, so it is usually reserved for cats with very low packed cell volume (less than 20%) that have clinical signs due to their anemia (Polzin, 1992).

Other cats with chronic kidney failure will have high blood pressure (hypertension). This may cause weakness, convulsions, mental confusion, coma, and visual problems or blindness. Drugs may be given to lower and stabilize the blood pressure.

Treatment of older cats with chronic renal failure can be as simple or complicated as you wish. Frequent monitoring, with measurement of electrolytes such as potassium, as well as tracking the cat's blood pressure and kidney-related serum metabolites, can be quite costly. In the beginning, the cat will need laboratory blood work at least monthly. Later, it can be checked every three to six months. It is the ideal treatment if you want that level of care. At the very least, the cat should be put on a specialized kidney diet with potassium supplementation, if needed. This can still buy a number of comfortable, reasonably healthy months of life for an older cat. A younger cat may have two or three years of quality life, especially if the disease is caught early.

MISCELLANEOUS KIDNEY PROBLEMS

The most common kidney tumor in cats is lymphosarcoma, usually caused by the feline leukemia virus (FeLV). About 90% of cats with this tumor will test negative for FeLV on standard blood tests. Cats with lymphoma or lymphosarcoma may have enlarged knobby kidneys. Signs may not appear until the cat goes into kidney failure. Lymphoma is confirmed by kidney biopsy, which also distinguishes it from feline infectious peritonitis. The prognosis for cats with renal lymphosarcoma is poor. With chemotherapy, cats may live from two or three months to three years.

Feline infectious peritonitis (FIP) is a disease caused by a coronavirus. Cats with the "dry" form of FIP often have seriously affected kidneys, but may not show outright signs of kidney disease. The cat may show weight loss, apathy, and fever (see Vaccinations Chapter).

Some family lines of Abyssinian cats have a type of kidney disease called renal amyloidosis. The disease is seen in cats between one and five years of age. Signs are those of uremia and chronic renal failure. The cat may have a poor appetite and weight loss, infected gums and fever. It may drink more water than usual and urinate excessively.

LIVER PROBLEMS

The liver is one of the largest organs in the body and has a considerable reserve. It must be extensively damaged before signs of disease are seen. Because many of its functions are similar to those of other organs in the body, signs of liver disease may resemble disease signs of other organs. Liver disease may also accompany disease processes such as pancreatitis, hyperthyroidism, and congestive heart failure.

Ascarids, tapeworm cysts, flukes, and toxoplamosis are among the parasites which can affect the liver. Diabetes mellitus and Cushing's syndrome (an excess of adrenal cortical hormone) cause liver damage. Toxins such as coal tars, cresols, dioxin, carbon tetrachloride, and excess vitamin D can cause liver damage. Feline infectious peritonitis, leukemia virus, and feline immunodeficiency virus also can involve the liver.

Because of its numerous functions, many signs are possible with liver disease. Icterus (also called jaundice) is one of the most common. This is a yellow coloration of the mucous membranes, caused by an accumulation of toxins which are no longer removed from the blood by the damaged liver. This causes the "white" of the eye to appear yellow. The gums also may look yellowish. Another sign of possible liver disease is fluid accumulation in the abdomen, seen as a widening of the lower part of the belly. In some liver diseases, brain and central nervous system abnormalities occur. Some cats have only vague symptoms, including a poor appetite, occasional vomiting, weight loss, and depression.

Laboratory tests are usually needed to determine the extent of liver disease. X-rays, ultrasound, and a liver biopsy may be necessary to confirm the diagnosis and determine the extent of the disease. Even these may not give a definite diagnosis.

Liver disease is difficult to diagnose and still more difficult to treat. When it is caused by another disease or abnormality, treatment will be aimed at that cause. Very little therapy is available when the liver itself is involved. About all that can be done is to try to lessen its work load by providing a diet with high-quality protein and carefully balanced vitamins and minerals. Drugs such as choline may be helpful in some cases.

Hepatic lipidosis, also called idiopathic hepatic lipidosis (IHL) or fatty liver syndrome, is a common liver disease in cats. Its cause is unknown, but it is more frequent in overweight, middle-aged cats. It may be due to metabolic, toxic, or nutritional causes, or to a lack of oxygen supply to the liver. It can occur with diabetes mellitus, and can be seen in cats that have been stressed by boarding, surgery, illness or being moved to a new home. It is sometimes seen in a cat that has been fed dry dog food. Fatty liver may occur in cats that have upper respiratory tract disease because of a high fever which uses reserves faster than is normal. Also, the cat may be unable to smell food because of its nasal congestion, and may have mouth ulcers which make eating painful.

The lipidosis occurs when an apparently susceptible cat eats little or no food for a couple of days to two or more weeks. It is not known whether the failure to eat causes the lipidosis, or if the lipidosis causes the lack of appetite. Once the liver becomes filled with fat, the cat seems to be unable to metabolize and remove it. The cat also seems unable to use stored body fat in this crisis; thus, its body uses muscle to provide protein. About 35% of cats that have hepatic lipidosis will die.

Signs of fatty liver include lack of appetite, often lasting several weeks, and weight loss, although the cat may still be noticeably overweight. It may be jaundiced, and vomiting, constipation, and intermittent salivation may be seen. The cat may be lethargic, dehydrated, and weak.

Cats with advanced hepatic lipidosis have enough liver damage that they cannot utilize protein and its amino acids. The cat may have little or no appetite, and will need a high-protein balanced diet. Your veterinarian may need to place a feeding tube in the cat. It then can be fed a mixture of high-quality cat food diluted half and half with water and pushed through the tube with a syringe. Nutrical® also can be used for feeding the cat. Human enteral feeding formulas do not have enough protein for cats, while human baby foods are either lacking in protein or have a severe calcium-phosphorus imbalance for cats. Fluids and electrolyte solutions also may be given via the tube, and added taurine may be necessary. The feeding tube will be removed when the cat is feeling better and wants to eat by itself. (See Viral Respiratory Disease section for more information on feeding cats at risk from hepatic lipidosis.)

Some cats that are supplemented with liquid diets may be unable to cope with the protein in these foods. If no signs of hepatic encephalopathy such as arching the neck backwards, head pressing, and tremor are seen, then the concentration of the diet can be increased. Be careful not to overfeed the cat with the liquid supplement. It may take three to six weeks of force-feeding for the cat's enzyme activity to return to normal and for its appetite to return. If you are willing to persist, there is a fairly good chance your cat eventually will return to normal.

Gallstones are rarely seen in cats, but are sometimes found incidentally when the cat is examined for another disease. A cat that does have symptoms may show icterus and dark yellow or orange urine. It may have poor appetite, weight loss, vomiting, and dehydration. Vomiting and intermittent icterus may occur over a period of several months or years when the stones have been present for a long time. Cats with a blocked bile duct may have clay-colored feces. The abdomen may bulge with fluid. Gallbladder problems which persist may eventually cause liver failure.

Some gallstones are diagnosed by radiographs of the abdomen or ultrasound examination. Others are discovered by examining fluid from the abdomen. The majority of cats with gallstones do not have any symptoms. Surgery should not be done on these animals—just keep an eye on the problem and operate if they cause illness in the future.

Cats with gallbladder disease (including gallstones) which causes symptoms must be hospitalized. They are treated with intravenous fluids and antibiotics. Surgery to remove gallstones or the entire gallbladder is usually done as soon as the cat is in stable condition.

The liver has great powers to regenerate, and managing the cat's diet will help the liver rest while it has a chance to heal. Many cases of hepatitis are acute, and only short-term management is needed. Long-term dietary are measures needed for a cat with chronic hepatitis. Dietary care for a cat with liver disease will include high-quality protein. Commercial cat foods such as Prescription Diet® Feline k/d® can be given. If the cat has diarrhea, it should be switched to Feline c/d®. Cats with liver problems should not be given shellfish, organ meat, or foods containing fish meal. These contain purines which metabolize to form uric acid, something the cat's damaged liver cannot process.

Chapter 17

LAMENESS AND BACK PROBLEMS

LAMENESS EXAMINATION

Your cat is limping. Where do you begin? If there is an obvious cut or fracture, administer first aid (see Emergency Chapter). Take the cat to a veterinarian or emergency clinic.

If no injury is obvious, start by observing the cat. Check it in a place with firm footing, such as short carpet. Have someone call the cat, or tempt it to cross the room for a treat so you can watch it as it walks. Is only one leg involved? Does the cat limp all the time, or only when it is turning? If the cat limps worse when making a left turn, for example, a leg on the left side is probably sore.

When no obvious limp is apparent, examine the cat carefully and systematically, beginning at its neck. Feel for spots that are swollen, damp, or warmer than other parts of the body. Compare each pair of legs, front and rear, to its mate. Is one a different size or shape than the other?

You can check feet and legs with the cat standing at a comfortable height on a table or counter. Or, ask someone to hold the cat lying on its side as you examine it. If a cat that is not normally allowed on the counter becomes upset when you put it there, examine it on the floor.

Begin at the foot. Check the bottom of the paw. Are the pads normal in size and color? Is anything caught in the web between the toes? Grass awns can lodge there, especially in long-haired cats. Use a fine comb or your fingers to comb the hair between the pads to eliminate any foreign objects.

Squeeze each claw from its sheath (gently!), checking for drainage or redness around its base. Move each joint separately. You should not feel any crackling or grating as you work it through its normal range of motion. If there is a grating sensation, one of the bones may be broken. As you move an injured area, the cat may show obvious signs of pain, crying out or trying to bite you or pull away from you. If this happens, go to the veterinary clinic.

Continue up the leg, feeling carefully for swelling or heat. All bones should appear in normal alignment. If you have any doubt about what you are finding, check to see if the opposite leg is the same. If so, it's probably normal.

If you don't find any obvious problems but the cat is still limping, you have two choices. You can take it directly to the clinic, or you can wait. If the cat has jumped out of a tree or off a piece of furniture, it may have sprained a ligament, from which it may recover in a day or two. If the cat shows other signs of illness, or has not improved in two or three days, have it examined.

FOOT PROBLEMS

Cut pads can occur when the cat steps on a sharp object such as a piece of glass or a jagged piece of ice in winter. If the wound is fresh, it may bleed profusely. These cuts are messy but not life threatening. The ideal treatment is to have it sutured by your veterinarian. Put a sterile pad over the cut, wrap it with a snug (but not tight!) bandage, and go to the clinic.

If this is not possible, you may be able to mend it with cyanomethacrylate glue ("Super Glue®"). Make the cat comfortable with someone holding it upside down, or roll the cat in a towel with the injured leg sticking out. Dab the area dry with a clean cloth or tissue. Cover it with a thin coating of the glue and hold the edges of the cut together until the glue is completely dry. You then can apply a second layer of glue, reinforcing it if you like, with a single thin layer of tissue or toilet paper. Be careful not to glue yourself to the cat!

Serious trauma to the lower part of the foot may injure the foot pad. Treatment should attempt to preserve the pad in its normal orientation. It may be necessary to splint the foot to give it time to heal. If the pad doesn't end up underneath, the cat may wear the side of its foot raw, causing severe pain. Amputation of the leg eventually may be necessary.

Foreign bodies often get caught between the toes, especially with long-haired cats. Grass awns (foxtails) can be removed with a pair of tweezers. Dab a bit of disinfectant on the spot and dry off the excess.

Abscesses are common on cats' feet. They usually result from one cat biting the other's foot as they fight. The first sign may be a swollen, hot, tender area. The cat may be reluctant to walk on the foot, and may protest when you touch it. As it progresses, the abscess will come to a point. This is a soft area at the top of the swelling, where the infected material (pus) is about to burst through the skin. The abscess can now be drained (see Abscesses, Skin Chapter). Do NOT bandage it. Keep it open and draining until it is healed, which may take one to two weeks.

If the abscess has already broken and drained, you may notice the cat constantly licking the area. Or, you may see damp, matted hair on the leg. It may be necessary to enlarge the opening so it will drain well. Otherwise, treatment is the same as for any abscess.

Fractured or dislocated toes can occur, and may be quite painful. They are usually stabilized with either a firm bandage or a splint. The cat may be confined to a small box or cage until it is healed. Dislocated toes may pop out of joint again and again, causing the animal to limp and show pain. If this continues to happen, the best cure is to have the toe amputated, allowing the foot to heal and removing the source of pain.

Cats may have extra toes or one or more deformed claws. These may snag in carpet or catch as the cat climbs a tree, causing tearing and pain. Your veterinarian easily can surgically remove the toes, ending the pain.

Cats' dewclaws should be trimmed along with the rest of the toenails, as a part of routine care. If this is not done, the nail on the dewclaw may curl around, grow into the skin on the inside of the leg, and become infected. If the problem persists, or if you are unwilling or unable to trim the nails, have the dewclaws removed.

Broken claws can be very painful. They may split across, lengthwise, or pieces may break off, leaving a red, raw area exposed. The open nail bed is easily infected. Pack the area with an antibiotic cream and bandage it lightly. Or, mend it with glue as discussed above.

FRACTURES

Fractures in the foot may occur when a cat is hit by a car, accidentally slammed in a door, or stepped on by a human foot. Fractures higher up the leg, especially of the tibia, happen when the cat jumps off a roof or out of a tree. In cities, cats can be severely injured when they fall or jump from the window of a high-rise building. Fractures also may occur from a dog bite or gunshot.

A compound fracture of a foot or leg is obvious—bones stick out through the skin. Put a sterile gauze pad over the open area, and take the cat to the clinic.

In simple fractures, the broken bone is still covered by undamaged skin. When the bone is broken completely through, the leg may hang limply at an odd angle. The cat will be in obvious pain, and may not put any weight on the leg. A greenstick fracture may fray the bone, breaking it partway through, but leaving it connected. There may be swelling over the break, and the cat may show pain but still limp on the leg. The severity of the problem may not be obvious until the leg is X-rayed.

Your veterinarian may suggest observing the cat overnight and repairing the fracture the next day. It is common practice to treat the animal for shock, give antibiotics, and allow its body to stabilize after the accident before subjecting it to the risk of anesthesia. The cat has a much better chance of surviving the fracture repair if it is not done immediately after the accident. Also, the surgeon has time to determine if there are other injuries, such as punctures to the chest or abdominal organs which were not evident on the initial examination.

Fractures in the foot or lower leg are sometimes easily stabilized by wrapping the limb to a splint on the back of the leg, often called a "spoon splint" because of its shape.

Further up the leg, the best method may be a pin down the inside of the bone (called an "intramedullary pin"). Or, a set of pins may be placed through the bone, at right angles to it. Usually, four pins are used, two on either side of the break. They are connected with tinker-toy-like brackets and rods. This is called a Kirschner apparatus. While it looks peculiar, it is comfortable for the animal. The cat may walk well, putting weight on the leg soon after surgery. Both methods can have good results, depending on the cat's healing capacity and your ability to keep the cat confined to a small area ("cage rest") while the bone heals. A disadvantage is that both are major surgical procedures and can be quite costly.

A Thomas splint can be used to stabilize some breaks that are too high in the leg to be held with a spoon splint. This is not as effective a method of repair as pinning for most cases, but is often used where cost is a problem because it is usually less expensive than the surgery involved in pinning. It can be used for fractures in both the front and hind legs. A Thomas splint is an aluminum rod frame fitted into the cat's armpit or groin. The cat is anesthetized. The bones are then put back into alignment, and the leg is pulled snugly against the framework to keep it immobile until healed. The leg is sandwiched into the splint using plenty of tape to hold it securely. Expect the cat to lose some hair when the splint is removed.

Any bandage or splint MUST be kept dry. If the cat is used to going outside for toilet functions, put a plastic bag over the splint before you let it out, and bring the cat inside as soon as it is finished. Be sure to remove the plastic while the cat is indoors or it may sweat, causing skin damage. Keep the cat indoors until the splint is removed. The cat may lick or chew at the splint. If the cat is persistent about it, there may be infection underneath, it may be too tight, or it may be rubbing or chafing. Return the cat to the clinic for a checkup.

Osteomyelitis is an infection in the bone. Usually caused by bacteria, especially *Staphylococcus*, it also can be caused by systemic fungus diseases. Osteomyelitis may occur after a fracture, or from a penetrating wound such as a bite, gunshot, or stab by a thorn or tree branch. It also can occur after surgery to mend a fracture or other injury, especially if the fracture is not completely immobilized. There is usually hard, bony swelling at the area. It may be painful, and the soft tissues also may be swollen. There may be a draining tract oozing pus out through the skin, and a foul odor.

Treatment of osteomyelitis may include long-term antibiotics (one to two months), surgical drainage, and removal of loose or separated bone pieces. The wound is often left open to allow drainage and cleaning. The cat usually will need strict cage rest during the recovery period. Some cats recover completely. In others, the disease will recur and necessitate bone grafting or amputation of the affected limb. A few die if the infection cannot be controlled.

ARTHRITIS

Arthritis may be seen in cats of any age when due to injury. This may occur when the cat is hit by a vehicle, falls from a tree or rooftop (or even the top of a refrigerator) or is bitten or mauled by another animal. Traumatic arthritis usually involves only one joint, which has obvious pain. It may be swollen. The cat should be examined by your veterinarian to make sure there are no fractures or torn ligaments or tendons which need surgical repair. These cats usually heal well with time and rest.

Septic arthritis is caused by a bacterial infection in the joint, usually because a bite or other injury penetrated the joint capsule. It also is seen when bacteria are carried in the blood from another site, such as an umbilical abscess in a kitten or uterine infection in a queen. Usually only one joint is involved, and it will be quite painful. It may feel hot to the touch compared to the surrounding tissue. The cat may have a fever and be droopy. Antibiotic treatment is needed. The joint may have to be drained surgically, and in the worst cases, the leg may have to be amputated. It is better for the cat to live in comfort with three legs than have four legs, one of which has the bones rubbing together because the joint surfaces have been destroyed.

Osteoarthritis is the common arthritis of elderly cats, just as it is in older humans. It occurs when the joint cartilage is torn or worn away as the animal ages. Spurs or lips of new bone form at the edges of the joint. These kinds of damage combine to cause pain. The cat may limp on one or more legs, or it may be less active than usual. Most arthritis in cats does not require treatment. If the cat is in severe pain, your veterinarian can prescribe drugs. They should be given only for short periods when the cat's pain is worst. Long-term treatment with these medications may cause severe health problems. Surgery usually is not helpful.

METABOLIC BONE DISEASES

Nutritional secondary hyperparathyroidism is also called juvenile or nutritional osteopenia. These words describe a disease caused by feeding an all-meat diet, which is severely unbalanced nutritionally. It is high in phosphorus and almost completely lacking in calcium. The kitten (or cat) cannot make strong bones without adequate calcium.

Kittens may limp and show stiffness and pain. They will have fractures without being injured because the bones are weak and brittle. The backbone may be kinked and deformed, and the kitten may become paralyzed. Kittens with spinal fractures should be euthanized as there is no chance of recovery to normal. Cats with fractures in the chest and pelvis may have trouble breathing, defecating, and, if female, would be unable to have kittens. If the disease is not too advanced and fractures are not in critical areas, the cat can sometimes be saved by putting it on a normal, nutritionally balanced diet.

Osteogenesis imperfecta is a hereditary bone disease with signs similar to nutritional osteopenia. It should be suspected when kittens have these signs but are fed a normal, balanced diet. Treatment is not usually successful. Because the disease is quite painful, the cat should be euthanized for humane reasons.

Kidney disease may cause similar symptoms in older cats, along with symptoms of chronic kidney failure (see Urinary Disease Chapter). The cat may appear to have pain in its bones, or they may fracture for no apparent reason. The jaw bone may be soft enough that it will feel rubbery and bend when pushed firmly with your thumb. Teeth may be loose or fall out. Treatment of the bone damage begins with treatment of the underlying kidney disease.

Cats that are fed excessive amounts of liver for a long time (two to three years) may have bony growths on the spine, especially over the neck and chest, and enlarged joints. The cat will show pain, lameness, and swelling in one or more joints, and may be very stiff. The coat may look ragged because the cat cannot turn around to groom itself. The damage may not be reversible after bony changes have occurred. Prevention is simple—feed a well-balanced diet.

RUPTURED CRUCIATE LIGAMENTS

The cruciate ligaments are a pair of ligaments that cross within the stifle joint. They stabilize that joint and help it function smoothly. Cats commonly tear them by hard landings, usually as they jump off a wall or fence, out of a tree, or off the top of the refrigerator. Keeping your cat indoors and off the top of high shelves and appliances will help avoid this problem.

If your cat has a hard landing from a high place and limps afterward, and continues to limp on a hind leg after several days have passed, it may have ruptured one of these ligaments. Take the cat to your veterinarian for a checkup. X-rays will not show any changes in the joint. The veterinarian will be able to move the lower part of the leg forward and back in relationship to the upper part, called "drawer motion." This is diagnostic for this particular injury. The cat may need to be anesthetized for the examination.

Surgery is the only cure for a ruptured cruciate ligament. It cannot be reattached, but is replaced by a fine piece of skin, fascia (the white, heavy covering over muscles), or an artificial material. After the cat heals, the limp will disappear and the leg motion should be normal or nearly so. This is often a very rewarding and successful surgery for everyone—you, your cat, and your veterinarian.

DISLOCATED HIP

Dislocated hips are occasionally seen in older cats, usually from being hit by a car or similar trauma. If the injury is not more than two or three days old, your veterinarian can probably replace it. A sling, holding the leg in a sort of frog-leg position, is used for one to two weeks.

A few dislocated hips will not stay in the socket after the sling is removed, or may pop out later. Surgery may be necessary, putting in a pin to hold the femur into the hip socket until it heals, usually one to two weeks. In severe cases where the head of the femur is damaged, it may be necessary to remove it. This sounds like a radical cure, but is not at all unusual. The majority of cats will walk without a limp after healing.

PELVIC FRACTURES

The pelvis is often fractured when the cat is hit by a car. The cat may drag its hind end or be paralyzed in one hind leg. X-rays usually are required to determine which cases need surgery. Most of them do not need treatment other than confining the cat to a small place for three to four weeks. A playpen is an ideal space. Put the cat's food and water and a litter box in it. The litter box can be made from a cardboard box cut down so that the sides are only an inch high, allowing the cat to get in and out easily. For the first few days after injury, put the playpen in a quiet area such as a bedroom, where the cat can rest comfortably. Then, it can be moved where the cat can see its family, such as in the living room.

Surgery is necessary for pelvic fractures when fragments are pushed inward, threatening to damage organs within the pelvis. In these cases, pins may be needed to pull the fragments into alignment and to hold the pieces in place until healing takes place.

During healing, constipation may be a problem. Give a stool softener or cat laxative according to the directions. Enemas may be necessary. The cat may need a careful diet for the rest of its life to prevent constipation.

Some cats will have enough damage after healing that the head of the femur has to be removed. This usually allows the cat to walk without pain. Surgery need not be done immediately after the injury—it can be done a month or two later if it becomes obvious that it is needed.

Damage may occur to the urinary tract or the nerves that control the hind legs. If the cat has not recovered urinary function after three to four weeks, chances of further recovery are nearly zero. Then, you will have to decide whether you can keep the animal healthy and happy with so severe a problem, or whether euthanasia is the kindest course.

If the cat with the fractured pelvis is a female that has not been spayed, this should be done as soon as the fractures have healed. Otherwise, there may be enough narrowing of the pelvis that if she becomes pregnant, there is not enough space for the kittens to come through the canal. An expensive Caesarean section may be needed to remove the kittens and save her life. If she is an outdoor cat and tries to give birth in seclusion, she may die.

Hip dysplasia, which is common in several large breeds of dogs, is occasionally seen in cats, especially those of Siamese heritage. Most cats do not have any clinical symptoms, or have minimal pain and live out their lives without needing treatment. Those that do show signs look similar to dysplastic dogs, including a crouching walk, intermittent hind leg lameness, reluctance to climb or jump, pain on defecation, and, sometimes, howling because of pain. If you move the hind legs, you may feel a crunching (called crepitus) in the hips. Surgery similar to that used in dogs can be done to provide relief in the worst cases.

RUPTURED ACHILLES TENDON

A cat's Achilles tendon may be torn when it is hit by a car or bitten by a dog. It may happen when a farm cat hides in a hay field and is cut by a mowing machine. The most common sign is that the affected hock drops to the floor on the injured side. The cat will be walking along with one hock in normal position, and one hitting the floor each time it takes a step. It will be unable to walk on its toes or stand on the injured leg. There will not be any crepitation (crunchy or crackly feeling) when the leg is palpated or moved, telling you there probably are no broken bones.

The "down on the hocks" posture can be seen with blood clots in the aorta. It also occurs with a ruptured gastrocnemius muscle. None of these problems will heal well without surgery. If your cat is walking this way, don't wait—get help within a few hours.

With surgery, including pinning any bone injury in the area and suturing damaged tendons, a ruptured Achilles tendon usually heals well. The cat usually can flex the leg normally in three to four weeks.

FORELEG PARALYSIS

Muscles served by the radial nerve may be paralyzed when the cat's front leg is injured, such as when it is hit by a car or bitten by a dog. The leg need not be broken—the nerve need only be damaged. Tumors in the nerve roots, especially lymphosarcoma, also cause paralysis of a single foreleg.

The cat drags the entire leg, often with the top of the paw folded backward, and with the hair, rather than the pad, dragging on the ground. This is because the cat is unable to pull the leg forward to place it into position for a normal step. Or, the cat may swing the leg forward, but be unable to pull the paw up into place to take a step. If the injury is severe, the cat may not have any feeling in the leg when a toe is pinched. If the paralysis has been present for some time, the muscles of the leg may atrophy (wither), leaving it thin and wasted when compared to the other leg.

In some cases, EARLY surgery may restore nerve function. Some cats regain partial use of the leg after several months, or learn to compensate for the damage with time. Other cats never regain any useful function of the leg. They are unable to compensate for the injury, and may be in continuous pain. Or, the foot may be dragged on the ground until it is raw and scraped. In these cases, amputation is the kindest treatment and will result in great relief (see below).

AMPUTATIONS

It's not pleasant to know that your beloved cat's leg should be amputated. However, for some injuries, this is the best cure. In many cases, removing the leg may be the only way to save the cat's life. Age is not a factor. If the cat is healthy enough to withstand surgery, it will adapt to the loss of the leg, usually without difficulty.

A cat may need to have a leg amputated for a number of reasons. It may have been hit by a car and the limb is shattered beyond repair. The accident may have damaged the blood supply so badly that the leg cannot be kept alive. The foot may have been caught in a fan belt or trap, or a heavy object may have been dropped on it, causing a severe crushing injury. The cat may have an infection in the bone or nerve damage so that it cannot control its foot. Do not hesitate to consider having the leg amputated if you love your cat and would like to have it around for years to come.

Any one leg may be lost without causing the cat much long-term trouble. If a human loses a leg, it removes 50% of the weight-bearing ability and perhaps 80% of balance. The cat loses 25% of its weight-bearing ability and only 10-15% of its balance. The cat becomes a tripod, which is very stable. A hind leg is little problem at all. A front leg is a little more of a challenge, but given a bit of time, the cat will learn to hop easily on the remaining front leg.

If your veterinarian believes amputation is necessary, please have it done. It is a relatively simple operation. Be sure your veterinarian removes the leg as close to the body as possible, even if only the foot is damaged. It may seem kinder to leave as much leg as possible, but it is not! If a stub is left, the cat doesn't know it needs to protect it. It will attempt to walk on it, keeping it raw, sore, and bleeding for the rest of its life. If the leg is taken off cleanly, near the body, the cat will learn do quite well without it.

You bring your cat home from the hospital after an amputation. What can you expect? For a week or two, the cat probably will be a bit tipsy and unbalanced. Give the cat love, attention, good nutrition, and let it find its balance. The cat is learning to walk all over again. If you have a yard and your pet is an outdoor cat, let it spend plenty of time outside if the weather is good. Play gently with the cat. It will gradually become accustomed to not having the leg, and will walk quite well without it. In time, most cats will run, play, and function much as they did before the accident. Some cats still will catch birds and mice and climb trees. Don't worry if the cat falls occasionally. It will be much less bothered by it than you are. Try not to laugh at the cat—it will be embarrassed enough as it is by falling down. Occasionally, a cat may experience phantom pain. One study found that nearly all the responding pet owners were satisfied with their pet after amputations were performed (Carberry, 1987).

It is especially important to keep your amputee at a normal weight. Excess weight can strain the remaining leg. After a while, the structure of the leg may break down and it will be necessary to euthanize the cat because of it.

One of my fondest memories is of a three-month-old calico named Tansy Ragwort jumping to play with a toy swinging from a string. She was reaching gaily up with her one front leg, only a few days after surgery. She never missed the other leg.

BACK PROBLEMS

Manx cats, which are either tailless or have stubby tails, are that way because of a dominant gene. This gene, sadly, is related to spina bifida, where the spinal canal does not close completely. In some cats, this leaves the spinal cord uncovered instead of being shielded by bone. The cat may become paralyzed because of this spinal deformity. This kills many kittens before or shortly after they are born. Even more common, many Manx have a lifetime of fecal incontinence. Some Manx cats normally have a bunny-hopping gait, but in others, this also may indicate abnormalities with the spinal cord.

Older cats of all breeds, especially those over 14 or 15 years of age, often have herniated intervertebral discs, usually without any physical symptoms. In the rare cat where symptoms do occur, they may include paralysis or dragging one or both hind legs. Disc injuries also can be caused by auto accidents or other impact injuries. They usually are treated with corticosteroids. Serious spinal problems also are seen with metabolic bone disease (see above).

Paralysis may occur when the cat's spinal cord is damaged by an accident. Many of these cats recover with cage rest, with or without a body cast.

Tumors in the spinal canal also may cause paralysis. Some animals recover with surgery accompanied by radiation or chemotherapy. An excess of vitamin A (usually due to feeding too much liver) may cause bony growths on the spine and other bones, leading to pain and problems with the nerves and paralysis.

TAIL PROBLEMS

Injury to the pelvis may include damage to the joint between the backbone and the tail (the sacrococcygeal joint). If the tail is totally paralyzed, or develops dry gangrene because blood circulation is inadequate, it should be amputated. This also should be done if the tail is continually soiled because the cat cannot get it out of the way when it urinates or defecates.

Tail amputation also is commonly needed after a cat is hit by a car or bitten by a dog, or the tail is accidentally slammed in a door. The blood supply to the tail is poor, and the bones are thin. In some cases, the vessels are irreparably damaged by the injury. If they are not damaged and the tail carefully splinted, it sometimes may heal. If not, the only treatment is amputation of the broken end. The tail usually heals well following surgery and looks good cosmetically. The end result is a bobtailed cat.

If the cat is a show cat or you particularly value its tail, your veterinarian may attempt to use plates or screws to stabilize the fracture during the healing period. This occasionally works, but does not work in all cases. Don't be surprised if it fails and amputation is necessary.

Chapter 18

THE BRAIN AND NERVOUS SYSTEM

- *Convulsions and Epilepsy*
- *Cerebellar Disease*
- *Miscellaneous*

Signs of brain and nervous system problems can include seizures, changes in behavior and attitude, depression, staggering or other abnormal gait, shaking or tremors, and a tilted head or rolling eyes. Nervous system ailments require careful veterinary diagnosis since many diseases or injuries can have the same signs—including rabies!

CONVULSIONS AND EPILEPSY

It can be quite upsetting when your cat has convulsions. It may be perfectly normal one minute, while writhing on the floor the next, twitching and jerking. Seizure disorders are far less common in cats than in dogs, but are occasionally seen. They occur when some area in the brain is overstimulated, producing an excessive electrical discharge. This in turn stimulates the muscles to twitch and spasm. Seizures are not a disease in themselves. They are a symptom of a problem somewhere in the central nervous system (brain or upper spinal cord), an injury, or an intoxication.

The first question: Is the cat an unspayed female? When a queen comes into heat, she may writhe and squirm on her side, rolling along the floor and meowing. This is normal, but it may look like a convulsion if you've never seen it.

Young cats that grow up alone may suddenly run around the house, often with eyes dilated, chasing imaginary prey or attacking persons. This is normal exuberant play behavior which would ordinarily be directed at another cat. If the cat's actions are a nuisance, behavior modification may be needed to change them. The easiest cure is to acquire another cat or a number of small toys to help use up some of this energy.

Most major (grand mal) seizures begin with a stage of anticipation. You may not recognize this the first time your cat has a seizure, but if it occurs frequently, you may become aware of it. The cat may sense that something is about to happen, and act in an unusual manner. It may be overly affectionate, or restless or anxious. Other cats do not change noticeably before convulsions occur. Grand mal seizures cause violent muscular activity; the cat falls on its side, becomes relatively immobile, and makes paddling movements with its feet. These running motions may

not stop even if the cat runs into an obstacle. The cat may salivate and/or lose control of its bowels or bladder.

Most seizures last only a few minutes. Don't pick up the cat or move it unless it is hurting itself or in an area like a stairway or balcony where it may fall and be injured. Don't try to shake the cat out of the seizure. Watch the cat to make sure it doesn't knock something onto itself, but don't worry if it doesn't recognize you. Lack of awareness is part of the seizure.

If the seizure lasts more than four or five minutes, take the animal to the nearest veterinarian. Seizures which last for a long time may damage the brain because of lack of oxygen, causing permanent injury or even death.

After the seizure, the cat may behave oddly for a period of time. It may be upset and confused, may refuse to eat, or cry out. The cat should be checked if this lasts more than a few minutes. There are a number of causes of convulsions.

Head injury may cause seizures. This may occur months or even years later when scar tissue in the brain contracts, putting pressure on some part of the brain. A diseased liver may fail to remove toxins from the cat's blood, leading to disorders in brain function.

Food allergies occasionally cause seizures. These may occur several hours after feeding—early in the morning, six to 10 hours after the cat's evening meal. Noting the relationship between the seizure and the cat's last meal may help in diagnosis. A different food may cure it completely.

Some toxins, such as organophosphate insecticides, can cause convulsions. A cat with this toxicity does not come out of the seizure, but continues to twitch and salivate profusely. Strychnine poisoning causes convulsions, usually with minimal salivation. Seizures also may be seen with antifreeze (ethylene glycol) poisoning. If you suspect any of these, take the cat to a clinic immediately.

Hypoglycemia (low blood sugar) can be seen in kittens fewer than eight weeks of age that have an inadequate or unbalanced diet. It also can be seen with diabetes or insulin treatment. Try to get the kitten to swallow some syrup, honey, or strong sugar water. This may stop the convulsions. Be careful, because the kitten may accidentally bite you. Make sure it does not inhale any of the liquid, and that the kitten is warmed to a normal body temperature. Have the kitten checked by your veterinarian as soon as possible.

Vitamin B1 (thiamine) deficiency can occur in cats that are fed nothing but fish. Some fish, such as catfish, smelt, saltwater herring, and carp, contain an enzyme called thiaminase which destroys thiamine. Adequate cooking inactivates the thiaminase—do not feed raw fish. Most commercial cat foods have added thiamine, but if they are stored for a long time, it can deteriorate. The cat may be unable to raise its head, be unaware of where it is, and lose weight. Incoordination, staggering, and convulsions may be seen. Thiamine deficiency can occur in young cats that have severe upper respiratory disease or other long-term illness. Giving thiamine can result in a dramatic cure. In severe cases, the cat may be permanently incoordinated, but may still be a good pet.

Stroke-like problems may occur when an artery in the brain begins to function abnormally. This can result in convulsions, and is fairly common in elderly cats. Some of them gain relief when treated with corticosteroids.

A disease called feline ischemic encephalopathy is seen on the East Coast of the United States, mostly during August. It does not occur elsewhere in the country. Affected cats are usually between one and three years of age. They may have a history of recent or current upper respiratory infection. The cat will have seizures, and may walk in circles. If the convulsions can be controlled, the cat usually recovers.

Feline infectious peritonitis (FIP) may attack the nervous system and other organs. The cat may have liver and kidney damage, as well as central nervous system involvement. Convulsions, tipped head, staggering, or paralysis may be the only visible symptoms, making diagnosis difficult. FIP is usually fatal.

The most common brain tumor in cats is meningioma, involving the membranes covering the brain. Most common in males over 10 years of age, these tumors are benign. However, if they grow for a long time, even slowly, they compress and destroy normal brain tissue. Signs of a brain tumor may be very subtle and hard to diagnose. If found early enough, the brain tumor may be removed surgically and the cat may return to normal or nearly so. In any case, the seizures are usually relieved. Radiation therapy and other treatments also are used, and may buy several more years of quality life for the cat.

Lysosomal storage disease is a rare condition seen in very young kittens. A hereditary defect allows fatty materials and proteins to build up throughout the body tissues. Brain function becomes progressively worse, with convulsions and blindness. There is no treatment for the disease, and the kitten eventually will die.

True epilepsy is quite rare in cats. However, when no cause can be found in the cat that has convulsions, a diagnosis of epilepsy may be made. In some cats that are fewer than three years-old, the problem may be hereditary. The cat may have attacks regularly, possibly every month or two, but is normal and healthy between them. These cats may sometimes be treated with phenobarbital. It is inexpensive and usually controls the seizures quite well.

Your cat's history will be important to diagnosis. Jot on your calendar when a seizure occurs and how long it lasts—time it with your watch or clock. Also note any unusual behaviors that occur before, during, or after the attack. It is possible that a cat can have one seizure for some unknown reason and never have another as long as it lives. Or, it may have them only every two or three months. If the cat appears otherwise healthy and normal within a day or so after the seizure, it may not be necessary to take it to your veterinarian. Wait and see if it has another one.

Many of the medications used to control seizures are somewhat sedative, but the cat will adjust to them in a short time. When a cat is placed on anticonvulsant medication, it is important to give the drug at the same time every day. This keeps a constant drug level in the bloodstream without large swings. Some cats respond to administration of a potassium bromide solution given by itself or in addition to anti-seizure medications.

A cat that has seizures more than once or twice, that has a seizure long enough to leave it exhausted, or that is otherwise ill should be checked by your veterinarian. The examination may include tests such as urinalysis and a blood chemistry panel, as well as a complete blood count (CBC) and chest X-rays. A thorough neurological examination is necessary. If no answers are found, your cat may be referred to a neurologist. An electroencephalogram (EEG) may be done to determine which part of the brain is involved. Diagnosis may include a computer assisted tomography (CAT!) scan and/or an MRI (magnetic resonance imaging). An electrocardiogram (EKG) is also a good idea in cats with seizures.

CEREBELLAR DISEASE

Cats that have a disease of the cerebellum often lose coordination of the limbs and head. Lysosomal storage disease (above) is one example.

Even more common is the brain damage caused when kittens are attacked by the panleukopenia (feline distemper) virus. Infection may occur while they are in the queen's uterus or shortly after birth, especially before three weeks of age. The kittens are partially protected by the mother's immunity so the virus does not kill them. However, it does infect the brain, stunting its development. This shows up as incoordination when the kittens begin to walk. They stagger and tip over, and may spread their feet abnormally far apart in an attempt to remain upright. Their heads may spasm or twist uncontrollably. There is no treatment—this part of the kitten's brain is simply not sufficiently developed to work properly and never will be. Some kittens that are mildly affected may be suitable pets for an understanding owner who will keep them indoors so they don't come to harm. This disease can be prevented by adequate vaccination of the queen. If she has a normal immune system, her kittens should be protected well past the critical first three weeks.

MISCELLANEOUS

Rabies infection initially causes behavioral changes in cats, followed by paralysis. Signs of rabies include an unusual expression in the eyes, increased or unusual cries or howls, and staggering or paralysis in the hind legs. Handle the cat with extreme care and have it examined as soon as possible. Rabies can be prevented by keeping the cat's vaccinations current.

Cats with obscure signs of brain or nervous system disease often are victims of feline leukemia. Unvaccinated cats should be treated for leukemia or lymphoma of the central nervous system until it is proven otherwise.

Hydrocephalus ("water on the brain") is sometimes seen in kittens. If it is severe, the kitten's skull may have an abnormal bulging dome on the front, above the eyes. This disease may cause convulsions. If the kitten lives, it will never be normal.

Vestibular disease involves the middle or inner ear or both. Symptoms include staggering, circling, or the head being held tipped to one side (see Ear Chapter).

Facial paralysis occurs when one side of the face is hit by a vehicle or otherwise injured. Or, it may occur with inflammation of the inner ear or problems within the brain. Facial paralysis also can be associated with tumors of the pituitary gland or lack of thyroid hormone. A cat with facial paralysis will have a drooping ear on the paralyzed side. The nose pulls to that side, and that eye may be wide open and unmoving. Keep the cat's eye moist if it is not blinking the lid; use any mild antibiotic eye ointment. Have the cat examined by your veterinarian. Food may pack inside the cheek on the affected side, so you may have to experiment with suitable foods until you find one the cat can eat easily. These cats usually need careful feeding for the rest of their lives. Depending on the cause and degree of damage, some cats may recover slight function over a LONG period of time. Other cats never recover, and may require eye drops or ointment to keep the eye moist. Facial paralysis is uncommon in cats.

Chapter 19

THE ENDOCRINE SYSTEM

- *Diabetes Mellitus*
- *Thyroid Problems*
- *Other Endocrine Disorders*

DIABETES MELLITUS

Diabetes mellitus (sometimes called sugar diabetes) occurs in cats, especially middle-aged and older animals. The cat's blood sugar is excessively high (hyperglycemia). The exact cause of diabetes is unknown, although many factors seem to trigger it. It can be treated, but there is no permanent cure.

Signs of diabetes can vary. One of the most common is the cat that drinks an excessive amount of water and urinates frequently. The cat may urinate in places other than its litter box because it cannot get there in time. It may have a ravenous appetite but lose weight, or a poor appetite. It may be weak, depressed, or lethargic. A cat that suddenly goes blind may do so from diabetic cataracts—have it checked within a day.

A blood test will show elevated amounts of glucose. This test is usually performed after a 12 to 24 hour fast, so if you suspect your cat may be diabetic, make an appointment for early morning. Remove all food after an early dinner the night before the visit. In some cases, it may be necessary to take blood glucose readings on three or four different days to confirm the diagnosis. This is because stress may raise the cat's blood glucose, causing a false diagnosis of diabetes on just one sample. The cat's urine glucose level also will be high.

Cats that have had pancreatitis are at greater risk for developing diabetes. Because the pancreas produces insulin, tumors, abscesses, or general inflammation of the organ can initiate diabetes. Peritonitis or other abdominal infection can also involve the pancreas, producing diabetes.

Obesity can also be a predisposing factor, as can poor diet, stress, and genetic predisposition. Cats that weigh more than 15 pounds (6.8 kg) were found to be twice as likely to develop diabetes than cats of normal size and weight (Panciera, 1990). Some cases of diabetes are due to overweight alone, and disappear when the cat's weight returns to normal.

Hormonal abnormalities and some medications also can push the cat into diabetes. Long-term administration of female hormones such as progesterone can trigger diabetes. Some cats that are treated with megestrol acetate (a drug used to keep dogs from coming into heat) may become diabetic, even with only one or a few doses.

Many of these cats no longer will be diabetic when the drug is discontinued, while others become permanently diabetic. Spayed female cats are far less likely to develop diabetes than are unspayed ones. Diabetes in cats is more common in males than in females.

Several different types of diabetes mellitus are seen. Insulin-dependent (juvenile or Type 1) diabetes is often inherited. It is rare, but when seen, occurs in younger cats and in cats with pancreatic disease. Juvenile diabetes is treated with regular insulin. These cats are very ill when first taken to the clinic, and it is sometimes difficult to get them to eat.

Insulin-resistant diabetes is usually found in fat, lazy, mature cats. The insulin they produce does not work adequately and their body cells do not utilize it well, resulting in less glucose than normal being taken up by the cells. It remains in the blood, giving high blood glucose. This diabetes also may be due to Cushing's disease (see below).

Insulin-resistant cats can be treated with injections of long-lasting insulin. Depending on the kind of insulin used, intramuscular injections may be needed once or twice daily. They are easy to give (see Nursing Chapter).

When giving injections day after day, it may help to pinch the skin before you insert the needle. The cat pays attention to the pinch, not the needle prick. Carefully shake the insulin before drawing it into the syringe. Make sure the insulin and the glucose test strips you use are not outdated. If a cat appears to be resistant to insulin, your technique should be checked to make sure you are injecting the drug correctly. Consistency in giving insulin and in diet and routine is very important for these cats. Insulin resistance also may be due to infection, allergic reaction against insulin, obesity, or an endocrine disorder. Further testing may be needed to determine the reason and how to treat it (Peterson, 1992).

Recent research under a Morris Animal Foundation grant has shown that as many as 50% of cats can be treated orally to regulate blood glucose. If your cat is one of the lucky ones with Type II (noninsulin-dependent) diabetes, it can live a relatively normal life with pills that are easily given (Nelson, 1993). Whatever insulin is used, the cost is only pennies per day. When your routine is established, treatment will take only a few minutes per day.

When diabetes is first diagnosed, it is necessary to find the appropriate dosage of insulin for your cat. Hospitalization may be needed for one to two weeks, and the cat will be stabilized on a suitable diet. Be aware that the insulin dosage probably will change when you bring the cat home. You may have to work with your veterinarian to get it just right. This is because the cat's activity and emotional state will be different from when in the hospital. Also, the pancreas of a cat with adult-onset diabetes may intermittently produce a small amount of insulin, making it difficult to regulate insulin needs. Diabetic cats may need supplemental potassium during stabilization.

You probably will need to test the cat's urine for glucose after you bring it home. This is easily accomplished using a litter box with a slotted bottom and special nonabsorbent litter (see Cat Care Chapter). This will supplement periodic glucose tests by your veterinarian. Or, newspaper can be used to line a freshly washed litter box, as it does not interfere with glucose tests. The glucose test is easily performed with testing sticks available from a pharmacy. The small plastic strips with chemically-treated areas change color in response to the amount of sugar present in the urine.

The blood glucose level needs to be kept between 100 milligrams per deciliter (mg/dl) and 200-250 mg/dl in any 24 hour period. This is difficult in many cats. When there is a problem, it is better for the sugar to be too high instead of too low. In some cats, it may be allowed to go as high as 300 mg/dl without problems, if recommended by your veterinarian.

When the diabetic cat is at home, report any behavior change to your veterinarian. Keep a chart of the urine glucose pattern, including the time of day the cat was fed, how much and what was fed, when the test was taken, and the glucose reading. Contact the veterinarian immediately if the cat has seizures, acts as if it is drunken, or goes into a coma. Check with your veterinarian within a day if the cat is depressed, does not have an appetite, or if you notice cataracts in the eyes.

Hypoglycemia (low blood sugar) can occur while the cat is being treated with insulin. Cats show low blood sugar by appearing mentally dull and lethargic, which easily may go undetected. They do not tend to have the seizures seen in dogs or humans. If untreated, the cat may go into coma and die. Reduce the amount of insulin and treat as below. If symptoms are mild, feed the cat its normal food.

An overdose of insulin may cause the sudden return of diabetes mellitus symptoms, and the cat may immediately go into convulsions. First aid consists of force-feeding honey (the best choice, as it is absorbed through the gums), Karo syrup or concentrated sugar water. Give two or three teaspoons per 10 pounds body weight unless directed otherwise by your veterinarian. Be careful to only give a few drops at a time, and be sure the cat swallows the liquid. Do not stick your fingers in the cat's mouth as you may be bitten accidentally. If the cat goes into complete collapse, massage honey or Karo syrup onto the gums. Contact your veterinarian immediately—this is a true EMERGENCY!

Any illness, especially one causing a lack of appetite or vomiting, may change the cat's insulin needs. Consult your veterinarian immediately. If the cat drinks more water than normal, the insulin dosage may need adjustment.

If the cat jumps when you give an injection or if you accidentally push the needle through the skin, some insulin may be lost. You won't know exactly how much was given. If you are unsure the cat received the full dose, do not repeat the injection or try to give a bit extra to make up for it. It is more hazardous to the cat to give too much insulin than not enough.

When cats with Type II (adult onset) diabetes are put on a high-fiber diet and the caloric intake is reduced, the high blood sugar level can sometimes be controlled. These cats are very sensitive to insulin, and need to be tested to determine if they need injections. Diet and weight control may be tried before starting insulin treatment. Or, after the cat's weight has stabilized, it may no longer need insulin. It is important when putting the cat on a reducing diet that the food is not so unpalatable that the energy and protein intake is suddenly changed. This may push a marginal case into full-blown diabetes.

Regulating diabetes is not easy in the cat. Several factors contribute to difficulty in blood sugar stabilization. Cats show great variability in how long insulin is effective and how many hours it takes for peak activity to occur in the body. Also, cats are small and the amount of insulin needed is very small. It is usually necessary to dilute the insulin, and it may be difficult to give an accurate dose. New low dose (30- and 50-unit) syringes are helpful.

The well-developed fight-or-flight response gives the cat a sharp, rapid rise in blood glucose when it is stressed. Cats that live in conflict with dogs or other cats may be difficult to regulate. Problems may occur with stress factors such as boarding, where smell, sight, and sound of other animals may make the cat stop eating. A cat that is physically active at home will be less active when boarded, greatly changing its insulin needs. You may notice a change in insulin needs when you go on vacation, if you have house guests, or when the cat is not eating normally.

The diabetic cat will need a cat food with an increased amount of fiber and a constant amount of fat, protein, and carbohydrates. This will allow a consistent dosage of insulin. Some commercial cat foods, especially the least expensive, are made with so-called "open" formulas. This means that the final analysis remains the same, but different ingredients may be used in each batch. Total caloric density may vary, making insulin dosage difficult.

Your cat should be stabilized on a high-quality food. This will insure that the ingredients are uniform in quality and quantity, making insulin dosage easier. The diet should contain about 10% fiber, which helps to even out the blood sugar level. If the cat is overweight and does not have other disease problems, it may be given a specialized diet such as Prescription Diet® Feline w/d®. If the cat has other medical problems, it may be put on another quality diet. Avoid commercial soft-moist foods, as they are high in simple sugars which may raise the cat's blood sugar.

The ideal feeding schedule for the diabetic cat is two to four measured meals per day, fed at the same times each day. It may be difficult to change a cat that is used to eating from its dish all day to meals only at certain times. Problems may occur with a cat that will only eat one or two foods. If the food needs to be changed, do so gradually, giving three-fourths of the old food and one-quarter of the new food, mixed together. After a few days, go to half and half, and then one-quarter and three-quarters. If you can't accomplish total change to the food your veterinarian recommends, even a partial switch may make a big difference. Careful dietary management and regularly spaced meals may allow the cat's insulin dosage to be reduced or even eliminated. Mixing a small amount of canned food with the cat's dry food several times a day may encourage it to eat.

Cats may spontaneously lose their need for insulin, even after being on it for several years. The cat may suddenly appear slow or dopey, and a veterinary checkup may show that the cat can do without insulin. Your veterinarian will gradually reduce the dosage until it is no longer given. The cat may be able to go without it permanently, or may need it again later. This "recovery" from diabetes is not seen in other animals. Diabetic cats that are obese may no longer need insulin when they reach normal weight. Also, some cats that are diagnosed with diabetes mellitus do not need insulin. They may have symptoms but be clinically stable for one or two years without treatment.

Kidney failure, thyroid problems, and liver disease may change the cat's need for insulin, raising or lowering it. Some cats may become immune to beef, pork, or human proteins found in insulin. If this occurs, the cat can be switched to a different type of insulin (Norsworthy, 1993). Treatment with corticosteroids also may change the cat's insulin needs.

Cats that have diabetes are more likely to have other health problems. They may have more infections, especially in the urinary tract and bladder. Injuries can be slow to heal. Intestinal problems, heart and kidney disease, nervous system problems and pancreatitis may be seen. Do NOT breed a female cat that has diabetes, as it may be impossible to control the disease during her pregnancy and you may lose her. A few cases of diabetes are first detected when the animal becomes pregnant. Hills Prescription Diet® has a very good free booklet on care of the diabetic pet. Ask your veterinarian for a copy.

THYROID PROBLEMS

Hyperthyroidism occurs with excessive secretion of thyroid hormones, resulting in an extremely high metabolic rate. Common in older cats, it should be considered in cats more than six years of age that are losing weight. In the early stages of the disease, most cats eat ravenously. Meanwhile, because the cat is not digesting the food well or not absorbing the nutrients from it, it becomes thin. The cat may be so restless and hyperactive that it doesn't sit or stand still. It may pace or howl in an unusual voice, and may appear agitated. The cat may have a personality change, becoming aggressive. There may be a fever. The cat may defecate or urinate in places other than the litter box. About half of hyperthyroid cats vomit frequently. About a third have large quantities of feces or diarrhea, which may be foamy-looking, grayish, or greasy. The cat may be unusually thirsty and have increased urine output. Less common is a ragged and unkempt hair coat, with patchy hair loss. The heartbeat may be fast and irregular. Later in the disease, the cat may have a poor appetite along with weight loss. This disease is usually diagnosed by blood and urine lab tests. Because the amount of

thyroid hormone in the bloodstream fluctuates, several tests may be needed to prove hyperthyroidism is the problem.

Treatment may include drugs that block the production of thyroid hormone to lower the amount circulating in the blood. Methimazole is one drug; side effects include vomiting, lethargy, liver dysfunction, and poor appetite. Possible serious side effects involve changes in blood cells. Still, this drug has fewer side effects than propylthiouracil, the other drug commonly used to treat hyperthyroidism. These treatments do not "cure" the disease but only control it. Symptoms will recur if the cat goes one to three days without medication. Most cats need treatment for the rest of their lives.

Other treatments include surgical removal of the thyroid gland and/or treatment with radioactive iodine to remove some of the glandular tissue, thus stopping overproduction of hormone. Radioactive iodine treatment, in particular, is highly effective and avoids the hazards of surgery. After surgery or irradiation, it is sometimes necessary to supplement the cat with replacement thyroid hormones. Because hyperthyroidism can recur, the cat should have its blood thyroid hormone level checked once or twice a year. After the cat is started on treatment, it is important to work with your veterinarian on follow-up tests and thyroid hormone measurements to make sure the cat is getting the proper dosage of medication and that the drug is working.

Hyperthyroidism cannot be cured by diet alone; you must consider the cat's tremendous energy and protein needs. Feed the cat all it can eat of a good quality, highly digestible cat food. After treatment, the cat may be much less active (and more mellow). Decrease the amount of food as needed.

Hypothyroidism, on the other hand, occurs when there is too little thyroid hormone in the cat's blood. It is rare in cats. If thyroid hormones are given to test whether it is the problem, the cat may show hair growth even though hypothyroidism may not be the problem. This is because its generally stimulates the body.

OTHER ENDOCRINE DISORDERS

Cushing's disease (hyperadrenocorticism) is due to overproduction of hormones from the cortex of the adrenal glands. It is rare in the cat, but when seen is most common in middle-aged or older females. The primary sign is hair loss on the cat's trunk, usually symmetrical from one side to the other. The skin is very thin and lacks elasticity. The cat may look pot-bellied and drink and urinate more than usual. She can have a ravenous appetite even though she is losing weight. Giving excess amounts of corticosteroid drugs (as for skin allergies) can cause the disease, especially if they are stopped suddenly or the cat is stressed. Many of these cats also are diabetic.

The opposite, hypoadrenocorticism is occasionally seen. Signs of insufficiency include poor appetite, weight loss, lethargy, dehydration, and weakness. Treatment may include fluids to stabilize the cat's blood volume and relieve dehydration. The cat will need hormone replacement therapy for the rest of its life. The prospect for a long and healthy life is good with continued treatment.

Chapter 20

TUMORS

Like humans, more cats are living long enough to develop tumors. The types of tumors seen in cats are similar to those in humans, dogs, and other animals. Because of this, they are of great interest to veterinarians. If a cure can be found for a particular type of tumor in cats or dogs, the same treatment may work for other animals as well as for humans. Similarly, treatments that work for humans are often scaled down for use on animals. While sure cures are not yet available for either humans or animals, many treatments can give additional years of comfortable life for pets.

When an elderly pet is affected, the increased fragility and lessened ability to deal with the powerful medications used to treat tumors must be balanced against the possibility of improvement. Other disease conditions such as kidney disease and heart failure must be considered. Consider the cat's future quality of life before you engage in expensive and long-term treatment. Making the animal more comfortable for its remaining time is a legitimate reason for treatment. When treated, signs previously attributed to "old age" may be strikingly reversed. Age, by itself, is not a reason to withhold treatment. Animals with cancer that has spread throughout the body are rarely cured. Cancer afflicts about 470 out of every 100,000 cats (Fox, 1993).

Tumors in cats, unfortunately, are more often malignant than benign. As many as 70-80% of them may be malignant. In contrast, less than one-third of canine tumors are malignant. For this reason, if you suspect your cat has a tumor, it is very important to obtain early diagnosis and treatment. Even a tiny "wart" should be checked. If it is malignant, it can be treated. If not, you will be relieved to know it is not serious. A "wait and see" approach is almost never appropriate in cats.

Common signs of cancer in animals, listed by the Veterinary Cancer Society, include: abnormal swellings that persist or continue to grow, sores that do not heal, loss of appetite, weight loss, bleeding or drainage from any body opening, offensive odor, difficulty eating or swallowing, hesitation to exercise or loss of stamina, persistent lameness or stiffness, and difficulty breathing, urinating or defecating (Kitchell, 1993).

You, the owner, are the first line of defense in watching (and feeling) for tumors on your pet. Keep an eye on any skin lumps, bumps, or swellings. They should be watched for change. Have them checked immediately if they become larger, bleed, or seem to annoy the cat.

Certain breeds and colors of cats may be more susceptible to cancer than others. Siamese and cats that are part Siamese may be more prone to tumors of the mammary glands, while they have fewer squamous cell carcinomas because their dark points protect against damage from the sun. Siamese cats also have more mast-cell tumors than do other breeds.

Cats that have white skin on their ears are susceptible to squamous cell carcinomas, much as are humans who are out in sunlight too much (see Ear Chapter). These lesions begin with a reddening, roughening, and thickening of the skin, and bleeding. The edges of the ears may become ragged and notched. Squamous cell carcinomas also are seen on the nose, eyelids, lips, and bridge of the nose when these areas are white. Surgical removal is the treatment of choice. It may be necessary to remove the entire ear or the end of the nose. While the treatment may not be pretty, it is usually quite successful if done early. Radiation may be used in some cases. Cryotherapy (freezing) is useful for tumors on the eyelid, where surgery might leave the lid unable to close. Keeping the cat out of the sun will help prevent these tumors. If you have an outdoor cat with white ears, allow it out only at night.

Basal cell tumors are the most common skin tumors found in the cat, especially in older animals. They are usually small, well-rounded, firm nodules which sharply raise the overlying skin. They are rarely malignant. Melanomas are extremely rare in cats.

Fibrosarcomas are a virus-caused skin tumor which often occur in cats infected with the feline leukemia virus. These may occur in cats as young as three or four months of age up to about seven years of age. They appear as a single mass or as small lumpy swellings along the legs, back and neck. They may feel rubbery and firm. Have the cat checked by your veterinarian.

When fibrosarcomas are seen in the flank area or on the ear and removed before they become too large, they usually do not recur and the cat probably will die from other causes. The same tumor on the legs, neck, or back usually recurs, with death in a few months. If the cat has only one fibrosarcoma, and it does not recur when removed, the cat probably will do well. If the area does not heal, a draining, open sore may remain. A few weeks later, more tumors may occur in the skin and muscles near where the original one was removed. Late in the course of the disease, the tumor may spread to the internal organs. If it recurs after removal or if there are multiple masses, the cat probably will not live more than a few months. Feline sarcomas can be prevented by preventing exposure to feline leukemia virus. The sarcomas, while caused by a virus, are not contagious from one cat to another. The virus is not contagious to humans.

In recent years, a number of tumors have been seen in skin areas at sites that are commonly used for injections of vaccine such as between the shoulder blades or on the upper shoulder and lower neck areas. Most of these are fibrosarcomas, although other types of tumors are seen. They are single slow-growing tumors thought to be due to inflammatory reactions to feline leukemia vaccine and/or killed rabies vaccine. The incidence is small, but may be one or two cats per 10,000 vaccinations. Tumors have been found following both intramuscular and subcutaneous injections. Fewer reactions seem to occur when these vaccinations are given in sites other than the lower neck or between the shoulder blades. Injections should be given further back along the ribs, as low as possible in the right hind leg, in the flank or intramuscularly, as directed. No one particular brand of vaccine is a problem. Usually, fibrosarcomas due to vaccine reactions do not recur after surgical removal.

Skin tumors are among the most easily seen, and on cats, they are frequently malignant. The good news is that they do not easily spread to other areas of the body. Tumors should be considered with many skin lumps, especially those that do not have any drainage. They may appear as small "warts" on the skin or larger lumps or swellings. Others may look like abscesses or draining wounds. Having the lesion removed is usually the safest course of treatment.

Your veterinarian usually will remove a large area around a skin tumor. This is to make sure all of it is removed (or as much as possible). Veterinarians call this "cut wide, cut deep." The first surgery for any cancer has the best chance of success. Tumors may be removed by heat (cautery), lasers, or standard surgical techniques. Freezing (cryosurgery) is sometimes used, but has a high rate of recurrence. With some tumors, lymph nodes in the area also will be removed to catch any cancer cells that have established themselves there, especially if the node is swollen or shows other signs of involvement. Ointment containing 5-fluorouracil (5-FU) should not be used in cats because it causes a fatal neurotoxicity (Ogilvie, 1995).

It is worth the cost to have the tissue examined by a pathology lab to learn exactly what it is and whether all of it has been removed. Knowing what type of tumor is present also will alert your veterinarian to watch for spread to other areas, such as the lungs.

Lymphoma is a tumor of the lymph nodes and lymphatic system. It is usually associated with feline leukemia virus infection. Occasionally, it may occur as a tumor of a single lymph node or several nodes. The most obvious lymph nodes on a cat are on the back of the hind leg opposite the stifle joint. You can feel them quite easily as small lumps lying under the skin. It is a good idea to check them every few months. If they become enlarged, have the cat checked. Lymphoma also can involve the skin, where it may show up as one or more lumps or masses. There may be pimples, plaques, or crusty or ulcerated areas, and hair may fall out.

Lymphoma also may occur within the abdomen if the lymph nodes there are affected. This form is most common in Siamese kittens and may be seen in cats as young as four months of age. Lymphoma within the chest cavity is also common. The liver may be involved in older cats, usually around eight years of age. This tumor can also occur in the cat's spleen, usually secondary to tumors elsewhere in the body. Abdominal lymphoma is difficult to treat because the lymph nodes are often quite large before the disease becomes apparent. Some cats respond well to chemotherapy.

Tumors of the bone are quite rare in cats. Any hard swelling which seems to be attached to a bone should be checked by your veterinarian.

Polyps may occur in the nose. They may be seen in young cats, and may occur a few weeks or months after the cat has had an upper respiratory tract infection. The cat may have trouble breathing. It may sneeze, snort, or breathe through its mouth, gag, and have a nasal discharge. Polyps may sometimes extend from the ear canal into the middle ear, then through the eardrum into the inner ear. Any growths in the ear should be biopsied. Surgery is often necessary to remove the polyps. These tumors are usually malignant, and the prognosis is poor. Fortunately, nasal tumors are rare.

Mammary tumors are the third most common tumor in cats, behind skin cancers and lymphoma. One major study found that 96% of them were malignant (Holzworth, 1987). They grow rapidly and may spread widely throughout the body from the starting point in the mammary glands (Jeglum, 1994). Mammary tumors can occur at any age, but are most common around 10 to 12 years of age. Spayed cats, especially those spayed before their first heat period, may have fewer mammary tumors than intact females. A higher number of mammary tumors may be seen in tri-color females and cats of Siamese origin. Because of the cat's thick fur, tumors may be far advanced before they are noticed. Any swelling or growth in the cat's breasts should be checked by your veterinarian. Treatment with megestrol acetate may cause mammary tumors in some cats.

Cats older than four to five years should have the breasts palpated at least once a month. This is especially important in long-haired cats where the tumors are not obvious. Feel for lumps or swellings, hardened areas or areas of unusual softness or sponginess. Lumpy, puckered, abnormally shaped glands are easily seen in shorthaired cats. A breast exam should be part of your routine care for the female cat.

Mammary tumors appear as firm flat thickenings or lumps in one or more of the glands. Others may be fluid-filled and soft. If not noticed early, the surface may become ulcerated. A red or gray sore or abscess draining pus or bloody material may be seen. It may be wet, matted, and foul-smelling. A single draining mammary tumor should not be mistaken for an abscess. Sometimes the nipple over a tumor-filled gland may ooze a bloody fluid or tan or yellowish pus if squeezed.

Non-lactating cats with swollen mammary glands should be examined by a veterinarian to distinguish between a tumor and a condition called fibroepithelial hyperplasia or feline mammary hypertrophy. These are fancy words for a massive overgrowth which is unique to cats. It can be seen in cats of both sexes after treatment with certain hormones, especially progestogens. It comes on suddenly, and the skin is discolored and may be ulcerated. A nursing cat also may have mastitis. Supportive care is given until the swelling goes down, at which time spaying (or castration) will give a permanent cure (Chisholm, 1993).

The prognosis for a cat with one or more mammary tumors is poor. This is due to the high degree of malignancy and because the tumors have been growing for some time before being discovered. The tumor may have spread to lymph nodes in the area, then to elsewhere in the body, especially the lungs, liver, and kidneys. Because these tumors are prone to spread to the lungs, a radiograph of the chest should be taken before treatment.

Surgical removal of all affected glands is the treatment of choice for mammary tumors. Prompt, aggressive treatment may give the cat several more years of quality life. Additional treatments such as radiation therapy, chemotherapy, and immunotherapy are sometimes used. Cats with mammary cancer often have tumors in the uterus or ovaries. If the cat is not spayed and can tolerate the surgery, she should be spayed as soon as possible. Spaying may help reduce hormonal factors leading to the development of further tumors.

Aftercare is also important. Feel the cat's entire belly at least twice a month, watching for the development of any new lumps. Ask your veterinarian to show you the lymph nodes in the area and check them for enlargement, lumps, or change in texture. At the first sign of any change, return the cat for examination. Incidentally, tumors of the prostate gland are very rare in cats.

Treatment of any cancer must begin with a diagnosis. This starts with a complete physical examination to evaluate the cat's overall health. It is especially important in the older cat, because one or more organs or systems may not be functioning normally. Then, your veterinarian will begin to determine what type of tumor is involved. Biopsy samples may be taken with a needle and sent to a laboratory. If the tumor is small, the veterinarian may remove the entire lesion for examination. With a larger tumor, the veterinarian may cut out a small piece, which is then sent to a laboratory. Knowing what kind of cells are involved helps predict the possibility of a cure and will help determine the appropriate treatment.

In general, local disease requires local treatment and systemic disease requires systemic treatment. Localized therapy includes surgery, cautery, cryotherapy (freezing), and, occasionally, radiation therapy. Systemic therapy includes hormonal therapy, chemotherapy, or immunotherapy. These are used with cancers that have spread throughout the body or with localized cancers which cannot be removed because of their size or location.

More cancer patients are cured by surgery than by any other method of treatment. Skin tumors are the most common kind of tumors seen in veterinary medicine. They are easily removed, which is a great advantage. Also, when the tumor begins, the cells remain localized for a period of time before they spread throughout the body. Thus, there is a good chance of completely removing the tumor if surgery is done early. Sometimes, lymph nodes in the area are removed, especially if they are enlarged, firm, or abnormally attached to the surrounding tissues.

Chemotherapy can be used for many types of tumors. It is important to understand that the goal of chemotherapy is to control the growth of the tumor; it rarely leads to a complete cure. Also, limitations in nursing care and facilities, along with financial constraints, will never allow veterinary medicine to have the same high remission rates or duration of remission seen in human medicine.

All chemotherapy drugs are potent poisons. The chance taken is that they will kill the tumor cells, which are susceptible because of their rapid growth, before they kill the cat. Bone marrow suppression is commonly seen. It is usually monitored as an indicator of the drug's toxicity to the animal's body. If the cat does not tolerate the anticancer drug, it may be necessary to go to a lower dosage or a less toxic agent. Cats on chemotherapy rarely suffer serious hair loss. Many lose their whiskers, and a few will lose some of the outer hairs, leaving the soft undercoat. These changes are reversible when treatment is stopped. Antibiotics may be given if the animal develops a fever.

Weight loss is common in cats that are infected with feline leukemia virus, and may occur with advanced tumors of other types. It may occur simply because the cat is not feeling well enough to eat. When the tumor involves the mouth, it may be too painful for the cat to eat. A tumor which involves the nasal passages can affect the cat's sense of smell so that it is not attracted to food. Chemotherapy or radiation can cause nausea, dry mouth, and inflammation of the mucous membranes in the mouth and digestive tract. As much as possible, it is important to keep the cat eating on its own. Appetite stimulants such as megestrol acetate (2.5 mg every day or two) may help the cat feel like eating and gain weight. It may help to give the cat canned food, which is usually tastier. Feeding a diet that the cat will eat is important, so use the food that your cat finds most tasty, no matter what its composition. Try a food with high fat and low fiber, such as a kitten or growth food. Do not feed the cat within four hours of radiation or chemotherapy, as it may develop an aversion to the food because of the nausea the treatment can cause.

Supportive care after cancer therapy is also important. Drugs, especially corticosteroids, may be given to manage the pain and make the cat more comfortable. These drugs also may have an anti-cancer effect on specific conditions, especially leukemia, lymphosarcoma, myeloma, and mast cell disease (Kitchell, 1993). They also stimulate the appetite and make the cat generally feel better. These benefits must be balanced against the possibility that the cat may not respond as well to future courses of chemotherapy after corticosteroid treatment.

Chapter 21

THE ELDERLY CAT

THE "OLD" CAT

Aging is a natural, normal part of the life process. Like humans, each cat ages differently. However, it is safe to consider the cat that is eight to 10 years of age or older to be "old." This is perhaps comparable to a 55- to 60-year-old human. One study estimated that about 13% of the cat population is 10 years of age or older. Some veterinarians consider any cat six years of age or older to be geriatric because subtle changes in function are beginning.

The average life span of a cat is about 12 to 14 years. Feral felines, exposed to hazards of the city or wilds, do well to survive three years. Barn cats and outdoor city cats rarely live beyond 10 years. Lucky cats, blessed with good health and good care (and usually living indoors) may live 15 to 20 years, and a few individuals live into their early or mid-20s. The oldest cat on record lived to be 36, according to the *Guinness Book of World Records*. Keeping the cat indoors will go a long way toward extending its life by keeping it away from cars, dogs, occasional human malice, disease, and parasites.

Some people say that one year of a cat's life is equivalent to seven years of a human's life. This isn't quite correct. The cat goes from infancy to adulthood in less than a year. Then, it doesn't change much for the next seven to nine years. When the cat finally "begins to show its age," the decline may appear to be quite rapid. Many purebred cats do not live as long as cats of less royal heritage, perhaps because of inbreeding. A cat that has been spayed or neutered early in life (especially before sexual maturity) may live five to seven years longer than a cat that remains intact.

Aging occurs in the last half of the cat's life span when it has a reduced ability to meet the demands of its environment. The cat gradually loses reserve in bodily organs. Age is not a disease condition; it is wear and tear on the body. How and when a cat ages is influenced by a number of factors, including its genetic background, the presence of internal disorders such as cancer and metabolic disease, and factors such as parasitism and trauma. The aging process is similar from one species to another, whether it's cats, cows, or humans. As many as 90% of geriatric cats may have detectable health problems.

As with humans, old age does not occur all at once. It may begin with a gradual slowing of activity. If you do not compensate by cutting the cat's food intake, it may become obese. Hairs may turn gray around the muzzle, face and ears, especially on black cats. This may begin as early as six years of age. The cat's attention span and mental facilities may become less acute.

Your cat may have run freely in its younger years, but certainly should not be allowed to do so in old age. Hearing and vision may be poor. The loss comes gradually, and causes little problem for a cat that lives indoors. In most cases the cat adapts before a human notices a problem. These losses may be fatal to an outdoor cat, as it may not notice an oncoming vehicle or dog that is chasing it. Even if it does see or hear it, the cat may be unable to hustle out of the way. If the cat is hit or attacked, age makes it less able to recover from the injury. An old cat may become confused, and if it wanders away it may be unable to find its way safely home. Also, the cat is prone to attack by other cats defending their territory (which may include YOUR yard!). An old, arthritic, nearly blind, and maybe toothless cat is defenseless. Take care of your cat and protect it.

The older cat's household environment also should be made safe. An older cat that has less awareness of the world around it should not have access to stairs. Block stairways with an accordion-style "kiddie gate". Any room where the cat might bump into objects which might fall on it should have the doors closed or the entry restricted.

Older cats are less tolerant of temperature changes. A heating pad (the kennel kind, not the drugstore kind) may make the indoor cat more comfortable, especially if it has arthritis. Purchase one with a thermostat so the heat can be controlled. At the very least, the cat should have a draft-free place. This will ease aching joints and muscles. If your cat has arthritis, you may choose old blankets, carpet, or rags which can be thrown away when they become soiled. If your cat has to climb stairs to reach its bed, make a second bed downstairs for naps.

Extremes of heat and cold are very hard on the older cat. Allowing the cat outdoors in the middle of a hot day may cause severe stress and could even be fatal. During the hottest part of the day, keep the cat indoors or in a cool, shady spot in your yard. Make sure plenty of fresh, clean water is available.

Stress and anxiety may cause your cat to age more rapidly or become ill. You can't keep everything from bothering your cat, but you can put it in a quiet room when you have a party or when children are visiting. If the cat wants to celebrate the holidays from under your bed or in the closet, allow it to do so. Don't drag your cat out and force it to face noise and strangers. Leave the poor old fellow alone! If you can't avoid change, try to make it as easy as possible.

The cat that is dribbling urine or that has reduced control of the bowels should be confined to a room which can be cleaned easily and sanitized, both for your peace of mind and to protect carpets in the rest of the house. Put down newspapers or washable rugs in places the cat is likely to soil. Place litter boxes in various parts of the house, especially if it is large or has several floors, so the cat does not have to go far to reach one. If the cat does have an accident, be understanding. Don't scold the cat for forgetting its housebreaking or for being unable to wait any longer. Your cat is at least as distressed about the accident as you are, and probably more so. The cat needs your understanding and care more now than at any other time of its life.

Older cats are at greater risk for arthritis and skeletal problems. They may have rear leg weakness because of loss of muscle tissue which does not regenerate. Arthritis pain is first seen as stiffness and lameness when the cat first moves around after sleeping. It will usually feel and move better after it has been moving for a while. There is no real cure for arthritis. Make sure the cat has a warm, comfortable place to sleep, and make sure the cat maintains its normal weight.

The cat may have a fading memory because of a poor supply of blood and oxygen to its brain. This is one reason the older cat may urinate or defecate in inappropriate places. It can't remember where it is supposed to go when it feels the urge. The cat also may forget where it is or where it was going. An outdoor cat may wander away from home and forget where it lives. It may forget to watch when it crosses the street. For these reasons, it is best for the elderly cat to live indoors.

An older cat may occasionally let out a loud howling meow. This may even happen in the middle of the night. Sometimes these are due to bladder or kidney infections, and in a male, it may mean the urethra is plugged. Make sure the cat is urinating and that the urine is normal. Some cats will howl if they are hypothyroid (have a low level of thyroid hormone). Other reasons may be aging processes within the brain or loss of hearing or vision. The cat may be disoriented or feel threatened, and cry out in distress. It may feel lost and alone and be crying out for physical contact. The cat may be reassured by having a warm bed in your bedroom. If there are no other signs of illness, don't worry about the crying. If it is accompanied by uncharacteristic behavior such as walking in circles or staggering, have the cat examined by your veterinarian.

The older cat may become grouchy or irritable. In many cases this is because it hurts. The cat may have a sore tooth, a muscle strain, or arthritis. This behavior may be associated with hypoglycemia, dehydration, anemia, lack of exercise or tumors. It may be seen with autointoxication because of inefficient elimination of waste products within the body, as with kidney or liver disease. It may be because of relative hypoxia, where the cells are simply not getting as much oxygen as they need. First look for a medical cause for the disposition change. In other cases, it may simply be because the animal is old and doesn't feel well. Your careful observation as to where and when the cat is grumpy may be crucial to help your veterinarian find the cat's problem. You are with the cat much more than the veterinarian. Your observations are valuable to the diagnosis!

An old cat that suddenly becomes hyperactive and runs around like a kitten may be hyperthyroid. Once diagnosed, it is easily controlled by medication.

Tom cats remain fertile as they age. Females continue to come into heat and may become pregnant if allowed to be with a tom. Pregnancy may be hazardous to an older queen's health, and she may have difficulty giving birth. Spaying at an advanced age also can be hazardous. If you have not had her spayed earlier in life, confine her when she is in heat to make sure she does not become pregnant. Older queens have smaller litters and tend to have more kittens with congenital defects.

Older cats may have color changes inside their eyes. The iris (colored part) may become lighter or develop dark spots. These changes come with the aging process and do not need treatment. Ask your veterinarian about them the next time you take the cat to the clinic. Cataracts are occasionally seen in older cats.

PHYSICAL EXAMINATION

A thorough annual physical examination is a good idea for the older cat. If it has continuing health problems, checkups should occur twice a year. The cat should have an annual fecal examination for internal parasites and be treated to remove worms if any are present.

Laboratory tests should be performed if needed. A CBC (Complete Blood Count) will tell the veterinarian that your cat's body is free of infections, is not anemic, and the blood cells are normal. A blood profile may be run to check liver and kidney function. These tests may include a BUN (Blood Urea Nitrogen test), which shows whether the cat's kidneys are functioning normally. A check for kidney function should be a standard part of a veterinary examination at least once a year for all older cats. As many as 80% of older cats have some degree of kidney dysfunction.

Liver tests may include alkaline phosphatase, SGPT, and bilirubin. A serum calcium test will help determine the health of the cat's bones. A blood sugar test will make sure the cat is not diabetic. Total protein will help find liver, kidney, or intestinal disease. These tests are important for early detection of ailments which may become life threatening if left untreated. This routine care can add to the quantity and quality of your cat's remaining years.

In some cases, your veterinarian may perform a panel of blood tests. There may be specific interest in only a few of the included tests, but it is often less expensive than doing them separately. Also, having test results on file will give baseline values for your cat so that changes can be noted as the cat ages. In some cases, the veterinarian may want to put your cat in a special cage in order to collect its urine for 24 hours to check protein and creatinine levels. The results from these two tests may detect early kidney disease even when the BUN is normal. It may be advisable to run a thyroid hormone test. A chest X-ray also may be a good idea, especially if your cat has been coughing or shows other signs of lung problems.

An electrocardiogram is an easy way to check for certain heart problems. If heart disease is detected early, the cat often can be treated before permanent damage occurs. Heart and kidney disease are perhaps the most common problems found on geriatric tests, and their treatment is among the most gratifying in terms of a healthy, long life for your pet.

Cats are not tolerant of pain in the mouth and may refuse to eat or drink if their gums or teeth hurt. Tartar deposits can accumulate any time from about five years of age onward. Gum disease is found in perhaps 60% of cats that are six years or older. Cats often lose their incisors (the tiny front teeth) as they age. This is relatively normal as long as the gums are not infected. Feeding dry food as long as the cat eats it readily will help keep the teeth clean. Tooth brushing, if you are willing to do it and have trained your cat to allow it, can significantly reduce gum problems and infection.

Many older cats need teeth cleaning two or three times per year. A period of treatment with antibiotics may be necessary before (and after) the cleaning if the cat has severe gum disease or infected tooth roots. Teeth cleaning should be done with anesthesia in all but the very oldest or sickest cats. It is difficult to get down under the gums and do an adequate job of cleaning without anesthetizing the cat. In human dentistry, this job is called "deep cleaning;" if you have ever had it done, you know it can sometimes hurt. Most veterinarians use an inhalant (gas) anesthetic to make sure the cat awakens as quickly and as smoothly as possible. If necessary, intravenous fluids may be given during the cleaning procedure to help the cat awaken more smoothly.

The cat's immunizations can be brought up to date at the same visit. Some people assume that when the cat becomes older, it acquires some sort of permanent immunity. This old wives' tale may be fatal to your cat. A disease such as feline distemper can easily cause the death of a cat whose defenses are weakened by age. Keep the annual vaccinations current! A cat that is kept STRICTLY indoors and has NO contact with other animals may do without rabies vaccinations. A cat that is upset by the trip to the clinic may be best served by a veterinarian who makes house calls.

GROOMING

The cat's coat may thin as it ages, and the skin may become dry and scaly. Daily brushing will help remove hair that the cat is unable to groom from its coat. Using a metal brush will help remove static electricity that contributes to fur mats. Grooming is very important in older cats to keep them from swallowing fur and forming hair balls. Feel all over the cat's skin two or three times a month to find lumps that are not visible. Growths on the skin should be checked soon, as most feline skin tumors are malignant. External parasites should be promptly treated. The cat may have a poor hair coat due to loss of sex hormones or vitamin and mineral deficiencies.

Older cats should need fewer baths than younger cats because they are less prone to getting into dirt. Avoid bathing the older cat, if possible, because it may lead to respiratory infections if the cat becomes chilled. If you need to bathe your cat, be sure to dry it carefully. Keep the cat warmer than normal for several hours after the bath. Nails which become too long may cause twisted toes, difficulty in walking, and joint problems in the elderly cat. If you are unable to trim its nails, have it done by your veterinarian or groomer.

Examine the cat's ears once a month if it does not have a history of ear problems. Check them every week or two if the cat has had (or has) ear mites or ear infections. Wrap a tissue around your finger and gently clean the outer parts of the ear.

SPECIAL DIET AND MEDICATIONS

The elderly cat needs basically the same nutrients as its younger counterpart, but in lesser quantities. It will need between 10% and 30% fewer calories than a younger, more active cat. The cat's metabolism is slower than it was in its younger years. If the cat is overweight, reduce the caloric intake by feeding less of a regular cat food or by feeding one of the "diet" cat foods.

The food should be of a high quality so it is easily digested. It should be palatable to tempt the cat's diminished senses of smell and taste. You may wish to give small treats from time to time to stimulate the cat's appetite if it is eating poorly. Try lean, cooked meat or fish, cooked eggs, or a tiny bit of yogurt. A few cats will eat vegetables or even fruit. Don't give too much of these goodies. They should never make up more than 20% of the diet. If the cat refuses to eat good, balanced cat food, stop feeding the "people food." Heating the food also can encourage the cat to eat it (Barrette, 1990). The cat should be fed fresh food at least twice a day.

Diets are available which are tailored specifically to the needs of the older cat, such as Waltham™ Formula Senior Diet (Waltham, (800)528-1838). Cats with kidney or heart problems may need veterinary prescription diets.

Constipation may be a problem in the older cat because of a decreased blood supply to the colon. Keep an eye on the cat's feces to make sure it is having normal bowel movements and that the material is not too hard for the cat to pass. Give a small amount of cat laxative daily when necessary, to maintain regularity. Be sure the cat always has fresh, clean water available. This will help lessen constipation problems and keep the kidneys healthy.

The elderly cat will need more fiber to compensate for lack of activity. It helps the food material move through the intestinal tract and avoids constipation. If megacolon (a large, expanded, inefficient colon) occurs or if your cat is chronically constipated, it may help to add a psyllium-seed product (such as Metamucil®) to the diet. Constipation occurs in the older cat because there is a less-active cat wrapped around a less-active digestive tract. If either constipation or diarrhea lasts longer than 48 hours, the cat should be examined by a veterinarian.

The kidney is one of the first organs to have reduced function with aging. Lower levels of phosphorus in the feed help prevent kidney disease. In the majority of cats, you cannot go wrong by treating the older cat as an animal with chronic kidney failure, even if you have not yet seen any signs (see Urinary Tract Chapter). A reduced sodium level in the cat food helps prevent congestive heart disease and high blood pressure, much as it does in humans. The cat will need extra water-soluble B-vitamins.

An older cat may suffer from potassium deficiency. It also may be seen with diabetes, diarrhea, vomiting, kidney failure, and some medications. Symptoms of potassium deficiency include a limp, lax neck, with the head turned downward. The cat may stagger in the hind end. Potassium supplementation works wonders for many of these cats (see also Feline Gourmet Chapter).

Choline supplements may help some elderly cats that have signs of senility. These cats may seem absent minded, and forget where they are or where they were going. This nutrient is supplied by giving a lecithin supplement such as Cholodin® (MVP Laboratories, Ralston, NE 68127). Some animals treated with this product seem to be more mentally alert and aware, and have a better appetite and seem to feel better.

Anabolic steroids such as stanozolol may be given to some older cats that are suffering poor appetite, nerve disorders or metabolic disease. These are the same drugs that are bad for young human athletes. In the elderly animal, however, anabolic steroids can increase muscle mass, improve well-being and appetite, increase the amount of muscle compared to the amount of body fat, improve nervous system function, and reverse some degenerative diseases by reducing the workload on the kidneys. These drugs should be given, if at all, after a complete physical examination, dental care if needed, and treatment of any disease problems. They can help as many as 80% of older cats, and very few side effects are seen. With a debilitated older cat, they are certainly worth a try. These drugs should not be used on a pregnant cat, as they may have a masculinizing effect on the kittens.

WATER

Water should be available at all times, indoors and out. This is especially important for the older cat because kidney problems are so common and it can be very difficult for them to be without water. When you travel with the cat, be sure to take water along and offer it in small quantities, frequently, especially when the weather is hot. Abrupt changes in the water quality may cause digestive upsets—take some water from home and gradually change to new water as you travel. Warm water should be provided in winter if the cat lives outdoors, and the water should be available at all times. If you have no way to keep it continuously unfrozen, offer warm water to the cat three or four (or more) times a day.

OBESITY

Because the cat is less active, and its metabolism has slowed, it probably will become obese if fed the same amount of the same food as earlier in its life. Obesity can be a serious problem in the elderly cat. Fat puts an extra burden on the heart, lungs, and other organs. In some cases, extra fat can cause severe respiratory distress because of pressure on the lungs and trachea, and because of the need to "aerate" a lot of fat. Coughing may accompany the respiratory distress. Obesity increases the probability that the cat will experience diabetes.

Extra weight can severely stress the joints and muscles. In some cases, it may result in total collapse of ligaments and tendons, with joints no longer able to support the cat's weight. In these cases, it is usually necessary to euthanize the cat for humane reasons, as it is not generally possible to keep it alive and comfortable long enough to lose weight and stand again. The obese cat will have less resistance to stress and disease. It is a poor risk for surgery, and its life expectancy may be reduced as much as 30-50%.

YOU have to be your cat's weight watcher. Start BEFORE the problem becomes severe—at the first sign of bulges or weight gain (see Obesity in Feline Gourmet Chapter).

TRAVEL

If your cat is accustomed to travel when young, it should not be a problem when it is old, especially if the cat is in good health. The cat will need more frequent stops to relieve itself or a handy litter box as you travel. Take along the cat's regular food if you are going to be gone during mealtime. Keep the cat from being overheated or chilled. NEVER leave the cat alone in a car. Even a sunny winter day can heat the inside of a car enough to severely stress a cat. A hot summer day may be fatal. This book is about cats, but I will mention that several children die each summer from being left in cars in the sun.

If your cat is not used to traveling, it is almost always better to leave it at home. If you can find a reliable friend or neighbor to come in once a day (or twice if possible) to feed and water the cat, it will appreciate not having to go to a kennel. If the person likes the cat and can spend a few minutes talking with it and petting it, that is even better.

If you can't find someone to care for the cat at home, try to find a kennel that gives personalized attention. This service may cost more, but will be worth it in terms of comfort for your cat and peace of mind for you. It is a good idea to board a cat in a kennel from time to time while it is younger so it can become accustomed to it. Once you have boarded the cat, stop worrying and enjoy your vacation. Most cats "tune out" situations they do not like. Your little friend may sleep through much of your vacation. This is certainly easier on the cat than having to cope with the stress, strangeness, and stimulation of travel.

WATCHING YOUR CAT

It is very important to observe your cat carefully in its old age. Small changes occur from day to day, so subtle that they are not easily noticed. At this stage of life, noticing small signs of trouble can prevent illness from becoming serious. Note how much the cat eats and drinks, how much and how often it urinates, and whether the bowel movements are normal. Changes in weight may signal problems, as can changes in the eyes, ears, and hair coat. Old cats have good days and bad days, so do not worry if it is different on one day. You are looking for trends and major changes.

A sudden increase in the frequency and quantity of urination (or drinking!) may signal kidney problems, which are common in older cats. Or, it may indicate diabetes or adrenal problems. Urinary incontinence can be a problem in the older cat, whether male or female. It is sometimes treatable—consult your veterinarian.

Many cats retain their normal personalities as they grow older. Others may become cranky or stubborn at times. Be as patient as you can, but do not allow the cat to get away with behavior that makes you feel uncomfortable or that you don't want the cat to do. The cat that has never been allowed on the sofa need not be there now. It should still be a pet, not a homeowner. Perhaps you could put a towel or cat bed at your feet or beside the sofa. The cat may come to you more often for love and touching and reassurance. Give it as long and as often as you can.

In some cases, acquiring a kitten will do an old cat a world of good. At first, the old cat will grump around, defending its territory and resenting the attention the intruder is receiving. If the cat is not extremely old or crippled, it eventually will begin to interact with the new cat. It may sleep less and take more interest in life. An additional advantage is that you, who may be contemplating the upcoming loss of your old and faithful friend, will have a new companion to help soften the loss when it inevitably comes. Of course, if your kids are grown and gone from home and you are looking forward to fewer responsibilities, a new kitten may not be a good idea.

EUTHANASIA

Your cat is a pet, and as such is meant to be a comfort and a pleasure to you. As it enters old age, it will sleep more and become gradually less active. The cat, however, still will be a loving and grateful friend.

As the cat goes through the years, it may no longer be comfortable. It may have urinary incontinence, or be unable to control its bowel movements. The cat's needs and care may become a burden. If you have had the cat examined by your veterinarian and you know the problems cannot be helped, it may be time to consider whether the cat is still a good pet. Consider the quality of life the cat is experiencing. If it is making a mess of your house and itself to the point where it is always miserable because of being soiled, it may be time to ask if the cat should be kept alive. A pet is supposed to be a pleasure, not a burden. If the animal has become a burden to you, it is time to consider euthanasia. Animals have no knowledge of the future as we do, and for that reason they do not fear death.

You may not feel your cat is very ill. It is important for an animal in the wild to mask the fact that it is hurt or sick. Your cat may be suffering from a terminal illness and yet your reaction may be "he's not acting very sick." In the wild, if the cat were to show signs of illness, chances are good that it would be eaten by another animal.

You may feel guilty about even considering "putting your pet to sleep." Other people may try to make you feel guilty. But, one of the advantages of a pet is that we CAN give it a kind death. We DO NOT HAVE TO keep it alive, in pain and misery and discomfort, totally without dignity at the end of its life. I try not to preach, but ask yourself: Is keeping the cat alive in misery the way to reward your pet for being a good friend and companion all those years? Give the cat the ultimate kindness, that of helping it die comfortably, kindly, and with dignity. It is not selfish for you to wish to euthanize the animal because it is causing you to have an hour's cleaning to do each night when you come home from work. The animal has become a burden, a job of work, not a pleasure. You will come to resent it—and the cat will know it. Incidentally, it's not a good idea to use the phrase "put him to sleep" around children. When the cat is later missing or dead, the child may fear going to sleep, afraid that something will happen to him or her. Phrases such as "eased into death" or "helped to die" may be more accurate and calming. This also is an opportunity to show that death is a natural end for all living things.

You may be torn by feelings of anger and helplessness. You may want to end the cat's suffering but be overwhelmed by feeling that you are "playing God." Choosing to euthanize your cat may be more difficult than dealing with its death. You may have the misguided notion that you owe it to the cat to keep it alive at all costs. Ask yourself what your cat would like you to do for it if it could talk.

It's not a matter, either, of "replacing" the pet. There WILL NEVER BE ANOTHER cat just like the one you are losing. The cat was its own individual self, just as you are different from your sister or brother or friend. While you may have another pet, you will never have another JUST LIKE this one. Even if you have another of the same breed, it will not be the same. And, if you are worried about comparing your new cat to your old one, change breeds, or get a different color or sex of cat.

When is euthanasia appropriate?

1) When the cat is unable to enjoy life. When it is so arthritic that it is unable to move well or to stand by itself. When it has urinary or bowel incontinence so that it is always soiled or cannot get to the litter box. When it is blind and deaf, and seems unaware of the world around it, or where it is and who it is with. When it has an advanced tumor or other disease process which makes it miserable, with no hope of cure. When it is in enough pain or discomfort that it is unkind or even inhumane to keep it alive.

2) When the owner is no longer able to enjoy the cat. Again, when the cleaning or upkeep is more than the owner can handle, or wishes to handle.

3) When a cat is vicious, whether toward humans or other animals. Cats of any age that are dispositionally or temperamentally unsuited to being pets should be euthanized for the protection of those around them, whether family or people in the neighborhood. A few cats are NOT suitable pets, no matter what is done with them or who their owners are. They do not work out for the family that currently owns them, and they will not work out for another family, no matter how well-meaning the people are. This is especially true of feral cats that are adopted after they are more than a couple of months old.

4) When the cat refuses to be housebroken. If you have a situation where the cat has to be kept in a house or apartment, even part of the time, it is not a suitable pet. While some people may hope that this animal might make a good pet for someone else, it is only suitable to be someone's barn cat.

In many cases, it is much kinder to a cat with a bad temperament or bad habit to simply euthanize it rather than to turn it in to a humane society, and have the cat placed with one or more other owners, during which it gets nuttier and nuttier, until it finally goes completely crazy. Giving the cat to a humane society or "no-kill shelter" to be placed may NOT be a kindness. It may, in fact, be a real cruelty.

Some veterinarians refuse to euthanize cats that they judge to be "normal" (i.e., not old or terminally diseased). I totally disagree with this—it is YOUR cat, and it is YOUR right to have it euthanized if you wish. If your veterinarian refuses to euthanize a temperamentally unsuitable cat, find another veterinarian. Keep looking until you find one who will do as you ask. And, ask to see the body after the job is done (even if you are leaving the body with the veterinarian for disposal) to confirm that it has been handled as you wish. Don't let a veterinarian make you feel guilty about euthanizing your cat. The cat is yours and the decision is yours.

5) When it is an economic decision. In some cases, people are unable to keep a perfectly suitable pet for economic reasons. Try to find a home for the cat with someone who can afford it. It is usually better to give the cat away than to try to sell it. You'll be more successful in finding a good home. If worse comes to worst, give the animal to a humane society so that it can try to place the cat. If the cat is registered, take its papers along—they may help the cat to find a home. Also, take along records of health care, immunizations, and any other information that may be helpful in placing the cat. Be honest with the people who will be placing the cat. Tell them if the cat is grouchy with children or prefers a quiet home. You need to know that if the cat is not adopted by someone, it will be euthanized.

Some veterinarians, unfortunately, have succumbed to the temptations rife in human medicine, to keep the animal alive at all costs. This may be because the veterinarian is unable to admit (to himself or to you) that there is no to help for your cat. It can be because the veterinarian

has the technology and skills to keep the cat alive, no matter how poor the cat's quality of life. For the veterinarian to advise you that the cat should be euthanized may be unpleasant and emotionally draining, and it may be tempting to avoid it by keeping the cat alive. And, keeping the cat alive can be very financially rewarding to the veterinarian; the temptation may be too much to resist. The result is torture for your pet, expense to your pocketbook, and an emotional mess for you (Hare, 1994).

What is the procedure for euthanasia? First, call to make sure your veterinarian will be there when you want to take the cat to the clinic. Some veterinarians make a specific appointment to make sure that time is set aside for your pet. If the cat is vicious or otherwise hard to handle, stop by the clinic in advance and get tranquilizers which can be fed to the cat an hour before you leave home. Take the cat in a carrier or pillowcase. A receptionist who is sensitive to your needs should take you to an examination room as soon as possible. Or, if you choose, you can leave the cat at the clinic for the veterinarian to euthanize when time is available. You may want to have someone go along with you to drive you home as you may be too upset to drive (it happens to all of us, myself included).

If you are a regular client, your veterinarian may be willing to come to your home to euthanize your cat if that is more comfortable for you. Be sure to offer to pay for the extra service that is involved. In some cities, small animal practitioners have mobile clinics that will come to your house. Again, this service may cost extra, but it may be worth it to you.

In most cases, you will be asked to sign a release form. This gives the veterinarian permission to euthanize the cat, and is a routine legal formality in most states. Read it thoroughly, and know what you are signing. The same form, or another form, may give the veterinarian permission to dispose of the body.

You may choose to dispose of the body yourself (check into the legality of this, depending on the state or city where you live), by burying it in your yard or another place which has meaning to you. Be sure to bury it deeply enough (three to four feet) so it will not be dug up by dogs or wild animals. You can take the body to a pet cemetery. You can have the veterinarian dispose of it, by burial, cremation, or whatever the normal method of disposal is. If you do not specify or discuss what is to be done with the body, the animal may end up in the daily trash. In fact, in most cities you may assume this to be the norm. If this bothers you, be sure to ask about other arrangements, or be prepared to make them yourself. If you are leaving the cat for euthanasia and disposal, your job is done.

If you want the veterinarian to euthanize the cat while you are present, you will be waiting with the cat. You may choose to stay and watch as the veterinarian gives the injection. Or, you may wish to stay in the waiting room until it is done. You can then see the body before you leave. I feel that this viewing is important for closure of your relationship with the animal. It also may be essential to assure yourself later that the cat was indeed dead. Please do it, even though you might not feel like it at the time.

The veterinarian may ask a few questions about why you are euthanizing the cat if he or she does not know you and the reason is not obvious. An assistant will hold the vein on the cat's leg or may put a tourniquet around it. The veterinarian will place a needle or catheter into the cat's vein and begin to inject the euthanasia solution. The cat may stiffen slightly, but in most cases will just relax and lie over to one side as though going to sleep (which it is). Euthanasia performed by most veterinarians is done by an overdose of an anesthetic agent. The cat feels no more than if it were being prepared for surgery. The cat may sigh once or twice, and then be gone—quickly, quietly, and kindly. An occasional cat may stiffen, stretch, or howl briefly, but that's all (this is a reflex, not a sign of pain). The veterinarian will usually check the cat with the stethoscope to be sure the heart has stopped.

Be prepared for the cat to possibly defecate and urinate after death. This is normal, and is due to the anal and urinary sphincter muscles relaxing. If you are leaving the body at the clinic, you may wish to spend a few minutes alone with your pet before you leave. Just ask the veterinarian to close the door and leave you alone for a bit. If you do not feel capable of driving home, don't hesitate to ask someone to call a taxi for you; or, call a friend to drive you. This is a very stressful time, and you should not be embarrassed to ask for help if you need it.

You may wish your cat to have a cemetery burial. Pets have been buried by humans since ancient times. Cat mummies have been found in Egypt, in their own graves. Burying the cat in a pet cemetery can allow you to formally participate in separation from your animal. It may comfort you to know where the animal is buried, and it will allow you to visit and quietly spend time with the cat if you wish. Interment in a pet cemetery may be simple or elaborate, and may vary from a few hundred to several thousand dollars. Many pet cemeteries have funds for perpetual care. Be sure to ask about this if it is important to you.

Group burial may be available and is much less costly. This is offered by some pet cemeteries or private humane organizations. Your pet will be buried with other animals. This will not affect its dignity. Individual or communal cremation may be available through your veterinarian, animal shelter, or pet cemetery. Again, the costs vary, with communal cremation being less expensive.

You may wish to bury your cat on your own property. This is especially easy if you live in a rural area. The cat should be placed in a thick liner bag and then in a wooden coffin-like box or similar container and buried three to four feet deep. This will keep animals from being attracted by the scent and digging up the body. You may wish to have a graveside service. If you are taking the cat home with you for burial, bring in a box or bag if you have one. Otherwise, the veterinarian may place the cat in whatever is handy. Take the cat home and bury it, and remember how it was your special friend.

If you have two cats that have lived together for a long period of time, the surviving partner may mourn. One of my cats, who had lived, slept, and groomed with another for six years, nearly quit living when the female suddenly died of kidney failure. The male sat on a heat register, seeming not to care if he lived or died. He only responded when we brought home two grown, homeless cats. His need to get up and defend his territory pushed him to get moving and eventually return to normal. He never formed as deep a bond with the new cats. Another cat sat unmoving for five days after her long-time companion vanished. She was a nearly wild outdoor cat, but she allowed me to brush and hold her. A few days of this treatment started her eating again, although she never regained her former cheer and bounce.

In an emergency, if you live in the country, it may be necessary to shoot a cat that has been slashed by a mower or otherwise is severely injured but not yet dead. Shooting is unpleasant, but entirely humane. When the shot is well placed, the cat is instantly unconscious, although muscle spasms and thrashing may persist for a short time. A .22 caliber pistol or rifle, or a .410 gauge shotgun can be used. Be sure that the cat is in a safe location, preferably close to a hill or dirt bank to absorb any stray shots. In some cases, the shot may pass through the cat's skull and out the other side. Be sure you look around to make sure there are no humans or animals in the line of fire. Because of their small size, it can be difficult to humanely shoot cats. Feral cats that have been trapped may be first given a tranquilizer or other sedative in their food. The cat can be wrapped in a towel or placed in a heavy sack, with only the head sticking out. Aim the firearm at the center of the cat's head, just below a line drawn between the bases of the ears (Longair, 1991).

THE MOURNING PROCESS

Don't be surprised if you enter a period of grieving, particularly if the cat was an old companion and friend. This can occur whether the cat died naturally or was euthanized. It is NORMAL to grieve for your pet. You have suffered the loss of an old friend, one who may have been with you longer than your children or friends or mate. It is normal to feel guilt, to feel that perhaps you should have done more for your pet, or taken it to a veterinarian sooner; that you SHOULD have done something else to make the cat well. Chances are good that you did all you could have done. Death is a reality of life. For most of us, whether animal or human, it should be a blessed relief, ending the pain and suffering of old age or disease which have been plaguing us.

Unfortunately, our society does not have a socially acceptable way to mourn a lost pet. Friends, even those who are well-meaning, may say "It's only a cat, you can get another one," or similar remarks. In most cases, these people mean well, but are not attached to an animal themselves and simply don't understand the depth of your loss. Their comments do little to help you in this time of emotional pain and crisis.

When someone close to us dies, we go through several stages of mourning. These stages are similar, whether the deceased loved one is human or a beloved cat.

The first stage of grief includes denial that the pet is gone. You may be depressed. Denial usually begins when we first learn about the animal's sudden death or its incurable illness. It is the mind's way of trying to protect us against the painful feelings we know will come.

Your second stage may be bargaining. When the veterinarian tells you that your cat has a malignant tumor, you may try to "make a deal," either with whatever you consider to be a higher power, or with the pet itself. This may be something such as "if you make it though this, I'll never put you in a kennel when I go on vacation again." This stage seems to be more common when a human loved one dies than when a person loses a pet.

Next, you may feel anger. This may show up as hostility or aggression. The anger is particularly difficult to handle, as we tend to lash out at those around us in our helplessness, our inability to do anything about a terminal illness or death of our beloved animal. Many veterinarians have been the brunt of this anger: "You didn't do all you could for him" or "You never really cared for him." It also falls on family members. It is particularly unfair to have this land on a child when a parent says, "If you'd just taken care of him, this wouldn't have happened." These outbursts relieve the owner's immediate pain, but at the expense of other persons.

The anger may turn inward, showing up as guilt. You may berate yourself with "If only . . ." regrets. "If only I had taken Kitty to the veterinarian last month instead of waiting." These recriminations only make you feel worse and do little to relieve your anger. Remember that the good and faithful care you have given the animal throughout its life is what enabled the cat to live to be this old.

The fourth stage is grief. This is when the true sadness takes over your emotions. Your cat is gone and your mind is realizing that it will never return. It will never curl up in your lap and purr for you again, will never beg as you fix its dinner in the kitchen. Only the emptiness remains. Now is when you most need the support of family and friends. It can be difficult to find. Some people find it hard to understand your loss. They don't understand how it can mean that much to lose your pet. This is especially true if they have never been closely attached to a pet. You are not alone in this sense of grief. It is normal and many other pet owners have experienced it.

The final stage is resolution. It is hard to believe while experiencing it, but the pain WILL go away in time. For some people who have had the pet for many years, the difficult period may last three to four months. If you have been extremely attached to the pet, or it was central to your life, the mourning may last longer. A sign that you are recovering from the loss of your pet is often a flood of pleasant memories about the pet, and an appreciation of the time the animal was able to spend with you. You may find yourself smiling quietly when you remember a long forgotten antic by your pet when it was a kitten. This also may be when you consider getting a new pet. If you want

to know more about the stages of grieving, consult Dr. Elizabeth Kubler-Ross' book, *On Death and Dying*.

For some people, it is helpful to acquire another pet right away. Some will want another "little yellow kitten just like Fluffy." Others who are concerned that they will expect the new pet to BE another "Fluffy," will choose a different color or sex of cat within the same breed. Yet other people will choose a completely different breed, or even a different pet: a dog or bird for a change. Acquire another pet ONLY if it is right for you.

Some people wait weeks, months, or even years until the time is right. Most people feel better waiting until they have resolved their grief and are completely at peace with the loss of the former pet. There will NEVER be another cat JUST like the one you have lost. But, there may be another (or several more) pet(s) in your life that will give you pleasure and share your company, each in its own special way.

You may wish to have your cat's memory live on by giving a donation to a worthy cat-related cause. Many veterinary schools will accept donations in your pet's honor. This money could go toward a scholarship, or to research on cat diseases to help other cats live longer, healthier lives. Humane organizations can always use money to care for homeless pets. The American Animal Hospital Association Foundation (Denver West Office Park, P.O. Box 15899, Denver, Colorado 80215-0899) accepts donations in memory of pets. These funds are used to further research into animal diseases and treatments for them.

Please, if you are having trouble coping with your pet's death, get professional help. Some veterinarians offer bereavement or grief counseling. Many of the veterinary colleges now have bereavement counselors. If you live near one of these institutions, contact it for assistance. Help may be available through a psychiatrist or local mental health center. In some larger cities, grieving classes are held and support groups are available. It is sometimes easier to deal with the process if you know something about it and can share your experiences with others. The Delta Society is a nonprofit, donor-based organization which can provide information on support groups throughout the country, as well as other information on dealing with the loss of your pet. Its address is: P.O. Box 1080, Renton, WA 98057-1080, (206) 226-7357.

Occasionally, some professionals may pooh-pooh your concern. If this occurs, keep looking until you find one who is sympathetic and sensitive to your feelings. Be aware that some of your friends and co-workers who have never lost a pet will not understand your feelings. Go to a friend or counselor who does. Cry a few tears. And, remember that the love you have given is never lost, whether for an animal or another human being. I have come to believe that our ability to grieve, like our ability to love, is one of the things that makes us human.

Chapter 22

TRAVELING WITH YOUR CAT

- *Moving With Your Cat*
- *The Lost Cat*

In the wild, adult cats live by themselves and are social only during kittenhood and adolescence. Pet cats usually remain social, like teenagers who never grow up. In the wild, a cat may travel considerable distances to find food, so forays are not totally alien. Pets depend completely on humans for their well being. Some cats are physically and emotionally stressed when away from their owners, while others are more disturbed by travel than by being left at home. If your cat is going to spend your whole vacation cowering under a strange bed, it would be much more comfortable in its own home or in a kennel. Cats normally don't need much in the way of exercise, so even staying in a cage for a couple of weeks can be more cozy than terrifying. It's much like a den to the cat.

Traveling with your cat can be a pleasant experience if the cat is accustomed to it. If not, it can be a miserable, unpleasant affair for all concerned. Train the cat when it is a kitten. Begin by starting the engine as you pet and praise the cat. Next, take the cat on short trips and not JUST to the clinic or groomer. A treat before and after the trip will help put a pleasant memory in the kitten's mind. Gradually make the trips longer. If you begin when the kitten is young, it probably will never have motion sickness. Some cats become eager travelers.

If your cat has a regular crate at home, this also can be its den or "home away from home" in the vehicle and in motels. If you don't have a crate and are just taking the cat to the veterinarian, put it in a cardboard box with ventilation holes punched in it. A bird cage also can be used. Ventilation and security are the prime considerations. Secure the crate with a seat belt so that it does not fly around if you must stop suddenly. If the cat is not confined, put a harness on it (not a collar!) and secure the leash so it doesn't get out if someone rolls down a window without thinking. In a pinch, cats travel perfectly well in a pillowcase with the top tied shut with a piece of string or twine.

If your cat is not a good traveler, plan on having a friend or petsitter come in to care for it while you are gone. Some cats learn to associate suitcases with being left alone and will use them for litter boxes. Or they will eliminate outside of the litter box when left alone. If the cat has this problem, it is best to board it in a kennel while you are gone. It may still be lonely and anxious, but as least your house will not be ruined. The American Boarding Kennels Association has a bill of rights for boarded pets. You can get a copy

from the ABKA at 4575 Galley Road, Suite 400A, Colorado Springs, CO, 80915. If you are moving, it will be necessary for the cat to travel, one way or another. You can get a quantity of tranquilizers or sedatives to help the cat travel without being upset. Or, you can send it ahead by plane—the cat still will need to be sedated.

Consider your cat when you are heading off on vacation. If it is adaptable and happy, it may enjoy the trip. Most cats, however, are both homebodies and creatures of habit. They are happiest when left at home. Leave a bowl of water, a dish of dry food, and a clean litter box. This may be quite enough if you are going to be gone only two or three days. If you are leaving the cat for a longer period of time, have someone come in to check the cat and give it some attention—daily if possible. The person can clean and refill the food and water, as well as making sure the animal is healthy, or taking it to a veterinarian if it becomes ill. (See Urinary Chapter for hazards of dry food for a cat who is unaccustomed to it.)

If your vacation includes a lot of sunbathing or sightseeing, your cat's "vacation" may mean many hours locked in a vehicle or abandoned in a motel room, which may not be pleasant. If you are visiting someone who has a cat, do the two animals get along well? If not, you may end up driving 1,000 miles, then kenneling your cat in a strange city when you arrive. The cat would have been better off left in a kennel at home. Are there children or dogs in the household that will make your cat's vacation a miserable experience? Some cats may travel well if they have their own familiar traveling crate. It can act as a "den," giving the cat a place where it feels safe. If you put the crate, a litter box, and food and water in a bedroom or motel room, the cat may be reasonably comfortable. It just depends on the cat.

Make sure your cat has a collar and identification tags with your name, address, and phone number. Do NOT put the cat's name on the tag. Calling the cat by name may be the only way to prove your ownership if it is lost, tags are removed, and it is not identified in any other way. For positive identification, you can have your veterinarian tattoo numbers or letters on the inside of the cat's ear flap or on the skin inside the thigh. Or, you can have an electronic microchip implant placed under the cat's skin. It is a good idea to take along some good photos of the cat for identification if it is lost.

Incidentally, having permanent identification on your cat is important even if your pet is strictly an indoor cat. You never know when it might slip out a door that is held open by a child or blown by the wind. Having identification helps to increase the probability that you can get it back.

If you are getting ready for a longer trip, pack for your cat as well as for yourself. Take its food dish, water bowl, and bed or blanket. If it has a delicate digestive system, take some of the water that it normally drinks. Also, take the cat's regular food—this is NOT the time to change diets. If you feed canned food, take small cans so that you can throw away leftover food, since it will spoil. It's a good idea to have a leash and harness. You can use a piece of light rope 10 or 12 feet long for country rest stops if you want to take the cat out for exercise or a toilet stop. Don't use a leash on a collar. It's too easy for a cat to slip out of a collar. Many cats learn to walk quite well on a leash, and can be taken for short walks. Pack a disposable litter box and some of the cat's favorite litter. You also will want cleaning materials such as paper towels, plastic bags, and cleaning spray. Take along a portable scratching post. If you're going to be gone for some time, take the cat's brush or comb, shampoo, and a toy or two. Flea powder or spray is useful, too. Your cat may never have had a flea, but if it picks up some on the trip, a quick dusting helps avoid bringing them home. The cat may get them when it stays at a house or motel where another animal has left the pests, or they may hop on during a walk.

DO NOT feed the cat for two to six hours before you leave. Plan for stops for your cat to exercise, relieve itself, and get a drink of water. Offer a little water every time you stop. Feed the cat at the last stop of the day or after you are through traveling for the day. If you take the cat out of your vehicle, remember that these are not normal surroundings for your pet. Be sure the cat is on a leash. Otherwise, if the cat panics and bolts, it might not be able to find its way back to you. The cat's collar also should have your name and new destination on it, so that it can be returned to you if it should escape for any reason. I have traveled quite happily with my cat by putting the airline crate on the right seat and a litter box on the right floor. When I stopped for fuel I put down a dish of water and a dish of food.

Car safety includes teaching the cat to stay in a given area (for example, on its bed in the back seat). Give the cat a comfortable, roomy place and train it to stay there so that it is not roaming all over the car. Otherwise, you may be paying attention to the cat's gyrations rather than the road, with fatal possibilities for both of you. If the cat will not stay put or at least move around slowly, it should be confined, both for the cat's safety and that of the driver and passengers. Do not leave a leash on the cat in a vehicle. The cat may become caught on a door handle and strangle itself. Pet harnesses are available that attach to a seat belt to keep the cat safely restrained. Keep the cat confined so that it does not leap out when you open the car door. Or, keep the cat safely in its crate for the entire trip.

Leaving a rear window open in a station wagon or van may allow exhaust fumes into the vehicle which could poison the cat (and you!). Never put a cat in the trunk of a car, even for a short period of time. Becoming too hot may quickly kill it, and the risk of carbon monoxide poisoning is considerable. If you put the cat on the floor of the back seat, be sure it is not over the catalytic converter, or the cat may die from overheating.

DO NOT leave the cat in a vehicle in hot weather, even with a window open. In some cities, it is legal for a passerby to shatter your car window if he or she believes the pet is in danger of heat stroke. And, do not underestimate the effects of the "greenhouse" effect in a closed vehicle. A day of only 70 degrees F (22 C) can still give a temperature over 100 degrees F (37.8 C) within the car. If you are leaving the cat, try to park in the shade if at all possible.

Remember that the angle of the sun changes. If your cat's "place" is on the side of the car where the sun is shining, either put something over the window for shade, or move it to the other side of the vehicle. A few cases of heat prostration are seen when the car is relatively cool inside but the sun is shining directly on the cat. Adequate ventilation WHILE you are traveling will make the trip more comfortable for the cat, as well as helping avoid motion sickness. A damp towel laid out on the seat or floor may help cool the cat. Carry cool (but NOT ice-cold) water for the cat to drink, and offer small amounts frequently. If you have to travel through a hot area in a vehicle without air conditioning, be extra careful that your cat does not overheat. Travel during the cooler times of the day, or even at night. Make sure the cat has fresh water available at all times. If necessary, sponge the cat with cool (not cold) water. When it evaporates, it will help cool the cat.

Cold weather may be no less hazardous to your cat. The temperature inside a parked car can drop quickly, and the animal can develop hypothermia. Cats (as well as dogs with short coats and toy dogs) are very susceptible to below normal body temperatures when they are confined in this manner. It is even more dangerous if the cat is damp when it is left in the cold, parked car.

Don't turn your cat loose when you reach your destination. Keep it confined to its carrier for a day or two. Then, let the cat loose in just one room until it is accustomed to the new premises. The cat can gradually be turned loose in the whole house. Be careful of opened doors. The cat may blindly flee in the unfamiliar neighborhood if it slips outside. Follow the same procedure when you arrive home. The cat needs time to become reacquainted with its home.

Be sure to take your cat's rabies vaccination certificate with you. Even more important than the rabies tag (which does not give the date of vaccination), it verifies that the cat is vaccinated if it bites someone. It may keep the cat from being impounded and quarantined, and will keep your travel plans from being disrupted.

Airline travel can be a convenient way to send your cat elsewhere or to take it with you. Call the airline WELL in advance of when you want to travel. Some airlines allow a cat to be carried in lieu of luggage if you are traveling at the same time. It may be much more expensive to send the cat by itself, and there may be a limit on how many pets are allowed on a given flight. Very small (and quiet!) cats may sometimes be taken as carry-on luggage. Be sure to check in EARLY. Some airlines allow one pet to a cabin on a first-come, first-served basis. Many airlines require a reservation for the cat much as they do for yourself. It sometimes happens that you will make reservations for your cat, be told that it can fly in the cabin, but then learn when you get to the airport that the cat must be put in the baggage compartment. Be prepared for that eventuality. If you are sending the cat by air freight, ask if the airline has a priority or express-freight service that will allow you to check your cat in at the last possible moment.

Airliner cargo areas are pressurized but not air-conditioned or heated. Federal regulations prohibit shipping pets if the outside temperature is below 45 degrees F (7.2 C) or above 80 degrees F (26.7 C). In most cases, cats must be at least eight-weeks-old for shipment. If you are flying during the summer, try to fly at night or early in the morning. Do not feed your cat for six to 12 hours before the flight. Small kittens have limited physical reserves; they should be fed as late as possible before the flight. Do not give them water within two hours of flight time except in hot weather. Be sure the cat is wearing a tag with your name and destination address, in case it escapes from the crate. If you are going to a foreign country, both the tag and the label on the crate should be written in that language.

Most airlines require a health certificate from your veterinarian, assuring them that the animal is in good health at the time of shipment. They also require a current rabies immunization if the cat is more than three months of age. While you are at the veterinarian's, have the rest of the cat's vaccinations brought up to date if they are not current. The examination should be scheduled about a week before you are going to travel in case your cat has a reaction to the vaccine, if that timing is acceptable to the airline. It is also a good idea to get copies of your cat's health records. These can be very helpful if it becomes ill while you are away from home.

If at all possible, try to get your cat on a nonstop flight. Discuss airline connections if the cat will transfer from one plane to another. Avoid peak travel periods when delays are longer. Plan the flight so that the cat does not arrive on a weekend, holiday, or during off-hours. Animals usually sleep during the flight, but may be upset during layovers. They also may be left in the sun or rain, depending on airport facilities. Some airports, such as JFK in New York and Los Angeles International have good kennel facilities, where the cat can be fed, watered, and attended.

Most airlines require an approved shipping crate. The crate will need a leak-proof bottom that you can cover with plenty of absorbent material. Use rags or disposable bedding. In addition, put something in the cage that has your scent on it. This can be comforting to the cat. The carrier should have a smooth, safe interior, and a sturdy handle or grip. It should have ample ventilation openings on opposite sides, and a strong, safe latch. It should be strong enough to avoid being crushed by shifting luggage. It should have sloping sides (wider at the middle than the top or bottom). This helps keep baggage from being stuffed around the cat and suffocating it. There should be a label that says "Live Animals," with arrows showing which side is up.

The crate should be large enough for the cat to lie down flat, turn around, and stand upright. Take the cat along when buying the crate so that you can try it out for size. If you buy it a couple of weeks before the trip, your cat will have a chance to become accustomed to it.

Some airlines will rent you a crate if you don't have your own. Try to get the crate ahead of time so that you can clean it with disinfectant and let the cat become accustomed to it. Request that the cat be hand-carried to the baggage area rather than being put on the conveyor belt.

Your name and the address and phone number of your destination should be securely attached so that they cannot be scraped off by adjacent luggage. Attach copies of the health and rabies certificates and destination instructions to the crate, but do NOT send originals if you can avoid it. They may be torn off by other pieces of luggage and lost. Make sure that someone can meet the cat on the other end. If you are moving, arrange for someone from a veterinary clinic or kennel to meet the cat at the plane and take it to the kennel to await your arrival.

If the trip is long, pack food and water dishes, as well as feed and instructions. A plastic bag of dry food, or a bag containing small pop-top cans of canned food can be securely tied to the top of the cage. If the cat is vicious, or bluffs well, don't bother to pack food for a short flight, as no one will try to feed it.

If your cat is prone to motion sickness or is excitable, obtain tranquilizers or a motion-sickness drug well before the trip. Some people seem to feel that it is wrong to tranquilize a cat for travel. But, if the cat does not travel well, or is sick all the time, it far kinder to sedate it than to have it afraid and miserable. The cat may have a "hangover" or be less than lively for several days after the trip. This is partly due to the drugs and partly due to fatigue and letdown after so much excitement. As long as it is not showing other signs of illness, let the cat sleep it off. If you travel frequently, keep track of what tranquilizer is used, which dosage, when you gave it, and how long it lasted. This will help you fine tune the dosage for future trips.

When you pick up your cat, take it to a quiet, secure place where it can rest from the trip. It may not eat, but be sure it has access to water, as it probably will be dehydrated from the airline trip.

Interstate bus lines do not allow cats or other pets except guide dogs for the blind. If you are traveling a short distance, it may be possible to do so on local bus lines, but the individual bus driver may make the decision as to whether or not the cat is allowed.

Amtrak trains do not allow animals other than Seeing Eye dogs, either in the passenger compartment or the baggage area. Other rail lines may allow the cat to travel in the baggage compartment. Baggage compartments are not heated or air-conditioned. Some oceangoing ships do allow cats, but require that they stay confined in special kennel areas. Pets are not allowed in cabin areas.

If you are staying in a motel or hotel, ask about their pet policy when you make reservations. Some will allow a cat, especially if it is quiet and stays in a crate. They may require a deposit to cover any damage. The law in

North Carolina does not allow pets in motel or hotel rooms. However, kennel facilities may be available. You may need to reserve the space in advance.

If you are traveling internationally with your cat, whether by plane or by vehicle, check with that nation's consulate WELL in advance (30-45 days) to learn the current requirements. It doesn't hurt to call the state veterinarian in your state (generally located in the state capitol), and ask for the information THEY have on the country where you are going. In some cases, you have to get an international health certificate form and allow time for it to go to both the state veterinarian's office and the consulate, to be countersigned, after it has been filled out by your veterinarian.

Some countries do not allow any entrance of any pets (such as Ecuador and the Soviet Union). England and some Caribbean countries have six-month quarantine periods, while Australia requires nine months. Hawaii has a 120-day quarantine period. In general, these countries and islands are free of rabies and want to be sure that it, as well as other diseases, are not introduced. And, some quarantine facilities are not of high quality. Also, if you are just landing at London on the way to another country and your plane is delayed more than four hours, for any reason, your pet may be seized and quarantined for six months. Of course, boarding during the quarantine period is at YOUR expense. Also, be sure of the requirements for bringing the cat back into the United States (if you are bringing it back), AND for the state to which you are returning. In some cases, it may be easier to have your pet shipped by a professional pet transport company that is familiar with the regulations and problems involved in moving animals across national borders. Bon voyage!

MOVING WITH YOUR CAT

Cats are somewhat territorial creatures of habit. They become accustomed to their surroundings and are bothered when things are changed. When the furniture starts moving and leaving, even the most settled of cats can be deeply disturbed. If at all possible, get the cat out of the house during the packing process. Send it to a kennel if it is familiar with it, or to stay with a friend until you are packed. Or, send the cat along to your new city, and have it boarded at a reliable kennel there. If you must keep the cat at home while you are preparing to leave, it should be shut securely in a room with its food, water, and litter box, along with any favorite toys that it might have and its own bed. Put a sign on the door warning people not to let the cat out. If the cat is running loose, it might get into one of the boxes and get packed. Recently, a cat spent more than a month packed in a reclining chair. It had been sleeping inside when the chair was closed up and loaded in the moving van. Or, the cat might slip outside in the confusion and become lost. In any case, make sure it is wearing a safety collar with your NEW address on it. This will help in returning the cat to you if it should become lost. A few cats have a good homing instinct, but it will usually take them to their old home, not the new.

Before you leave your home, have copies of your cat's medical records to take with you or make arrangements with your veterinarian to forward them to a clinic near your new home. If you have your cat's records with you, these can be helpful if it becomes ill en route to your new home.

When you reach your new location, keep the cat securely caged until you are completely moved in and the doors can be kept closed. Otherwise, the cat may escape in the confusion. You can keep the cat in one room with all its familiar utensils and bed, as above. Then, gradually let the cat into one more room at a time until it is acquainted with the entire house. Even if the cat is normally an outdoor cat, do not allow it outside for two to three weeks so that it is completely familiar with its new home. Otherwise, the cat may become confused and try to return to its old home. If you do have to take the cat outdoors, use a harness and leash. It is also a good idea to walk the cat on a leash until you are sure it knows the area and will stay. Then, allow the cat outside and stay with it until it seems familiar with the surroundings. An old story says the cat will stay at the new home if you butter the pads of its feet. Might be worth a try!

THE LOST CAT

Take every precaution possible to insure that your cat does not escape while you are traveling. This includes making sure it is in its crate and that it is securely latched before anyone in the vehicle opens a door or window. Or, make sure the cat is wearing its harness and leash, and that one person is responsible for keeping track of it. If the cat is lost in a strange place, it does not know where to return.

If the cat becomes lost and runs away, start by searching the immediate vicinity. Call for the cat in the tone of voice that you normally use, even though you may feel ridiculous doing it. Tell everyone you meet that you have lost your cat. If you can't find it within a couple of hours, notify the local humane society and/or animal shelter. Make up a flyer with the photos you brought from home. You can go to a copy shop, stick the photos on a piece of paper, and write the information with a pen. Make copies to give to the postman, any delivery drivers who work in the area (such as the UPS), and residents in the area. Leave signs at stores, at intersections, and at places like the post office and laundromat. Put an ad in the lost-and-found column of the local newspaper. The radio station may have a public notice program which will let people know of your loss.

Whatever happens, don't give up. The lost cat may be confused. It may go for a week or more without coming near humans, especially if it is in a neighborhood where people leave food out for their pets, where it can bum or steal a meal without seeing anyone. It may be several weeks before the cat makes contact with anyone. If you have to leave, make arrangements for an animal shelter employee or motel clerk to get in touch with you if the cat is found. Some pets have been returned to their owners after four to six months, or even a year after they have been lost.

- Grandma Kitty (yellow SH tabby) who brought me three mice, chortling gently in the early hours when I slept out in the yard as a child.
- Greenie (brown SH tabby) who sat on the porch chair, face raised to the morning sun.
- Squirrely (black SH, white shoes), my kitten who was squashed by the tractor.
- Scooter James (calico-splashed SH tabby) who bit my ankles with tiny kitten teeth in the mornings, rolled walnuts under the refrigerator, and loved me through lonely times.
- Kitter (the cover cat, brown SH tabby) who lifted his nose to sniff the autumn breeze. With sightless eyes and head held high, he strode forth into the crackling leaves. He hugged my neck and bit my hair and is buried near the pinnacle beneath the wild poppies.
- Kitty Mudder (black SH, white socks) who hunted at the farm and hid on the bridge, racing her plump body before vehicles into the night.
- Chubby (black SH, white shoes), my rolling-in-the-dirt cat.
- Tiggy Tomcat (brown SH tabby, white shoes and tie). His bold racing stripes strolled onto the farm one day and stayed, all muscles and love.
- Mangy Alice (brown SH tabby) who came to cheat death and stayed to hunt, coming home before the first snow flew each fall, remembering sadly when it was once warm.
- Lert (brown butterfly-pattern SH tabby), the space cat-det who drooled with love.
- Spot (black SH with white shoes) and Julie (tortoise shell) who were inseparable. He shouted to her deafness and stayed close, even far from the sheltering barn.
- Camouflage (calico-tabby SH) "Cammy" who jogged down the canal bank with me, her injured raccoon-tail flopping behind as if chasing her. I gave her away and she walked ten miles across the coyote-filled prairie back to the farm. She stayed.
- Pooh Bear (black SH, white shoes). A plump giant who balanced on the porch rail and climbed the corner of the three-story house to sleep like a fat fur pillow on the skylight.
- Tara (black SH, white shoes). A shy gentle unhappy soul who was so afraid. Dear Tara, I did the best that I knew.
- Kangaroo (chocolate point Siamese). A rotund scraggle-eared, cross-eyed, rasp-voiced teddy bear cat who saved four lives by waking his family when their home was burning.
- Schwartz the Magnificent (black SH). A huge cat who slept upside-down, trusting, in my arms.

When I was a child, I wanted a cat. My father wouldn't allow me to have one. Our farm was overrun with mice. Finally, he said that I would have to earn the cat by trapping 25 mice in the barn. It took all of a day and a half for me to run my trapline and earn my first feline. Since, then, I have loved many a cat, both mine and others—these are only a few which have come to mind.

- Gilligan (tabby-point Siamese). A special blue-eyed giant.
- Sambo (black SH), a loving character cat who adventured by the pond.
- Ginger (black SH, faint tabby stripes), the "Miss Kitty" with a lame leg and brave personality who hunts game large and small and tries to keep Sharon well fed.
- Pinkie (black, silver undercoat LH) who rules a farm with simple elegance.
- Francoise (silver tabby SH), my friend the "Fuzzois" who went from little wildcat to cuddly lover boy.
- Peanut Butter (light tan SH tabby). "Nutty Butter" was a truly memorable friend.
- Pyewacket (sealpoint Siamese). A large and special beast.
- Kit Kat (gray and tan calico SH, white trim). A plump funny-face cat with a mind of her own.
- Tinker (gray/brown tabby half-white SH), the original "elderkatz" who finally wore out.
- Sam (orange tabby SH, white trim). Brian's knee-grabber.
- Fernobulax (tabby-point Siamix). "Nobs," an imperious, elegant giant.
- Nuke (yellow tabby LH), the "new kid on the block," who came home the long way.
- Buddha (long-haired bluepoint Siamix, white trim and snow-shoe feet) who loved quietly.
- Ashtar (racing-model Abby) with the intelligent grace of an Egyptian queen.
- Nada (fat-footed brown tabby LH) who chased the Sheltie down the stairs.
- Bartlett (bluepoint Siamese) who helped us through the rough school days.
- Old Blue (bluepoint Siamix with white ends, whiskers and necktie), the eater of mousies who ran Animal Clinic.
- Ocelot and Ocelittle, companions of Rona of Marble Canyon.
- Slim (black SH with white trim), a special devoted pal who ran Walworth Quarter Horses.
- Colombo (golden-yellow with racing stripes), a plump sweetie who chased the mice from Howard's haystack.
- K.C. (bluepoint Siamese). Sue's lean little lover.
- Tucker (yellow SH) who came home from the post office and stayed.
- The Fur Person at Falcon Field (bluepoint Siamese) who owned the hangar—everyone else just worked there.
- Hey Cat (black SH with white trim), she meowed from the rooftops and came when called, chortling from under the bushes.
- Squatita (gray and white SH), a friendly, lumpy ghost in the night.
- Yitten (yellow tabby, white trim) who attacks my legs as I cut the grass.

REFERENCES AND NOTES

Alishouse, H.F., Personal communication, 1996.

August, J.R., Cat Scratch Disease, *Journal of the American Veterinary Medical Association, (JAVMA)* Vol. 193, No. 3, 1 August 1988, pp. 312-314.

Barrette, D., Feeding Older Cats and Dogs, *Canadian Veterinary Journal (Can Vet J)*, Vol. 31, November 1990, pp. 784-785.

Barr, M.C., in Wilford, C.L., Feline Immunodeficiency Virus Transmission, *Veterinary Forum*, March 1995, p. 46.

Beaver, B.V., Effectiveness of Products in Eliminating Cat Urine Odors from Carpet, *JAVMA*, Vol. 194., No. 11, 1 June 1989, pp. 1589-1590.

Beaver, B.V., *Feline Behavior: A Guide for Veterinarians*, W.V. Saunders Co., Philadelphia, 1992. This is a thoroughly researched and well-written guide. It covers normal feline behavior and briefly discusses clinical cases to show how some behavioral problems can be corrected.

Brown, R.G., Fiber in Cat Diets, *Can Vet J.*, Vol. 30, March 1989, pp. 258-259.

Buck, W.B., and P.M. Bratich, Activated Charcoal: Preventing Unnecessary Death by Poisoning, *Veterinary Medicine (Vet Med)*, January 1986, pp. 73-77.

Buck, W.B., Clarification on Use of Chlorpyrifos, Letters, *JAVMA*, Vol. 199, No. 12, 15 December 1991, p. 1682.

Buck, W.B., A Poison Control Center for Animals: Liability and Standard of Care, *JAVMA*, Vol. 203, No. 8, 15 October 1993, p. 1119.

Burrows, C.F., et.al., Experts Discuss Feline Nutritional Needs, *DVM Newsmagazine*, November 1989, pp. 25-33.

CDC, Centers for Disease Control and Prevention, *Plague Surveillance*, Volume 3, No. 1, June 1993.

Cappucci, D.T., Puerto Rico and Rabies, *JAVMA*, Vol. 205, No. 3, 1 August 1994, p. 402.

Carberry, C.A., and H.J. Harvey, Owner Satisfaction with Limb Amputation in Dogs and Cats, *(Journal of the*

American Animal Hospital Association (JAAHA), Vol. 23, March/April 1987, pp. 227-232.

Chisholm, H., Massive Mammary Enlargement in a Cat, *Can Vet J*, Vol. 34, May 1993, p. 315.

Clark, K.A., Rabies (Zoonosis Update), *JAVMA*, Vol. 192, No. 10, 15 May 1988, pp. 1404-1406.

Connaught Labs, Inc., *Rabies: What To Do In An Emergency*, Connaught Laboratories, Inc., Swiftwater, PA, 1992.

Davidson, A.P., E.C. Feldman, and R.W. Nelson, Treatment of Pyometra in Cats, Using Prostaglandin F2 alpha: 21 cases (1982-1990), *JAVMA*, Vol. 200, No. 6,15 March 1992, pp. 825-828.

DeBoer, D.J., and K.A. Moriello, Inability of Two Topical Treatments to Influence the Course of Experimentally Induced Dermatophytosis in Cats, *JAVMA*, Vol. 207, No. 1, 1 July 1995, pp. 52-57.

Delack, J.B., Hereditary Deafness in the White Cat, *Compendium of Continuing Education*, Vol. 4, pp. 609-617, 1984.

Dhein, C.R., *Feline Nutrition, Animal Nutrition Series 2*, Kal Kan Foods, Inc., 1986.

Dhupa, Nishi, Hypothermia in Dogs and Cats, *Compendium on Continuing Education*, Vol. 17, No. 1, January 1995, pp. 61-68.

Donner, G.S., Treating Chylothorax—Some New Ideas For an Old Disease, Vol. 33, No. 10, 1991, pp. 19-20.

Dryden, M.E., G.R. Long, and Gaafar, S.M., et al., Effects of Ultrasonic Flea Collars on *Ctenocephalides felis* in Cats, *JAVMA*, Vol. 195, 15 December 1989, pp. 1717-1718, 1989.

Espada, Y., A. Prats and F. Abo, Feline Hemobartonellosis, in *Friskies Veterinary International*, Vol. 3 No. 1, 1991, pp. 34-40.

Fadok, V.A., Three Dermatologic Syndromes and Their Relationship to Allergy, in *Waltham Feline Medicine Symposium*, 1995, pp. 29-30.

Fischer, C.A., Ocular Feline Herpesvirus, *Veterinary Forum*, July 1995, pp. 48-50.

Fishbein, D.B., and S. Arcangeli, Rabies Prevention in Primary Care: A Four-Step Approach, *Postgraduate Medicine*, McGraw-Hill, Inc., N.Y., Vol. 82, No. 3, September 1, 1987.

Fleming, E.J., D.L. McCaw, J.A. Smith, G.M. Burning, and C. Johnson, Clinical, Hematologic and Survival Data from Cats Infected With Feline Immunodeficiency Virus: 42 Cases (1983-1988), *JAVMA*, Vol. 198, 1991, pp. 913-916.

Fogelman, V., and H.R. Fischman, J.T. Horman, and J.K. Grigor, Epidemiologic and Clinical Characteristics of Rabies in Cats, *JAVMA*, Vol. 202, No. 11, 1 June 1993, pp. 1829-1833.

Fox, L., in Researchers Study Drug to Treat Feline Mouth Cancer, *DVM Newsmagazine*, August 1993, p. 28.

Freiman, H.S., Protocol for Treating Feline Indolent Ulcers, *Veterinary Forum*, March 1991.

Frischke, H., and L. Hunt., Suspected Ivermectin Toxicity in Kittens, *Can Vet J.*, Vol. 32, April 1991, p. 245.

Fyfe, J.C., Glycogen Storage Disease in Cats, *JAVMA*, Vol. 206, No. 3, 1 February 1995, p. 286.

Gionfriddo, J.R., Recognizing and Managing Acute and Chronic Cases of Glaucoma, *Vet Med*, March 1995, pp. 265-275.

Greene, R.T., Feline Coccidioidomycosis, *Proceedings 12th American College of Veterinary Internal Medicine Forum*, San Francisco, 1994.

Greene, R.T., and G.C. Troy, Coccidioidomycosis in 48 Cats: A Retrospective Study (1984-1993), *Journal of Veterinary Internal Medicine*, Vol. 9, No. 2 (March/April) 1995, pp. 86-91.

Gunther, R.L., J. Felice, R.K. Nelson, and A.M. Franson, Toxicity of a Vitamin D3 Rodenticide to Dogs, *JAVMA*, Vol. 193, No. 1, July 1, 1988, pp. 211-214.

Halliwell, R.E.W., Ineffectiveness of Thiamine As a Flea Repellent in Dogs, *JAAHA*, 1982. Vol. 18, p. 423.

Harai, J., S. Gustafson, and K. Meinkoth, Dental Bacteremia in Cats, *Feline Practice*, Vol. 19, No. 4., 1991, pp. 27-29.

Harbour, D.A., P.E. Howard, and R.M. Gaskell, Isolation of Feline Calicivirus and Feline Herpesvirus From Domestic Cats from 1980 to 1989, *Veterinary Record*, Vol. 128, 1991, pp. 77-80.

Hare, D., Le Droit de Mourir (The right to die), *Can Vet J.*, Vol. 35, February 1994, pp. 69-70.

Harvey, D.E., and W.E. Alston, Dental Disease in Cat Skulls Acquired Before 1960, in *Proceedings, 4th Veterinary Dental Forum*, 1990, p. 41.

Hendrick, M.J., Shofer, F.S., Goldschmidt, M.H., Haviland, J.C., Schelling, S.H., Engler, S.J., and Gliatto, J.M., Comparison of Fibrosarcomas That Developed at Vaccination Sites and at Nonvaccination Sites in Cats: 239 Cases (1991-1992), *JAVMA*, Vol. 205, No. 10, 15 November 1994, pp.1425-1429.

Holmes, R.A., Feline Heartworm Disease, *Compendium on Continuing Education*, Vol. 15, No. 5., May 1993, pp. 687-695.

Holmstrom, S.E., Does Close Up Home Care Turn Your Clients Off? *Veterinary Forum*, July 1992, p. 38.

Hoskins, J.D., Congenital Defects of Cats, *Compendium on Continuing Education*, Vol. 17, No. 3, March 1995, pp. 385-405.

Houpt, K.A., Ingestive Behavior: The Control of Feeding in Dogs and Cats, *Compendium of Continuing Education for the Practicing Veterinarian*, Vol. 1, No. 8., pp. 587-594, 1979.

Houpt, K.A., and Smith, S.L., Taste Preferences and Their Relation to Obesity in Dogs and Cats, *Can Vet J.*, Vol. 22, 1981, pp. 77-81.

Hornfeldt, C. S., Chocolate Toxicity in Dogs, *Modern Veterinary Practice*, December, 1987, pp. 552-553.

James, R.B., Notes on Blindness in Cats, *Vet Med*, May 1982, pp. 776-778.

Jarrett, O., Overview of Feline Leukemia Virus Research, *JAVMA*, Vol. 199, No. 10, 15 November 1991, pp. 1279-1280.

Jarrett, O., A.M. Pacitti, M.J. Hosie and G. Reid, Comparison of Diagnostic Methods for Feline Leukemia Virus and Feline Immunodeficiency Virus, *JAVMA*, Vol. 199, No. 10, 15 November 1991, pp. 1362-1371.

Jeglum, K.A., Solid Tumors in Cats, in *Waltham Feline Medicine Symposium*, Jan. 1994.

Johnson, B.W., Congenitally Abnormal Visual Pathways of Siamese Cats, *Compendium on Continuing Education*, Vo. 13, No. 3, March 1991, pp. 374-377.

Johnston, S.D., Questions and Answers on the Effects of Surgically Neutering Dogs and Cats, *JAVMA*, Vol. 1998, No. 7, 1 April 1991, pp. 1206-1213.

Kane, E., Texture, Odor, and Flavor Important in Determining Feline Food Preference, *DVM Newsmagazine*, June, 1987.

Kane, E., J.B. Morris, and Q.A. Rogers, Acceptability and Digestibility by Adult Cats of Diets Made With Various Sources and Levels of Fat, *Journal of Animal Science*, Vol. 53, 1977, pp. 1526-1523.

Kitchell, B.E., Cancer Therapy for Geriatric Dogs and Cats, *JAAHA*, Vol. 29, January/February 1993, pp. 41-48.

Koehler, J.E., C.A. Glaser, and J.W. Tappero, *Rochalimaea henslae* Infection: A New Zoonosis with the Domestic Cat as a Reservoir, *Journal of the American Medical Association*, Vol. 271, No. 7, 1994, pp. 531-535.

Krebaum, P., Formula for Deodorizing a Skunk Afflicted Pet, *Chemical and Engineering News*, 18 October 1993, p. 90.

Krebs, J.W., T.W. Strine, J.S. Smith, C.E. Rupprecht, and J.E. Childs, Rabies Surveillance in the United States During 1993, *JAVMA*, Vol. 205, No. 12, 15 December 1994, pp. 1695-1709.

Lewis, L., Three Factors Critical in Cause, Prevention of Troublesome FUS, *DVM Newsmagazine*, 1987, pp. 39-53.

Longair, J., G.G. Finley, M. Laniel, C. MacKay, K. Mould, E.D. Olfert, H. Rowsell, and A. Preston, Guidelines for Euthanasia of Domestic Animals by Firearms, *Can Vet J.*, Vol. 32, December, 1991, pp. 724-726.

Lovell, R.A., Ivermectin and Piperazine Toxicoses in Dogs and Cats, *Veterinary Clinics of North America, Small Animal Practice*, Vol. 20, pp. 453-468, 1990.

Lynch, M.J. et. al., An Evaluation of Live *Toxoplasma gondii* Vaccine in Tammar Wallabies (*Macropus eugenii*), *Australian Veterinary Journal*, Vol. 70, No. 9, September 1993, pp. 352-353.

Mandelker, L., Uncovering Many New Psychotherapeutic Agents, *Veterinary Forum*, August 1990, p. 28.

McGill, L.D., Vaccine Associated Sarcomas, *Veterinary Forum*, June 1993, pp. 26-28.

McKeown, D., A. Luescher and M. Machum, The Problem of Destructive Scratching by Cats, *Can Vet J.*, Vol. 29, December 1988, pp. 1017-1018.

Melman, Steven A., *Skin Diseases of Dogs and Cats: A Guide for Pet Owners and Professionals.* DermaPet®, Inc., P.O. Box 59713, Potomac, MD 20859, 1994. This book is a good overview of skin diseases in pets, more for dogs than cats. It has good photos of many problems but may be a bit technical for many pet owners.

Miller, W.H., Efficacy of Chlorpheniramine Maleate for Management of Pruritis in Cats, *JAVMA*, Vol. 197, No. 1, 1 July 1990, pp. 67-69.

Nelson, R.W., E.C. Feldman, S.L. Ford and O.P. Roemer, Effect of an Orally Administered Sulfonylurea, Glipizide, for Treatment of Diabetes Mellitus in Cats, *JAVMA*, Vol. 203, No. 6, 15 September 1993, pp. 821-827.

Norsworthy, G.D., The Difficulties in Regulating Diabetic Cats, *Vet Med*, April, 1993, pp. 342-348.

Ogilvie, G.K., Mysteries of Feline Skin Tumors, in *Waltham Feline Medicine Symposium*, 18 January 1995, p. 40.

Otto, G.F., L.A. Jachowski, Jr., Mosquitoes and Canine Heartworm Disease, *Proceedings of 1992 Heartworm Symposium* (G.F. Otto, ed.), Veterinary Medicine Publishing Co., Edwardsville, KS, 1981, pp. 17-32.

Panciera, et al., *JAVMA*, 1990, Vol. 197, pp. 1504-1508.

Papich, M.G., Absorption of Salicylate from an Antidiarrheal Preparation in Dogs and Cats, *JAAHA*, Vol. 23, March/April 1987, pp. 221-226.

Peterson, M.E., Insulin-resistant Diabetes Mellitus in Cats, in *Waltham Feline Medicine Symposium*, Kal Kan Foods, Inc., 15 January 1992, pp. 44-54.

Polzin, D.J., et al., Chronic Renal Failure in Cats: Diagnosis and Management, in *Waltham/OSU Symposium, Nephrology and Urology*, Kal Kan Foods, Inc., October 1992, p. 36.

Prescott, C.W., Clinical Findings in Dogs and Cats with Lead Poisoning, *Australian Veterinary Journal*, Vol. 60, pp. 270-271, 1983.

Rhone-Merieux, Human Deaths from Rabies Rise Dramatically in 1994: Are You Protected, *The Rabies Monitor*, Vol. 3, No. 1, Summer, 1995.

Ross, L.A., Feline Urologic Syndrome: Understanding and Diagnosing This Enigmatic Disease, *Vet Med*, November 1990, pp. 1194-1203.

Rosser, W.W., Bubonic Plague, *JAVMA*, Vol. 191, No. 4, 15 August 1987, pp. 406-409.

Rude, T.A., Product Complaints Associated with the Use of Veterinary Biological Products, *Veterinary Forum*, Feb. 1995, pp. 44-45.

Schantz, P.M., Of Worms, Dogs, and Human Hosts: Continuing Challenges for Veterinarians in Prevention of Human Disease, *JAVMA*, Vol. 204, No. 7, 1 April 1994.

Seawright, A.A., and J. Hrdlicka, Severe Retardation of Growth with Retention and Displacement of Incisors in Young Cats Fed a Diet of Raw Sheep Liver High in Vitamin A., *Australian Veterinary Journal*, Vol. 50, 1974, p. 306.

Sellon, R.K., Feline Immunodeficiency Virus Transmission: An Update, *Proceedings, 12th Annual Veterinary Medical Forum of the American College of Veterinary Internal Medicine*, 1004, pp. 116-118.

Shelton, G.H., M.L. Linenberger, M.T. Persik and J.L. Abkowitz, Prospective Hematologic and Clinicopathologic Study of Asymptomatic Cats with Naturally Acquired Feline Immunodeficiency Virus Infection, *Journal of Veterinary Internal Medicine*, Vol. 9, No. 3, May/June 1995, pp. 133-140.

Sosna, C.B., and Medleau, L., Treating Parasitic Skin Conditions, *Vet Med*, June 1992, p. 573.

Stewart, A.F., Pancreatitis in Dogs and Cats: Cause, Pathogenesis, Diagnosis and Treatment, *Compendium on Continuing Education*, Vol. 16, No. 11, November 1994, pp. 1423-1430.

Swaim, S.F., and A.H. Lee, Topical Wound Medications: A Review, *JAVMA*, Vol. 190, No. 12, 15 June 1987, pp. 1588-1592.

Vet-Kem, *Treatment of Suspected Organophosphorus and Carbamate Insecticide Toxicosis in Small Animals*, Vet-Kem, 12200 Denton Drive, Dallas, Texas, 75234, 1992.

Watson, A., Diet and Periodontal Disease in Dogs and Cats, *Australian Veterinary Journal*, Vol. 71, No. 10, October 1994, pp. 313-317.

Werner, A.H., and B.E. Werner, Feline Sporotrichosis, Vol. 15, No. 9, September 1993, pp. 1189-1197.

Whitford, R.F., Practice Tips, *Veterinary Forum*, 1989.

Whitney, W.O., and C.J. Mehlhaff, High-rise Syndrome in Cats, *JAVMA*, Vol. 191, No. 11, 1 December 2987, pp. 1399-1403.

Wills, J., and A. Wolf, Eds., *Handbook of Feline Medicine*, Pergamon Press, New York, 1993. This book is detailed, concise and well-written. It is a veterinary text but would be suitable for readers who want information in greater depth and detail than I have given, especially if they are familiar with medical terminology. It is filled with helpful charts and lists of symptoms and causes.

Wolf, A.M., Systemic Mycotic and Protozoal Infections in Cats, in *Friskies Veterinary International*, Vol. 3, No. 1, 1991, p.17.

Wolfran, G., J. Eckart, B. Walther, and N. Zullner, Factors Influencing Essential Fatty Acid Requirements in Total Parenteral Nutrition (TPN), *Journal Parenteral Nutrition*, Vol. 2, pp. 634-639, 1978.

Zaunbrecher, K.I., and R.E. Smith, Neutering of Feral Cats as an Alternative to Eradication Programs, *JAVMA*, Vol. 203, No. 3, 1 August 1993, pp. 449-452.

INDEX

About The Author

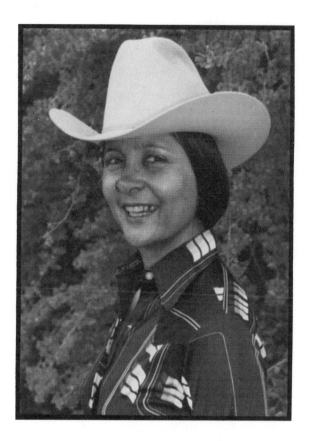

Ruth B. James, DVM

Dr. James took her preveterinary training at the
University of Denver and graduated from the College
of Veterinary Medicine at Colorado State University.
She replaced veterinarians who were on vacation,
working for over fifty veterinarians in five western states.
During this time, her work included cats, dogs, horses,
and numerous farm animals. Later, she established
a successful veterinary practice in Casper, Wyoming.
She has emphasized preventive medicine for her
clients, preferring to prevent problems rather than to
treat them, and has given health clinics and seminars,
and classes for 4-H members. Dr. James pilots a Super Cub
airplane. Her other interests include hiking and
backpacking, tracking, trail riding, snorkeling
and scuba diving, rock hunting, and travel.

Do-It-Yourself Veterinary Guides for ANIMAL OWNERS

These books cover the latest breakthroughs and newest treatements, as well as tried-and-true remedies that really work!

TOPICS INCLUDE . . .

- Choosing a Dog
- Housebreaking
- Common Behavioral Problems
- Worms and Worming
- External Parasites
- The Canine Gourmet
- Skin Diseases
- Emergency Care
- Care of the Elderly Dog
- Puppy Care

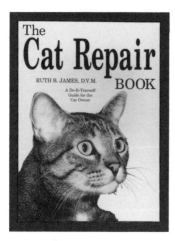

ISBN 0-9615114-2-7   288 pp. $19.95

- Feline First Aid
- Cat Care and Training
- Traveling with Your Cat
- Parasites, Inside and Out
- The Feline Gourmet
- Vaccinations and Disease Prevention
- Skin Diseases
- Eye and Ear Problems
- Reproduction and Kitten Care
- Heart and Lung Problems
  . . . and MORE!

You'll know how to give your own injections, saving time and money. Most importantly, you'll know when you should call your vet, and when you can take care of a problem yourself.

ISBN 0-9615114-1-9   256 pp. $18.95

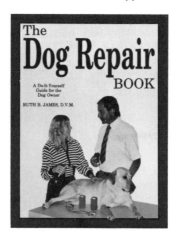

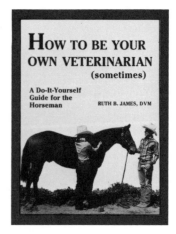

ISBN 0-9615114-0-0   356 pp. $19.95

- Medications
- Bandages and Bandaging
- Lameness and Soundness
- Back Problems
- Restraint and Safety
- Common Sense Horse Feeding
- Reproduction and Foaling
- Skin Problems
  . . . and MORE!

Dr. James, a respected veterinary practitioner, has written these books in the same easy-to-read style as her many articles in the Vet's Corner of *WESTERN HORSEMAN*.

100% Money-Back Guarantee for One Full Year!

If for ANY reason, you are not satisfied with this book, return it within 1 year from date of purchase for a full, courteous refund. Also available at better feed stores, tack shops, and bookstores. *Dealer Inquiries Invited.*

A Wealth of Money-Saving Information. SEND TODAY!

Each book is shipped in a custom mailing package.
Please send:

_____ The Cat Repair Book at $19.95 each	$_____
_____ How To Be Your Own Veterinarian (Sometimes) at $19.95 each	$_____
_____ The Dog Repair Book at $18.95	$_____

**Add $2.50 postage and handling per order, please.
(Canadian and foreign orders payable in U.S. funds.)
Wyoming residents only, add 5% sales tax.** $_____

Total Enclosed $_____

❑ Check Enclosed ❑ MasterCard ❑ VISA

Card No. _____ Exp. Date _____

Card Holder's Signature _____

MasterCard
VISA

SHIPPING LABEL
SPECIAL 4th CLASS BOOK RATE

FROM: **ALPINE PRESS**
P.O. Box 1930, Dept. M-26
Mills, WY 82644

TO:

Mr./Mrs./Ms. _____

Address _____

City _____

State _____ Zip _____

We Hope...
   You've enjoyed reading this book as much as we've enjoyed writing and publishing it.

Please...
   Help us to help others keep their cats healthy and save money on cat care.
   Give this page to a neighbor or friend, or use it to order a copy for a gift.

Please complete and include the following if this book is a gift or institutional purchase:

- -

Shall we enclose a gift card?   ☐ Yes.   Person sending gift:

Occasion _____   Name _____
         (Christmas, Birthday, Graduation, Mothers'
         or Fathers' Day, Valentines, etc.)   Address _____

         Schools or Libraries: City _____
         Purchase Order No. _____

         State _____ Zip _____

- -

Each book is shipped promptly in a custom mailing package.
Please send:

_____ The Cat Repair Book at $19.95   _____

_____ The Dog Repair Book at $18.95   _____

_____ How To Be Your Own Veterinarian
         (Sometimes): A Do-It-Yourself Guide
         for the Horseman at $19.95   _____

(Canadian and foreign orders payable
   in U.S. funds)

Postage and handling per order $2.50   _____

Wyoming residents only add 5% sales tax   _____

                  Total Enclosed   _____

☐ Check Enclosed   ☐ MasterCard   ☐ VISA

Card No. _____

Expiration Date _____

_____
Card Holder's Signature

SHIPPING LABEL
Special 4th Class Book Rate
_____

From: **ALPINE PRESS**
        P.O. Box 1930
        Mills, WY 82644

TO:

Name _____

Address _____ Apt. _____

City _____

State _____ Zip _____

Our Guarantee

We are convinced that this book will help you to care for your cat(s), and that the information contained in it will help you avoid problems and save money.

If, for any reason, during ONE YEAR following the date of purchase, you are not satisfied with this book, you may return it for a full, courteous refund. Send it, with the receipt with purchase price circled, to:

Alpine Press
P.O. Box 1930
Mills, Wyoming 82644

Sincerely,

Lynn Wilson
Production Assistant